MOSBY'S COMPREHENSIVE REVIEW OF NURSING

MOSBY'S
COMPREHENSIVE REVIEW OF NURSING

NINTH EDITION

THE C. V. MOSBY COMPANY

Saint Louis 1977

NINTH EDITION

Copyright © 1977 by The C. V. Mosby Company

All rights reserved. No part of this book may be reproduced in any manner without written permission of the publisher.

Previous editions copyrighted 1949, 1951, 1955, 1958, 1961, 1965, 1969, 1973

Printed in the United States of America

Distributed in Great Britain by Henry Kimpton, London

Library of Congress Cataloging in Publication Data

Mosby (C. V.) Company.
  Mosby's Comprehensive review of nursing.

  (Mosby's comprehensive review series)
  Includes bibliographies and index.
    1. Nursing—Examinations, questions, etc.
2. Nursing—Outlines, syllabi, etc. I. Title.
II. Title: Comprehensive review of nursing.
RT55.M6   1977   610.73′076   76-26682
ISBN   0-8016-3529-2

CB/CB/B   9   8   7   6   5   4   3   2

Editorial panel

EDITOR

Dolores F. Saxton, R.N., B.S. in Ed., M.A., Ed.D.
Professor of Nursing, Nassau Community College, Garden City,
New York

ASSISTANT EDITORS

Patricia M. Nugent, R.N., A.A.S., B.S., M.S.
Clinical Specialist, Mercy Hospital, Rockville Center, New York

Phyllis K. Pelikan, R.N., A.A.S., B.S., M.A.
Associate Professor of Nursing, Nassau Community College,
Garden City, New York

CONTRIBUTING AUTHORS

BIOLOGICAL AND PHYSICAL SCIENCES

John Joy, A.B., M.A., Ph.D., Professor of
Biology, Kingsboro Community College,
City University of New York, Brooklyn,
New York

Peter Pilchman, B.A., Ph.D., Assistant Professor of Biology, Kingsboro Community
College, City University of New York,
Brooklyn, New York

NUTRITIONAL SCIENCE

Sue Rodwell Williams, B.S., M.R.Ed.,
M.P.H., Ph.D., Chief, Nutrition Program,
Kaiser-Permanente Medical Center, Oakland, California

BEHAVIORAL SCIENCE

Phyllis W. Haring, R.N., A.A.S., B.S., M.S.,
M.Ed., Ed.D., Professor of Nursing, Nassau
Community College, Garden City, New
York

Dolores F. Saxton, R.N., B.S. in Ed., M.A.,
Ed.D., Professor of Nursing, Nassau Community College, Garden City, New York

PHARMACOLOGY AND DRUG THERAPY

Marjorie P. Johns, R.N., B.S., M.S., Coordinator, Medical-Surgical Nursing, Baccalaureate Program, College of Nursing,
Northeastern University, Boston, Massachusetts

HISTORY AND TRENDS IN NURSING

Mildred L. Montag, R.N., B.A., B.S., M.A.,
Ed.D., LL.D., L.H.D., Professor Emeritus,
Teachers College, Columbia University,
New York, New York

Mary Sirotnik, Reg. N., B.Sc.N., Year II Coordinator, Mack Centre of Nursing Education, Niagara College of Applied Arts and
Technology, St. Catharines, Ontario, Canada

FUNDAMENTALS OF NURSING

Phyllis K. Pelikan, R.N., A.A.S., B.S., M.A.,
Associate Professor of Nursing, Nassau
Community College, Garden City, New
York

FAMILY-CENTERED NURSING

Josephine Iorio, R.N., B.S., M.A., M.Ed., Professor of Nursing, College of Nursing, Seton Hall University, South Orange, New Jersey

Donna Wong, R.N., B.S., M.A., Assistant Professor of Nursing, College of Nursing, Seton Hall University, South Orange, New Jersey

PSYCHIATRIC NURSING

Dolores F. Saxton, R.N., B.S. in Ed., M.A., Ed.D., Professor of Nursing, Nassau Community College, Garden City, New York

Phyllis W. Haring, R.N., A.A.S., B.S., M.S., M.Ed., Ed.D., Professor of Nursing, Nassau Community College, Garden City, New York

MEDICAL-SURGICAL NURSING

Patricia A. Hyland, R.N., B.S., M.S., M.Ed., Professor of Nursing and Chairperson, Department of Nursing, Nassau Community College, Garden City, New York

Patricia M. Nugent, R.N., A.A.S., B.S., M.S., Clinical Specialist, Mercy Hospital, Rockville Center, New York

Phyllis K. Pelikan, R.N., A.A.S., B.S., M.A., Associate Professor of Nursing, Nassau Community College, Garden City, New York

Dolores F. Saxton, R.N., B.S. in Ed., M.A., Ed.D., Professor of Nursing, Nassau Community College, Garden City, New York

Mary Sirotnik, Reg. N., B.Sc.N., Year II Coordinator, Mack Centre of Nursing Education, Niagara College of Applied Arts and Technology, St. Catharines, Ontario, Canada

REHABILITATION NURSING

Patricia M. Nugent, R.N., A.A.S., B.S., M.S., Clinical Specialist, Mercy Hospital, Rockville Center, New York

CONTRIBUTORS OF ADDITIONAL TEST QUESTIONS

Norma Ercolano, R.N., B.S., M.S., Assistant Professor of Nursing, Nassau Community College, Garden City, New York

JoAnn V. Festa, R.N., A.A.S., B.S.N., Staff Nurse I.C.U. and C.C.U., Brunswick Hospital Center, Amityville, New York

Rosemarie E. Fraund, R.N., B.S., M.Ed., Instructor, Hunter College, City University of New York, New York, New York

Marion Gooding, R.N., B.S.N., M.A., Director, Department of Nursing Education, Tennessee State University, Nashville, Tennessee

Judith Green, R.N., A.A.S., B.A., M.A., Professor of Nursing, Nassau Community College, Garden City, New York

Marilouise Kelly, R.N., B.S., M.S., Assistant Professor of Nursing, Nassau Community College, Garden City, New York

Nancy Schultz Latterner, R.N., A.A.S., B.S., M.A., Assistant Professor of Nursing, Nassau Community College, Garden City, New York

Donald McDermitt, B.S., M.S., Biology Department, Essex County College, Newark, New Jersey

Wendy Ann McNabb, R.N., A.A., A.A.S., Staff Nurse, Gynecological Service, Mercy Hospital, Rockville Center, New York

Geri Scaramuzzo, R.N., A.A.S., B.S., Coordinator of Nursing, Nassau Center for Emotionally Disturbed Children, Woodbury, New York

Irene S. Pagel, R.N., B.S., M.A., M.Ed., Ed.D., Professor of Nursing, Adelphi University, Garden City, New York

Lenore D. Reilly, R.N., A.A.S., B.A., M.A., Assistant Professor of Nursing, Nassau Community College, Garden City, New York

Shirley M. Riley, R.N., B.A., M.A., Assistant Chairman, Nursing Department, Essex County College, Newark, New Jersey

Elaine M. Wittman, R.N., B.S., M.A., M.Ed., Ed.D., Professor of Nursing, Adelphi University, Garden City, New York

STATISTICAL CONSULTANT

Francis P. Hughes, B.S., M.A., Ph.D., Supervisor for Educational Testing, New York State Regents External Degree Program, Albany, New York

Preface

The previous material in *Mosby's Comprehensive Review of Nursing* has undergone major revision for this, the ninth edition. The addition of an introduction and the progression of subject matter in each area reflect the consistent approach that has been utilized throughout the book. The information that has been selected for inclusion incorporates the latest knowledge, newest trends, and current practices in the profession of nursing.

The material in the section on supportive areas is specific to nursing and is utilized to develop the scientific foundations of care. Superfluous material has been deleted from all of these sections, and a section on physics has been added. The behavioral science and history and trends sections have been totally revised, and Canadian nursing has been included.

The nursing areas have all been revised, reorganized, and updated, with the sections on psychiatric nursing, medical-surgical nursing, and rehabilitation nursing being rewritten from an entirely different approach. Maternity and pediatrics have been combined with additional material on parent-child health to form the family-centered nursing section.

This edition features a unique approach to the *Comprehensive Review's* long-standing excellence in providing questions for study. Test questions were submitted by the contributing authors as well as by other outstanding educators and practitioners of nursing. Initially, the editorial panel reviewed all questions, selecting the most pertinent for inclusion in a mass field-testing project. Graduating students from baccalaureate, associate degree, and diploma nursing programs in various locations in the United States and Canada provided a diverse testing group. The results were statistically analyzed. This analysis was utilized in the selection of questions for inclusion in the book and to provide the reader with a general idea of each question's level of difficulty. Letters indicating the difficulty of the questions appear next to the answers in the answer book. The letter *a* signifies that more than 75% of the students answering the question answered it correctly; *b* signifies that between 50 and 75% of the students answering the question answered it correctly; and *c* signifies that between 25 and 50% of the students answering the question answered it correctly.

We would like to take this opportunity to express our sincere appreciation to Mr. Frank Saxton and the many other people who contributed their time and energies to assist us, especially Mrs. Dianne Caruso and Mrs. Arlene Pelliccia, who, with the assistance of Mrs. Sally Festa and Mrs. Irene Elber, so carefully typed the manuscript; Mrs. Joan Schmidt and Mrs. Nancy Schultz Latterner, who assisted with proofreading; and, last but not least, our families, who supported our efforts.

DOLORES F. SAXTON
PATRICIA M. NUGENT
PHYLLIS K. PELIKAN

Contents

PART ONE
SUPPORTIVE AREAS

Anatomy and physiology

Physical science

Microbiology

Nutritional science: community and
clinical nutrition

The behavioral sciences

Pharmacology and drug therapy

History and trends in nursing and
nursing education in the United States
and Canada

CHAPTER 1

Anatomy and physiology

Anatomy and physiology are the study of the components of the human body and their functions. A thorough knowledge of the normal is necessary before there can be an understanding of the pathology associated with disease.

The basic concepts begin at the level of the cell and progress through the tissues, organs, and systems. The systems are discussed as singular entities as well as interrelated components of body functioning.

Structure and function are related to pathologic conditions where possible to demonstrate the application of the biologic sciences to nursing. A brief review of the development of the individual from fertilization to parturition has been included. A summary of the factors in human heredity and the traits associated with the genes is outlined.

This complex material is presented in a simple, concise manner to assist the reader in reviewing the basic information necessary for progression.

CONCEPTS AND DEFINITIONS
Basic concepts

A. Organization a prime characteristic of both structure and function of the body; because of organization, the body is a structural and functional unit and not merely a chaotic collection of countless smaller units
B. Four kinds of smaller units organize to form the body
   1. Cells—smallest units that can maintain life and reproduce
   2. Tissues—organizations of many similar cells with nonliving intercellular substance between them
   3. Organs—organizations of several different kinds of tissues so arranged that they can perform more complex functions than any individual tissue
   4. Systems—organizations of different kinds of organs so arranged that they can perform more complex functions than any individual organ
C. Structure determines function
D. Body structure and function are changed gradually in many ways throughout life

E. Survival—the body's prime function is survival of the individual and of the species
F. Each cell performs self-serving functions to maintain its own life and also specializes in some body-serving function to help maintain the body's life
G. Body functions change in response to changes in the environment; usually the responses are adaptive and they maintain or quickly restore balance

Definition of terms

A. Directional terms for the human body
   1. Cranial—toward the head end of the body
   2. Caudal—toward the tail end of the body
   3. Superior—upper portion or surface
   4. Inferior—under portion
   5. Anterior or ventral—front of the body
   6. Posterior or dorsal—back of the body
   7. Medial or mesial—toward the midline of the body
   8. Lateral—away from the midline of the body

9. Proximal—toward or nearest the trunk or the point of origin
10. Distal—away from or farthest from the trunk or the point of origin

B. Planes of the body
1. Sagittal—a lengthwise plane running from front to back; divides the body or any of its parts
2. Median—sagittal plane through midline
3. Frontal or coronal—a lengthwise plane running from side to side; divides the body or any of its parts into anterior and posterior portions
4. Transverse or horizontal—a crosswise plane; divides the body or any of its parts into upper and lower parts

BASIC STRUCTURES OF THE HUMAN BODY

CELLS
Structure

See Fig. 1 and Table 1-1

Functions

A. Movement of substances through cell membrane, accomplished by physical and physiologic processes; main physical processes are diffusion and osmosis; main physiologic processes are active transport mechanisms, phagocytosis, pinocytosis; energy for physical processes comes from random, never-ceasing movements of atoms, ions, and molecules; energy for physiologic processes comes from chemical reactions of catabolism carried on by living cells
1. Diffusion—movement of solutes and water in all directions within a fluid and in both directions through membrane; net movement of each substance, however, occurs from area where that substance is more concentrated into one in which it is less concentrated; hence, net diffusion of solute across a membrane is from more to less concentrated solution, but net diffusion of water is from less to more concentrated solution (because water molecules are more concentrated in less concentrated solution); tends to equilibrate concentrations of two solutions separated by membrane—e.g.,

water and oxygen diffuse through cell membranes
2. Osmosis—diffusion of water through a membrane that maintains at least one concentration gradient across the membrane; direction of net osmosis: more water osmoses out of the more dilute solution into the more concentrated one than osmoses in the opposite direction; pressure developed in a solution, a result of net osmosis into it, called osmotic pressure; net osmosis occurs into a hypertonic solution from a solution that is hypotonic to it
   a. Hypertonic solution—has greater potential osmotic pressure because it has higher concentration of solute particles than solution to which it is hypertonic
   b. Hypotonic solution—has lower potential osmotic pressure and lower solute concentration than solution to which it is hypotonic
   c. Isotonic solution—has equal concentration of solute particles on each side of a membrane
3. Dialysis—a process of separating small particles (crystalloids) from larger particles (colloids) by the more rapid diffusion of small molecules through a semipermeable membrane; the process of dialysis is used to mechanically remove impurities from the blood during kidney failure
4. Active transport mechanisms ("pumps")—devices that move ions or molecules through cell membranes against their concentration gradients (i.e., in direction opposite from net diffusion or net osmosis; energy supplied by catabolism of cell)
5. Phagocytosis—the engulfment of bacteria, cells, cell fragments, and foreign particles by white blood cells and phagocytic cells found in various areas of the body
6. Pinocytosis—physiologic process similar to phagocytosis, except that pinocytosis moves fluid into cell whereas phagocytosis moves particles

B. Cell metabolism—consists of two processes, catabolism and anabolism
1. Catabolism—complex process that releases energy stored in food molecules; part of this energy is released

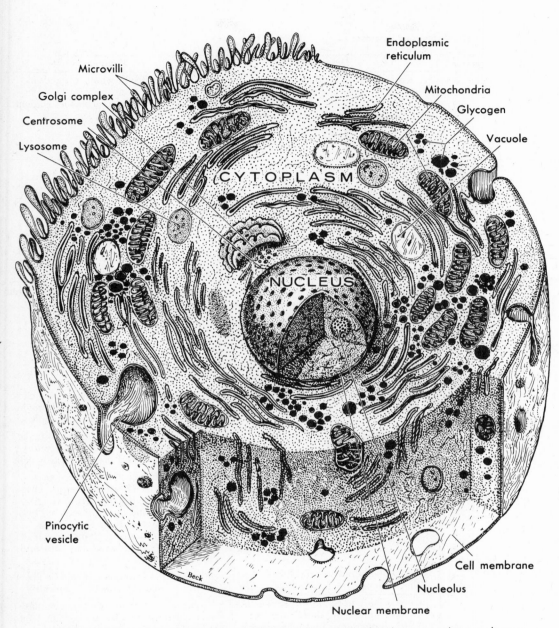

Fig. 1. Modern diagram of a generalized cell, based on what is seen under an electron microscope. The mitochondria are the sites of the oxidative reactions that provide the cell with energy. The dots that line the endoplasmic reticulum are ribosomes, the sites of protein synthesis. (From Anthony, C. P., and Kolthoff, N. J.: Textbook of anatomy and physiology, ed. 9, St. Louis, 1975, The C. V. Mosby Co.)

Table 1-1. Cell structures and functions

Name of structure	Description	Function
1. Cell membrane	1. About 3/10,000,000 inch thick 2. Consists, according to triple-layer hypothesis, of inner and outer layers of protein molecules with double layer of lipid molecules between them 3. Few tiny pores or openings in membrane	1. Maintains cell's wholeness and organization 2. Determines what substances can enter and leave cell

2. Cytoplasm	1. Body of cell, exclusive of nucleus
	2. Contains thousands of organelles ("little organs")
	  a. Membranous organelles: endoplasmic reticulum, Golgi apparatus, mitochondria, lysosomes
	  b. Nonmembranous organelles: ribosomes, centrosome	

3. Cytoplasmic organelles		
a. Endoplasmic reticulum (ER)	Complicated network of canals, extending through cytoplasm and opening at cell's surface	Serves as cell's circulatory system, in that some substances are transported through ER
b. Golgi apparatus	Membranous vesicles near nucleus	Synthesizes large carbohydrate molecules, combines them with proteins, secretes products
c. Mitochondria	Sacs whose walls consist of outer and inner membranes separated by fluid; enzyme molecules attach to these membranes	Serve as cell's "powerhouses"; enzymes of mitochondria catalyze series of chemical reactions known as the citric acid cycle and these reactions provide about 95% of cell's energy supply
d. Lysosomes	Membranous sacs; contain enzymes	Enzymes in lysosomes digest substances that enter them; under some conditions, digest and thereby destroy cells
e. Ribosomes	Tiny granules, large numbers of which dot surfaces of endoplasmic reticulum; others scattered through cytoplasm	Cell's "protein factories"; ribosomes attached to ER synthesize proteins, which move through ER to Golgi apparatus and then are secreted by cell; ribosomes lying free in cytoplasm synthesize proteins for cell's own use (its enzymes and structural proteins)
f. Centrosome (centrosphere)	Spherical body near center of cell (i.e., the nucleus)	Plays part in formation of spindle fibers during cell reproduction (mitosis)
4. Nucleus	Spherical body in center of cell; enclosed by pore-containing membrane; contains *chromosomes* and *nucleoli;* segments of DNA molecule called *genes;* chromosomes composed mainly of DNA molecules; genes are segments of DNA molecules; nucleoli composed mainly of RNA	Genes determine heredity by complex mechanism that transcribes DNA into RNA and then translates RNA into proteins; each of thousands of kinds of proteins synthesized performs specific function

as heat but a little more than half of it is immediately put back in storage in unstable, high-energy bonds of ATP molecules; as cells need energy, the bonds break down rapidly, supplying the energy that does all kinds of cellular work; consists of two series of chemical reactions—glycolysis and the citric acid cycle

   a. Glycolysis—anaerobic (nonoxygen-utilizing) reactions that convert 1 glucose molecule to 2 pyruvic acid molecules and yield a small amount of ATP and heat

   b. Citric acid cycle—series of aerobic reactions that use oxygen to oxidize 2 pyruvic acid molecules to 6 carbon dioxide molecules and 6 water molecules and yield about 95% of the ATP and heat formed during catabolism

  2. Anabolism—series of chemical reactions by which cell synthesizes complex chemical compounds (enzymes, structural proteins, secretions); anabolism is one kind of cellular work for which catabolism supplies energy via ATP

C. Cell reproduction—accomplished by mitosis, process in which chromosomes (DNA molecules) duplicate themselves before cell divides to form 2 new cells, each of which receives a full set of chromosomes; 46 chromosomes in normal human cells other than mature ova and sperm, which contain 23 chromosomes

D. Malignant cells—when cell growth and differentiation are no longer regulated, a malignant cell results that may be differentiated from normal cells in several ways

  1. Slides of malignant cells show many more mitotic figures than normal tissue cells; in addition, there are many abnormal mitotic figures

  2. Malignant cells have enlarged nuclei and an increased amount of chromatin material within the nucleus

  3. Malignant cells have a rapid growth rate

  4. Tissue cultures of malignant cells from the liver and kidney lack selective "stickiness" in contrast to normal cells, which have a tendency to group into specific tissue

  5. Tissue cultures of malignant cells from the liver and kidney lack contact inhibition; this feature of normal cells limits their growth

TISSUES

See Table 1-2 for names of 4 main kinds of tissues, some subtypes of each, and examples of location and function

SKELETAL SYSTEM
Functions

A. Furnishes supporting framework

B. Affords protection for viscera, brain, etc.

C. Provides levers for muscles to pull on to produce movements

D. Hemopoiesis by red bone marrow—formation of all kinds of blood cells except lymphocytes and monocytes

Structure of long bones

See Fig. 2

Names and numbers of bones

See Table 1-3

Differences between male and female skeletons

A. Male skeleton larger and heavier than that of female

B. Male pelvis deep and funnel-shaped with narrow pubic arch; female pelvis shallow, broad, and flaring with wider pubic arch

Age changes in skeleton

A. From infancy to adulthood, not only do bones grow, but also their relative sizes change; head becomes proportionately smaller, pelvis relatively larger, legs proportionately longer, etc.

B. From young adulthood to old age, bone margins and projections change gradually; bone piles up along them (marginal lipping and spurs), thereby restricting movement

Joints

A. Types

  1. Diarthroses (freely movable joints)—most joints of body are of this type; many subtypes; e.g., ball-and-socket, hinge, pivot

Table 1-2. Tissues

Tissues	Main locations	Functions
1. Epithelial		
a. Simple squamous (single layer flat cells)	1. Alveoli of lungs	1. Diffusion of gases between air and blood
b. Stratified squamous (several layers of cells)	1. Outer layer of skin (epidermis)	1. Protection
c. Simple columnar	1. Secreting cells of glands	1. Secretion
2. Muscle		
a. Skeletal (voluntary or striated)	1. Attached to bones 2. Extrinsic eyeball muscles 3. Upper one third of esophagus	1. Movement of bones 2. Eye movements 3. First part of swallowing
b. Visceral (involuntary or smooth)	1. In walls of tubular viscera 2. In walls of blood vessels and large lymphatics 3. In ducts of glands 4. Intrinsic eye muscles (iris and ciliary body) 5. Arrector muscles of hairs	1. Movement of substances along tubes 2. Changes in size of blood vessels 3. Movement of substances along ducts 4. Changes in size of pupils and in shape of lens 5. Erection of hairs (gooseflesh)
c. Cardiac (branching)	1. Wall of heart	1. Contraction of heart
3. Connective Most widely distributed of all tissues		
a. Areolar (loose connective tissue)	1. Between other tissues 2. Between organs 3. Superficial fascia	1. Cement various parts of body together
b. Adipose (fat)	1. Subcutaneous 2. Padding at various points	1. Protection 2. Insulation 3. Support 4. Reserve food
c. Dense fibrous	1. Tendons 2. Ligaments 3. Aponeuroses 4. Deep fascia 5. Scars 6. Capsule of kidney, etc.	1. Furnish flexible but strong connection
d. Hemopoietic (1) Myeloid	1. Bone marrow	1. Forms red blood cells, most white blood cells (i.e., neutrophils, eosinophils, basophils), and platelets
(2) Lymphatic or lymphoid	1. Lymph nodes 2. Spleen 3. Thymus gland 4. Tonsils and adenoids	1. Form lymphocytes, monocytes, and plasma cells; filter lymph 2. Forms lymphocytes, monocytes, and plasma cells; filters blood 3. Forms lymphocytes 4. Form lymphocytes and plasma cells
e. Bone	1. Skeleton	1. Support 2. Protection
f. Cartilage (1) Hyaline	1. Part of nasal septum 2. Covering articular surfaces of bones 3. Larynx 4. Rings in trachea and bronchi	1. Furnish firm but flexible support

Table 1-2. Tissues—cont'd

Tissues	Main locations	Functions
f. Cartilage—cont'd		
(2) Fibrocartilage	1. Discs between vertebrae 2. Symphysis pubis	
(3) Elastic	1. External ear 2. Eustachian (auditory) tube	
4. Nervous	1. Brain 2. Spinal cord 3. Nerves	1. Receive and transmit stimuli

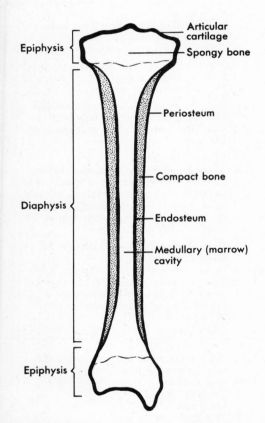

Fig. 2. Diagram to show structure of long bone as seen in longitudinal section. (From Anthony, C. P., and Kolthoff, N. J.: Textbook of anatomy and physiology, ed. 9, St. Louis, 1975, The C. V. Mosby Co.)

Labels in figure:
- Epiphysis
- Articular cartilage
- Spongy bone
- Periosteum
- Diaphysis
- Compact bone
- Endosteum
- Medullary (marrow) cavity
- Epiphysis

2. Synarthroses
  a. Cartilaginous type—slightly movable joints; e.g., intervertebral discs between bodies of vertebrae
  b. Fibrous type—immovable joints; e.g., sutures between skull bones

B. Structure of 2 types of joints
  1. Diarthroses—joint cavity or space between articular surfaces of 2 bones united by joint, thin layer of hyaline cartilage covering articular surfaces of joining bones; bones held together by fibrous capsule lined with synovial membrane and ligaments
  2. Synarthroses—no joint cavity, no capsule; joining bones held together by fibrous tissue (sutures of skull) or cartilage (between bodies of vertebrae)

C. Kinds of movement possible at diarthrotic joints
  1. Flexion—bending one bone upon another; e.g., bending forearm on upper arm
  2. Extension—stretching one bone away from another; e.g., straightening lower arm out from flexed position
  3. Abduction—moving bone away from body's midline; e.g., moving arms straight out from sides
  4. Adduction—moving bone back toward body's midline; e.g., bringing arms back to sides of body from outstretched or abducted position
  5. Rotation—pivoting bone upon its axis; e.g., partial rotation such as turning head from side to side
  6. Circumduction—describing surface of cone with moving part; e.g., moving arm around so that hand describes circle
  7. Special movements
    a. Supination—forearm movement turning palm forward

Table 1-3. Bones of the body

Part of body	Name of bone	Number	Description

1. Axial skeleton
  a. Skull
    (1) Cranium
	1. Frontal
	2. Parietal
	3. Temporal
	
	4. Occipital
	
	5. Sphenoid
	6. Ethmoid
		1
		2
		2
		
		1
		
		1
		1
			1. Forehead bone
			2. Bulging bones that form top sides of cranium
			3. Form lower sides of cranium and part of cranial floor
			4. Forms posterior part of cranial floor and walls
			5. Forms mid portion of cranial floor
			6. Composes part of anterior portion of cranial floor; lies anterior to sphenoid, posterior to nasal bones

(2) Face	1. Nasal 2. Maxillary 3. Zygomatic (malar) 4. Mandible 5. Lacrimal 6. Palatine 7. Inferior conchae (turbinates) 8. Vomer	2 2 2 1 2 2 2 1	1. Form upper part of bridge of nose 2. Upper jaw bones 3. Cheek bones 4. Lower jaw bone 5. Fingernail-shaped bones posterior and lateral to nasal bones, in medial wall of orbit 6. Form posterior part of hard palate 7. Thin scroll of bone along inner surface of side wall of nasal cavity 8. Lower, posterior part of nasal septum
(3) Ear ossicles	1. Malleus (hammer) 2. Incus (anvil) 3. Stapes (stirrups)	2 2 2	Tiny bones in middle ear cavity in temporal bone; resemble, respectively, miniature hammer, anvil, and stirrups
b. Hyoid bone		1	U-shaped bone in neck between mandible and upper part of larynx; only bone in body that forms no joints with any other bones
c. Vertebral column	1. Cervical vertebrae 2. Thoracic vertebrae 3. Lumbar vertebrae 4. Sacrum 5. Coccyx	7 12 5 1 1	1. Upper 7 vertebrae 2. Next 12 vertebrae, ribs attached to these 3. Next 5 vertebrae, located in "small" of back 4. In embryo, 5 separate vertebrae, but fused in adult into 1 wedge-shaped bone 5. In embryo, 4 or 5 separate vertebrae, but fused in adult into 1 bone
d. Ribs and sternum	1. True ribs 2. False ribs 3. Sternum	7 pairs 5 pairs 1	1. Upper 7 pairs fastened to sternum by costal cartilages 2. Do not attach to sternum directly; upper 3 pairs of false ribs attached by means of costal cartilage of seventh ribs; last 2 pairs not attached at all and therefore called "floating" ribs 3. Breast bone
2. Appendicular skeleton a. Upper extremities	1. Clavicle 2. Scapula 3. Humerus 4. Radius 5. Ulna 6. Carpals 7. Metacarpals 8. Phalanges	2 2 2 2 2 16 10 28	1. Collar bone; shoulder girdle fastened to axial skeleton by articulation of clavicle with sternum 2. Shoulder blade 3. Long bone of upper arm 4. Thumb side of forearm 5. Little finger side of forearm 6. Wrist bones; arranged in 2 rows at proximal end of hand 7. Long bones; form framework of palm of hand 8. Miniature long bones of fingers; 3 in each finger, 2 in each thumb

Table 1-3. Bones of the body—cont'd

Part of body	Name of bone	Number	Description
b. Lower extremities	1. Os coxae, or pelvic bone	2	1. Large hip bones; lower extremities attached to axial skeleton by articulation of pelvic bones with sacrum
	2. Femur	2	2. Thigh bone
	3. Patella	2	3. Kneecap
	4. Tibia	2	4. Shin bone
	5. Fibula	2	5. Long, slender bone of lateral side of lower leg
	6. Tarsals	14	6. "Ankle" bones; form heel and proximal end of foot
	7. Metatarsals	10	7. Long bones of feet
	8. Phalanges	28	8. Miniature long bones of toes
	Total	206*	

*Sesamoid bones (rounded bones found in various tendons) have not been counted except for patellae, which are largest sesamoid bones; number of these bones varies greatly between individuals. Wormian bones (small islets of bones in some cranial sutures) have not been counted because of variability of occurrence.

b. Pronation—forearm movement turning back of hand forward
c. Inversion—ankle movement turning sole of foot inward
d. Eversion—ankle movement turning sole of foot outward
e. Protraction—moving part, such as lower jaw, forward
f. Retraction—pulling part back; opposite of protraction

Ossification

A. Process that replaces cartilage or fibrous tissue with bony tissue; skeleton originally formed of fibrous membranes and hyaline cartilage, most of which undergoes ossification before birth; ossification not completed, however, until about age 25; two processes accomplish ossification: formation of bone matrix and then its calcification
   1. Formation of bone matrix (the intercellular substance of bone, made up of collagen fibers and a cementlike substance)—osteoblasts (bone-forming cells) synthesize collagen and cement substance from proteins provided by the diet; vitamin C promotes formation of bone matrix; exercise and estrogens act in some way to stimulate osteoblasts to form bone matrix
   2. Calcification of bone matrix—calcium salts deposited in the bone matrix; vitamin D promotes calcification

B. Growth
   1. In length—by continual thickening of epiphyseal cartilage followed by ossification; as long as bone growth continues, epiphyseal cartilage grows faster than it can be replaced by bone; therefore, line of cartilage persists between diaphysis and epiphyses and can be seen on x-ray film; during adolescence cartilage is completely transformed into bone, at which time bone growth is complete
   2. In diameter—osteoclasts destroy bone surrounding medullary cavity, thereby enlarging the cavity; at same time, osteoblasts add new bone around outer surface of the bone

Bone pathology

A. Fractures
   1. Simple fracture—bone breaks but does not pierce the skin
   2. Compound fracture—bone breaks and pierces the skin
   3. Partial fracture—incomplete break in the bone
   4. Comminuted fracture—the bone is splintered into fragments
   5. Greenstick fracture—a break in one side of a long bone with a bending of the opposite side

B. Bone disorders
   1. Osteomalacia—demineralization of bone caused by vitamin D deficiency

2. Osteomyelitis—infectious disease of the bone marrow and periosteum
3. Osteoporosis—a decrease in bone strength usually caused by hormone change
4. Rickets—condition in children produced by vitamin D deficiency

MUSCULAR SYSTEM
Functions

A. Movement
B. Posture
C. Heat production—metabolism in muscle cells produces relatively large share of body heat

Types of muscles and neural control

A. Striated—controlled by voluntary nervous system via somatic motoneurons in spinal and some cranial nerves
B. Smooth—controlled by autonomic nervous system via autonomic motoneurons in autonomic, spinal, and some cranial nerves; not under voluntary control (with rare exceptions)
C. Cardiac—control is identical to smooth muscle

Basic principles of skeletal muscle action

A. Skeletal muscles contract only if stimulated; a skeletal muscle and its motor nerve function as a physiologic unit; either is useless without the other's functioning; for this reason anything that prevents impulse conduction to a skeletal muscle paralyzes the muscle
B. Most skeletal muscles attach to at least 2 bones; as a muscle contracts and pulls on its bones, it moves the bone that moves most easily; the bone that moves is called the muscle's insertion bone, and the bone that holds stationary is its origin bone
C. Bones serve as levers, and joints as fulcrums of these levers; a muscle's contraction exerts a pulling force on its insertion bone at the point where the muscle inserts, pulling that point nearer the muscle's origin bone
D. Skeletal muscles almost always act in groups rather than singly; members of groups are classified as follows:
  1. Prime movers—the muscle or muscles whose contraction actually produces the movement
  2. Synergists—muscles that contract at the same time as the prime mover, helping it produce the movement or stabilizing the part; i.e., holding it steady, so the prime mover can produce a more effective movement
  3. Antagonists—muscles that relax while the prime mover is contracting (exception: antagonist contracts at the same time as the prime mover when a part needs to be held rigid, as the knee joint does in standing); antagonists usually have directly opposite locations with reference to bones they move; e.g., muscle that flexes lower arm lies on anterior surface of upper arm bone, whereas that which extends lower arm lies on posterior surface of upper arm
E. The body of a muscle usually does not lie over the part moved by the muscle; instead it lies above or below, or anterior or posterior to, the part; thus the body of a muscle that moves the lower arm will not be located in the lower arm but in the upper arm; e.g., biceps and triceps brachii muscles
F. Contraction of a skeletal muscle either shortens the muscle, producing movement, or increases the tension (tone) in the muscle; contractions are classified according to whether they produce movement or increase muscle tone as follows:
  1. Tonic contractions—produce muscle tone; do not shorten the muscle so do not produce movements; only a few fibers contract at one time and this produces a moderate degree of muscle tone; in the healthy, awake body, all muscles exhibit tone
  2. Isometric contractions—increase the degree of muscle tone; do not shorten the muscle so do not produce movements; daily repetition of isometric contractions gradually increases muscle strength
  3. Isotonic contractions—muscle shortens, thereby producing movement; all movements are produced by isotonic contractions

Origins, insertions, and functions of main skeletal muscles

Grouped according to functions (Table 1-4)

Table 1-4. Origins, insertions, and functions of main skeletal muscles

Part of body moved	Movement	Muscle	Origin	Insertion
Upper arm	Flexion	Pectoralis major	Clavicle (medial half) Sternum Costal cartilages of true ribs	Humerus (greater tubercle)
	Extension	Latissimus dorsi	Vertebrae (spines of lower thoracic, lumbar, and sacral) Ilium (crest) Lumbodorsal fascia	Humerus (intertubercular groove)
	Abduction	Deltoid	Clavicle Scapula (spine and acromion)	Humerus (lateral side on deltoid tubercle)
	Adduction	Latissimus dorsi contracting with Pectoralis major	See above See above	See above See above
Shoulder	Shrugging, elevating	Trapezius	Occipital bone Vertebrae (cervical and thoracic)	Scapula (spine and acromion) Clavicle
	Lowering	Pectoralis minor Serratus anterior	Ribs (second to fifth) Ribs (upper 8 or 9)	Scapula (coracoid) Scapula (anterior surface)
Lower arm	Flexion (With forearm supinated)	Biceps brachii	Scapula (supraglenoid tuberosity) Scapula (coracoid)	Radius (tubercle at proximal end)
	(With forearm pronated)	Brachialis	Humerus (distal half, anterior surface)	Ulna (front of coronoid process)
	(With forearm semisupinated or semipronated)	Brachioradialis	Humerus (above lateral epicondyle)	Radius (styloid process)
	Extension	Triceps brachii	Scapula (infraglenoid tuberosity) Humerus (posterior surface—lateral head above radial groove; medial head, below)	Ulna (olecranon process)
Thigh	Flexion	Iliopsoas (iliacus and psoas major)	Ilium (iliac fossa) Vertebrae (bodies of twelfth thoracic to fifth lumbar)	Femur (small trochanter)
		Rectus femoris	Ilium and anterior, inferior iliac spine	Tibia (by way of patellar tendon)
	Extension	Gluteus maximus	Ilium (crest and posterior surface) Sacrum and coccyx (posterior surface) Sacrotuberous ligament	Femur (gluteal tuberosity) Iliotibial tract
		Hamstring group (see below)	Ischium (tuberosity) Femur (linea aspera)	Fibula (head of) Tibia (lateral condyle, medial condyle, and medial surface)
	Abduction	Gluteus medius and minimus	Ilium (lateral surface)	Femur (greater trochanter)
		Tensor fasciae latae	Ilium (anterior part of crest)	Iliotibial tract

Continued.

Table 1-4. Origins, insertions, and functions of main skeletal muscles—cont'd

Part of body moved	Movement	Muscle	Origin	Insertion
Thigh— cont'd	Adduction	Adductor group Brevis Longus Magnus	Pubic bone	Femur (linea aspera)
Lower leg	Flexion	Hamstring group Biceps femoris Semitendinosus Semimembranosus	Ischium (tuberosity) Femur (linea aspera)	Fibula (head of) Tibia (lateral condyle, medial condyle, and medial surface)
		Gastrocnemius	Femur (condyles)	Tarsal bone (calcaneus by way of tendo calcaneus)
	Extension	Quadriceps femoris group Rectus femoris Vastus lateralis Vastus medialis Vastus intermedius	Ilium (anterior, inferior spine) Femur (linea aspera and anterior surface)	Tibia (by way of patellar tendon)
Foot	Flexion (dorsiflexion)	Tibialis anterior	Tibia (lateral condyle)	First cuneiform tarsal Base of first metatarsal
	Extension (plantar flexion)	Gastrocnemius	Femur (condyles)	Calcaneus, by way of tendo calcaneus
		Soleus	Tibia	Same as gastrocnemius, but underneath
Head	Flexion	Sternocleidomastoid	Sternum Clavicle	Temporal bone (mastoid process)
	Extension	Trapezius	Vertebrae (cervical) Scapula (spine and acromion) Clavicle	Occiput
Abdominal wall	Compress abdominal cavity; therefore assists in straining, defecation, forced expiration, childbirth, posture, etc.	External oblique	Ribs (lower 8)	Innominate bone (iliac crest and pubis by way of inguinal ligament) Linea alba
		Internal oblique	Innominate bone (iliac crest, inguinal ligament) Lumbodorsal fascia	Ribs (lower 3) Pubic bone Linea alba
		Transversus	Ribs (lower 6) Innominate bone (iliac crest, inguinal ligament) Lumbodorsal fascia	Pubic bone Linea alba
		Rectus abdominis	Innominate bone (pubic bone and symphysis pubis)	Ribs (costal cartilage of fifth, sixth, seventh)
Chest wall	Elevate ribs, thereby enlarging anteroposterior and anterolateral dimensions of chest and causing inspiration	External intercostals	Ribs (lower border of all but twelfth)	Ribs (upper border of rib below origin)

Table 1-4. Origins, insertions, and functions of main skeletal muscles—cont'd

Part of body moved	Movement	Muscle	Origin	Insertion
Chest wall —cont'd	Depress ribs	Internal intercostals	Ribs (inner surface, upper border of all except first)	Ribs (lower border of rib above origin)
	Pull floor of thorax downward, thereby enlarging vertical dimension of chest and causing inspiration	Diaphragm	Lower circumference of rib cage	Central tendon of diaphragm
Trunk	Flexion	Iliopsoas	Femur (small trochanter)	Ilium Vertebrae (bodies of twelfth thoracic to fifth lumbar)
	Extension	Sacrospinalis Iliocostalis (lateral) Longissimus (medial)	Vertebrae (posterior surface of sacrum, spinous processes of lumbar and last 2 thoracic)	Ribs (lower 6) Vertebrae (transverse processes of thoracic) Ribs
			Ilium (posterior part of crest)	Vertebrae (spines of thoracic)
		Quadratus lumborum	Ilium (posterior part of crest) Vertebrae (lower 3 lumbar)	Ribs (twelfth) Vertebrae (transverse processes of first 4 lumbar)

Weak places in abdominal wall where hernias may occur

A. Inguinal rings—right and left internal, right and left external
B. Femoral rings—right and left
C. Umbilicus

Bursae

A. Definition—small sacs lined with synovial membrane and containing synovial fluid
B. Locations—wherever pressure is exerted over moving parts
   1. Between skin and bone
   2. Between tendons and bone
   3. Between muscles or ligaments and bone
C. Names of bursae that frequently become inflamed (bursitis)

1. Subacromial—between deltoid muscle and head of humerus and acromion process
2. Olecranon—between olecranon process and skin; inflammation called "student's elbow"
3. Prepatellar—between patella and skin; inflammation called "housemaid's knee"
D. Function—act as cushions, relieving pressure between moving parts

Tendon sheaths

A. Definition and location—tube-shaped structures that enclose certain tendons, notably those of wrist and ankle; made of connective tissue lined with synovial membrane
B. Function—facilitate gliding movements of tendon

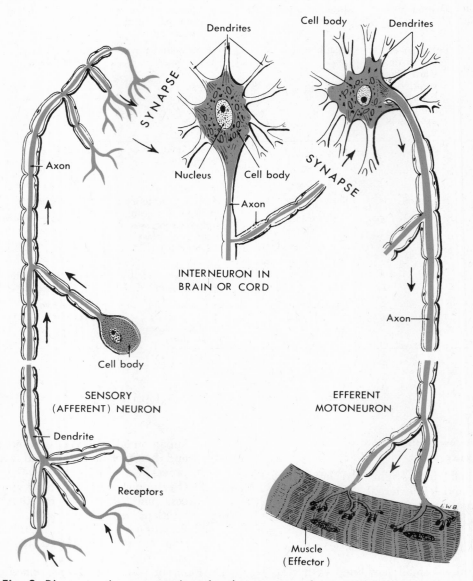

Fig. 3. Diagrammatic representation of a three-neuron reflex arc. Note that each neuron has three parts: a cell body and two extensions, dendrite(s) and an axon. (From Anthony, C. P., and Kolthoff, N. J.: Textbook of anatomy and physiology, ed. 9, St. Louis, 1975, The C. V. Mosby Co.)

INTEGRATION AND CONTROL OF THE BODY

NERVOUS SYSTEM
Cells

A. Neuroglia (glial cells)—specialized cells that serve as connective tissue for the central nervous system; these cells are far more numerous than the neurons; they consist of several types having different shapes and functions; specializations range from ciliated cells of the central canal to the Schwann cells that produce myelin; many have supporting networks that surround neurons, others are attached to blood vessels; they are clinically important because they give rise to many tumors of the nervous system

B. Neurons (nerve cells)
1. Types
   a. Sensory (afferent) neurons—transmit impulses to spinal cord or brain
   b. Motoneurons (motor or efferent neurons)—transmit impulses away from brain or spinal cord toward or to muscles or glands
      (1) Somatic motoneurons—transmit impulses from cord or brainstem to skeletal muscle
      (2) Visceral or autonomic motoneurons—transmit impulses from cord or brainstem to smooth muscle, cardiac muscle, or glands
   c. Interneurons (internuncial or intercalated neurons)—transmit impulses from sensory neurons to motoneurons
2. Structure (Fig. 3)
   a. Main structural difference from other cells is that threadlike structures called dendrites, axons, or nerve fibers extend out from opposite ends of neuron cell bodies; this unique structural feature makes neuron well suited to its special function of transmitting impulses over distances

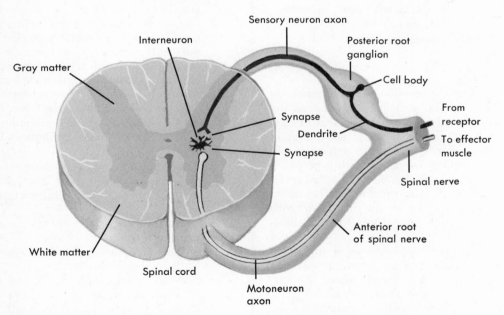

Fig. 4. Three-neuron ipsilateral reflex arc, consisting of a sensory neuron, an interneuron, and a motoneuron. Note the presence of two synapses in this arc: (1) between sensory neuron axon terminals and interneuron dendrites and (2) between interneuron axon terminals and motoneuron dendrites and cell bodies (located in anterior gray matter). Nerve impulses traversing such arcs produce many spinal reflexes. Example: withdrawing the hand from a hot object. (From Anthony, C. P., and Kolthoff, N. J.: Textbook of anatomy and physiology, ed. 9, St. Louis, 1975, The C. V. Mosby Co.)

b. Dendrites—fibers that conduct impulses to neuron cell body; most neurons have several dendrites

c. Receptors—the beginnings of dendrites of sensory neurons, the part that receives stimuli; impulse conduction normally begins in receptors

d. Axons—fibers that conduct impulses away from neuron cell bodies; each neuron has only 1 axon, but this may have 1 or more branches

e. Myelin sheath—segmented covering around nerve fiber

f. Neurilemma—continuous sheath around segmented myelin sheath; essential for nerve fiber regeneration; absent from brain and spinal cord fibers; these are not known to regenerate if destroyed by disease or injury

g. Synapse—contact points between endings of axon of one neuron and dendrites or cell body of another neuron

h. Effector—structure in which motoneuron axons terminate; specifically, either muscle or gland

3. Function—impulse conduction

Nerve impulse

A. Definitions

1. Resting potential—the difference in electric charge that exists between the outer and inner surfaces of a neuron cell membrane when it is resting, in other words, when the neuron is not conducting impulses; resting potential normally equals about 70 to 90 millivolts, with the outside of the membrane positive to the inside or with the inside negative to the outside

2. Action potential—synonym for nerve impulse; a self-propagating wave of negativity that travels along the surface of a neuron's membrane

B. Basic route of impulse conduction—the reflex arc

1. Description—impulse conduction
   a. Starts in receptors
   b. Continues over reflex arc(s)
   c. Terminates in effectors (muscles and glands)
   d. Results in a reflex—a response by muscles or glands in which impulse terminates; a reflex, therefore, is either contraction of muscle or secretion by gland

   e. Not all impulses result in reflexes; many are inhibited at some point along the reflex arc

2. Types of reflex arcs
   a. Two-neuron (monosynaptic) reflex arc—simplest arc possible; consists of at least 1 sensory neuron, 1 synapse, and 1 motoneuron; synapse is region of contact between axon terminals of one neuron and dendrites or cell body of another neuron

   b. Three-neuron arc (Fig. 4)—consists of at least 1 sensory neuron, synapse, interneuron, synapse, and motoneuron

   c. Complex, multisynaptic neural pathways also exist; many not yet clearly mapped

C. Conduction across synapses

1. When impulse reaches axon terminals, a chemical (acetylcholine or norepinephrine) is ejected into the microscopic synaptic space

2. Chemical released from many axon terminals has a stimulating effect on adjacent neurons (presumably this stimulating chemical is either acetylcholine or norepinephrine); chemical released from other axon terminals has an inhibitory effect on adjacent neurons; gamma-aminobutyric acid (GABA) is one inhibitory chemical

3. Axons that release acetylcholine called cholinergic fibers; those that release norepinephrine called adrenergic fibers

4. Termination of action of chemical transmitters
   a. Acetylcholine inactivated in synapses by cholinesterase
   b. Most norepinephrine leaves synapses to reenter axons, where some of it is again stored in small vesicles, and some is inactivated by monoamine oxidase in mitochondria; some norepinephrine inactivated in synapses by catechol-O-methyl transferase (COMT)

D. Speed of impulse conduction
   1. The larger the diameter of an axon

the faster it conducts impulses; largest, fastest-conducting fibers; e.g., axons of somatic motoneurons transmit impulses at speed of about 100 meters per second (more than 200 miles per hour)

2. The smaller an axon's diameter, the slower it conducts impulses; smallest, slowest-conducting fibers transmit impulses at speed of about 1 mile per hour

Organs of nervous system

A. Central nervous system (CNS)—spinal cord and brain
B. Peripheral nervous system (PNS)—nerves and ganglia
C. Definitions
1. White matter—bundles of myelinated nerve fibers
2. Gray matter—clusters of mainly neuron cell bodies
3. Nerves—bundles of myelinated nerve fibers located outside CNS
4. Tracts—bundles of myelinated nerve fibers located within CNS
5. Ganglia (singular, ganglion)—microscopic structures consisting of neuron cell bodies; mainly located outside CNS

Spinal cord

A. Location—in spinal cavity, from foramen magnum to first lumbar vertebra
B. Structure
1. Deep groove (anterior median fissure) and more shallow groove (posterior median sulcus) incompletely divide cord into right and left symmetric halves
2. Inner core of cord consists of gray matter shaped like a three-dimensional letter H
3. Long columns of white matter surround the cord's inner core of gray matter; namely, right and left anterior, lateral, and posterior columns; composed of numerous sensory and motor tracts (Fig. 5)
C. Functions
1. Sensory tracts conduct impulses up cord to brain; motor tracts conduct impulses down cord from brain
2. Gray matter of cord contains reflex centers for all spinal cord reflexes

Brain—divisions of brain named in ascending order—medulla, pons, midbrain, cerebellum, diencephalon, and cerebrum

A. Medulla
1. Part of brain formed by enlargement of cord as it enters cranial cavity
2. Consists mainly of white matter (sensory and motor tracts); also contains reticular formation (mixture of gray and white matter); some important reflex centers located in reticular formation: cardiac, vasomotor, respiratory, and swallowing centers
3. Functions—contains centers for vital heart, blood vessel diameter (blood pressure), and respiratory reflexes; also centers for vomiting, coughing, swallowing, etc.; conducts impulses between cord and brain (both sensory and motor)
B. Pons
1. Part of brain located just above medulla; consists mainly of white matter (sensory and motor tracts) interspersed with gray matter (reflex centers)
2. Conducts impulses between cord and various parts of brain and contains reflex centers for cranial nerves V, VI, VII, and VIII
C. Midbrain
1. Part of brain located between the pons which lies below it, and the diencephalon and cerebrum, which lie above it; consists mainly of white matter with scattered bits of gray matter
2. Conducts impulses between cord and various parts of brain and contains reflex centers for cranial nerves III and IV (thus for pupillary reflexes and eye movements)
D. Diencephalon—thalamus and hypothalamus are major parts of the diencephalon
1. Thalamus
a. Large rounded mass of gray matter in each cerebral hemisphere, lateral to third ventricle
b. Functions—conscious recognition of crude sensations of pain, temperature, and touch; relays almost all sensory impulses to cerebral cortex; responsible for emotional com-

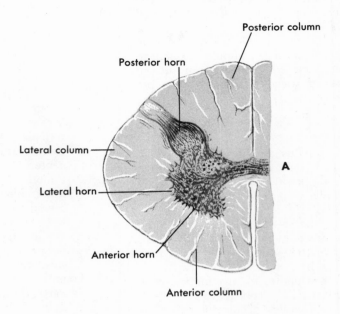

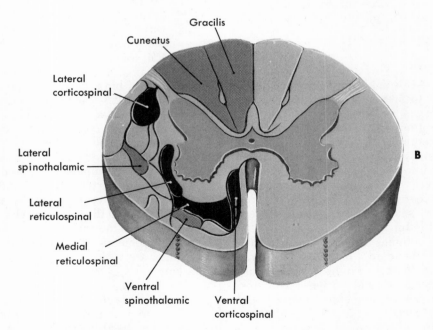

Fig. 5. A, Distribution of gray matter (horns) and white matter (columns) in a section of the spinal cord at the thoracic level. **B,** Location in the spinal cord of some major projection tracts. Black areas, descending motor tracts. Shaded areas, ascending sensory tracts. (From Anthony, C. P., and Kolthoff, N. J.: Textbook of anatomy and physiology, ed. 9, St. Louis, 1975, The C. V. Mosby Co.)

ponent of sensations; e.g., feelings of pleasantness or unpleasantness associated with them

2. Hypothalamus
   a. Gray matter that forms floor of third ventricle and lower part of its lateral walls
   b. Functions
      (1) Contains many higher autonomic reflex centers; these centers integrate autonomic functions by sending impulses to each other and to lower autonomic centers; they form a crucial part of the neural path by which emotions and other cerebral functions can alter vital, automatic functions such as the heartbeat, blood pressure, peristalsis, and secretion by glands and, thereby, produce psychosomatic diseases; neural path for psychosomatic disease—impulses from cerebral cortex to autonomic centers in hypothalamus, to lower autonomic centers in brainstem and cord, to visceral effectors; e.g., heart, smooth muscle, glands
      (2) Helps control both the anterior pituitary gland and the posterior pituitary gland; certain neurons in hypothalamus release secretions into the pituitary portal veins, which transport them to the anterior pituitary gland where they influence secretion of various important hormones; e.g., hypothalamic neurons secrete CRF (corticotropin-releasing factor) into pituitary portal veins, which stimulates the anterior pituitary gland to secrete ACTH into the blood; neurons in the supraoptic nucleus of the hypothalamus synthesize ADH (antidiuretic hormone); from the cell bodies of these neurons, ADH migrates down their axons into the posterior pituitary gland, from which it is released into the blood; in short, hypothalamic neurons

make ADH, but the posterior pituitary gland secretes it
      (3) Certain hypothalamic neurons serve as an appetite center and others function as a satiety center; together these centers regulate appetite and food intake
      (4) Certain hypothalamic neurons serve as heat-regulating centers by relaying impulses to lower autonomic centers for vasoconstriction, vasodilation, and sweating, and to somatic centers for shivering
      (5) Maintains waking state; constitutes part of the arousal or alerting neural pathway

E. Cerebrum
   1. Hemispheres, fissures, and lobes—longitudinal fissure divides cerebrum into 2 hemispheres connected only by corpus callosum; each cerebral hemisphere divided by fissures into 5 lobes: frontal, parietal, temporal, occipital, and island of Reil (insula)
   2. Cerebral cortex—outer layer of gray matter arranged in ridges called convolutions or gyri
   3. Cerebral tracts—bundles of axons compose white matter in interior of cerebrum; ascending projection tracts transmit impulses toward or to brain; descending projection tracts transmit impulses down from brain to cord; commissural tracts transmit from one hemisphere to the other; association tracts transmit from one convolution to another in same hemisphere
   4. Basal ganglia (or cerebral nuclei)—masses of gray matter embedded deep inside white matter in interior of cerebrum; caudate, putamen, and pallidum; putamen and pallidum constitute lenticular nucleus
   5. Functions—in general, all conscious functions; e.g., analysis, integration, and interpretation of sensations, control of voluntary movements, use and understanding of language, and all other mental functions

F. Cerebellum
   1. Structure—second-largest part of human brain; surface marked with sulci (grooves) and very slightly raised, slender convolutions; internal white

matter forms pattern suggestive of veins of leaf

2. Functions
   a. The cerebellum exerts synergic control over skeletal muscles; this means that impulses conducted by cerebellar neurons coordinate skeletal muscle contractions to produce smooth, steady, and precise movements
   b. Because it coordinates skeletal muscle contractions, the cerebellum plays an essential part in producing normal postures and maintaining equilibrium

G. Cord and brain coverings
   1. Bony—vertebrae around cord; cranial bones around brain
   2. Membranous—called meninges; consist of three layers
      a. Dura mater—white fibrous tissue, outer layer
      b. Arachnoid membrane—cobwebby middle layer
      c. Pia mater—innermost layer of meninges; adheres to outer surface of cord and brain; contains blood vessels

H. Cord and brain fluid spaces
   1. Subarachnoid space around cord and extending beyond the cord into the fourth and fifth lumbar vertebrae
   2. Subarachnoid space around brain
   3. Central canal inside cord
   4. Ventricles and cerebral aqueduct inside brain; 4 cavities within brain
      a. First and second (lateral ventricles) —large cavities, one in each cerebral hemisphere
      b. Third ventricle—vertical slit in cerebrum beneath corpus callosum and longitudinal fissure
      c. Fourth ventricle—diamond-shaped space between cerebellum and medulla and pons; is expansion of central canal of cord

I. Formation and circulation of cerebrospinal fluid
   1. Formed by plasma filtering from network of capillaries (choroid plexus) in each ventricle
   2. Circulates from lateral ventricles to third ventricle, cerebral aqueduct, fourth ventricle, central canal of cord, subarachnoid space of cord and brain;

returns to blood via venous sinuses of brain

Cranial nerves—12 pairs

See Table 1-5

Spinal nerves—31 pairs

A. Each nerve attaches to cord by 2 short roots, anterior and posterior; posterior roots marked by swelling, namely, spinal ganglion
B. Branches of spinal nerves form plexuses or intricate networks of fibers; e.g., brachial plexus from which nerves emerge to supply various parts of skin, mucosa, and skeletal muscles
C. All spinal nerves are mixed nerves composed of both sensory dendrites and motor axons and function in both sensations and movements

Sensory neural pathways—conduction

A. Sensory pathways to the cerebral cortex from the periphery consist of relays of at least 3 neurons, which are identified by Roman numerals
   1. Sensory neuron I—conducts from the periphery to the cord or to the brainstem
   2. Sensory neuron II—conducts from the cord or brainstem to the thalamus
   3. Sensory neuron III—conducts from the thalamus to the general sensory area of the cerebral cortex
B. Crude awareness of sensations occurs when impulses reach the thalamus
C. Full consciousness of sensations with accurate localization and discrimination of fine details occurs when impulses reach the cerebral cortex
D. Most sensory neuron II axons decussate; so one side of the brain registers most of the sensations for the opposite side of the body
E. The principle of divergence applies to sensory neural pathways; each sensory neuron synapses with many neurons and therefore impulses may diverge from any sensory neuron and be conducted to many effectors
F. Impulses that produce pain and temperature are conducted up the cord to the thalamus by the lateral spinothalamic tracts
G. Impulses that produce touch and pressure sensations are conducted up the

Table 1-5. Distribution and function of cranial nerve pairs

Name and number	Distribution	Function
Olfactory (I)	Nasal mucosa, high up along the septum especially	Sense of smell (sensory only)
Optic (II)	Retina of eyeball	Vision (sensory only)
Oculomotor (III)	Extrinsic muscles of eyeball, except superior oblique and external rectus; also intrinsic eye muscles (iris and ciliary)	Eye movements; constriction of pupil and bulging of lens, which together produce accommodation for near vision
Trochlear (IV) (smallest cranial nerve)	Superior oblique muscle of eye	Eye movements
Trifacial (V) (or trigeminal) largest cranial nerve	Sensory fibers to skin and mucosa of head and to teeth; muscles of mastication (sensory and motor fibers)	Sensations of head and face; chewing movements
Abducens (VI)	External rectus muscle of eye	Abduction of eye
Facial (VII)	Muscles of facial expression; taste buds of anterior two thirds of tongue; motor fibers to submaxillary and sublingual salivary glands	Facial expressions; taste; secretion of saliva
Auditory (VIII) (acoustic)	Inner ear	Hearing and equilibrium (sensory only)
Glossopharyngeal (IX)	Posterior one third of tongue; mucosa and muscles of pharynx; parotid gland; carotid sinus and body	Taste and other sensations of tongue; secretion of saliva; swallowing movements; functions in reflex arcs for control of blood pressure and respiration
Vagus (X) (or pneumogastric)	Mucosa and muscles of pharynx, larynx, trachea, bronchi, esophagus; thoracic and abdominal viscera	Sensations and movements of organs supplied; for example, slows heart, increases peristalsis and gastric and pancreatic secretion; voice production
Spinal accessory (XI)	Certain neck and shoulder muscles (muscles of larynx, sternocleidomastoid, trapezius)	Shoulder movements; turns head; voice production; muscle sense
Hypoglossal (XII)	Tongue muscles	Tongue movements, as in talking; muscle sense

Note: The first letters of the words in the following sentence are the first letters of the names of the cranial nerves, and many generations of anatomy students have used it as an aid to memorizing the names: "On Old Olympus Tiny Tops, A Finn and German Viewed Some Hops." (There are several slightly different versions of this sentence.)

cord to the thalamus by the following 2 pathways

1. Impulses that result in discriminating touch and pressure sensations (such as stereognosis, precise localization, and vibratory sense) are conducted by the tracts of the posterior white columns of the cord to the medulla and from there are transferred to the thalamus
2. Impulses that result in crude touch and pressure sensations are conducted up the cord to the thalamus by fibers of the ventral spinothalamic tracts

H. Sensory impulses that result in conscious proprioception or kinesthesia (sense of position or movement of body parts) are conducted over the same pathway as are impulses that result in discriminating touch and pressure sensations

I. Sensory impulses, in addition, are also conducted to the cerebral cortex via complex multineuron pathways known as the reticular activating system; spino-

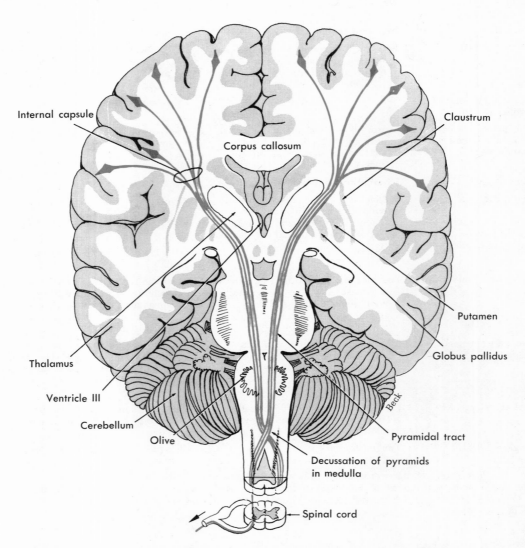

Fig. 6. The crossed pyramidal tracts (lateral corticospinal), the main motor tracts of the body. Axons that compose pyramidal tracts come from neuron cell bodies in the cerebral cortex. After they descend through the internal capsule of the cerebrum and the white matter of the brainstem, about ¾ of the fibers decussate—cross over from one side to the other—in the medulla, as shown here. Then they continue downward in the lateral corticospinal tract on the opposite side of the cord. Each lateral corticospinal tract, therefore, conducts motor impulses from one side of the brain to skeletal muscles on the opposite side of the body. (From Anthony, C. P., and Kolthoff, N. J.: Textbook of anatomy and physiology, ed. 9, St. Louis, 1975, The C. V. Mosby Co.)

reticular tracts relay sensory impulses up the cord to the brainstem reticular gray matter, and from there other neurons relay them to the hypothalamus, thalamus, and probably other parts of the brain, then finally to the cerebral cortex; conduction by the reticular activating system is essential for producing and maintaining consciousness; presumably, general anesthetics produce unconsciousness by inhibiting conduction by the reticular activating system; conversely, amphetamines and norepinephrine are thought to produce wakefulness by stimulating the reticular activating system

Motor neural pathways to skeletal muscles

A. Principle of the final common path— the final common path for impulse conduction to skeletal muscles consists of anterior horn neurons (i.e., motoneurons whose dendrites and cell bodies lie in the anterior gray columns of the cord and whose axons extend out through the anterior roots of spinal nerves and their branches to terminate in skeletal muscles); besides being referred to as the final common path and as anterior horn cells, these neurons are also called lower motoneurons and somatic motoneurons
B. Principle of convergence—axons of many neurons converge on (i.e., synapse with) each anterior horn motoneuron
C. Motor pathways from the cerebral cortex to anterior horn cells are classified according to the route by which the fibers enter the cord:
   1. Pyramidal tracts (corticospinal tracts) —axons of neurons whose dendrites and cell bodies lie in the cerebral cortex; axons descend from cortex through internal capsule, pyramids of medulla, and spinal cord; a few of these axons synapse with anterior horn cells, but most of them synapse with internuncial neurons that synapse with anterior horn cells; conduction by pyramidal tracts is necessary for willed movements to occur; hence one cause of paralysis is interruption of pyramidal tract conduction
   2. Extrapyramidal tracts—all tracts that conduct between the motor cortex and the anterior horn cells, except the pyramidal tracts; upper extrapyramidal tracts relay impulses between the cortex, basal ganglia, thalamus, and brainstem; reticulospinal tracts (the main lower extrapyramidal tracts) relay impulses from the brainstem to the anterior horn cells in the cord; impulse conduction via extrapyramidal tracts is essential for producing large, automatic movements (e.g., walking, swimming) and for producing facial expressions and movements that characterize many emotions
D. The motor conduction pathway from the primary motor area of the cerebral cortex to skeletal muscles via pyramidal tracts consists of a two-neuron relay; an upper motoneuron conducts impulses from cerebrum to cord and a lower motoneuron (anterior horn cell) conducts from cord to skeletal muscle (Fig. 6)
E. The motor conduction pathway from the cerebral cortex via extrapyramidal tracts consists of complex multineuron relays; several upper motoneurons relay impulses through basal ganglia, thalamus, brainstem, and down the cord to the lower motoneuron
F. Motor pathways from the cerebral cortex to anterior horn cells are classified according to their influence on anterior horn cells as follows:
   1. Facilitatory tracts—conduct impulses that have a facilitating or stimulating effect on anterior horn cells; main facilitatory tracts are the pyramidal tracts and the facilitatory reticulospinal tracts
   2. Inhibitory tracts—conduct impulses that have an inhibiting effect on anterior horn cells; main inhibitory tracts are the inhibitory reticulospinal tracts; interruption of inhibitory reticulospinal tracts results in spasticity and rigidity
G. The ratio of facilitatory and inhibitory impulses impinging on anterior horn cells determines their activity (whether they are facilitated, stimulated, or inhibited)

Autonomic nervous system

A. Definition—the division of the nervous system that conducts impulses from the brainstem or cord out to visceral effectors; visceral effectors are cardiac muscle, smooth muscle, and glandular tissue
B. Divisions—autonomic nervous system consists of 2 divisions: the sympathetic

(thoracolumbar) system and the parasympathetic (craniosacral) system

1. Sympathetic system
   a. Sympathetic ganglia—2 chains of 21 or 22 ganglia located immediately in front of the spinal column, one chain to the right, one to the left
   b. Collateral ganglia—located a short distance from the cord; e.g., celiac ganglia (solar plexus), superior and inferior mesenteric ganglia
   c. Sympathetic nerves—e.g., splanchnic nerves, cardiac nerves
2. Parasympathetic system
   a. Parasympathetic ganglia—located at a distance from the spinal column, in or near visceral effectors; e.g., ciliary ganglion in posterior part of the orbit, near the iris and ciliary muscle
   b. Parasympathetic nerves—e.g., vagus nerve, called the great parasympathetic nerve of the body

C. Neurons
   1. Preganglionic sympathetic neurons—dendrites and cell bodies lie in lateral gray columns of thoracic and lumbar segments of cord; axons conduct from cord to sympathetic ganglia or to collateral ganglia
   2. Postganglionic sympathetic neurons—dendrites and cell bodies lie in sympathetic ganglia or in collateral ganglia; axons conduct to visceral effectors
   3. Preganglionic parasympathetic neurons—dendrites and cell bodies of some of these neurons lie in gray matter of brainstem and others lie in gray matter of sacral segments of cord; conduct impulses from brainstem or cord to parasympathetic ganglia
   4. Postganglionic parasympathetic neurons—dendrites and cell bodies lie in parasympathetic ganglia; axons conduct to visceral effectors

D. Some principles about the autonomic nervous system
   1. Dual autonomic innervation—both sympathetic and parasympathetic fibers supply most visceral effectors
   2. Single autonomic innervation—only sympathetic fibers supply sweat glands and probably the smooth muscles of hairs and of most blood vessels; preganglionic sympathetic fibers terminate in adrenal medulla (not postganglionic fibers as in other glands)
   3. Autonomic chemical transmitters—all preganglionic axons are cholinergic fibers, as are most (or perhaps all) parasympathetic postganglionic axons and a few sympathetic postganglionic axons (to sweat glands, external genitalia, and smooth muscle in walls of blood vessels located in skeletal muscles); sympathetic postganglionic axons are the only adrenergic (i.e., norepinephrine-releasing) fibers; but, as just mentioned, a few of them are cholinergic
   4. Autonomic antagonism and summation—sympathetic and parasympathetic impulses tend to produce opposite effects; algebraic sum of two opposing tendencies determines response made by doubly innervated visceral effector
   5. The principle of parasympathetic dominance of the digestive tract—normally, parasympathetic impulses to digestive tract glands and smooth muscle dominate over sympathetic impulses to them; dominance of parasympathetic impulses promotes digestive gland secretion, peristalsis, and defecation
   6. The principle of sympathetic dominance in stress—under the condition of stress, sympathetic impulses to visceral effectors usually increase greatly and dominate over parasympathetic impulses; however, in some individuals under stress, parasympathetic impulses via the vagus nerve to glands and smooth muscle of the stomach greatly increase, causing increased hydrochloric acid secretion and increased gastric motility that eventually cause peptic ulcer, a condition that may aptly be called the great parasympathetic stress disease
   7. In general, when the sympathetic system dominates control of visceral effectors, it causes them to function in ways that enable the body to expend maximum energy as is necessary in strenuous exercise and other types of stress; see Table 1-6 for sympathetic effects on specific effectors
   8. Principle of nonautonomy—autonomic nervous system neither anatomically

Table 1-6. Autonomic functions

Visceral effectors	Parasympathetic (cholinergic) effects	Sympathetic (adrenergic or cholinergic) effects
Cardiac muscle	Slows heart rate; decreases strength of contraction	Accelerates heart rate; increases strength of contraction
Smooth muscle of blood vessels Skin blood vessels	No parasympathetic fibers	Adrenergic sympathetic fibers → stimulate → constrict skin vessels
Skeletal muscle blood vessels	No parasympathetic fibers	Adrenergic sympathetic fibers → stimulate → constrict skeletal muscle vessels Cholinergic sympathetic fibers → inhibit → dilate skeletal muscle vessels
Blood vessels in cerebrum, abdominal viscera, and genitalia	Parasympathetic fibers → inhibit → dilate vessels in cerebrum, abdominal viscera, and genitalia	Adrenergic sympathetic fibers → stimulate → constrict vessels in cerebrum and abdominal viscera Cholinergic sympathetic fibers → inhibit → dilate vessels in external genitalia
Smooth muscle of hollow organs and sphincters Bronchi	Stimulates → bronchial constriction	Inhibits → bronchial dilation
Digestive tract	Stimulates → increased peristalsis	Inhibits → decreased peristalsis
Anal sphincter	Inhibits → opens sphincter for defecation	Stimulates → closes sphincter
Urinary bladder	Stimulates → contracts bladder	Inhibits → relaxes bladder
Urinary sphincters	Inhibits → opens sphincters for urination	Stimulates → closes sphincters
Eye Iris	Stimulates circular fibers → constriction of pupil	Stimulates radial fibers → dilation of pupil
Ciliary	Stimulates → accommodation for near vision (bulging of lens)	Inhibits → accommodation for far vision (flattening of lens)
Hairs (pilomotor muscles)	No parasympathetic fibers	Stimulates → "goose pimples" (piloerection)
Glands Sweat	No parasympathetic fibers	Cholinergic sympathetic fibers stimulate sweat glands
Digestive (salivary, gastric, etc.)	Stimulates secretion of saliva and gastric juice	Decreases secretion of saliva and gastric juice
Pancreas, including islets	Stimulates secretion of pancreatic juice and insulin	Decreases secretion of pancreatic juice and insulin
Liver	No parasympathetic fibers	Stimulates glycogenolysis, which tends to increase blood sugar
Adrenal medulla	No parasympathetic fibers	Stimulates epinephrine (and some norepinephrine) secretion which tends to increase blood sugar, blood pressure, and heart rate and to produce many other sympathetic effects

From Anthony, C. P., and Kolthoff, N. J.: Textbook of anatomy and physiology, ed. 9, St. Louis, 1975, The C. V. Mosby Co.

Table 1-7. Receptors

Kinds	Locations	Stimulated by	Functions
Exteroceptors	Skin, mucosa, ear, eye	Changes in external environment (e.g., pressure, heat, cold, light waves, sound waves)	Initiate reflexes Initiate sensations of many kinds (e.g., pressure, heat, cold, pain, vision, hearing)
Visceroceptors (interoceptors)	Viscera	Changes in internal environment (e.g., pressure, chemical)	Initiate reflexes Initiate sensations of many kinds (e.g., hunger, sex, nausea, pressure)
Proprioceptors	Muscles, tendons, joints, semicircular canals of inner ear	Pressure changes	Initiate reflexes Initiate muscle sense, or sense of position and movement of parts; also called kinesthesia

Table 1-8. Eye muscles

Location	Kind of muscle	Names	Functions
Extrinsic—attached to outside of eyeball and to bones of orbit	Skeletal (voluntary, striated)	Superior rectus Inferior rectus Lateral rectus Mesial rectus Superior oblique Inferior oblique	Move eyeball in various directions
Intrinsic—within eyeball	Visceral (involuntary, smooth)	Iris Ciliary muscle	Regulates size of pupil Controls shape of lens, making possible accommodation for near and far objects

nor physiologically independent of rest of nervous system; all parts of nervous system work together as single functional unit; e.g., dendrites and cells of all preganglionic neurons located in gray matter of brain stem or cord (lower autonomic centers) and influenced by impulses conducted to them from higher autonomic centers, notably in hypothalamus

9. Importance of autonomic nervous system—autonomic system plays major role in maintaining physiologic balance; under usual conditions, autonomic impulses regulate activities of visceral effectors so that they maintain or quickly restore this balance; under highly stressful conditions, problems may occur

Sense organs

Millions of receptors distributed widely throughout skin, mucosa; muscles, tendons, joints, and viscera are sense organs of body (Table 1-7)

Sense organs of skin and mucosa

Consist of receptors for spinal or cranial nerve branches; different types of receptors for different sensations such as heat, cold, pain, touch, and pressure; receptors unevenly distributed through skin and mucosa, joints, internal organs, etc.

Sense organs of muscles, tendons, and joints (proprioceptors)

Several types; e.g., muscle and tendon "spindles," stimulated by so-called "stretch stimuli"; pressure on spindles caused by stretching of muscles or tendons during movements initiates stretch reflexes

Eye

A. Highly specialized receptor
B. Anatomy
   1. Coats of eyeball

a. Outer coat—sclera proper and cornea
b. Middle coat—choroid proper, ciliary body, suspensory ligament holding lens, and iris
c. Inner coat—retina
2. Cavities and humors of eyeball
a. Anterior cavity with an anterior and posterior chamber; both chambers contain aqueous humor
b. Posterior cavity has no divisions and contains vitreous humor
3. Muscles of the eye (Table 1-8)
4. Refractory media of eye
a. Cornea
b. Aqueous humor
c. Crystalline lens (has greatest refractive power)
d. Vitreous humor
5. Accessory structures of eye
a. Eyebrows and lashes
b. Eyelids or palpebrae—lined with mucous membrane (conjunctiva) that continues over surface of eyeball; corners of eyes, where upper and lower lids join, called inner and outer canthus
c. Lacrimal apparatus—lacrimal glands, ducts, sacs, and nasolacrimal ducts
C. Physiology of vision
1. Formation of image on retina accomplished by
a. Refraction—bending of light rays as they pass through eye
b. Accommodation—bulging of lens for viewing near objects
c. Constriction of pupils—occurs simultaneously with accommodation and in bright light
d. Convergence of eyes for near objects in order that light rays from object may fall on corresponding points of 2 retinas; necessary for single binocular vision
2. Stimulation of retina—dim light causes breakdown of chemical rhodopsin present in rods, thereby initiating impulse conduction by rods; bright light causes breakdown of chemicals in cones; rods considered receptors for night vision and cones for daylight and color vision
3. Conduction to visual area in occipital lobe of cerebral cortex by fibers of optic nerves and optic tracts; vision occurs when impulses reach visual area

Ear
A. External ear—consists of auricle (or pinna) and external acoustic meatus (ear canal)
B. Middle ear—separated from external ear by tympanic membrane; middle ear contains auditory ossicles (malleus, incus, stapes) and openings from auditory (eustachian) tubes, mastoid cells, external ear, and internal ear (fenestra rotunda and ovalis); auditory tube is collapsible, lined with mucosa and extends from nasopharynx to middle ear; equalizes pressure on both sides of eardrum, as when tubes open during yawning or swallowing
C. Inner ear (or labyrinth)—composed of a bony labyrinth that has a membranous labyrinth inside it; parts of the inner ear
1. Bony vestibule that contains the membranous utricle and saccule, each of which, in turn, contains a sense organ called the macula; vestibular nerve (branch of eighth cranial nerve) supplies the maculae; maculae are sense organs for 3 sensations: equilibrium, position of the head, and acceleration and deceleration
2. Bony semicircular canals that contain the membranous semicircular canals in which are located the crista ampullaris, the sense organ for sensations of equilibrium and head movements; vestibular nerve supplies the crista as well as the macula
3. Bony cochlea that contains the membranous cochlear duct in which is located the organ of Corti, the hearing sense organ; cochlear nerve (branch of eighth cranial nerve) supplies the organ of Corti
D. Physiology of hearing
1. Sound waves moving through air enter ear canal and move down it to strike against the tympanic membrane, causing it to vibrate
2. Vibrations of tympanic membrane move the malleus, whose handle is attached to the membrane
3. Movement of the malleus moves the incus, to which the head of the malleus attaches
4. Incus attaches to the stapes; so as the

incus moves, it moves the stapes against the oval window into which it fits; as the stapes presses inwardly on the perilymph around the cochlear duct, it starts a ripple in the perilymph

5. Movement of the perilymph is transmitted to the endolymph inside the cochlear duct and stimulates the organ of Corti, which projects into the endolymph

6. Cochlear nerve conducts impulses from the organ of Corti to the brain; hearing occurs when impulses reach the auditory area in the temporal lobe of the cerebral cortex

Olfactory sense organs

Consist of receptors for first cranial nerve; located in nasal mucosa high along septum; highly sensitive to chemical stimuli, but easily fatigued

Gustatory sense organs

Consist of receptors for cranial nerves VII and IX; called taste corpuscles or taste buds; located in papillae of tongue; taste buds sensitive to sweet are most numerous at the

Table 1-9. Endocrine glands—locations and hormones

Endocrine glands	Location	Hormones
Anterior pituitary (adeno-hypophysis)	Cranial cavity, in sella turcica of sphenoid bone	Growth hormone (GH, somatotropin, somatropic hormone, STH) Thyrotropin (thyroid-stimulating hormone or TSH) Adrenocorticotropic hormone (ACTH, adrenocorticotropin) Follicle-stimulating hormone (FSH) Luteinizing hormone (LH) in female; interstitial cell–stimulating hormone (ICSH) in male Prolactin (lactogenic hormone) Melanocyte-stimulating hormone (MSH)
Posterior pituitary (neuro-hypophysis)	In sella turcica of sphenoid bone	Antidiuretic hormone (ADH, vasopressin, Pitressin)* Oxytocin
Thyroid	Overlays the thyroid cartilage below the larynx	Thyroid hormones (thyroxine and triiodothyronine) Thyrocalcitonin
Parathyroids	Usually 4 beads on posterior wall of the thyroid	Parathyroid hormone (PTH, parathormone)
Adrenal cortex	Rest upon the medial anterior surface of the kidney	Glucocorticoids (mainly cortisol and corticosterone) Mineralocorticoids (mainly aldosterone) Sex hormones (small amounts of androgens and estrogens)
Adrenal medulla		Epinephrine (mainly) Norepinephrine
Islands of Langerhans	In isolated area of the pancreas	Insulin (secreted by beta cells) Glucagon (secreted by alpha cells)
Ovaries Graafian follicles Corpus luteum	Pelvic cavity (female)	Estrogens Progesterone
Testes Interstitial cells of testes	Scrotum (male)	Testosterone

*ADH and oxytocin are synthesized in the hypothalamus but are secreted by the posterior pituitary gland. Synthesis occurs in cell bodies of neurons of the supraoptic and paraventricular nuclei. From here they migrate down the neurons' axons into the posterior pituitary gland, which secretes them into the blood.

Table 1-10. Functions of anterior pituitary hormones

Hormones	Functions	Hyposecretion effects	Hypersecretion effects
Growth hormone (GH)	Promotes protein anabolism (hence essential for normal growth)	Dwarfism (well-formed type) before skeletal growth is completed	Giantism (if occurs before skeleton full-grown)
	Promotes fat mobilization and catabolism; i.e., causes shift from carbohydrate catabolism to fat catabolism	Simmond's disease after skeletal maturity	Acromegaly (if occurs in adult)
	Slows carbohydrate metabolism; has anti-insulin, hyperglycemic, diabetogenic effect		Hyperglycemia; chronic excess GH may cause diabetes mellitus
TSH	Stimulates synthesis and secretion of thyroid hormones	Hypothyroidism: cretinism in early life, myxedema in adults	Hyperthyroidism (exophthalmic goiter, various other names)
ACTH	Stimulates adrenal cortex growth and secretion of glucocorticoids	Atrophy of adrenal cortex and hyposecretion (e.g., Addison's disease) Increased skin pigmentation	Hypertrophy of adrenal cortex and hypersecretion (Cushing's syndrome)
FSH	Stimulates primary graafian follicle to start growing and to develop to maturity Stimulates follicle cells to secrete estrogens In male, FSH stimulates development of seminiferous tubules and spermatogenesis by them	Failure of follicle and ovum to grow and mature; sterility	
LH	Essential for bringing about complete maturation of follicle and ovum Causes ovulation; therefore, LH also known as the ovulating hormone Causes formation of corpus luteum in ruptured follicle following ovulation; hence the name, luteinizing hormone Stimulates corpus luteum to secrete progesterone In male, LH is called ICSH (interstitial cell–stimulating hormone) because it stimulates interstitial cells of testes to secrete testosterone		
Prolactin	Promotes breast development during pregnancy Initiates milk secretion after delivery of baby	Failure to lactate	
MSH (melanocyte-stimulating hormone)	Postulated to increase skin pigmentation by stimulating formation and dispersion of melanin granules in humans, as it is known to do in lower animals		

tip of the tongue, those sensitive to sour and salt are most numerous at the tip and sides of the tongue, and those sensitive to bitter are most numerous at the back of the tongue; all tastes except sweet, sour, salt, and bitter result from fusion of two or more of these tastes plus olfactory stimulation

ENDOCRINE SYSTEM
Functions

A. Communication, control, and integration of body
B. Carries out same general functions as nervous system
C. Glands secrete hormones
D. Hormones enter blood directly since glands are ductless

Organs—location and hormones

See Table 1-9

Anterior pituitary gland

A. Hormones—functions and effects (Table 1-10)
B. Mechanisms influencing secretion of anterior pituitary hormones
   1. Hypothalamus—certain neurons of hypothalamus synthesize and secrete chemicals into blood vessels (i.e., the hypothalamico-hypophyseal portal system), which transport them to the anterior pituitary, where they either stimulate or inhibit secretion of specific hormones; names of these chemicals and their effects are:
      a. GH-RF (growth hormone–releasing factor) stimulates growth hormone secretion by anterior pituitary

   b. TRF (thyrotropin-releasing factor) stimulates thyrotropin secretion by anterior pituitary
   c. CRF (corticotropin or ACTH-releasing factor) stimulates ACTH secretion by anterior pituitary
   d. FSH-RF (follicle-stimulating hormone–releasing factor) stimulates FSH secretion by anterior pituitary
   e. LH-RF (luteinizing hormone–releasing factor) stimulates LH secretion by anterior pituitary
   f. PIF (prolactin-inhibiting factor) inhibits prolactin secretion by anterior pituitary; after childbirth, PIF secretion ceases, thereby allowing prolactin secretion and lactation
   g. MIF (melanocyte-stimulating hormone–inhibiting factor) inhibits MSH secretion by anterior pituitary
   2. Negative feedback mechanisms
      a. Between thyroid hormones and TSH; high blood levels of thyroid hormones inhibit TSH secretion by anterior pituitary directly by inhibiting the anterior pituitary gland or indirectly by inhibiting the hypothalamus' secretion of TRF, or perhaps by both actions
      b. Between corticoids and ACTH; high blood levels of corticoids inhibit ACTH secretion by anterior pituitary either directly or indirectly by inhibiting CRF secretion by hypothalamus
      c. Between progesterone and LH; high blood levels of LH directly

Table 1-11. Functions of posterior pituitary hormones

Hormones	Functions	Hyposecretion effects	Hypersecretion effects
ADH (antidiuretic hormone; vasopressin)	Increases water reabsorption by kidney's distal and collecting tubules, thereby producing antidiuresis (less urine volume; name based on this effect)	Diuresis (polyuria); diabetes insipidus	Antidiuresis (oliguria)
Oxytocin (the "quick-birth hormone")	Stimulates powerful contractions by pregnant uterus; name oxytocin from Greek for "swift childbirth" Stimulates milk ejection from alveoli (milk-secreting cells) of lactating breasts into ducts; essential before milk can be removed by suckling		

or indirectly inhibit LH secretion by anterior pituitary

    d. Between estrogens and FSH; high blood levels of estrogens directly or indirectly inhibit FSH secretion by anterior pituitary

3. Other mechanisms such as

    a. Stress and low blood sugar increase growth hormone secretion

    b. Suckling increases prolactin secretion

Posterior pituitary gland

A. Hormones—functions and effects (Table 1-11)

B. Mechanisms influencing secretion of posterior pituitary hormones

1. ADH (antidiuretic hormone) secretion is controlled chiefly by the osmotic pressure and volume of the extracellular fluid; a decrease in extracellular fluid volume and/or an increase in its osmotic pressure stimulates hypothalamic neurons in supraoptic nuclei to synthesize more ADH and, as a result, the posterior pituitary secretes more ADH

2. Oxytocin secretion is increased by stimulation of mother's nipples during nursing

Thyroid gland

A. Hormones—functions and effects (Table 1-12)

B. Mechanisms influencing secretion of thyroid hormone

1. TRF (thyroid-releasing factor) from hypothalamus stimulates anterior pituitary secretion of TSH (thyroid-stimulating hormone), which stimulates thyroid secretion of thyroxine and triiodothyronine

2. Blood level of calcium ions controls thyroid secretion of thyrocalcitonin;

Table 1-12. Functions of thyroid and parathyroid hormones

Hormones	Functions	Hypofunction effects	Hyperfunction effects
Thyroid hormones Thyroxine Triiodothyronine	Stimulate metabolic rate; therefore, essential for normal physical and mental development Inhibit anterior pituitary secretion of TSH	Cretinism, if occurs early in life; myxedema, if occurs in older children or adults	Hyperthyroidism
Thyrocalcitonin	Quickly decreases blood calcium concentration if it increases about 20% above normal level; presumably accelerates calcium movement from blood into bone		
Parathyroid hormone Parathormone	Increases blood calcium concentration by accelerating following three processes:	Decreased blood calcium (hypocalcemia), which causes increased neural excitability and tetany	Increased blood calcium (hypercalcemia), which causes decreased neural excitability and muscle weakness
	Breakdown of bone with release of calcium into blood Calcium absorption from intestine into blood Kidney tubule reabsorption of calcium from tubular urine into blood, thereby decreasing calcium loss in urine		Bone "softening"— decalcification
	Decreases blood phosphate concentration by slowing its reabsorption by kidney tubules and thereby increasing phosphate loss in urine	Increased blood phosphorus (hyperphosphatemia)	Hypophosphatemia

Table 1-13. Functions of adrenal cortex hormones

Hormones	Functions	Hypofunction effects (e.g., in Addison's disease)	Hyperfunction effects (e.g., in Cushing's syndrome)
Glucocorticoids (GC's), mainly cortisol (hydrocortisone) and corticosterone	In general, a normal blood concentration of glucocorticoids promotes normal metabolism of all three kinds of foods and a high blood concentration produces various stress responses, e.g.:		
	Accelerates mobilization and catabolism of fats; i.e., causes shift from usual utilization of carbohydrates for energy to fat utilization		
	Accelerates tissue protein mobilization and catabolism (tissue proteins hydrolyzed to amino acids, which enter blood and are carried to liver for deamination and gluconeogenesis)		Muscle atrophy and weakness; osteoporosis
	Accelerates liver gluconeogenesis; i.e., formation of glucose from mobilized proteins (hyperglycemic effect)		Hyperglycemia
	Causes atrophy of lymphatic tissues, notably thymus and lymph nodes		Lymphocytopenia
	Decreases antibody formation (immunosuppressive, antiallergic effect)		Decreased immunity Decreased allergy
	Slows the proliferation of fibroblasts characteristic of inflammation (anti-inflammatory effect)		Spread of infections; slower wound healing
	Mild acceleration of sodium and water reabsorption and potassium excretion by kidney tubules		High blood sodium (hypernatremia; sodium retention); also water retention; low blood potassium (hypokalemia)
	Decreases ACTH secretion		
Mineralocorticoids (MC's), mainly aldosterone	Marked acceleration of sodium and water reabsorption by kidney tubules	Low blood sodium (hyponatremia); dehydration	High blood sodium (hypernatremia); water retention, edema
	Marked acceleration of potassium excretion by kidney tubules	High blood potassium (hyperkalemia)	Low blood potassium (hypokalemia)

high blood concentration of calcium stimulates thyroid secretion of thyrocalcitonin

Parathyroid glands

A. Hormone—functions and effects (Table 1-12)
B. Mechanisms influencing secretion of parathyroid hormone

1. Low blood calcium concentration stimulates parathyroids to secrete parathyroid hormone; high blood calcium concentration inhibits parathyroid hormone secretion
2. Parathyroids, unlike most other endocrine glands, are not controlled by an anterior pituitary hormone

Table 1-14. Functions of sex hormones (ovarian and testicular)

Hormones	Functions
Estrogens (secreted by graafian follicle and corpus luteum)	Stimulate proliferation of epithelial cells of female reproductive organs; e.g., thickening of endometrium, breast development Stimulate uterine contractions Accelerate protein anabolism (including bone matrix synthesis) so promote growth; but also promote epiphyseal closure so limit height Mildly accelerate sodium and water reabsorption by kidney tubules; increase water content of uterus High blood estrogen concentration inhibits anterior pituitary secretion of FSH and prolactin but stimulates its secretion of LH Low blood estrogen concentration after delivery of baby stimulates anterior pituitary secretion of prolactin
Progesterone (secreted by corpus luteum)	Name "progesterone" indicates hormone's general function, "favoring pregnancy," e.g.: Stimulates secretion by endometrial glands, thereby preparing endometrium for implantation of fertilized ovum Inhibits uterine contractions, thereby favoring retention of implanted ovum Promotes development of alveoli (secreting cells) of estrogen-primed breasts; necessary for lactation Protein-catabolic and salt- and water-retaining effects similar to corticoids but milder; increases water content of endometrium
Testosterone (secreted by interstitial cells of testes)	Growth and development of male reproductive organs; promotes "maleness" Marked stimulating effect on protein anabolism, including synthesis of bone matrix; hence, promotes growth; however, it also tends to limit height by promoting epiphyseal closure Mild acceleration of kidney tubule reabsorption of sodium chloride and water Inhibits secretion of ICSH by anterior pituitary

Cortex of adrenal glands

A. Hormones—functions and effects (Table 1-13)
B. Mechanisms influencing secretion of adrenal cortex hormones
   1. Glucocorticoid secretion
      a. Some factor stimulates hypothalamus to increase secretion of CRF (corticotropin-releasing factor) into hypothalamico-hypophyseal portal veins
      b. High concentration of CRF in blood carried to anterior pituitary gland
      c. CRF stimulates ACTH (corticotropin) secretion by anterior pituitary gland
      d. High blood concentration of ACTH stimulates the secretion of glucocorticoid hormone by adrenal cortex
   2. Aldosterone secretion
      a. Some factor decreases arterial pressure in the kidneys
      b. This stimulates the juxtaglomerular apparatus of the kidneys to release renin into blood
      c. This enzyme converts angiotensinogen to angiotensin I, which is converted by another enzyme into angiotensin II
      d. Angiotensin II stimulates the adrenal cortex to increase the secretion of aldosterone

Female sex glands (ovaries)

A. Hormones and functions (Table 1-14)
B. Mechanisms influencing secretions of ovarian hormones
   1. Estrogen secretion (Fig. 7)
   2. Progesterone secretion—high blood concentration of LH (luteinizing hormone) stimulates progesterone secretion

Male sex glands (testes)

A. Hormone and functions (Table 1-14)
B. Mechanism influencing secretion of testicular hormone
   1. High blood concentration of ICSH (interstitial cell–stimulating hormone, analogous to luteinizing hormone in the female) stimulates testosterone secretion

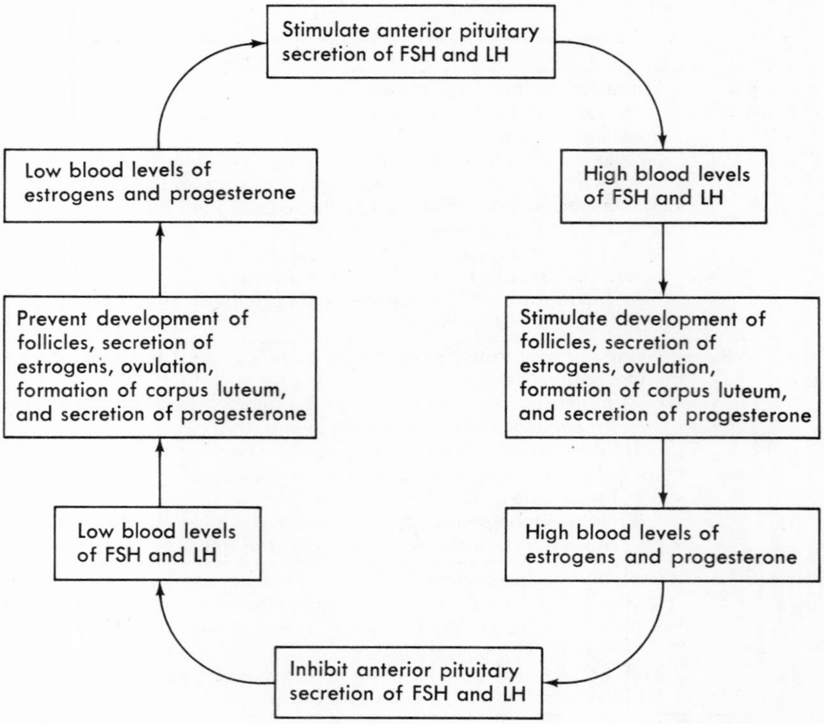

Fig. 7. A negative feedback mechanism that controls anterior pituitary secretion of follicle-stimulating hormone (FSH) and ovarian secretion of estrogens. A high blood level of FSH stimulates estrogen secretion, whereas the resulting high estrogen level inhibits FSH secretion. (From Anthony, C. P., and Kolthoff, N. J.: Textbook of anatomy and physiology, ed. 9, St. Louis, 1975, The C. V. Mosby Co.)

2. Testosterone is secreted by the interstitial cells of the testes

Other glands
A. Pineal gland
   1. Located in the roof of the third ventricle of the brain
   2. Secretions
      a. Melatonin, which inhibits ovarian function
      b. Adrenoglomerulotropin, which stimulates aldosterone secretion
B. Thymus gland
   1. Located between the lungs and above the diaphragm
   2. Believed to secrete a hormone that enables the plasma cells to produce antibodies

Prostaglandins
A. Discovered as secretions of the prostate gland, however present information indicates that they are secreted by many cells of the body
B. Prostaglandins modify the action of hormones and the activities of many of the cells in which they are synthesized
C. Some effects—stimulation of inflammation; regulation of blood flow to particular organs; control of ion transport across some membranes; modulation of synaptic transmission

MAINTAINING THE METABOLISM OF THE BODY

CIRCULATORY SYSTEM
Functions

A. Primary function—transportation of various substances to and from body cells
B. Secondary functions—contributes to all of body's functions: metabolism, water balance, homeostasis of pH and tempera-

Table 1-15. Blood cells

Cells	Number	Function	Formation (hemopoiesis)	Destruction
Red blood cells (erythrocytes)	4.5 to 5.5 million/mm^3 total of approximately 30 trillion in adult body)	Transport oxygen and carbon dioxide	Red marrow of bones (myeloid tissue)	Reticuloendothelial cells in lining of blood vessels in liver, spleen, and bone marrow phagocytose old red cells; live about 120 days in bloodstream
White blood cells (leukocytes)	Usually about 5000 to 9000/mm^3	Play important part in producing immunity —e.g., phagocytosis by neutrophils; lymphocytes form cellular antibodies; some lymphocytes become plasma cells, cells that form circulating antibodies	Granular and nongranular leukocytes in red marrow; lymphocytes formed in thymus gland of fetus; postnatally, most lymphocytes and monocytes formed in lymph nodes and other lymphatic tissues	Not known definitely; probably some destroyed by phagocystosis
Platelets (thrombocytes)	150,000 to 300,000/mm^3	Initiate blood clotting	Red marrow	Unknown

From Anthony, C. P., and Kolthoff, N. J.: Textbook of anatomy and physiology, ed. 9, St. Louis, 1975, The C. V. Mosby Co.

ture, defense against microorganisms, etc.

Structures

Blood

A. Blood cells
  1. Kinds of cells
    a. Red blood cells (erythrocytes)
    b. White blood cells (leukocytes)
      (1) Neutrophils—constitute 65% to 75% of total white count
      (2) Eosinophils—constitute 2% to 5% of total white count
      (3) Basophils—constitute 0.5% to 1% of total white count
      (4) Lymphocytes—constitute about 20% to 25% of total white count
      (5) Monocytes—constitute 3% to 8% of total white count
  2. Number, function, formation, and distribution of cells (Table 1-15)
B. Blood types
  1. Names—indicate type antigens on or in red cell membrane; e.g., type A blood means that red cells have A antigens; type O means that red cells have no antigens

  2. Every person's blood belongs to one of the 4 blood groups—type A, type B, type AB, or type O—and is either Rh-positive or Rh-negative
  3. Plasma—normally contains no antibodies against antigens present on its own red cells but does contain antibodies against other A or B antigens not present on its red cells; e.g., type A plasma does not contain antibodies against A antigen but does contain antibodies against B antigen
  4. Blood does not normally contain anti-Rh antibodies; Rh-positive blood never contains them; Rh-negative blood will contain anti-Rh antibodies if the individual has been transfused with Rh-positive blood or has carried an Rh-positive fetus
  5. The potential danger in transfusing blood is that the donor's blood may be agglutinated (clumped) by the recipient's antibodies
C. Blood plasma
  1. Definition—liquid part of blood (whole blood minus cells); constitutes about 55% of total blood volume; remaining percentage of whole

blood volume is composed of red blood cells (hematocrit)

2. Composition of plasma—about 90% water, 10% solutes (electrolytes, foods, gases, hormones, antibodies)

D. Blood clotting
1. Purpose—to plug up ruptured vessels and prevent bleeding
2. Mechanism—swift, complex mechanism for changing soluble blood protein, fibrinogen, into insoluble protein, fibrin
   a. The trigger that sets in operation the blood clotting mechanism is the appearance of a rough spot in the lining of a blood vessel; e.g., patchlike deposits of a cholesterol-lipid substance as in atherosclerosis, or a cut wall of a vessel
   b. Within a second or so, clumps of platelets adhere to the rough spot and their membranes rupture, releasing chemicals called "platelet factors," which act as the chemical trigger for starting a series of chemical reactions to follow in quick succession and bring about coagulation
3. Some facts about the blood proteins essential for clotting
   a. Liver cells synthesize prothrombin and fibrinogen (as they do various other blood proteins); adequate amounts of vitamin K must be present in blood for the liver to make normal amounts of prothrombin
   b. Normal blood prothrombin content—10 to 15 mg. per 100 ml. of plasma
   c. Normal blood fibrinogen content—350 mg. per 100 ml. of plasma
   d. Both prothrombin and fibrinogen are soluble proteins normally present in blood in adequate amounts for clotting to occur at the normal rapid rate
   e. Fibrin is an insoluble protein formed from the soluble protein fibrinogen, in the presence of the enzyme thrombin; fibrin appears as a tangled mass of threads having a jellylike texture; blood cells become enmeshed in these threads, and red cells give the clot its red color

4. Clinical applications
   a. Hemophilia—hereditary disease characterized by defect in clotting ability of blood caused by lack of a blood protein essential for clotting
   b. Thrombosis—partial or complete occlusion of a blood vessel, caused by presence of a stationary clot (thrombus)
   c. Embolism—partial or complete occlusion of a blood vessel by a moving clot (embolus)
   d. Atherosclerosis—plaques of lipoid material deposited in endothelium act as rough spots, causing platelet disintegration and thrombus formation
   e. Sluggish blood flow causes thrombus formation; frequent moving of a bed patient helps prevent sluggish blood flow, and thrombus formation

Heart

A. Location—in mediastinum with apex on diaphragm and pointing to left (apical beat may be counted by placing stethoscope in fifth intercostal space on line with left midclavicular point); two thirds of bulk of heart lies to left of midline of body, one third to right

B. Covering—pericardium
1. Structure
   a. Fibrous pericardium—loose-fitting, inextensible sac around heart
   b. Serous pericardium—consists of 2 layers
      (1) Parietal layer—lines inner surface of fibrous pericardium
      (2) Visceral layer (epicardium)—adheres to outer surface of the heart; pericardial space, lying between parietal and visceral layers, contains a few drops of lubricating pericardial fluid
2. Function—protects heart against friction by providing well-lubricated, smooth sac for heart to beat in

C. Structure of heart
1. Heart wall
   a. Myocardium—composed of cardiac muscle cells
   b. Endocardium—delicate endothelial lining of myocardium

2. Cavities
   a. Upper 2 called atria
   b. Lower 2 called ventricles
3. Valves and openings
   a. Openings between atria and ventricles known as atrioventricular orifices
      (1) Guarded by cuspid valves
         (a) Tricuspid on right
         (b) Mitral (bicuspid) on left
      (2) Valves consist of 3 parts
         (a) Flaps or cusps
         (b) Chordae tendineae
         (c) Papillary muscles
   b. Opening from right ventricle into pulmonary artery guarded by pulmonary semilunar valves
   c. Opening from left ventricle into great aorta guarded by aortic semilunar valves
4. Blood supply to myocardium (heart muscle)
   a. By way of only 2 small vessels: the right and left coronary arteries, the first branches of the aorta
   b. Both coronary arteries send branches to both sides of the heart
   c. Right coronary branches supply right side of heart mainly, but also carry some blood to left ventricle
   d. Left coronary branches supply left side of heart mainly but also carry some blood to right ventricle
   e. Most abundant blood supply of all goes to the myocardium of the left ventricle
   f. Relatively few anastomoses (branches from one artery to another artery) exist between the larger branches of the coronary arteries; hence, if one of these vessels becomes occluded, little or no blood can reach the myocardial cells supplied by that vessel; deprived of an adequate blood supply, cells soon die (myocardial infarction)
5. Nerve supply to heart
   a. Sympathetic fibers (in cardiac nerves) and parasympathetic fibers (in vagus nerves) form cardiac plexuses
   b. Fibers from cardiac plexuses terminate mainly in sinoatrial (SA) node

   c. Sympathetic impulses tend to accelerate and strengthen heartbeat
   d. Parasympathetic (vagal) impulses slow the heartbeat
6. Conduction system of heart
   a. Sinoatrial node (SA node)—a cluster of cells located in the right atrial wall near the opening of the superior vena cava
   b. Atrioventricular node (AV node)—a small mass of special conducting cells located in the right atrium at the top of the interventricular septum
   c. AV bundle of His—special conducting fibers that originate in the AV node and extend by 2 branches down the 2 sides of the interventricular septum
   d. Purkinje fibers—special conducting fibers that extend from the AV bundle throughout the wall of the ventricles
   e. Normally a nerve impulse begins its course through the heart in the heart's own pacemaker, the SA node; it quickly spreads through both atria, via special conducting fibers, to the AV node; after a short delay at this node, the impulse is conducted by 2 branches of the AV bundle of His down both sides of the interventricular septum; from there, the impulse travels over Purkinje fibers to the lateral walls of the ventricles
   f. Impulse conduction through heart generates tiny electric currents that spread through surrounding tissues to the skin, from which visible records of conduction can be made with the electrocardiograph or oscillograph; conduction from the SA node through the atria causes atrial contraction and gives rise to the so-called P wave of the electrocardiogram; conduction from the AV node down the bundle of His and out the Purkinje fibers causes ventricular contraction and gives rise to the QRS wave
D. Physiology of heart
   1. Function—to pump varying amounts of blood through vessels as needs of cells change
   2. Cardiac cycle

a. Consists of systole (contraction) and diastole (relaxation) of atria and of ventricles; atria contract and as they relax ventricles contract
b. Time required—about 4/5 second from one cardiac cycle; so 70 to 80 cycles or heartbeats per minute

Blood vessels

A. Kinds
1. Arteries—vessels that carry blood away from heart (all arteries except pulmonary artery carry oxygenated blood); arteries branch into smaller and smaller vessels called arterioles that branch into microscopic vessels, the capillaries
2. Veins—vessels that carry blood toward heart (all veins except the pulmonary veins carry deoxygenated blood)
3. Capillaries—microscopic vessels that carry blood from arterioles to venules; capillaries unite to form small veins or venules, which, in turn, unite to form veins; exchange of substances between blood and interstitial fluid occurs in capillaries
B. Structure of blood vessels (Table 1-16)
C. Names of main blood vessels
1. Arteries (Fig. 8)
2. Veins (Fig. 9)—deep veins lie close to bones and many of them bear same name as corresponding artery; superficial veins lie near surface; veins in

cranial cavity formed by dura mater called sinuses
D. Fetal circulation—structures essential for fetal circulation but normally cease to exist after birth
1. Umbilical arteries—2 extensions of hypogastric arteries (internal iliacs) carry fetal blood to placenta
2. Placenta—attached to uterine wall
3. Umbilical vein—extends from placenta back to fetus' body; returns oxygenated blood from placental to fetal circulation; 2 umbilical arteries and 1 umbilical vein constitute umbilical cord
4. Ductus venosus—small vessel that connects umbilical vein with inferior vena cava in fetus
5. Foramen ovale—opening in fetal heart septum between right and left atria
6. Ductus arteriosus—small vessel connecting pulmonary artery with descending thoracic aorta
7. Only 2 fetal blood vessels carry oxygenated blood—umbilical vein and ductus venosus; as soon as blood enters inferior vena cava from ductus venosus it becomes mixed with venous blood

Physiology of circulation

A. Definitions
1. Circulation—blood flow through circuit of vessels
2. Systemic circulation—blood flow from

Table 1-16. Structure of the blood vessels

	Arteries	Veins	Capillaries
Coats	Lining (tunica intima) of endothelium Middle coat (tunica media) of smooth muscle, elastic, and fibrous tissues; this coat permits constriction and dilatation Outer coat (tunica adventitia or externa) of fibrous tissue; its firmness makes arteries stand open instead of collapsing when cut	Same 3 coats, but thinner and fewer elastic fibers; veins collapse when cut; semilunar valves present at intervals	Only lining coat present; therefore capillary wall only 1 cell thick
Blood supply	Endothelial lining cells supplied by blood flowing through vessels; cells of middle and outer coats supplied by tiny vessels known as the vasa vasorum or "vessels of the vessels"		
Nerve supply	Smooth muscle cells of middle coat innervated by autonomic fibers controlled by vasomotor center of medulla; able to cause either vasoconstriction or vasodilatation		
Abnormalities	Arteriosclerosis—hardening and thickening of walls of arteries Aneurysm—saclike dilatation of an artery wall Varicose veins—stretching of walls, particularly around semilunar valves Phlebitis—inflammation of vein; "milk leg"; phlebitis of femoral vein of women after childbirth		

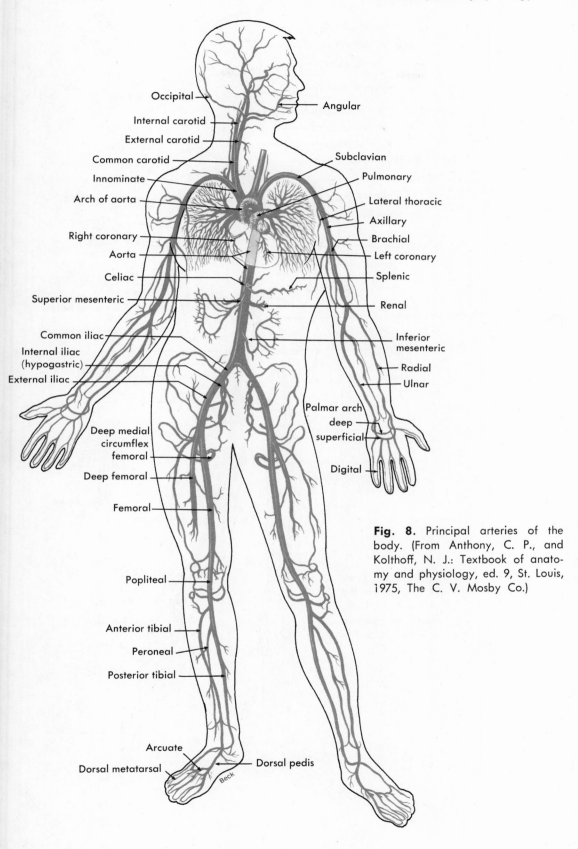

Occipital

Internal carotid

External carotid

Common carotid

Innominate

Arch of aorta

Right coronary

Aorta

Celiac

Superior mesenteric

Common iliac

Internal iliac
(hypogastric)

External iliac

Deep medial
circumflex
femoral

Deep femoral

Femoral

Popliteal

Anterior tibial

Peroneal

Posterior tibial

Arcuate

Dorsal metatarsal

Angular

Subclavian

Pulmonary

Lateral thoracic

Axillary

Brachial

Left coronary

Splenic

Renal

Inferior
mesenteric

Radial

Ulnar

Palmar arch
deep
superficial

Digital

Dorsal pedis

Beck

Fig. 8. Principal arteries of the body. (From Anthony, C. P., and Kolthoff, N. J.: Textbook of anatomy and physiology, ed. 9, St. Louis, 1975, The C. V. Mosby Co.)

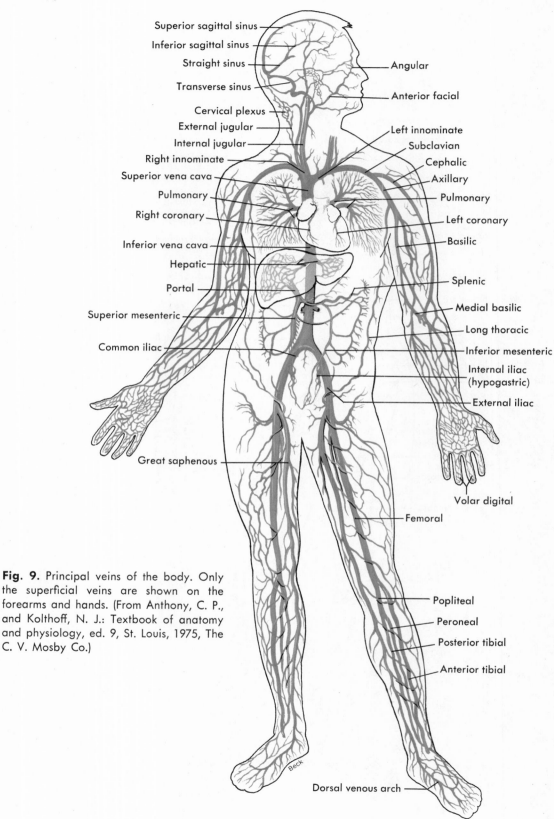

Fig. 9. Principal veins of the body. Only the superficial veins are shown on the forearms and hands. (From Anthony, C. P., and Kolthoff, N. J.: Textbook of anatomy and physiology, ed. 9, St. Louis, 1975, The C. V. Mosby Co.)

left ventricle into aorta, other arteries, arterioles, capillaries, venules, and veins to right atrium of heart

3. Pulmonary circulation—blood flow from right ventricle to pulmonary artery to lung arterioles, capillaries, and venules, to pulmonary veins, to left atrium

4. Portal circulation—blood flow from capillaries, venules, veins of stomach, intestines, and spleen into portal vein, liver arterioles, liver capillaries, to hepatic veins, to inferior vena cava

B. Principles of circulation

1. Blood circulates because a blood pressure gradient exists in its vessels; like all fluids, blood moves from regions where its pressure is greater to regions where pressure is less; because blood pressure is highest in aorta and successively lower in arteries, arterioles, capillaries, venules, veins, and lowest in the central veins (venae cavae), blood flows through vessels in this order

2. Normally systemic blood pressure gradient and mean arterial blood pressure about equal; reason—systemic blood pressure gradient equals mean arterial pressure minus central venous pressure

3. Volume of blood circulating each minute varies directly with systemic blood pressure gradient and inversely with resistance opposing blood flow (peripheral resistance)

4. Arterial pressure determined directly by volume of blood in arteries; when arterial blood volume increases, arterial pressure tends to increase; when arterial blood volume decreases, arterial pressure tends to decrease

5. Arterial blood volume varies directly with cardiac minute output (rate × systolic discharge); anything that increases the heart rate or systolic discharge, therefore, tends to increase cardiac minute output, arterial volume, arterial pressure, systemic blood pressure gradient, and volume of blood circulating per minute

6. Heart rate is regulated mainly by pressoreflexes; increase in arterial pressure stimulates baroreceptors in aorta and carotid sinus, which leads to increased parasympathetic impulses

to heart via vagus nerve, which slow the heart rate; a decrease in arterial pressure inhibits baroreceptors in aorta and carotid sinus and thereby leads to decreased parasympathetic impulses and increased sympathetic impulses to heart, which in turn causes a faster heart rate

7. Systolic discharge of heart is regulated mainly by ratio of sympathetic-parasympathetic impulses to it and by concentration of epinephrine in the blood; sympathetic dominance and a high blood epinephrine concentration increase systolic discharge; parasympathetic dominance decreases systolic discharge

8. Peripheral resistance varies directly with blood viscosity and inversely with diameter of arterioles; anything that increases blood viscosity tends to increase peripheral resistance, whereas anything that increases diameter of arterioles (dilates them) tends to decrease peripheral resistance; converse also true

9. Blood viscosity varies directly with blood protein concentration and number of blood cells; decrease in either tends to decrease blood viscosity; converse also true

10. Arteriole diameter is controlled mainly by vasomotor baroreflexes and chemoreflexes; in general, a decrease in arterial pressure initiates reflex vasoconstriction of small vessels in the so-called blood reservoirs (skin and abdominal viscera); conversely, an increase in arterial pressure initiates reflex vasodilation in the skin and abdominal organs; hypoxia and hypercapnia cause vasoconstriction in the skin and abdominal organs but vasodilation in skeletal muscles, heart, and brain

11. Increase in peripheral resistance tends to decrease circulation; at same time, however, an increase in peripheral resistance also tends to produce opposite effect; reason—increased peripheral resistance hinders blood flow out of arteries into arterioles, so more blood remains in arteries, and this tends to increase arterial pressure and circulation; summarizing, an increase in peripheral re-

sistance may decrease volume of blood circulating per minute, increase it, or not change it at all

C. Pulse
   1. Definition—alternate expansion and recoil of blood vessel
   2. Cause—variations in pressure within vessel caused by intermittent injections of blood from heart into aorta with each ventricular contraction; pulse can be felt because of elasticity of arterial walls
   3. Pulse can be felt wherever artery lies near surface and over firm background such as bone; some of those most easily palpated are:
      a. Radial artery—at wrist
      b. Temporal artery—in front of ear, or above and to outer side of eye
      c. Common carotid artery—along anterior edge of sternocleidomastoid muscle, at level of lower margin of thyroid cartilage
      d. Facial artery—at lower margin of lower jaw bone, on line with corners of mouth, in groove in mandible about one third of way forward from angle of bone
      e. Brachial artery—at bend of elbow, along inner margin of biceps muscle
      f. Posterior tibial artery—behind medial malleolus (inner "ankle bone")
      g. Dorsalis pedis—on anterior surface of foot, just below the bend of the ankle
   4. Venous pulse—in large veins only; produced by changes in venous pressure brought about by alternate contraction and relaxation of atria rather than of ventricles as in arterial pulse

Lymphatic system
Lymphatic vessels

A. Structure—lymph capillaries similar to blood capillaries in structure; larger lymphatics similar to veins but are thinner walled, have more valves, and have lymph nodes in certain places along their course
B. Names—largest lymphatic known as thoracic duct; drains lymph from entire body except upper right quadrant into left subclavian vein (where it joins the internal jugular); right lymphatic ducts drain lymph from upper right quadrant into right subclavian vein

C. Functions
   1. Lymphatics return fluid and proteins to blood from interstitial fluid; about 60% of fluid filtered out of blood capillaries returns to circulation via lymphatics rather than by osmosis into venous ends of capillaries; about 50% of total blood proteins leak out of capillaries per day; since the only way these large molecules can return to blood is via lymphatics
   2. Adequate lymph return is essential for maintaining homeostasis of blood proteins and, therefore, of blood volume
   3. Interference with the return of proteins to the blood results in edema caused by the loss of protein and changes in hydrostatic pressure

Lymph nodes

A. Structure—lymphatic tissue, separated into compartments by fibrous partitions; afferent lymphatic vessels enter each node; 1 (usually) efferent vessel drains lymph out of node
B. Location—usually in clusters; some of more important groups, from nursing viewpoint, listed below
   1. Submental and submaxillary groups in floor of mouth; lymph from nose, lips, and teeth drains through these
   2. Superficial cervical nodes in neck, along sternocleidomastoid muscle; lymph from head and neck drains through these nodes
   3. Superficial cubital nodes at bend of elbow; lymph from hand and forearm drains through these nodes
   4. Axillary nodes in axilla; lymph from arm and upper part of chest wall, including breast, drains through these nodes (frequently removed during mastectomy for carcinoma)
   5. Inguinal nodes in groin; lymph from legs and external genitals drains through these nodes
C. Functions
   1. Help defend body against injurious substances (notably, bacteria and tumor cells) by filtering them out of lymph and thereby preventing their entrance into bloodstream; phagocytes in lymph nodes destroy many of these substances by phagocytosis
   2. Lymphatic tissue of lymph nodes carries on process of hemopoiesis; specif-

ically, it forms 2 types of white blood cells—lymphocytes and monocytes; some lymphocytes now thought to produce antibodies and some to become transformed into plasma cells, which, in turn, produce antibodies, thus lymph nodes help defend the body in another way; they also function as an important part of the immune response

Lymph
A. Lymph—fluid in lymphatics
B. Source of lymph is interstitial fluid that has entered the lymphatic capillaries
  1. Interstitial fluid is the fluid in the microscopic tissue spaces
  2. Interstitial fluid is formed by plasma filtering out of the blood capillaries into the tissue spaces

Spleen
A. Location—left hypochondrium, above and behind cardiac portion of stomach
B. Structure—lymphatic tissue, similar to lymph nodes; size varies; contains numerous spaces filled with venous blood
C. Functions
  1. Defense—phagocytosis of particles such as microbes, red cell fragments, and platelets by reticuloendothelial cells of spleen (reticuloendothelial system—phagocytic cells, located mainly in liver, spleen, bone marrow, and lymph nodes; also, macrophages of connective tissue and microglia in brain and cord); antibody formation by plasma cells of spleen
  2. Hemopoiesis—lymphatic tissue of spleen, like that of the lymph nodes, forms lymphocytes and monocytes
  3. Spleen serves as blood reservoir; sympathetic stimulation causes constriction of its capsule, squeezing out an estimated 200 ml. of blood into general circulation within 1 minute

RESPIRATORY SYSTEM
Functions
A. To make possible exchange of gases between blood and air
B. To make possible cellular respiration

Organs
Nose
A. Structure

1. Portions
  a. Internal—in skull, above roof of mouth
  b. External—protruding from face
2. Cavities
  a. Divisions—right and left
  b. Meati—superior, middle, and lower; named for turbinates located above each meatus
  c. Openings
    (1) To exterior—the anterior nares
    (2) To nasopharynx—the posterior nares
  d. Conchae (turbinates)
    (1) Superior and middle processes of ethmoid bone; inferior conchae, separate bones
    (2) Conchae partition each nasal cavity into 3 passageways or meati
  e. Floor—formed by palatine bones and maxillae; these also act as roof of mouth
3. Lining—ciliated mucosa
4. Sinuses draining into nose (paranasal sinuses)
  a. Frontal
  b. Maxillary (antrum of Highmore)
  c. Sphenoidal
  d. Ethmoidal
B. Functions
  1. Serves as passageway for incoming and outgoing air, filtering, warming, moistening, and chemically examining it
  2. Organ of smell (olfactory receptors located in nasal mucosa)
  3. Aids in phonation

Pharynx
A. Structure—composed of muscle with mucous lining
  1. Divisions
    a. Nasopharynx—behind nose
    b. Oropharynx—behind mouth
    c. Laryngopharynx—behind larynx
  2. Openings
    a. In nasopharynx—4 openings: 2 auditory (eustachian) tubes and 2 posterior nares
    b. In oropharynx—1 opening: fauces, archway into mouth
    c. In laryngopharynx—2 openings: into esophagus and into larynx
  3. Organs in pharynx

a. In nasopharynx—pharyngeal tonsils (adenoids)
b. In oropharynx—palatine and lingual tonsils
B. Functions
1. Serves as passageway and entrance to both respiratory and digestive tracts
2. Aids in phonation

Larynx
A. Location—at upper end of trachea, just below pharynx
B. Structure
1. Cartilages—9 pieces arranged in box-like formation; thyroid largest of cartilages, "Adam's apple"; epiglottis, "lid" cartilage; cricoid, "signet ring" cartilage
2. Vocal cords
a. False cords—folds of mucous lining
b. True cords—fibroelastic bands stretched across hollow interior of larynx; glottis is opening between true cords
3. Lining—ciliated mucosa
C. Functions
1. Voice production—during expiration, air passing through larynx causes vocal cords to vibrate; vibration of short, tense cords produces high pitch; long, relaxed cords, low pitch
2. Serves as part of passageway for air; entrance to lower respiratory tract

Trachea
A. Structure
1. Walls—smooth muscle; contain C-shaped rings of cartilage at intervals; these keep tube open at all times
2. Lining—ciliated mucosa
3. Extent—from larynx to bronchi; about 4½ inches long
B. Function—furnishes open passageway for air going to and from lungs

Lungs
A. Structure
1. Size—large enough to fill pleural divisions of thoracic cavity
2. Shape—cone-shaped, with base downward
3. Location—in pleural divisions of thorax; extend from slightly above clavicle to diaphragm; base of each lung rests on diaphragm

4. Divisions
a. Lobes—3 in right lung, 2 in left
b. Root—consists of primary bronchus, pulmonary artery and veins bound together by connective tissue
c. Hilum—vertical slit on mesial surface of lung, through which root structures enter lung
d. Apex—pointed upper part of lung
e. Base—broad, inferior surface of lung
5. Bronchial tree—consists of following:
a. Bronchi—right and left bronchi formed by branching of trachea; right bronchus slightly larger and more vertical than left; each primary bronchus branches, upon entering lung, into secondary bronchi
b. Bronchioles—small branches off secondary bronchi
c. Alveolar ducts—microscopic branches off bronchioles
d. Alveoli—microscopic sacs composed of single layer of simple squamous epithelial cells; each alveolar duct terminates in cluster of alveoli often likened to bunch of grapes; each alveolus enveloped by network of lung capillaries
6. Covering of lung—visceral layer of pleura
B. Function—place where air and blood can come in close enough contact for rapid diffusion of gases to occur
1. Bronchi, bronchioles, alveolar ducts—lower part of airway through which air moves into and out of alveoli
2. Alveoli—microscopic sacs in which gases are exchanged very rapidly between air and blood; membranous walls of the millions of alveoli provide surface area large enough and thin enough to make possible rapid gas exchange

Physiology of respiration
A. Mechanism of inspiration
1. Respiratory muscles contract
2. Thorax increases in size
3. Intrathoracic pressure decreases
4. Lungs increase in size
5. Intrapulmonic pressure decreases
6. Air rushes from positive pressure in atmosphere to negative pressure in alveoli

7. Inspiration is completed
B. Mechanism of expiration
    1. Respiratory muscles relax
    2. Thorax decreases in size
    3. Intrathoracic pressure increases
    4. Lungs decrease in size
    5. Intrapulmonic pressure increases
    6. Air expelled from higher pressure in the lung to lower pressure in the atmosphere
    7. Expiration is completed
C. Amount of air exchanged in breathing
    1. Directly related to gas pressure gradient between atmosphere and alveoli and inversely related to resistance opposing air flow; the greater the difference between atmospheric pressure and alveolar pressure, the greater the amount of air exchanged in breathing; the greater the resistance opposing air flow to or from the lungs, the less air exchanged
    2. Measured by apparatus called spirometer
    3. Tidal air—average amount expired after normal inspiration; approximately 500 ml.
    4. Expiratory reserve volume (ERV)—largest additional volume of air that can be forcibly expired after a normal inspiration and expiration; normal ERV 1000 to 1200 ml.
    5. Inspiratory reserve volume (IRV)—largest additional volume of air that can be forcibly inspired after a normal inspiration; normal IRV 3000 to 3300 ml.
    6. Residual air—that which cannot be forcibly expired from lungs; about 1200 ml.
    7. Minimal air—that which can never be removed from alveoli if they have been inflated even once, even though lungs are subjected to atmospheric pressure that squeezes part of residual air out
    8. Vital capacity—approximate capacity of lungs as measured by amount of air that can be forcibly expired after forcible inspiration; varies with size of thoracic cavity, which is determined by various factors; e.g., size of rib cage, posture, volume of blood and interstitial fluid in lungs, size of heart
D. Diffusion of gases between air and blood

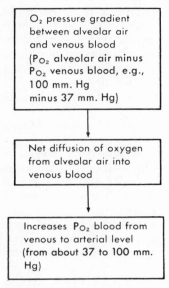

Fig. 10. Mechanism of oxygen diffusion.

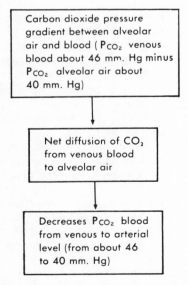

Fig. 11. Mechanism of carbon dioxide diffusion.

occurs across alveolar-capillary membranes; i.e., in lungs between air in alveoli and venous blood in lung capillaries

1. Direction of diffusion
   a. Oxygen—net diffusion toward lower oxygen pressure gradient; i.e., from alveolar air to blood
   b. Carbon dioxide—net diffusion toward lower carbon dioxide pressure gradient; i.e., from blood to alveolar air
2. Mechanism of oxygen diffusion (Fig. 10)
3. Mechanism of carbon dioxide diffusion (Fig. 11)

E. How blood transports oxygen
   1. As solute—about 0.5 ml. of oxygen is dissolved in 100 ml. of blood; produces the blood P_{O_2} (pressure of oxygen in the blood)
   2. As oxyhemoglobin—each gram of hemoglobin can combine with 1.34 ml. of oxygen; hence, with normal hemoglobin content (e.g., 15 g.* per 100 ml. of blood) and 100% oxygen saturation, about 20 ml. (15 × 1.34) of oxygen is transported as oxyhemoglobin
   3. Various factors influence rate at which oxygen associates with hemoglobin to form oxyhemoglobin including:
      a. Increasing pressure of oxygen in the blood
      b. Decreasing pressure of carbon dioxide in the blood
   4. Various factors influence rate at which oxygen dissociates from hemoglobin including:
      a. Decreasing pressure of oxygen in the blood
      b. Increasing pressure of carbon dioxide in the blood
      c. Increased blood temperature

F. How blood transports carbon dioxide
   1. As solute—small amount dissolves in plasma
   2. As bicarbonate ion—more than half of CO_2 in blood is present in the plasma as bicarbonate ion, formed by ionization of carbonic acid as follows:

$$CO_2 + H_2O \leftrightarrows H_2CO_3$$
$$\downarrow$$
$$H^+ + HCO_3^-$$

   3. As carbhemoglobin—less than one third of CO_2 is transported in combination with hemoglobin

G. Diffusion of gases between arterial blood and tissues occurs in tissue capillaries
   1. Oxygen—net diffusion of dissolved O_2 out of blood into tissues because of lower P_{O_2} there (perhaps 30 mm. Hg compared with arterial P_{O_2} of 100 mm. Hg); diffusion of dissolved oxygen out of blood lowers blood P_{O_2} from arterial to venous level (from 100 to 40 mm. Hg); decreasing P_{O_2} as blood moves through tissue capillaries causes oxygen to dissociate from hemoglobin, thereby releasing more oxygen for diffusion out of blood to tissue cells
   2. Carbon dioxide—net diffusion of CO_2 into blood because of lower P_{CO_2} there (40 mm. Hg compared with probably over 50 mm. Hg in tissues); diffusion of CO_2 into tissue capillaries increases blood P_{CO_2} from arterial to venous level (from 40 to 46 mm. Hg); increasing P_{CO_2}, like decreasing P_{O_2}, tends to accelerate oxygen dissociation from hemoglobin

Control of respirations

A. Usual regulators of respirations are arterial blood P_{CO_2} and pH; increase in arterial P_{CO_2} or decrease in its pH has stimulating effect on respirations and is followed by hyperventilation (increased rate and depth of respirations), whereas decrease in arterial P_{CO_2} or increase in its pH leads to hypoventilation; presumably, increase in arterial P_{CO_2} or decrease in arterial blood pH stimulates neurons of respiratory center in two ways—directly and indirectly via stimulation of carotid and aortic chemoreceptors
B. The P_{O_2} of the arterial blood has both a direct and an indirect effect upon the control of respirations

DIGESTIVE SYSTEM
Functions

A. Digestion of food, essential preparation for absorption and metabolism
B. Absorption of digested food
C. Elimination of wastes of digestion

---

*Instead of Gm., the abbreviation more traditional in nursing, this book uses g. as the abbreviation for gram. This form, as part of the International System of Units, is rapidly becoming universal in use.

Coats composing wall of alimentary canal

A. Mucous lining
B. Submucous coat of connective tissue containing main blood vessels
C. Muscle coat
D. Fibroserous coat

Organs

Mouth (buccal cavity)

A. Cheeks
B. Hard palate—formed by 2 palatine bones and palatine processes of maxillae
C. Soft palate—formed of muscle in shape of arch that forms partition between mouth and nasopharynx; fauces, archway, or opening, from mouth into oropharynx; uvula, conical shaped process suspended from midpoint of soft palate arch

Tongue

A. Papillae—many rough elevations on tongue's surface
B. Taste buds—specialized receptors of cranial nerves VII and IX; located in papillae
C. Frenum (or frenulum)—fold of mucous membrane that helps anchor tongue to mouth floor

Salivary glands

A. Parotid—below and in front of ear
B. Submandibular—posterior part of floor of mouth

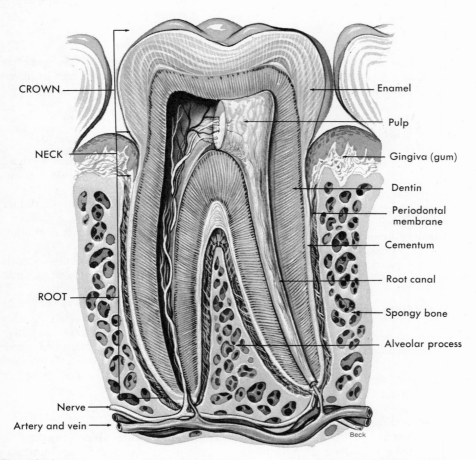

Fig. 12. A molar tooth, sectioned to show its bony socket and details of its three main parts: crown, neck, and root. The pulp contains nerves and blood vessels. (From Anthony, C. P., and Kolthoff, N. J.: Textbook of anatomy and physiology, ed. 9, St. Louis, 1975, The C. V. Mosby Co.)

C. Sublingual—anterior part of floor of mouth, under tongue

Teeth

A. Deciduous or "baby teeth"—10 in each jaw or 20 in set
B. Permanent—16 per jaw or 32 in set
C. Eruption
    1. Deciduous—first one erupts usually at 6 months of age; rest follow at intervals of 1 or more months; however, great individual variation in time of eruption of teeth; deciduous teeth shed between 6 and 13 years of age
    2. Permanent—usually between 6 years and about 17 years; third molars (wisdom teeth) last to erupt
D. Structure of tooth (Fig. 12)

Pharynx

See p. 45

Esophagus

A. Location and extent
    1. Posterior and extent
    2. Extends from pharynx through diaphragm to stomach—distance of approximately 10 inches
B. Structure—collapsible, muscle tube

Stomach

A. Size, shape, position
    1. Size—varies in different persons and according to degree of distention
    2. Shape—elongated pouch, with greater curve forming lower, left border
    3. Position—in epigastric and left hypochondriac portions of abdominal cavity
B. Divisions
    1. Fundus—portion above esophageal opening
    2. Body—central portion
    3. Pylorus—constricted, lower portion
C. Curves
    1. Lesser—upper, right border
    2. Greater—lower, left border
D. Sphincters
    1. Cardiac—guarding opening of esophagus into stomach
    2. Pyloric—guarding opening of pylorus into duodenum
E. Glands of stomach—secrete gastric juice composed of mucus, hydrochloric acid, and enzymes

    1. Simple columnar epithelial cells form surface of gastric mucosa and secrete mucus
    2. Millions of microscopic gastric glands embedded in gastric mucosa composed of different types of cells; mainly chief cells (zymogen cells), that secrete gastric juice enzymes, and parietal cells that secrete hydrochloric acid

Small intestine

A. Size—approximately 1 inch in diameter, 20 feet in length when relaxed
B. Divisions
    1. Duodenum—joins pylorus of stomach; about 10 inches in length; C-shaped
    2. Jejunum—middle section about 8 feet in length
    3. Ileum—lower section about 12 feet in length; no clear boundary between jejunum and ileum

Large intestine

A. Size—approximately 2½ inches in diameter, but only 5 or 6 feet in length when relaxed
B. Divisions
    1. Cecum—the first 2 or 3 inches of large intestine
    2. Colon
        a. Ascending—extends vertically along right border of abdomen up to level of liver
        b. Transverse colon—extends horizontally across abdomen, below liver and stomach and above small intestine
        c. Descending colon—extends vertically down left side of abdomen to level of iliac crest
        d. Sigmoid colon—S-shaped part of large intestine curving downward below iliac crest to join rectum; lower part of sigmoid curve which joins rectum bends toward left
    3. Rectum—last 7 or 8 inches of intestines

Liver

A. Location and size—occupies most of right hypochondrium and part of epigastrium; largest gland in body
B. Lobes—divided into lobules by blood vessels and fibrous partitions
    1. Right lobe—subdivided into 2 smaller

lobes (caudate and quadrate) and right lobe proper
2. Left lobe—single lobe
C. Ducts
1. Hepatic duct—from liver
2. Cystic duct—from gallbladder
3. Common bile duct—formed by union of hepatic and cystic ducts in Y formation; drains bile into duodenum at hepato-pancreatic papilla
D. Functions—liver is one of most vital organs because of its role in metabolism of proteins, carbohydrates, and fats
1. Carbohydrate metabolism by liver cells
   a. Glycogenesis—conversion of glucose to glycogen for storage; insulin tends to promote liver glycogenesis
   b. Glycogenolysis—conversion of glycogen to glucose and release of glucose into blood; epinephrine and glucagon accelerate glycogenolysis
   c. Gluconeogenesis—formation of glucose from proteins or fats; glucocorticoids (hydrocortisone, corticosterone) have accelerating effect on gluconeogenesis
2. Fat metabolism by liver cells
   a. Ketogenesis—first step in fat catabolism occurs mainly in liver cells; consists of series of reactions by which fatty acids are converted to ketone bodies (acetoacetic acid, acetone, beta-hydroxybutyric acid)
   b. Fat storage
3. Protein metabolism by liver cells
   a. Anabolism—synthesis of various proteins, notably blood proteins; e.g., prothrombin, fibrinogen, albumins, most globulins
   b. Deamination—first step in protein catabolism; chemical reaction by which amino group is split off from amino acid to form ammonia and a keto acid
   c. Urea formation—liver cells convert most of the ammonia formed by deamination to urea
4. Secretes bile, substance important in digestion and absorption of fats, and as vehicle for excretion of cholesterol and bile pigments
5. Detoxifies various harmful substances; e.g., drugs

Gallbladder

A. Size, shape, location—approximately size and shape of small pear; lies on undersurface of liver

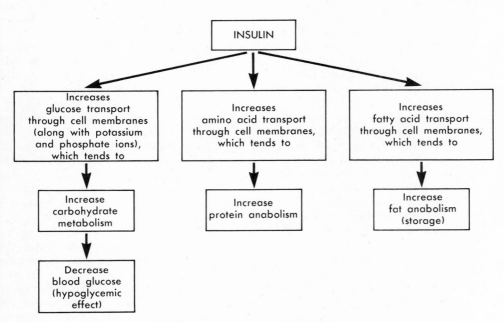

Fig. 13. Major insulin effects.

B. Structure—sac made of smooth muscle, lined with mucosa arranged in rugae (expandable longitudinal folds)
C. Function—concentrates and stores bile

Pancreas

A. Size, shape, location—larger in men than in women, but considerable individual variation; fish-shaped, with body, head, and tail, located in C-shaped curve of duodenum
B. Structure—both duct and ductless gland
 1. Pancreatic cells—pour secretion, pancreatic juice, into duct that runs length of gland and empties into duodenum at hepato-pancreatic papilla
 2. Islands of Langerhans (or islet cells)—clusters of cells not connected with pancreatic ducts; 2 main types of cells compose islets, namely, alpha and beta cells; constitute endocrine glands
C. Functions
 1. Pancreatic cells connected with pancreatic ducts secrete pancreatic juice, enzymes of which help digest all three kinds of foods
 2. Islet cells constitute endocrine gland
  a. Alpha cells secrete hormone glucagon, which accelerates liver glycogenolysis; hence, tends to increase blood sugar
  b. Beta cells secrete insulin, one of most important metabolic hormones, which exerts profound influence over the metabolism of carbohydrates, proteins, and fats
   (1) Insulin accelerates active transport of glucose (along with potassium and phosphate ions) through cell membranes; therefore, it tends to decrease blood glucose (hypoglycemic effect) and to increase glucose utilization by cells either for catabolism or for anabolism (Fig. 13)
   (2) Insulin stimulates liver cell glucokinase; therefore, it promotes liver glycogenesis, another effect that tends to lower blood glucose
   (3) Insulin inhibits liver cell phosphatase and therefore inhibits liver glycogenolysis
   (4) Insulin accelerates rate of amino acid transfer into cells, so promotes protein anabolism within them
   (5) Insulin accelerates rate of fatty acid transfer into cells, promotes fat anabolism (also called fat desposition or lipogenesis), and inhibits fat catabolism

Vermiform appendix

A. Size, shape, location—about size and shape of large angleworm; blind-end tube off cecum just beyond ileocecal valve
B. Structure—same coats as compose intestinal wall

Digestion

A. Definition—all changes that food undergoes in alimentary canal
B. Purpose—conversion of foods into chemical and physical forms that can be absorbed and metabolized
C. Kinds
 1. Mechanical digestion—all movements of alimentary tract that:
  a. Change physical state of foods from comparatively large solid pieces into minute dissolved particles
  b. Propel food forward along alimentary tract, finally eliminating digestive wastes from body
   (1) Deglutition—swallowing
   (2) Peristalsis—wormlike movements that squeeze food downward in tract
   (3) Mass peristalsis—entire contents moved into sigmoid colon and rectum; usually occurs after meal
   (4) Defecation—emptying of rectum, so-called bowel movement
  c. Churn intestinal contents so all become well mixed with digestive juices and all parts of contents come in contact with surface of intestinal mucosa to facilitate absorption
 2. Chemical digestion—series of hydrolytic processes dependent upon specific enzymes; hydrolysis, decomposition of complex compound into two or more simple compounds by means of chemical reaction with water (Table on chemistry of digestion, p. 98)
D. Control of digestive gland secretion

1. Secretion of saliva—neural control of this reflex results from parasympathetic impulses to glands, initiated by taste, smell, and sight of food
2. Gastric juice
   a. Neural control similar to that of salivary glands
   b. Hormonal control—partially digested proteins cause gastric mucosa to release hormone (gastrin) into blood; gastrin stimulates gastric mucosa to secrete juice with high pepsin and hydrochloric acid content
3. Pancreatic juice
   a. Hormonal control—hydrochloric acid in chyme entering duodenum from stomach causes intestinal mucosa to release hormone (secretin) into blood; secretin stimulates pancreatic cells to secrete juice high in sodium bicarbonate content to neutralize hydrochloric acid but low in enzymes; products of protein digestion (e.g., proteoses, peptones, and amino acids) cause intestinal mucosa to release another hormone, pancreozymin, which stimulates pancreatic cells to secrete enzymes
   b. Neural control—reflex secretion of pancreatic juice results from parasympathetic impulses via vagus nerve
4. Bile
   a. Although bile is secreted continuously, secretin increases amount of bile secreted
   b. Presence of fats in intestine causes intestinal mucosa to release hormone, cholecystokinin, into blood; cholecystokinin stimulates smooth muscle of gallbladder to contract, ejecting bile into duodenum
5. Intestinal juice—control obscure but believed to be both reflex and hormonal; food in small intestine causes mucosa to release hormone (enterocrinin) into blood; enterocrinin stimulates intestinal glands to secrete

Absorption

A. Definition—passage of substances through intestinal mucosa into blood or lymph
B. Accomplished mainly through active transport by intestinal cells; makes it possible for both water and solutes to move through intestinal mucosa in direction opposite that expected in osmosis and diffusion
C. Absorption occurs from small intestine, with exception of alcohol, certain drugs, and some water, which are absorbed from stomach; largest amount of water absorbed from large intestine
D. Absorption of protein, carbohydrate, and fat (Table 1-17)

Metabolism—includes catabolism and anabolism

A. Catabolism
   1. Consists of complex series of chemical reactions that take place inside cells and yield energy, carbon dioxide, and water; about half of energy released from food molecules by catabolism is put back in storage in unstable, high-energy bonds of ATP molecules and the rest is transformed to heat; energy

Table 1-17. Absorption of protein, carbohydrate, and fat

Substance	Structures into which absorbed	Circulation
Protein—amino acids	Into blood in intestinal capillaries	Portal vein, liver, hepatic vein, inferior vena cava to heart, etc.
Carbohydrate—monosaccharides (glucose and fructose)	Same as amino acids	Same as amino acids
Fat—glycerol and fatty acids; fatty acids are insoluble and must first combine with bile salts to form water-soluble substance	Chiefly into lymph in intestinal lacteals; some into blood	During absorption while in epithelial cells of intestinal mucosa, glycerol and fatty acids recombine to form microscopic particles of fats (chylomicrons); lymphatics carry them by way of thoracic duct to left subclavian vein, superior vena cava, heart, etc.

in high-energy bonds of ATP can be released as rapidly as needed for doing cellular work

2. Two processes involved; glycolysis and Krebs' citric acid cycle
3. Purpose—to continually provide cells with utilizable energy

B. Anabolism
1. Synthesis of various compounds from simpler compounds
2. Cellular work that uses some of energy made available by catabolism

C. Metabolism of carbohydrates
1. Consists of the following processes
   a. Glucose transport through cell membranes and phosphorylation
      (1) Insulin promotes this transport through cell membranes
      (2) Glucose phosphorylation— conversion of glucose to glucose-6-phosphate, catalyzed by enzyme glucokinase; insulin increases activity of glucokinase and promotes glucose phosphorylation, which is essential prior to both glycogenesis and glucose catabolism
   b. Glycogenesis—conversion of glucose to glycogen for storage; occurs mainly in liver and muscle cells
   c. Glycogenolysis
      (1) In muscle cells glycogen is changed back to glucose-6-phosphate, which is then catabolized in the muscle cells
      (2) In liver cells glycogen is changed back to glucose; enzyme, glucose phosphatase, is present in liver cells and catalyzes final step of glycogenolysis, the changing of glucose-6-phosphate to glucose; glucagon and epinephrine accelerate liver glycogenolysis
   d. Glucose catabolism
      (1) Glycolysis—series of anaerobic reactions that break 1 glucose molecule down into 2 pyruvic acid molecules with conversion of about 5% of energy stored in glucose to heat and ATP molecules
      (2) Krebs' citric acid cycle—series of aerobic chemical reactions by which 2 pyruvic acid molecules (from 1 glucose molecule) are broken down to 6 carbon dioxide and 6 water molecules with release of some energy as heat and some stored again in ATP; citric acid cycle releases about 95%, and glycolysis only about 5% of energy stored in glucose; citric acid cycle occurs in the mitochondria of cells

   e. Gluconeogenesis—sequence of chemical reactions carried on in liver cells; process converts protein or fat compounds into glucose
   f. Principles of normal carbohydrate metabolism
      (1) Principle of preferred energy fuel—cells first catabolize glucose, sparing fats and proteins; when their glucose supply becomes inadequate, they next catabolize fats, sparing proteins; and finally, when fats are used up, they catabolize their own cell proteins
      (2) Principle of glycogenesis— glucose in excess of about 120 to 140 mg. per 100 ml. blood brought to liver by portal veins enters liver cells where it undergoes glycogenesis and is stored as glycogen
      (3) Principle of glycogenolysis— when blood glucose decreases below midpoint of normal, liver glycogenolysis accelerates and tends to raise blood glucose concentration back toward midpoint of normal
      (4) Principle of gluconeogenesis —when blood glucose decreases below normal or when amount of glucose entering cells is inadequate, liver gluconeogenesis accelerates and tends to raise blood glucose concentration
      (5) Principle of glucose storage as fat—when blood insulin content is adequate, glucose in excess of amount used for catabolism and glycogenesis is

converted to fat and stored in fat depots

D. Control of metabolism—primarily by hormones
1. Pancreatic hormones
   a. Insulin—exerts predominant control over carbohydrate metabolism but also affects protein and fat metabolism; in general, insulin accelerates carbohydrate metabolism by cells, thereby decreasing blood glucose
   b. Glucagon secreted by alpha cells of islands of Langerhans—accelerates liver glycogenolysis only
2. Anterior pituitary hormones
   a. Growth hormone tends to
      (1) Accelerate protein anabolism; hence promotes growth of skeleton and soft tissues
      (2) Accelerate fat mobilization from adipose cells, which tends to bring about a shift from use of glucose to use of fats for catabolism
      (3) Accelerate liver gluconeogenesis from fats, which tends to increase blood glucose
      (4) Stimulate glucagon secretion, which, in turn stimulates liver glycogenolysis and glucose release into blood
   b. ACTH (adrenocorticotropic hormone)—stimulates adrenal cortex secretion, especially of glucocorticoids
3. Adrenal cortex hormones—glucocorticoids mainly cortisol and corticosterone tend to
   a. Accelerate fat mobilization and catabolism, thereby promoting shift to fat catabolism from glucose catabolism whenever latter is inadequate for energy needs
   b. Accelerate tissue protein mobilization (catabolism)
   c. Accelerate liver gluconeogenesis; presumably secondary effect; results from protein mobilization and tends to increase blood sugar
4. Adrenal medulla hormones—the catecholamines, epinephrine and norepinephrine, tend to accelerate both liver and muscle glycogenolysis with release of glucose from liver into circulation; therefore tend to increase blood sugar

5. Male sex gland hormone—testosterone, secreted by interstitial cells of testes, tends to accelerate protein anabolism

E. Metabolic rate—calories of heat energy produced and expended per hour or per day
1. Basal metabolic rate (BMR)—calories of heat produced when individual is awake but resting in a comfortably warm environment 12 to 18 hours after last meal
   a. Factors determining basal metabolic rates
      (1) Size—BMR is directly related to square meters of surface area of body; the larger the surface area, the higher the BMR
      (2) Sex—5% to 7% higher in male than in female of same size and age
      (3) Age—BMR inversely related to age; as age increases BMR decreases
      (4) Amount of thyroid hormones secreted; thyroid hormones accelerate BMR
      (5) Body temperature—BMR directly related to body temperature; 1° C. increase in body temperature above normal is accompanied by about 13% increase in BMR
      (6) Miscellaneous factors such as sleep (decreases BMR), pregnancy, and emotions (increase BMR)
   b. Measurement
      (1) Determined by measuring the amount of oxygen inspired in a given time
      (2) Reported as normal or as a definite percentage above or below normal
2. Total metabolic rate—calories of heat energy expended per day; equal to basal metabolic rate plus number of calories of energy used for muscular work, eating and digesting food, and adjusting to cool temperatures
3. Some principles about the metabolic rate and its relation to body weight
   a. For body weight to remain constant except for variations in water content, energy balance must be maintained; body weight remains con-

stant when energy input equals energy output

b. Whenever energy input (food intake) is greater than the energy output (total metabolic rate) body weight increases

c. Whenever energy input (food intake) is less than the energy output (total metabolic rate), body weight decreases

Maintenance of body temperature

A. To maintain body temperature, heat production must equal heat loss

B. Heat is produced only by catabolism especially in skeletal muscles and liver

C. Heat lost from the body
1. By the physical processes of evaporation, radiation, conduction, and convection about 80% of the total heat lost from the body occurs through the skin
2. Through mucosa of respiratory, digestive, and urinary tracts, in warming cool inspired air, and cooling ingested foods and liquids

D. Thermostatic control of heat production and loss
1. The human thermostat consists of neurons located in the anterior part of the hypothalamus, which serve as thermal receptors
2. Heat-dissipating mechanism
a. Set in operation by an increase in blood temperature above the threshold of stimulation of thermal receptors in hypothalamus
b. Responses
(1) Increased sweating, which increases heat loss from skin by evaporation
(2) Dilatation of skin blood vessels, which increases heat loss from skin by radiation
3. Heat-gaining mechanism
a. Mechanism is activated by a decrease in blood temperature
b. Responses
(1) Skin blood vessel constriction, which decreases heat loss from skin
(2) Shivering, which increases heat production

E. Skin thermal receptors—stimulation of these receptors give rise to sensations of heat or cold and often initiates voluntary movements to reduce these sensations;

e.g., fanning oneself to cool off or exercising to warm up

URINARY SYSTEM
Functions

A. Secrete urine

B. Eliminate urine from body (urination, micturition, or voiding) to:
1. Excrete various normal and abnormal metabolic wastes
2. Regulate composition and volume of blood and blood pressure; especially important in maintenance of fluid and electrolyte balance and acid-base balance

Organs
Kidneys

A. Gross anatomy
1. Size, shape, and location—about 4 × 2 × 1 inch; shaped like lima beans; lie against posterior abdominal wall, behind peritoneum at level of last thoracic and first 3 lumbar vertebrae; right kidney slightly lower than left
2. External structure
a. Hilum—concave notch on mesial surface; blood vessels and ureter enter kidney through this notch
b. Renal capsule—protective capsule of fibrous tissue that envelops kidney
3. Internal structure
a. Cortex—outer layer of kidney substance; composed of renal corpuscles, convoluted tubules, and adjacent parts of loops of Henle
b. Medulla—inner portion of kidney; composed of loops of Henle and collecting tubules
c. Pyramids—triangular wedges of medullary substance that have striped appearance
d. Papillae—apices of pyramids; collecting tubules open into renal pelvis here
e. Columns—inward extensions of cortex between pyramids

B. Microscopic anatomy of kidney
1. Glomerulus—cluster of capillaries invaginated in Bowman's capsule
2. Bowman's capsule—funnel-shaped upper end of urinary tubules
3. Renal corpuscle—composed of Bowman's capsule and the glomerulus invaginated in it

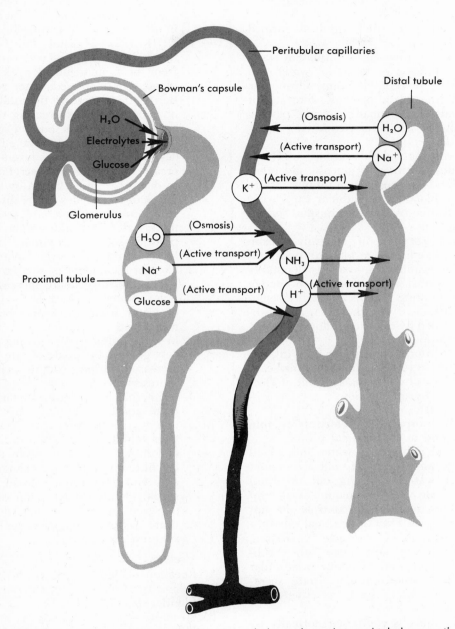

Fig. 14. Diagram showing glomerular filtration, tubular reabsorption, and tubular secretion—the three processes by which the kidneys secrete urine. In the proximal tubule, note that water is reabsorbed from the tubular filtrate into blood by osmosis, but sodium and glucose are reabsorbed mainly by active transport mechanisms. Note, too, that water and sodium are also reabsorbed from the distal tubule. Potassium and hydrogen ions and ammonia, in contrast, are secreted into the tubule from the blood. (From Anthony, C. P., and Kolthoff, N. J.: Textbook of anatomy and physiology, ed. 9, St. Louis, 1975, The C. V. Mosby Co.)

4. Nephron—physiologic unit of kidney that consists of renal corpuscle plus tubules

C. Mechanism by which urine is formed (Fig. 14)
1. In glomerulus—urine formation starts with process of filtration; water and solutes (except albumins, fibrinogen, and other blood proteins) filter out of blood into Bowman's capsule, passing through glomerular-capsular membrane
2. In proximal tubule and loop of Henle
   a. Reabsorption of glucose and other food molecules from tubular filtrate to blood in peritubular capillaries; mainly by active transport mechanisms
   b. Reabsorption of electrolyes from tubule filtrate to blood in peritubular capillaries; cations (notably sodium) are reabsorbed by active transport; anions (notably chlorides and bicarbonate) are reabsorbed by diffusion following cation transport
   c. Reabsorption of water from tubular filtrate to blood in peritubular capillaries by osmosis as result of electrolyte reabsorption
3. In distal tubule
   a. Reabsorption of electrolytes into blood as in proximal tubule
   b. Reabsorption of water into blood by osmosis; ADH controls amount of water osmosing out of distal tubule whereas amount of electrolytes reabsorbed controls amount of osmosis out of proximal tubule
   c. Secretion of hydrogen, potassium, ammonia, and some other substances from blood in peritubular capillaries to tubular filtrate; secretion accomplished by active transport mechanism

D. Urine volume is controlled normally by mechanisms that regulate the amount of water reabsorbed by the kidney tubules; only under abnormal conditions does the glomerular filtration rate influence urine volume
1. The ADH mechanism—neurons in the hypothalamus (mainly in the supraoptic nucleus) produce the antidiuretic hormone and the posterior pituitary gland secretes it into the blood; ADH secretion is stimulated by two conditions, an increase in the osmotic pressure of extracellular fluid or a decrease in the volume of extracellular fluid; ADH acts on distal and collecting tubules, causing more water to osmose from the tubular filtrate back into the blood; this increased water reabsorption tends to increase the total volume of body fluid by decreasing the urine volume; ADH has both a water-retaining and an antidiuretic effect
2. The aldosterone mechanism—an increase in aldosterone secretion tends to decrease urine volume by stimulating kidney tubules to reabsorb primarily more sodium and secondarily more water; thus aldosterone tends to produce sodium retention, water retention, and a low urine volume
3. Control by amount of solutes in tubular filtrate; in general, increase in tubular solutes causes decreased osmosis of water from proximal tubule back into blood and therefore an increase in urine volume; e.g., in diabetes, excess glucose in tubule filtrate leads to increased urine volume (polyuria, diuresis)
4. Glomerular filtration rate normally is quite constant at about 125 ml. per minute, it does not vary enough to alter volume of urine produced, but in certain pathologic conditions glomerular filtration rate may change markedly and alter urine volume; e.g., in shock, glomerular filtration decreases or even ceases, causing decreased urine volume (oliguria) or urinary suppression (anuria)

Ureters
A. Location—behind parietal peritoneum; extend from kidneys to posterior part of bladder floor
B. Structure—ureter expands as it enters kidney to form renal pelvis; subdivided into calyces, each of which contains renal papilla; ureter walls composed of smooth muscle with mucosa lining and fibrous outer coat
C. Function—collect urine secreted by kidney cells and drain it into bladder

Urinary bladder
A. Location—behind symphysis pubis, below parietal peritoneum

B. Structure—collapsible bag of smooth muscle lined with mucosa arranged in rugae; 3 openings—2 from ureters and 1 into the urethra

C. Functions
1. Reservoir for urine until sufficient amount accumulated for elimination
2. Expulsion of urine from body by way of urethra

Urethra

A. Location
1. Female—behind symphysis pubis, in front of vagina
2. Male—extends through prostate gland, fibrous sheet, and penis
B. Structure—musculomembranous tube lined with mucosa; opening to exterior called urinary meatus
C. Functions
1. Female—passageway for expulsion of urine
2. Male—passageway for expulsion of both urine and male reproductive fluid

Urine

A. Normal chemical composition—urine consists of approximately 95% water, which contains the following main substances:
1. Wastes
   a. From protein metabolism—urea, uric acid, creatinine, etc.
   b. Miscellaneous; e.g., hippuric acid formed in liver from detoxication of benzoates (in some foods)
2. Salts (electrolytes)
   a. Cations—sodium is most abundant; also potassium, ammonium, and others
   b. Anions—chlorides most abundant; also bicarbonate, phosphate, and others
3. Pigments—urochrome is principal one
4. Hormones and products of their metabolism
   a. Pituitary gonadotropins
   b. Chorionic gonadotropins (in pregnancy, secreted by placenta; presence of chorionic gonadotropins in urine is basis for pregnancy tests)
   c. 17-Ketosteroids from metabolism of corticoids and androgens
B. Abnormal constituents—glucose, albumin, red blood cells, casts, calculi, etc.

FLUID AND ELECTROLYTE BALANCE

Basic concepts

A. Total volume of fluid and total amount of electrolytes in body normally remain relatively constant
B. Volume of blood plasma, interstitial fluid, and intracellular fluid and the concentration of electrolytes in each remain relatively constant
C. Fluid balance and electrolyte balance are interdependent

Principles of fluid balance

A. Intake must equal output
B. Fluid and electrolyte balance maintained primarily by mechanisms that adjust output to intake; secondarily by mechanisms that adjust intake to output
C. Fluid balance also maintained by mechanisms that control movement of water between fluid compartments

Avenues by which water enters and leaves body

A. Water enters body through digestive tract both in liquids and in foods
B. Water is formed in body by metabolism of foods
C. Water leaves body via kidneys, lungs, skin, and intestines

Mechanisms that maintain total fluid volume

A. The mechanism that regulates the amount of fluid lost by way of the urine, increasing or decreasing it to make the total fluid output volume equal the total fluid intake volume
B. Various factors such as hyperventilation, hypoventilation, vomiting, diarrhea, and circulatory failure may alter the volume of fluid lost
C. Regulation of fluid intake
1. Mechanism by which intake adjusted to output not completely known
2. One controlling factor seems to be degree of moistness of mucosa of mouth—if output exceeds intake, mouth feels dry, sensation of thirst occurs, and individual ingests liquids

Mechanisms that maintain fluid distribution

A. Comparison of plasma, interstitial fluid, and intracellular fluid

1. Plasma and interstitial fluid constitute extracellular fluid, which is the internal environment of body
2. Intracellular fluid volume is the largest and constitutes about 40% of body weight; interstitial fluid about 16%; plasma about 4%
3. Chemically, plasma and interstitial fluid are almost identical except that plasma contains slightly more electrolytes, considerably more proteins, somewhat more sodium, and fewer chloride ions than interstitial fluid
4. Chemically, extracellular fluid and intracellular fluid are strikingly different; sodium is the main cation of extracellular fluid, potassium is the main cation of intracellular fluid; chloride is the main anion of extracellular fluid, phosphate is the main anion of intracellular fluid; protein concentration is much higher in intracellular fluid than in interstitial fluid

B. Control of movement of liquid between blood and interstitial fluid
 1. Four pressures are involved
   a. Blood hydrostatic pressure
   b. Blood osmotic pressure
   c. Interstitial fluid hydrostatic pressure
   d. Interstitial fluid osmotic pressure
 2. Blood hydrostatic pressure and interstitial fluid osmotic pressure tend to move fluid out of the blood in the capillaries into the interstitial fluid
 3. Blood osmotic pressure and interstitial fluid hydrostatic pressure tend to move fluid back into the capillary blood from the interstitial fluid
 4. Starling's law of the capillaries states that equal amounts of water move back and forth between blood and interstitial fluid only when blood hydrostatic pressure plus interstitial fluid osmotic pressure equals blood osmotic pressure plus interstitial fluid hydrostatic pressure; under these conditions fluid balance exists between blood and interstitial fluid
 5. Corollaries of Starling's law of the capillaries
   a. Blood gains liquid from interstitial fluid whenever blood hydrostatic pressure plus interstitial fluid osmotic pressure is less than blood osmotic pressure plus interstitial fluid hydrostatic pressure
   b. Blood loses liquid to interstitial fluid whenever blood osmotic pressure plus interstitial fluid hydrostatic pressure is less than blood hydrostatic pressure plus interstitial fluid osmotic pressure
   c. Control of the movement of liquid through cell membrane
     (1) Primarily by relative osmotic pressures of extracellular fluid and intracellular fluid
     (2) Osmotic pressure depends mainly upon:
       (a) Sodium concentration of extracellular fluid
       (b) Potassium concentration of intracellular fluid

ACID-BASE BALANCE
General principles

A. Healthy survival depends upon the body's maintaining a state of acid-base balance; more specifically, healthy survival depends upon the maintenance of a relatively constant, slightly alkaline pH of blood and other fluids
B. When the body is in a state of acid-base balance, it maintains a stable hydrogen ion concentration in body fluids; specifically, blood pH remains relatively constant between 7.35 and 7.45
C. The body has three devices or mechanisms for maintaining acid-base balance; named in order of the speed with which they act they are the buffer mechanism, the respiratory mechanism, and the renal or urinary mechanism
D. A state of uncompensated acidosis exists if blood pH decreases below 7.35
E. A state of uncompensated alkalosis exists if blood pH increases above 7.45

Buffer mechanism for maintaining acid-base balance

A. The buffer mechanism consists of chemicals called buffers, which are present in the blood and other body fluids and which combine with relatively strong acids or bases to convert them to weaker acids or bases; hence, buffers function to prevent marked changes in blood pH when either acids or bases enter the blood
B. A buffer is often referred to as a buffer

pair because it consists of not one but two substances; the chief buffer pair in the blood consists of the weak acid, carbonic acid (H_2CO_3), and its basic salts, collectively called base bicarbonate ($B \cdot HCO_3$); sodium bicarbonate ($NaHCO_3$) is by far the most abundant base bicarbonate present in blood plasma

C. When the body is in a state of acid-base balance, blood contains 27 mEq. base bicarbonate per liter and 1.35 mEq. carbonic acid per liter; usually this is written as a ratio, referred to as the base bicarbonate/carbonic acid ratio:

$$\frac{27 \text{ mEq. } B \cdot HCO_3}{1.35 \text{ mEq. } H_2CO_3} = \frac{20}{1}$$

D. Whenever the base bicarbonate/carbonic acid ratio of blood equals 20/1, blood pH equals 7.4

E. Base bicarbonate buffers nonvolatile acids that are stronger than carbonic acid; it reacts with them to convert them to carbonic acid and a basic salt

F. Some facts about the changes in capillary blood produced by the buffering of blood by base bicarbonate
1. Buffering does not prevent blood pH from decreasing, but it does prevent it from decreasing as markedly as it would without buffering
2. Buffering removes some sodium bicarbonate from blood and adds some carbonic acid to it; this necessarily decreases the base bicarbonate/carbonic acid ratio, which in turn necessarily decreases the pH of blood as it flows through capillaries (from its arterial level of about 7.4 to its venous level of about 7.38)

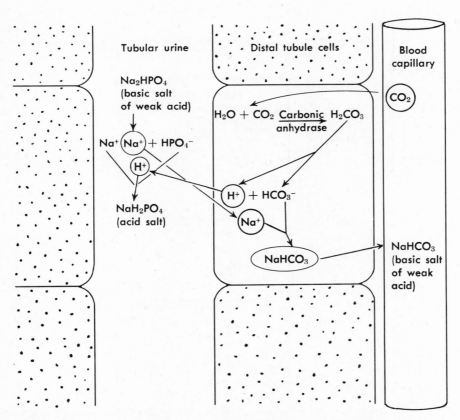

Fig. 15. Acidification of urine and conservation of base by distal renal tubule excretion of H ions into the urine and reabsorption of Na ions into the blood in exchange for the H ions excreted from it. (From Anthony, C. P., and Kolthoff, N. J.: Textbook of anatomy and physiology, ed. 9, St. Louis, 1975, The C. V. Mosby Co.)

3. Anything that decreases blood's base bicarbonate/carbonic acid ratio necessarily decreases blood pH, hence tends to produce acidosis; the corollary is also true: anything that increases the base bicarbonate/carbonic acid ratio necessarily increases blood pH, hence tends to produce alkalosis

Respiratory mechanism for controlling acid-base balance

A. Venous blood enters lung capillaries and as it flows through them, carbon dioxide moves out of the blood into the alveolar air and is blown out of the body in the expired air; this means that the arterial blood leaving the lung capillaries contains less carbon dioxide than does the venous blood entering them

B. Whenever blood's carbon dioxide content decreases, its hydrogen ion concentration also decreases, and therefore its pH increases because a decrease in the amount of carbon dioxide in blood decreases the number of hydrogen ions remaining in the blood

C. The carbon dioxide content of blood and its hydrogen ion concentration are always directly related to each other; any increase in blood's carbon dioxide content drives the reactions to the right and so increases blood's hydrogen ion concentration (decreases its pH); any decrease in blood's carbon dioxide decreases its hydrogen ion concentration (increases its pH)

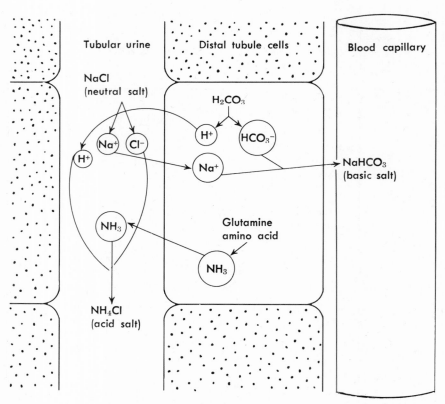

Fig. 16. Acidification of urine by tubule excretion of ammonia (NH_3). An acid (glutamine) leaves the blood, enters a tubule cell, and is deaminized to form ammonia that is excreted into urine, where it combines with hydrogen to form NH_4 ion. In exchange for NH_4 ion, the tubule cell reabsorbs Na ion. (From Anthony, C. P., and Kolthoff, N. J.: Textbook of anatomy and physiology, ed. 9, St. Louis, 1975, The C. V. Mosby Co.)

Renal or urinary mechanism for maintaining acid-base balance

A. The renal mechanism is the most effective device the body has for maintaining acid-base balance; unless it operates adequately, acid-base balance cannot be maintained

B. The renal mechanism for maintaining acid-base balance makes the urine more acid and the blood more alkaline; the mechanism consists of two functions performed by the distal renal tubule cells, both of which remove hydrogen ions from blood to urine and in exchange reabsorb sodium ions from tubular urine to blood
   1. Distal tubule cells secrete hydrogen ions and reabsorb sodium ions (Fig. 15)
   2. Distal tubule cells form ammonia, which combines with hydrogen ions they have secreted to form ammonium (NH_4) ions, which are excreted in the urine in exchange for sodium ions, which are reabsorbed into the blood (Fig. 16)

C. The distal tubule functions produce the following results:
   1. They increase blood's sodium bicarbonate content and decrease its carbonic acid content, thereby increasing the base bicarbonate/carbonic acid ratio and blood pH
   2. They acidify urine (decrease urine pH)

MAINTAINING THE SPECIES

REPRODUCTIVE SYSTEM
Male reproductive organs
   Glands

A. Main male sex glands (gonads) are the testes
   1. Structure—fibrous capsule covers each testis and sends partitions into interior of gland, dividing it into lobules composed of tiny tubules called seminiferous tubules, embedded in connective tissue containing interstitial cells; few ducts emerge from top of gland to enter head of epididymis
   2. Location—in scrotum, 1 testis in each of 2 compartments of scrotum
   3. Functions
      a. Seminiferous tubules carry on sper-matogenesis; that is, they form spermatozoa, the male sex cells or gametes
      b. Interstitial cells secrete testosterone, the main androgen or male hormone (see Table 1-14 for testosterone functions)
   4. Structure of spermatozoon—consists of head, middle piece, and whiplike tail that propels sperm; microscopic in size

B. Accessory glands
   1. Seminal vesicles
      a. Location—on posterior surface of bladder
      b. Structure—convoluted pouches, mucous lining
      c. Function—secrete nutrient-rich fluid estimated to constitute about 30% of semen
   2. Prostate gland
      a. Location—encircles urethra just below bladder
      b. Structure—doughnut-shaped gland with ducts opening into urethra
      c. Function—secretes estimated 60% of semen; prostatic secretion is alkaline in reaction since acid lessens sperm motility; prostatic secretion contains abundance of enzyme, acid phosphatase; therefore, blood level of this enzyme increases in metastasizing cancer of prostate
   3. Bulbourethral glands (Cowper's)
      a. Location—just below prostate gland
      b. Structure—small, pea-shaped structures with duct leading into urethra
      c. Function—secrete alkaline fluid that forms part of semen

   Ducts

A. Epididymis
   1. Location—lies along top and side of each testis
   2. Structure—each epididymis consists of single, tightly coiled tube enclosed in fibrous casing
   3. Function—conducts seminal fluid (semen) from testes to vas deferens; secretes small part of semen; stores semen prior to ejaculation, sperm becoming motile during this period

B. Vas deferens (seminal ducts)
   1. Location—extend through inguinal canal into abdominal cavity, over top and down posterior surface of bladder to join ducts from seminal vesicles

2. Structure—pair of tubes or ducts
3. Function—conduct sperm and small amount of semen from each epididymis to an ejaculatory duct
4. Clinical application—vasectomy is the surgical procedure in which a short section of each vas is cut out and its separated ends tied off; as a result, sperm cannot enter the ejaculatory ducts and be ejaculated; vasectomy produces only one important physiologic change—semen from a vasectomized male contains no sperm; hence vasectomy sterilizes a man (makes him infertile); it does not render him impotent; it does, however, slightly decrease the amount of semen ejaculated

C. Ejaculatory ducts—formed by union of each vas with duct from seminal vesicle; pass through prostate gland to terminate in urethra; function—ejaculate semen into urethra
D. Urethra—described under urinary system

Supporting structures

A. External—scrotum and penis
  1. Scrotum—skin-covered pouch suspended from perineal region; divided into 2 compartments, each one containing testis, epididymis, and first part of seminal duct
  2. Penis—made up of 3 cylindrical masses of erectile tissue that contain large vascular spaces; filling of these with blood causes erection of penis; 2 larger and upper cylinders named corpora cavernosa; smaller, lower one contains urethra, called corpus cavernosum; glans penis—a bulging structure at distal end of penis, over which double fold of skin, prepuce or foreskin, fits loosely
B. Internal—spermatic cords are fibrous tubes located in each inguinal canal; serve as casing around each vas deferens and its accompanying blood vessels, lymphatics, and nerves

Female reproductive organs
Ovaries—female gonads

A. Location—behind and below uterine tubes, anchored to uterus and broad ligaments
B. Size and shape of large almonds

C. Microscopic structure—each ovary of newborn female consists of several thousand graafian follicles embedded in connective tissue; follicles are epithelial sacs in which ova develop; usually, between years of menarche and menopause, 1 follicle matures each month, ruptures surface of ovary and expels its ovum into pelvic cavity
D. Functions
  1. Oogenesis—formation of mature ovum in graafian follicle
  2. Ovulation—expulsion of ovum from follicle into pelvic cavity
  3. Secretion of female hormones—maturing follicle secretes estrogens; corpus luteum secretes progesterone and estrogens (see Table 1-14 for hormone functions)

Uterine tubes (fallopian tubes, oviducts)

A. Location—attached to upper, outer angles of uterus
B. Structure—same 3 coats as uterus; distal ends fimbriated and open into pelvic cavity; mucosal lining of tubes and peritoneal lining of pelvis in direct contact here (facilitates spread of infection from tubes to peritoneum)
C. Function—serve as ducts through which ova travel from ovaries to uterus; fertilization normally occurs in tube

Uterus

A. Location of uterus—in pelvic cavity between bladder and rectum
B. Structure
  1. Shape and size—pear-shaped organ approximately the size of a clenched fist
  2. Divisions
    a. Body—upper and main part of uterus; fundus bulging upper surface of body
    b. Cervix—narrow, lower part of uterus; projects into vagina
  3. Walls—composed of smooth muscle (myometrium), lined with mucosa (endometrium)
  4. Cavities
    a. Body cavity—small and triangular in shape with 3 openings into it; 2 from uterine tubes, 1 into cervical canal

b. Cervical cavity—canal with constricted opening, internal os into body cavity and another, external os, into vagina
C. Position of uterus—flexed between body and cervix portions with body portion lying over bladder, pointing forward and slightly upward; cervix joins vagina at right angles; ligaments of uterus hold uterus in position
   1. Broad ligaments (2)—a double fold of parietal peritoneum that forms a kind of partition across pelvic cavity, suspending uterus between its folds
   2. Uterosacral ligaments (2)—foldlike extensions of peritoneum from posterior surface of uterus to sacrum, 1 on each side of rectum
   3. Posterior ligament (1)—fold of peritoneum between posterior surface of uterus and rectum; forms deep pouch, cul-de-sac of Douglas (or rectouterine pouch); this pouch lowest point in pelvic cavity and, therefore, place where pus accumulates in pelvic inflammations; can be drained by posterior colpotomy (incision at top of posterior vaginal wall)
   4. Anterior ligament (1)—fold of peritoneum between uterus and bladder; forms shallow cul-de-sac
   5. Round ligaments (2)—fibromuscular cords from upper, outer angles of uterus, through inguinal canals, terminating in labia majora
D. Functions of uterus
   1. Menstruation
   2. Pregnancy
   3. Labor

Vagina

A. Location—between rectum and urethra
B. Structure—collapsible, musculomembranous tube, capable of great distention; outlet to exterior protected by fold of mucous membrane called hymen
C. Functions
   1. Receives semen from male
   2. Constitutes lower part of birth canal
   3. Acts as excretory duct for uterine secretions and menstrual flow

Vulva

Consists of numerous structures that together constitute external genitals

A. Mons veneris—hairy, skin-covered pad of fat over symphysis pubis
B. Labia majora—hairy, skin-covered lips
C. Labia minora—small lips covered with modified skin
D. Clitoris—small mound of erectile tissue, below junction of two labia minora
E. Urinary meatus—just below clitoris; opening into urethra
F. Vaginal orifice—below urinary meatus; opening into vagina; hymen, fold of mucosa, partially closes orifice
G. Skene's glands—small mucous glands whose ducts open on either side of the urinary meatus
H. Bartholin's glands—2 small, bean-shaped glands; duct from each gland opens on either side of the vaginal orifice; both Bartholin's glands and Skene's glands have clinical interest because they frequently become infected (especially by the gonococci)

Breasts, or mammary glands

A. Location—just under skin, over pectoralis major muscles
B. Size—depends on deposits of adipose tissue rather than amount of glandular tissue
C. Structure—divided into lobes and lobules that, in turn, are composed of racemose glands; excretory duct leads from each lobe to open in nipple; circular, pigmented area, the areola, borders nipples
D. Function—secrete milk (lactation)
   1. Shedding of placenta causes marked decrease in blood levels of estrogens and progesterone, which, in turn, stimulates anterior pituitary to increase prolactin secretion; high blood level of prolactin stimulates alveoli of breast to secrete milk
   2. Suckling controls lactation in 2 ways; by acting in some way to stimulate anterior pituitary secretion of prolactin and to stimulate posterior pituitary secretion of oxytocin, which stimulates release of milk out of alveoli into ducts from which infant can remove it by suckling (letdown reflex)

Menstrual cycle

A. *Menstrual cycle* refers mainly to changes in the uterus and ovaries, which recur cyclically from the time of the menarche to the menopause

B. Length of cycle—usually 28 days although considerable variations occur
C. Hormonal control of menstrual cycle (see Fig. 7)
1. Menses—brought on by marked decrease in blood levels of progesterone and estrogens at about cycle day 25
2. Growth of new follicle and ovum—the low blood concentration of estrogens present for a few days before and during the menses stimulates the anterior pituitary gland to secrete follicle-stimulating hormone (FSH); the resulting high blood concentration of FSH stimulates 1 or more primitive graafian follicles and their ova to start growing and also stimulates the follicle cells to secrete estrogens; this leads to a high blood concentration of estrogens, which, in turn, has a negative feedback effect on FSH secretion by the anterior pituitary gland
3. Endometrial thickening—in preovulatory phase is caused by proliferation of endometrial cells stimulated by the increasing concentration of estrogens in blood; the premenstrual phase is caused partly by endometrial cell proliferation and partly by fluid retention caused by increasing progesterone concentration
4. Ovulation—brought on by high LH concentration
D. Clinical applications
1. Contraceptive pills contain synthetic preparations of estrogen-like and/or progesterone-like compounds
2. Most commonly used contraceptive pills prevent pregnancy by preventing ovulation

DEVELOPMENT OF THE INDIVIDUAL
The formation of gametes
A. The egg and spermatozoan each have 1 set of chromosomes (23); this is in contrast to other cells of the body that have 2 sets or 46 chromosomes (23 pairs)
B. The production of ova (eggs) and spermatozoa (sperm) requires a special type of nuclear division (meiosis) in which the chromosome number is reduced from 2 sets (46 chromosomes) to 1 set (23 chromosomes)

Fertilization
A. Spermatozoa are deposited in the vagina
B. Fertilization occurs in the uterine tube when the egg is about one third of the way down the tube; usually this is about 24 hours after ovulation
C. Sperm must be in the genital tract 4 to 6 hours before they are able to fertilize an egg; during this period the enzyme hyaluronidase is activated; this enzyme is able to dissolve the cement substance (hyaluronic acid) that holds together the cells that surround the ovum
D. The male nucleus enters the cytoplasm of the egg and several events follow
1. A fertilization membrane forms around the egg that prevents the entrance of other sperm
2. The sperm tail is lost and the male nucleus (male pronucleus) moves toward the female nucleus (female pronucleus)
E. Fertilization proper occurs when the male pronucleus unites with the female pronucleus; thus, the chromosome number is restored to 2 sets (46 chromosomes)

Cleavage
A. In a short time after fertilization the zygote undergoes rapid division to produce a mass of cells (morula) that descends in the uterine tube
B. As it descends it also divides to form a hollow ball referred to as the blastocyst

Implantation
A. The blastocyst implants in the uterine wall
1. The blastocyst is differentiated into an inner cell mass, a blastocoel (internal cavity)
2. An outer covering of cells, the trophectoderm, which becomes trophoderm and will form the fetal portion of the placenta
3. Seven to 8 days after fertilization implantation occurs
B. During implantation, cells of trophoderm secrete enzymes that eat into the endometrium and absorb nutrients necessary for embryo growth

Embryonic period
A. First 2 months, after this period it is called a fetus

B. The inner cell mass differentiates into germ layers
  1. Ectoderm—outer layer of skin and mouth cavity and nervous tissue
  2. Mesoderm—connective tissue, including blood and muscle tissue
  3. Endoderm—linings of the alimentary tract, respiratory system, and several glands
C. About the twelfth day after fertilization a fetal membrane, the amnion, forms around the embryo; another membrane, the yolk sac, develops beneath the embryo
D. Later an allantois develops that will supply placental blood vessels
E. A chorion surrounds the embryo; this will eventually form the major part of the placenta; fingerlike projections of the chorion called chorionic villi grow into the endometrium

Umbilical cord

A. Consists of an outer layer of amnion
B. Contains 2 umbilical arteries and 1 umbilical vein

Fetal growth

A. Differentiation of cells occurs
B. Development of organs progresses from anterior to posterior in the growing fetus

Hormones

A. During pregnancy the chorion of the placenta secretes a hormone, chorionic gonadotropin, which seems to maintain the corpus luteum and the secretion of progesterone which is necessary for attachment
B. Chorionic gonadotropin reaches a peak in the third month and then drops
C. Estrogen and progesterone increase and continue to be secreted during the last 6 months of pregnancy
D. In the last month uterine contents shift downward so that the fetus is in contact with the cervix; this contact induces oxytocin secretion by the posterior pituitary
E. The secretion of oxytocin, which stimulates uterine contractions, coupled with the drop in progesterone brings about labor; uterine contractions increase in frequency and intensity

HEREDITY
Chromosomes

A. Humans have 23 pairs of homologous chromosomes
B. In males the sex chromosomes (the X and Y) are not equal in size
C. Homologous chromosomes carry sets of matching genes (alleles) in which one may be dominant and the other recessive or they may have blending expressions

Sex determination in humans

A. Genetic females have 2 sets of autosomes (nonsex chromosomes) and 2 X chromosomes, whereas genetic males have 2 sets of autosomes and 1 X chromosome and 1 Y chromosome
B. All eggs produced by females will have 1 set of autosomes and 1 X chromosome; spermatozoa produced by a male will have a set of autosomes and either an X or a Y chromosome
C. If an X-bearing spermatozoon fertilizes an egg a female will result; if a Y-bearing spermatozoon fertilizes an egg a male will result

Genes

A. Sex-linked genes—genes carried on the X chromosome are called sex-linked genes that are always expressed in the male even though they may be recessive; examples of such genes cause hemophilia and color blindness
B. Multiple genes—many different genes may combine to produce cumulative effects such as the degree of pigmentation or height
C. Multiple alleles—an example of human traits controlled by multiple alleles are the genes controlling normal blood types; the genes for type O are dominated by the genes for type A or type B; the genes for A and B are both expressed

Genes	Blood type
OO	O
AO	A
AA	A
BO	B
BB	B
AB	AB

D. The following are some other human traits controlled by genes

Dominant	Recessive
Brown eyes	Blue eyes
Normal blood clotting	Hemophilia (sex-linked)
Normal color vision	Color blind (sex-linked)
Normal pigmentation	Albinism
Rh positive (multiple alleles)	Rh negative
Normal red blood cell development	Sickle cell trait

Chromosomal alterations

A. In rare cases additional sex chromosomes may appear and produce abnormal individuals
   1. X chromosome and no Y chromosome —Turner's syndrome
   2. Two or more X chromosomes and a Y chromosome—Klinefelter's syndrome
B. Translocation of chromosome—a cytogenetic abnormality such as trisomy 21 (Down's syndrome)
C. Mutations
   1. Changes in the DNA are mutations; there may also be chromosomal changes
   2. The frequency of mutations may be increased by certain agents such as ultraviolet radiation, x-ray films, radioactive radiation, and certain chemical substances

REVIEW QUESTIONS FOR ANATOMY AND PHYSIOLOGY

1. Which of the following are derived from mesoderm?
   1. Bone
   2. Lining of the digestive tract
   3. Liver
   4. Nervous tissue
2. In an adult, red blood cells are formed mainly in the
   1. Bone marrow
   2. Pancreas
   3. Liver
   4. Lymph nodes
3. Fragments of cells in the bloodstream that break down on exposure to injured tissue and begin the chain reaction leading to a blood clot are known as
   1. Red blood cells
   2. Platelets
   3. Leukocytes
   4. Erythrocytes
4. The protein of blood involved with immune responses is
   1. Hemoglobin
   2. Albumin
   3. Globulin
   4. Thrombin
5. Blood plasma is chiefly composed of
   1. Hemoglobin
   2. Fibrinogin
   3. Water
   4. The antibody component
6. Agglutinogens involved in determination of blood compatability are
   1. Found as soluble components of the blood serum
   2. Part of the leukocytes
   3. Functional only outside the body
   4. Located on the surface of red blood cells
7. A cell can still live in a healthy condition without performing which one of the following functions?
   1. Active transport
   2. Anabolism
   3. Catabolism
   4. Mitosis
8. White blood cells that are the chief phagocytes are
   1. Neutrophils
   2. Eosinophils
   3. Lymphocytes
   4. Basophils
9. The scientific name for bone-forming cells is
   1. Haversian cells
   2. Osteoblasts
   3. Osteoclasts
   4. Osteocytes
10. Cilia are
    1. Found in all epithelial cells
    2. Seldom seen in human structures
    3. Hairlike structures that move
    4. The secreting portion of glands
11. Anabolism is
    1. The derivation of energy
    2. Building up of molecules
    3. Breaking down of cells
    4. Eating members of the same species
12. Large complex molecules are subdivided chemically into smaller simpler components by the process known as
    1. Synthesis
    2. Condensation
    3. Hydrolysis
    4. Diffusion
13. Glucose is an important molecule to a cell because this molecule is used for
    1. The building of cell membranes
    2. The synthesis of proteins
    3. Extraction of energy
    4. Building the genetic material
14. The large molecules called starch and proteins are made of smaller molecules called
    1. Fatty acids and alcohols
    2. Carbon dioxide and methane
    3. Acetic acid and glucose
    4. Simple sugars and amino acids
15. The relay center for sensory impulses is the
    1. Medulla oblongata
    2. Hypothalamus
    3. Cerebellum
    4. Thalamus
16. The basic function of all receptor structures of the nervous system is to
    1. Produce muscle contractions
    2. Stimulate secretions from the endocrine glands
    3. Transform stimuli into nerve impulses
    4. Coordinate nerve impulses

17. Nerve fibers of the brain or spinal cord that are destroyed do not regenerate because they lack
    1. A myelin sheath
    2. A neurilemma
    3. Nissl bodies
    4. Nuclei
18. Impulses travel in one direction because
    1. Polarization occurs laterally
    2. Only axons secrete acetylcholine
    3. Sodium pump doesn't work in reverse
    4. Cholinesterase acts all along the axon
19. Visual impulses are received in the
    1. Temporal lobe
    2. Occipital lobe
    3. Frontal lobe
    4. Parietal lobe
20. The part of the brain that controls respiration is the
    1. Medulla
    2. Cerebral cortex
    3. Hypothalamus
    4. Cerebellum
21. The medulla has centers for
    1. Control of sexual development
    2. Fat metabolism, temperature, water balance
    3. Voluntary movements, taste, skin sensations
    4. Control of breathing, heart beat, blood vessels' size
22. The internal organs of humans, such as the bladder and the esophagus, are under the control of the
    1. Peripheral nervous system
    2. Central nervous system
    3. Autonomic nervous system
    4. Spinal cord
23. Acetylcholine is produced
    1. In the nerve cell body
    2. At dendrite ends
    3. At axon ends
    4. All along the neuron
24. Coordination of skeletal muscles and equilibrium is controlled by the
    1. Medulla oblongata
    2. Hypothalamus
    3. Cerebellum
    4. Thalamus
25. Stimulation of the vagus nerve results in
    1. Tachycardia
    2. Dilatation of the bronchioles
    3. Slowing of the heart
    4. Coronary artery vasodilatation
26. An arterial anastomosis present at the base of the brain is the
    1. Volar arch
    2. Brachiocephalic
    3. Circle of Willis
    4. Brachial plexus
27. The foramen magnum is located
    1. In the mandible
    2. Within the sacrum
    3. In fetal hearts only
    4. Completely within the occipital bone
28. Crushing of the spinal cord above the level of the phrenic nerve origin will result in
    1. Ventricular fibrillation
    2. Activity counter to that indicated by control of the vagus nerve
    3. Spinal shock and paralysis of the lower extremities
    4. Respiratory paralysis and stopping of diaphragmatic contractions
29. An injury or infection that would cause nerve deafness would most likely be to the
    1. Cochlear nerve
    2. Vestibular nerve
    3. Trigeminal nerve
    4. Vagus nerve
30. The function of the ciliary muscle of the eye is
    1. To distinguish between light and dark objects
    2. To distinguish different colors
    3. To regulate the amount of light entering the eye
    4. To focus the lens
31. The ear bones that transmit vibrations to the basilar membrane of the cochlea are found in the
    1. Outer ear
    2. Inner ear
    3. Middle ear
    4. Eustachian tube
32. The optic chiasm
    1. Receives nerve impulses from the optic tracts
    2. Is the space posterior to the lens, with the consistency of jelly
    3. Is a crossing of some optic nerves in the cranial cavity
    4. Is the cavity in which the eyeball is fixed
33. Smooth muscle
    1. Is located in the heart
    2. Is located in arteries
    3. Is a voluntary muscle
    4. Has cross-striations
34. The type of membrane that lines the knee joint is called the
    1. Serous
    2. Synovial
    3. Mucous
    4. Epithelial
35. The layman's name for the clavicle is the
    1. Collar bone
    2. Kneecap
    3. Shin bone
    4. Shoulder blade
36. The scientific name for the shin bone is the
    1. Femur
    2. Fibula
    3. Patella
    4. Tibia
37. What term describes the location of the upper arm muscles with reference to the lower arm?
    1. Caudal
    2. Distal
    3. Dorsal
    4. Proximal
38. With an "oxygen debt," muscle shows
    1. High levels of calcium
    2. Low levels of lactic acid
    3. High levels of glycogen
    4. Low levels of ATP
39. Lacunae and haversian canals are important

structural features that help to microscopically identify
1. Skeletal muscle
2. Nerve cells
3. Cartilage tissue
4. Osseous tissue

40. When the femur is articulated, its head moves in the
1. Acetabulum
2. Vertebral foramen
3. Transverse foramen
4. Glenoid cavity

41. A fracture of the talus bone would necessarily produce difficulty with
1. Speech
2. Breathing
3. Hand articulation
4. Walking

42. The rate of oxidation in all the body cells is regulated primarily by which gland?
1. Pituitary
2. Thyroid
3. Adrenal
4. Pancreas

43. Rapid adjustments made by the body during an emergency are associated with the increased activity of which gland?
1. Pituitary
2. Thyroid
3. Adrenal
4. Pancreas

44. Underactivity of which gland is associated with the appearance of sugar in the urine?
1. Pituitary
2. Thyroid
3. Adrenal
4. Pancreas

45. Which of the following secretes an anti-diuretic substance important for maintaining fluid balance?
1. Anterior pituitary
2. Adrenal cortex
3. Adrenal medulla
4. Posterior pituitary

46. Removal of the parathyroids causes
1. Tetany and death
2. Adrenal cortex stimulation
3. Myxedema
4. Acromegaly

47. Underproduction of thyroxin produces
1. Myxedema
2. Acromegaly
3. Cushing's disease
4. Tetany and death

48. The pituitary hormone that stimulates the secretion of milk from the mammary glands is
1. Prolactin
2. Oxytocin
3. Progesterone
4. Estrogen

49. Aldosterone is a
1. Sex hormone
2. Regulator of fluid and electrolytes
3. Growth regulator
4. Thyroid gland stimulus

50. Parathyroid hormone tends to
1. Accelerate bone breakdown with the release of calcium to the blood

2. Decrease blood calcium concentration
3. Decrease blood phosphate concentration
4. Increase calcium absorption into bone

51. Vitamin K is essential for normal blood clotting because it promotes
1. Ionization of blood calcium
2. Platelet disintegration
3. Fibrinogen formation by liver
4. Prothrombin formation by liver

52. Arteries have
1. Thinner walls than veins
2. Walls without muscle fibers
3. Thick elastic walls with muscle fibers
4. Walls without elastic fibers

53. In general, valves in the circulatory system
1. Permit blood to enter or leave the circulatory system
2. Prevent blood from flowing in the wrong direction
3. Prevent blood from moving too rapidly
4. Stop circulation whenever necessary

54. The muscle of the heart is known as the
1. Myocardium
2. Pericardium
3. Epicardium
4. Endocardium

55. Dissolved organic nutrients are normally transported in the blood by the
1. Erythrocytes
2. Leukocytes
3. Lymphocytes
4. Plasma

56. Hemoglobin is most closely associated with
1. Blood clotting
2. Hormone formation
3. Food transport
4. Oxygen transport

57. What part of the heart does blood enter when returning from the lungs?
1. Left atrium
2. Left ventricle
3. Right atrium
4. Right ventricle

58. The portal vein can be identified as the one that
1. Brings blood away from the liver
2. Brings venous blood from the intestinal wall to the liver
3. Enters the superior vena cava from the cranium
4. Is located superficially on the anteromedial surface of the thigh

59. Blood samples from the right atrium, right ventricle, and pulmonary artery are analyzed for their oxygen content during cardiac catheterization. Normally
1. All contain about the same amount of oxygen
2. All contain less CO_2 than pulmonary vein blood
3. Pulmonary artery blood contains more oxygen than the other samples
4. All contain more oxygen than pulmonary vein blood

60. The coronary arteries
1. Carry low-oxygen-content blood to the lungs

2. Carry blood from the aorta to the myo-cardium
3. Supply blood to the endocardium
4. Carry high-oxygen-content blood from the lungs toward the heart

61. Which chamber of the heart ejects oxygenated blood into the general systemic circulation?
   1. Left atrium
   2. Left ventricle
   3. Right atrium
   4. Right ventricle

62. A pacemaker is used in some patients to perform the function normally performed by the
   1. Accelerator nerves in the heart
   2. Atrioventricular node
   3. Bundle of His
   4. Sinoatrial node

63. Each of the following are structural components of fetal circulation. Which one should not be functionally obliterated after birth?
   1. Umbilical vein
   2. Ductus venosus
   3. Ductus arteriosus
   4. Celiac artery

64. Which chamber of the heart receives most of the returning venous blood?
   1. Left atrium
   2. Left ventricle
   3. Right atrium
   4. Right ventricle

65. The vein present in the human umbilical cord carries
   1. Deoxygenated blood to the fetus
   2. Wastes from the fetus
   3. Oxygenated blood to the fetus
   4. Glucose from the fetus

66. The ductus arteriosus
   1. Shunts blood away from the fetal lungs
   2. Shunts blood away from the fetal liver
   3. Is present in adults as well as in the fetus
   4. Carries venous blood

67. If breathing is deliberately stopped in a person
   1. The individual will soon die of suffocation
   2. Rising oxygen concentrations will stimulate the breathing center
   3. Accumulated CO_2 will force resumption of breathing
   4. Increased N_2 concentration will have a toxic effect

68. Air rushes into the alveoli as a result of
   1. The rising pressure in the alveoli
   2. The rising pressure in the pleura
   3. The lowered pressure in the chest cavity
   4. The relaxation of the diaphragm

69. Tidal air is the amount of air
   1. Exhaled normally after a normal inspiration
   2. Exhaled forcibly after a normal inspiration
   3. Forcibly inspired over and above a normal inspiration
   4. Trapped in the alveoli that cannot be exhaled

70. The poisonous nature of carbon monoxide results from
   1. Its preferential combination with hemoglobin
   2. Its tendency to block CO_2 transport
   3. Its inhibitory effect on vasodilation

4. The bubbles it tends to form in blood plasma

71. The common passageway for food and air is the
   1. Nasopharynx
   2. Oropharynx
   3. Larynx
   4. Trachea

72. One of the main functions of bile is to
   1. Produce an acid condition
   2. Provide vitamins
   3. Emulsify fats
   4. Split protein

73. The end products of lipid digestion are
   1. Starches
   2. Amino acids
   3. Glycerol and fatty acid
   4. Simple sugars

74. The end products of carbohydrate digestion are
   1. Starches
   2. Amino acids
   3. Fats
   4. Simple sugars

75. The end products of protein digestion are
   1. Starches
   2. Amino acids
   3. Fats
   4. Simple sugars

76. A bilirubin level above 2 mg. per 100 ml. blood volume could be indicative of
   1. Anemia
   2. Low oxygen carrying capacity of erythrocytes
   3. Achlorhydria or pernicious anemia
   4. Increased rate of red cell destruction

77. Progesterone is secreted by which of the following structures?
   1. Corpus luteum
   2. Adrenal cortex
   3. Endometrium
   4. Pituitary gland

78. The chief function of progesterone is
   1. The establishment of secondary male sex characteristics
   2. The rupturing of follicles for ovulation to occur
   3. The development of female reproductive organs
   4. To prepare the uterus to receive a fertilized ovum

79. High levels of estrogen in the blood
   1. Cause ovulation
   2. Inhibit output of FSH
   3. Predispose to osteoporosis
   4. Stimulate lactation

80. Ovulation occurs when
   1. The blood levels of FSH and LH are high
   2. The endometrial wall is "sloughed off"
   3. Progesterone level is high
   4. Oxytocin level is high

81. Spermatogenesis occurs in the
   1. Vas deferens
   2. Epididymis
   3. Seminiferous tubules
   4. Seminal vesicles

82. Human sperm and ova are similar because
    1. About the same number of each is produced
    2. They have the same number of chromosomes in their nuclei
    3. They have the same amount of cytoplasm in their cells
    4. They have the same type of locomotion
83. Pregnancy tests are possible because in early pregnancy the urine contains
    1. Prolactin
    2. Chorionic gonadotropin
    3. Estrogen
    4. Luteinizing hormone
84. The inner membrane that provides fluid medium for the embryo is
    1. Amnion
    2. Yolk sac
    3. Chorion
    4. Allantois
85. The outer-most membrane that helps form the placenta is
    1. Amnion

    2. Yolk sac
    3. Chorion
    4. Allantois
86. A normal woman who had a hemophilic father is mated to a man with normal blood clotting. What is the probable phenotype of the offspring?
    1. All children are hemophiliacs
    2. One-half the male children are hemophiliacs
    3. All male children are hemophiliacs
    4. All children are normal
87. A substance that acts to resist a change in pH is called
    1. A salt
    2. An acid
    3. A buffer
    4. An electrolyte
88. Mineralocorticoids
    1. Control the electrolytic balance
    2. Produce progesterone
    3. Stimulate the adrenal cortex
    4. Cause tetany and death

2

Physical science

Science is the knowledge about any subject that can be acquired and explained through use of the scientific method. The basic branches of science include life sciences and physical sciences.

The scientific method is an effective way to explore and understand a topic. The steps of the method include: recognizing or defining a problem; gathering as many facts about the problem as possible; forming a hypothesis or educated guess as to the possible solution; testing the hypothesis by experimenting and collecting data; and comparing the experimental results (data) with the original hypothesis, and keeping, discarding, or changing the original hypothesis according to the experimental facts. Many scientific discoveries have been made without using the steps of the scientific method. But even scientists making discoveries through luck or chance observations have embodied the spirit of the scientific method by maintaining an open mind when presented with the facts.

Chemistry is the study of the composition and properties of matter. The science of chemistry studies the nature of chemical changes and the laws governing them. The study of chemistry is divided into inorganic chemistry (compounds other than carbon) and organic chemistry (carbon compounds).

Physics is the study of matter and energy and their relationships to each other. Since matter and energy are fundamental to everything known to science, physics is really fundamental to both life sciences and physical sciences.

The principles of chemistry and physics underlie the study of nursing. A basic understanding of these principles will broaden and deepen a nurse's knowledge of the human body and the techniques used to treat the human body. Most importantly, the nurse approaches work from both a technical and a professional point of view since the nurse must understand why something is done as well as how it is done.

CHEMISTRY

BASIC CONCEPTS
All chemical reactions involve energy changes

 See pp. 103-106 in Physics section

Matter occupies space, has mass, and possesses inertia

A. Properties of matter
 1. Physical—color, odor, taste, melting point, density, etc.

  2. Chemical—the tendencies of a substance to undergo chemical change
B. Changes in matter
 1. Chemical change—one in which the chemical and physical properties are changed and a new substance is formed; e.g., iron plus oxygen is called rust, a new substance
 2. Physical change—one in which the physical properties are changed but

the chemical nature remains unchanged; e.g., liquid water freezing into ice or boiling into steam
C. States of matter
1. Solid—definite size and shape, particles tightly compact
   a. Crystalline—as in crystals of sodium chloride (table salt) or sucrose (cane sugar)
   b. Amorphous—such as glass or pitch
2. Liquid—mobility of particles, assumes shape of container while maintaining definite volume; e.g., water, rubbing alcohol
3. Gas—no fixed shape, particles move independently of each other; e.g., air, steam, oxygen
   a. Compressible
   b. Expandable
   c. Fills container into which it is placed
4. Plasma—hot gases composed of electrically charged ions and electrons; e.g., the ionized mercury vapor of a fluorescent bulb, the ionized neon gas in a glowing advertising sign, and the hot glowing surface of the sun
D. Classes of matter
1. Elements—substances that cannot be decomposed by chemical means into more simple substances, each element having a specific place in the periodic table of elements; e.g., hydrogen, helium, iron, uranium
2. Compounds—2 or more elements chemically combined in definite proportion by weight into a new substance having chemical properties different from those of the elements uniting to form it; e.g., water, ethyl alcohol, ether
3. Mixtures—physical combinations of 2 or more substances not chemically united; e.g., air (a mixture of oxygen, nitrogen, carbon dioxide, and other gases); blood plasma (a mixture of salts, sugars, proteins, lipids, and other substances)
E. Structure of matter
1. Atom—the smallest fundamental unit of an element and the particle of an element that takes part in chemical change
2. Atomic weight unit of mass (a.w.u.) —approximately the weight of one hydrogen atom (lightest known element)

3. Subatomic particles
   a. Electron—negligible weight, 1 negative electric charge
   b. Proton—1 atomic weight unit of mass, 1 positive electric charge
   c. Neutron—1 atomic weight unit of mass, no electric charge
4. Nucleus of the atom
   a. Bulk of weight of atom here, composed of protons and neutrons in approximately equal numbers
   b. Number of protons in the nucleus of atom is the same as the atomic number; e.g., carbon—6 protons and atomic number 6
   c. Enough neutrons in nucleus to make up the difference between the atomic number and the atomic weights; e.g., carbon, having an atomic weight of 12 a.w.u., an atomic number of 6, and 6 neutrons
   d. A powerful force in nature, the *nuclear force*, exists in the nucleus of atoms, which
      (1) Binds proton to proton, neutron to neutron, and proton to neutron
      (2) Overcomes the electric force of nature (also existing in the nucleus) that repels protons away from each other (since they have like charges)
   e. Isotope—an atom of an element, having the same number of protons and electrons as other atoms of that element but possessing a different number of neutrons and a different atomic weight; some isotopes are radioactive
5. Outer energy orbitals of the atom
   a. Electrons are here
   b. Chemical properties determined by number and arrangement of electrons in outer orbital
   c. Arrangement of electrons: maximum of 2 in first orbital, maximum of 8 in second orbital, maximum of 18 in third orbital, maximum of 32 in fourth orbital, etc.
   d. Element having 8 electrons in the outer orbital of its atom is a chemically inert element; exception is helium, which is inert and has 2 electrons in its first and only orbital
6. Number of protons always equal to number of electrons, so an atom is always electrically neutral

7. Recent discoveries show electrons in atom assume more complex spacing
   a. Electrons occupy certain fixed areas away from nucleus
   b. Energy required to move to other fixed areas farther from nucleus
      (1) Energy absorbed in packets called "quanta"
      (2) Absorbing quanta results in electrons' moving farther from nucleus
      (3) Electrons returning to original areas release energy
8. Difference between an atom of one element and an atom of another element is a result of the difference in number and arrangement of the subatomic particles in the respective atoms
9. Weight of an atom (mass number of atom) is the sum of all of the subatomic particles in that atom
10. By convention, the weight of an atom of the most plentiful carbon isotope is taken as 12 atomic weight units and all other atomic weights are based on this standard
11. Molecule—the smallest unit of a compound is formed by union of 2 or more atoms of different elements; a molecule of an element may be formed from 2 or more atoms of that element

   a. Molecular weight—sum of all of the atomic weights of the atoms making up the molecule
   b. Ion—an atom or molecule that has lost or gained an electron (or electrons) and thus has gained an electric charge (positive or negative)
12. Valence—the electric charge on an ion; also used to indicate the combining power of atoms that do not ionize
13. Radical—a group of 2 or more atoms or ions, chemically united and acting as a unit; has its own valence, which is the sum of the valences of the atoms or ions making up the radical (Table 2-1)
F. Chemical symbol—abbreviation for name of element, first letter always capitalized; e.g., Ca (calcium) stands for 1 atom of calcium
G. Formula—abbreviation of name of a compound, made up of chemical symbols for the atoms making up the molecule of the compound, with subscripts to show proportion of each element; e.g., $CaCl_2$ (calcium chloride) stands for 1 atom of calcium and 2 atoms of chlorine for each molecule of calcium chloride
H. Catalyst—substance entering into a reaction, speeding up or slowing down the

Table 2-1. Valences shown by common elements and radicals

1+	2+	3+
Ammonium, NH_4^+	Barium, Ba^{++}	Aluminum, Al^{+++}
Copper (I), Cu^+	Calcium, Ca^{++}	Chromium (III), Cr^{+++}
Mercury (I), Hg^+	Copper (II), Cu^{++}	Iron (III), Fe^{+++}
Potassium, K^+	Iron (II), Fe^{++}	
Silver, Ag^+	Lead (II), Pb^{++}	
Sodium, Na^+	Magnesium, Mg^{++}	
Hydronium, H_3O^+	Mercury (II), Hg^{++}	
	Nickel (II), Ni^{++}	
	Zinc, Zn^{++}	
1−	**2−**	**3−**
Acetate, $C_2H_3O_2^-$	Carbonate, $CO_3^=$	Phosphate, $PO_4^{\equiv}$
Bicarbonate, HCO_3^-	Chromate, $CrO_4^=$	
Bisulfate, HSO_4^-	Oxide, $O^=$	
Bromide, Br^-	Peroxide, $O_2^=$	
Chlorate, ClO_3^-	Sulfide, $S^=$	
Chloride, Cl^-	Sulfite, $SO_3^=$	
Fluoride, F^-	Sulfate, $SO_4^=$	
Hydroxide, OH^-		
Iodide, I^-		
Nitrite, NO_2^-		
Nitrate, NO_3^-		

reaction; catalyst is unchanged by the reaction; needed in small amounts

I. Enzyme—organic catalyst found in all living things

Atoms are linked together by chemical bonds

A. Electrovalent (ionic)—type of bonding characterized by exchange of electrons between atoms of different elements
1. The atoms losing electrons become positively charged ions; atoms of metals form positive ions
2. The atoms gaining electrons become negatively charged ions; atoms of non-metals form negative ions
3. Molecules of compounds are then formed by attractions between oppositely charged ions
4. Elements whose atoms can form either positive or negative ions are called amphoteric

B. Covalent—type of bonding common in atoms that do not lose or gain electrons readily; such atoms form molecules of compounds by sharing electrons, the shared electrons forming bonds between the atoms

C. Metallic bonding—similar to covalent bonding except that specific atoms do not share specific electrons
1. Electrons are free to migrate through the arrangement of atoms
2. These "roaming" electrons make up the flow of charge (electricity) when a voltage difference is applied to the ends of a metal (like a copper wire)
3. Energetic movements and collisions of these electrons also account for heat transfer through the metal; thus the conductivity of heat and electricity in metals is caused by metallic bonding

D. Van der Waals bonds—attractive forces between atoms that exist when the atoms come extremely close to each other
1. Not based on permanent charge differences between atoms (as in ionic bonds) but on induced electric charge differences that occur when atoms approach each other
2. Thought to be important in bonding together antigens and antibodies

E. Hydrogen bonds—the attractive force between a covalently bound hydrogen atom possessing a positive charge and another atom (such as nitrogen, N, or oxygen, O) possessing a negative charge
1. Help hold large protein molecules in specific shapes such as helices or sheets
2. Loosely bond liquid water molecules together
3. Account for the solubility of many organic molecules (like sugars and amino acids) in water; these molecules form hydrogen bonds with water molecules; this is as opposed to molecules like benzine or octane (gasoline) that will not mix or dissolve in water; these molecules cannot form any weak bonds (hydrogen bonds) with water molecules
4. Hold the 2 strands of the DNA double helix together
a. The weakness of the hydrogen bonds is extremely important since this weakness permits the easy unravelling of the double helix for such critical cellular functions as replication of genes and transcription of the genetic code onto messenger RNA molecules
b. One theory of aging suggests an impairment of the ability of DNA to unravel and direct normal cellular function resulting from covalent bonds (very strong bonds) cross-linking the DNA strands; thus weak hydrogen bonds are essential for normal cellular functioning

Matter can undergo chemical change

A. Rules regulating chemical change
1. Law of conservation of energy—in any chemical reaction energy is neither created nor destroyed but only changed from one form of energy to another
2. Law of conservation of matter—in a chemical reaction matter is neither created nor destroyed but only changed in form; the weight of the products equals the weight of the reactants
3. Law of definite composition—any given compound always contains same elements in same proportions by weight and united in the same manner

4. Law of multiple proportion—when 2 elements form more than 1 compound with each other, simple whole-number relationships exist in proportions of the elements whose amounts vary
5. Avogadro's hypothesis—equal volumes of gases under similar conditions of temperature and pressure contain the same number of molecules
6. Avogadro's number—at standard temperature ($0°C.$) and pressure (1 atmosphere) 22.4 liters of any gas contains 6.02×10^{23} molecules

B. Chemical equation
1. Function—symbolic expression of a chemical reaction
   a. Tells what elements or compounds react
   b. Tells what elements or compounds are formed
   c. Tells the amounts of reactants and products
2. Writing an equation
   a. On the left side are written symbols representing the reactants
   b. On the right side are written symbols representing the products
   c. For each element the number of atoms on left must equal the number of atoms on right
   d. In the formula of a compound, the positive valences must equal the negative valences
   e. An arrow shows direction of the reaction
   f. If more than 1 atom of an element is needed to balance valences in a molecule of a compound, small subscripts are used to indicate the number of atoms in the molecule; e.g., $CaCl_2$
   g. When a radical is used in a compound, the elements composing the radical are enclosed in parentheses if more than 1 particle of the radical is needed to balance valences; e.g., ammonium carbonate— $(NH_4)_2CO_3$

C. Kinds of chemical reactions
1. Combination or synthesis

$$C \quad + \quad O_2 \quad \rightarrow \quad CO_2$$

| Carbon | Oxygen | Carbon dioxide |

2. Decomposition or analysis

$$2HgO \quad \rightarrow \quad 2Hg \quad + \quad O_2$$

| Mercuric oxide | Mercury | Oxygen gas |

3. Replacement or substitution

$$Zn \quad + \quad H_2SO_4 \quad \rightarrow \quad ZnSO_4 \quad + \quad H_2$$

| Zinc | Sulfuric acid | Zinc sulfate | Hydrogen gas |

4. Double replacement

$$AgNO_3 + HCl \quad \rightarrow \quad AgCl + HNO_3$$

| Silver nitrate | Hydro-chloric acid | Silver chloride | Nitric acid |

5. Irreversible reactions—if one of the products of a chemical reaction is a gas that can escape, a substance that is insoluble, or a substance that ionizes poorly, the reaction is irreversible; all other reactions are to some extent reversible
6. When the products of a reversible reaction are being formed at the same rate as the reactants are being reformed, the reaction is said to be in equilibrium; e.g., $2NaNO_3 + K_2SO_4 \rightleftharpoons Na_2SO_4 + 2KNO_3$

THE PERIODIC TABLE
General information

A. Chemical nature of elements depends on the number and position of electrons in orbitals outside nucleus
B. Reactivity of elements depends especially on the number and position of electrons in the outermost electron orbital
C. Relationship exists between elements having same number of electrons in the outermost electron orbital
   1. Sodium has 11 electrons with 1 electron in the outermost orbital
   2. Potassium has 19 electrons with 1 electron in the outermost orbital
   3. Chemically sodium and potassium react similarly, since each has 1 electron in the outermost orbital
D. Chemical relationship is the basis of the periodic table
E. Elements in vertical columns of table are similar to one another and are called families of elements
F. Knowing the chemical nature of one member of a family, you can predict the chemical nature of the rest of the family

G. The outer orbital of electrons in an atom is responsible for the following characteristics of substances; taste, texture, appearance, color, freezing and boiling temperatures, and electrical and magnetic properties

Important elements in periodic table

A. Oxygen
1. Physical properties
   a. Colorless, odorless, and tasteless gas
   b. Heavier than air
   c. Slightly soluble in water
   d. Liquifies and solidifies only at very low temperatures and high pressures
2. Chemical properties
   a. Member of Group VI in periodic table
   b. Has 8 electrons, 6 in the outermost orbital
   c. Tends, in chemical reaction, to gain 2 electrons to complete outer orbital
      (1) Becomes a negatively charged particle
      (2) Reacts as a nonmetal
   d. Can also form covalent bonds
   e. Will not burn
   f. Supports combustion
   g. Unites with many elements to form oxides
      (1) Oxides of metals are basic anhydrides; if put into water, they form bases
      (2) Oxides of nonmetals are acid anhydrides; if put into water they form acids
      (3) Many elements form more than 1 oxide; e.g., H_2O—water, and H_2O_2—hydrogen peroxide
      (4) The uniting of a substance with oxygen is called "oxidation"
3. Importance of oxygen
   a. Forms about 21% of air
   b. Forms about 50% of earth's crust
   c. Is present in water—89% by weight, 33% by volume
   d. Is present in foods, plant tissue, and animal tissue
   e. Oxidation of organic compounds results in production of carbon dioxide, water, and energy
      (1) Oxidation of foods takes place in the cytoplasm and mitochondria of cells and supplies the energy for life
      (2) Oxidation of wood, coal, and other fuels supplies the energy for heat, functioning of machinery, movement of cars and buses, etc.
      (3) Some oxidation is harmful
         (a) The rusting of iron can be prevented by coating the iron with material that reacts poorly with oxygen
         (b) Certain drugs are useless when oxidized; prevention lies in keeping bottles tightly closed to shut out air
4. Medical uses of oxygen
   a. Oxygen therapy used in many instances
      (1) Lung congestion
      (2) Cardiac failure
      (3) Carbon monoxide poisoning
      (4) In combination with anesthetics
      (5) Newborn infants' breathing problems
      (6) During and following operations, as a supportive measure
      (7) To test for rate of cellular oxidation in basal metabolism test
5. Other uses of oxygen
   a. High-altitude aircraft
   b. Space capsules
   c. Oxyacetylene torches for welding
   d. Bleaching
   e. Antiseptic action
6. Preparation of oxygen
   a. Natural—green plants form oxygen as a product of photosynthesis
   b. Commercial
      (1) Fractional distillation of liquid air
      (2) Electrolysis of water
   c. Laboratory—heating an oxide to decompose it; e.g., potassium chlorate ($KClO_3$) with manganese dioxide as a catalyst decomposes to potassium chloride (KCl) and oxygen
7. Forms of oxygen
   a. Free

(1) Usually oxygen is found as a diatomic molecule (O_2), as is common to most gases

(2) Occasionally a triatomic molecule of oxygen (O_3) occurs; this is called ozone and represents an especially active form of oxygen

b. Combined—oxygen forms many compounds called oxides

B. Hydrogen
   1. Physical properties
      a. Odorless, tasteless, colorless gas
      b. Slightly soluble in water
      c. Lightest element
   2. Chemical properties
      a. Is a member of Group IA or VIIA elements
      b. Has only 1 electron in its outer orbital—its only electron
      c. Usually loses this lone electron to become a positively charged ion (a metal) in chemical reaction
      d. Occasionally can gain an electron and become a negatively charged ion (a nonmetal) in chemical reaction
      e. By sharing its electron, can form covalent bond
      f. Burns with explosive force
      g. Does not support combustion
   3. Importance of hydrogen
      a. Forms about 11% of water by weight, 66% by volume
      b. Is present in acids and in bases
      c. Is present in organic substances such as fuels and oils and other hydrocarbons
      d. Is present in foods and in cells of plants and animal tissues
      e. Uniting with nitrogen, hydrogen forms ammonia and amino acids (proteins)
      f. Acting as a reducing agent (opposite of oxidation), hydrogen removes oxygen from many oxides; e.g.,

$$FeO \ + \ H_2 \ \rightarrow \ Fe \ + \ H_2O$$
Iron **Hydro-** **Iron** **Water**
oxide **gen**

      g. Added to liquid fat, hydrogen forms solid fat by process of hydrogenation
   4. Preparation of hydrogen
      a. Naturally—in volcanic eruptions
      b. Commercially—electrolysis of water
      c. Laboratory
         (1) Reaction of active metal with water

$$2Na \ + \ 2H_2O \ \rightarrow \ H_2 \ + \ 2NaOH$$
Sodium **Water** **Hydro-** **Sodium**
gen **hydroxide**

         (2) Reaction of acids with metals

$$2HCl \ + \ Zn \ \rightarrow \ H_2 \ + \ ZnCl_2$$
Hydro- **Zinc** **Hydro-** **Zinc**
chloric **gen** **chloride**
acid

C. Group IA—the alkali metals
   1. Sodium
      a. Important metal ion in plasma and intercellular fluids
         (1) Sodium ions help to regulate the size of body cells; the flow of water into cells caused by osmotically active proteins of the intracellular fluid is balanced by the outward flow of water from the cells into the interstitial fluid caused by the osmotic "pull" of sodium ions present in high concentration in the interstitial fluid
         (2) Sodium ions of the extracellular fluid are responsible for action potentials of nervous and muscular tissues; after some stimulus, it is the diffusion of Na^+ from the interstitial fluid into the intracellular fluid of neurons and muscle fibers that brings about depolarization; thus sodium ions are basic to the functioning of the body's communication system, the nervous system, and all muscular movements
      b. Basic forming element; forms antacid compounds
      c. With chlorine forms NaCl (table salt)
   2. Potassium
      a. Important metal in body; found in intracellular fluid
      b. The resting polarization of neurons, all types of muscle fibers (smooth, cardiac, and striated), and most

cells of the body is caused by the continual diffusion of K^+ from the intracellular fluid to the interstitial fluid; similarly, repolarization of neurons and muscle fibers is caused by the outward diffusion of K^+ to the interstitial fluid from the intracellular fluid

c. A number of important cellular enzymes functioning in glucose and amino acid metabolism require K^+ as a cofactor

d. In nursing, recognition of signs of hypokalemia (below normal levels of K^+ in the extracellular fluid) and hyperkalemia (above normal levels of K^+ in the extracellular fluid) are vitally important; e.g., hypokalemia may occur in any one of a number of common medical situations such as prolonged diarrhea, intestinal drainage, polyuria, starvation or dietary deficiencies, and prolonged corticosteroid therapy

D. Group IIA—the alkali earth metals
1. Magnesium
    a. Forms part of the chlorophyll molecule
    b. Activator for many enzymes
    c. Present in bones
2. Calcium
    a. Gives hardness to bones and teeth by forming phosphate, carbonate, and fluoride salts
    b. A cofactor in the formation of prothrombin activator and thrombin
    c. Important in muscle contraction; ATP must combine with Ca^{++} before its energy can be used to slide actin and myosin filaments together
    d. Extracellular Ca^{++} concentration must be precisely regulated (through the parathyroid glands) for normal body functioning; hypocalcemia can result in tetany; hypercalcemia can result in depression of the nervous system
    e. Needed for lactation
3. Strontium
    a. May substitute for calcium in body
    b. Radioactive isotope (strontium 90) can be a health hazard, forming pockets of radiation in tissues

4. Barium—used for outlining intestinal tract for x-ray studies
5. Radium—radiotherapy

E. Group IIIA
1. Boron—antiseptic, dentifrice, washing powders
2. Aluminum—alum, antacids, metal containers

F. Group IVA
1. Carbon—fuel (coal, coke), hydrocarbons, carbohydrates
2. Silicon—sandstone, sand, glass
3. Tin—tinfoil, dishes
4. Lead—piping, paint (some lead compounds poisonous)

G. Group V
1. Nitrogen—forms 80% of air; found in amino acids and proteins
2. Phosphorus
    a. The phosphate ions, $H_2PO_4^-$ and $HPO_4^=$, are part of the phosphate buffer system that helps to maintain the correct pH of the body fluids (between 7.35 and 7.45)
    b. Functions in cellular energy metabolism; the phosphorylation of ADP with phosphate ion during cellular respiration results in the formation of the high-energy molecule, ATP; ATP then functions in such diverse cellular, energy-requiring activities as active transport, muscle contraction, ciliary beating, and the synthesis of proteins, carbohydrates, lipids, and nucleic acids
    c. Phosphate ions in combination with Ca^{++} help give hardness to bones and teeth
    d. Phosphates are part of the structure of the genetic information molecules, DNA and RNA
3. Arsenic—poison
    a. Used in medication
    b. Used to kill pests and vermin

H. Group VI
1. Oxygen—essential to life; the body's need for oxygen results from the need for a final oxidizing agent (electron acceptor) in the mitochondrion during the release of energy from foods (cellular respiration)
2. Sulfur—vulcanizing rubber; local medication in skin diseases

I. Group VIIA—the halogens

1. Fluorine—to etch glass, to prevent tooth decay when added to water supply
2. Chlorine—bleach, poison gas, disinfectant, water purifier
3. Bromine—nerve medicine, photography
4. Iodine—local antiseptic, part of the thyroid hormone (thyroxine)

J. Group IB
   1. Copper—wire, electric fixtures
   2. Silver—filling for teeth, surgical mending of bone, photography
   3. Gold—filling for teeth

K. Inert gases
   1. Helium
      a. Lighter-than-air craft (will not burn)
      b. Used with oxygen in therapy for breathing difficulties
   2. Neon—electric signs

OXIDATION AND REDUCTION

Definitions

A. Uniting of oxygen with a substance results in oxidation
B. Uniting of hydrogen with a substance results in reduction

Basis of oxidation and reduction— transfer of electrons

A. Removal of an electron from an atom of an element results in oxidation of that atom; e.g.,

$$Na \quad - \quad e^- \quad \rightarrow \quad Na^+$$

Sodium   Electron   Sodium
atom   ion

B. Addition of an electron to an atom of an element results in reduction of that element, e.g.,

$$Cl_2 \quad + \quad 2e^- \quad \rightarrow \quad 2Cl^-$$

Chlorine   Electrons   Chlorine
                                 ions

C. Substance that causes removal of an electron from an atom is called an oxidizing agent
D. Substance that adds an electron to an atom is called a reducing agent
E. Substances other than oxygen can act as oxidizing agents; e.g., chlorine—more effective than oxygen in removing electrons in many reactions
F. Substances other than hydrogen can act

as reducing agents; e.g., carbon and carbon monoxide

G. In an oxidation-reduction reaction, the oxidizing agent is itself reduced and the reducing agent is itself oxidized; e.g.,

$$O_2 \quad + \quad 2H_2 \quad \rightarrow \quad 2H_2O$$

Oxidizing   Reducing   Water
agent   agent

The hydrogen becomes oxidized and the oxygen becomes reduced

Oxidation-reduction reactions in the body

A. Important in body chemistry as a source of energy through cellular oxidation of foods in mitochondria
B. Oxygen is the usual oxidizing agent in cells
C. Some forms of life (anaerobes) can use substances other than oxygen for cellular oxidation

IONIZATION
Ion

A. When an atom loses or gains an electron (electrons), it is no longer a neutral atom but a charged particle—an ion
B. The charge on this particle depends upon whether electrons are lost (+) or gained (−) and the number of electrons lost or gained
C. An electron is a negative particle; the loss of 1 electron makes ion positive (less negative) by 1; with loss of 2 electrons, ion is 2+, etc.
D. The gain of 1 electron makes ion negative by 1; with 2 electrons gained, the ion is 2−, etc.

Overall reaction

In any chemical reaction the number of electrons lost by 1 atom is equal to gain by another atom; overall reaction neutral

Ionization and water

A. When certain compounds are placed in water, the polar water molecules dissociate the molecules of the compound into ions—a process called ionization
B. A substance that will ionize when placed in water is called an electrolyte
C. A substance that will ionize in water (an electrolyte) will allow the passage of an electric current through its solution

D. Certain other compounds will dissolve in water but will not form ions
  1. These substances are called nonelectrolytes
  2. Their solutions will not allow the passage of an electric current

Acids, bases, and salts as electrolytes

A. They will ionize in water
B. Their water solutions will conduct an electric current

Electrolytes in water solutions

A. Characterized by very rapid reactions
B. Ions are free in solution to react

Factors affecting strength or weakness of electrolytes

A. Amount of electrolyte present in solution
B. How well the electrolyte dissociates in solution—degree of ionization
  1. So-called "weak" electrolytes are substances that dissociate into ions to only a slight degree
  2. So-called "strong" electrolytes are substances that dissociate into ions to a larger degree

Electrolytes in the human body

A. The most important electrolytes in the human body include sodium (Na^+), potassium (K^+), magnesium (Mg^{++}), calcium (Ca^{++}), chloride (Cl^-), bicarbonate (HCO_3^-), and phosphates ($H_2PO_4^-$ and $HPO_4^=$)
B. See pp. 166-169 in Chapter 4 for important functions of specific electrolytes in the human body

WATER

General information

A. A chemical combination of oxygen and hydrogen
B. Most abundant compound
C. Essential to life
D. Useful in many phases of living

Physical properties

A. Colorless, tasteless, odorless liquid
B. Exists chiefly as ice at low temperatures, liquid at moderate temperatures, and gas at elevated temperatures
  1. Water changes from liquid to solid at the freezing point (0°C. or 32°F.)
  2. Water changes from liquid to gas at the boiling point (100°C. or 212°F.)

3. These transition points in the physical states of water are the basis of the Celsius and Fahrenheit temperature scales
4. Conversion from one temperature scale to the other is accomplished by using the formula

$$C.° = \frac{5}{9} (F.° - 32)$$

Chemical properties

A. Water molecule is a polar molecule
  1. The water molecule has a special shape with a concentration of electrons in one area
  2. This gives the water molecule positive and negative poles; e.g.,

$$+H—O -$$
$$|$$
$$H$$
$$+$$

  3. Because of this molecular shape, water is an excellent solvent for ionic or slightly ionic substances
B. Water is a very stable compound; dissociates very slightly to H^+ and OH^- ions under normal conditions
C. Electrolysis can dissociate water into its components, hydrogen and oxygen
  1. Electrolysis gives 2 volumes of hydrogen for each volume of oxygen
  2. Electrolysis gives hydrogen and oxygen released from water in the ratio of 1 to 8 by weight
D. Many chemical reactions need water as a solvent before reaction will occur
E. Process of splitting a substance with the addition of water is called hydrolysis
F. Crystals formed with water in their molecule are called hydrates
  1. Water held in hydrates is called the water of crystallization
  2. When a hydrate loses the water of crystallization, it is called an anhydride

Occurrence

A. Five sevenths of the earth is covered with water
B. Present in atmosphere, in crust of earth, in all plant and animal life
C. Sixty percent of the average adult human body weight is water; this percentage may be as high as 80% in infants and as low as 40% to 50% in the aged

D. All food and most materials used in everyday living contain some water

Importance

A. Necessary for life
B. Essential for many chemical reactions
C. Needed for digestion (hydrolysis) of food
D. Forms large percentage of plant and animal tissue
E. Necessary for circulation of blood; plasma is a water solution
F. Necessary for elimination; urine, sweat, feces contain water
G. Lubricating fluid at joints (synovial fluid) contains water

Evaporation

A. Change of liquid water to water vapor
B. Occurs at all temperatures but is rapid and complete at boiling point

Solidification

A. Change of liquid water to solid ice at freezing point
B. Causes expansion; ice occupies larger volume than water that forms it
C. Freezing water can break pipes and vessels in which it is contained
D. Because of expansion, ice is lighter than water and floats on top of unfrozen water

Humidity

Amount of water vapor in the air

Heat absorption

A. Water has a great capacity for absorbing heat or giving off absorbed heat
B. Makes water (and ice) useful in ice packs, hydrotherapy, and hot compresses

Water as a standard

A. Thermometer scales—the freezing and boiling points of water are used to standardize Celsius and Fahrenheit scales
B. Specific gravity—compares the density of a volume of water to the density of the same volume of another substance
C. Weight—1 g. is the weight of 1 ml. of water at 4°C.
D. Calorie—the heat needed to raise 1 g. of water 1°C.
E. pH—water acts as neutrality point on acid-base scale

Purifying water

A. Source of pure water necessary for health
B. Methods of purifying
   1. Filtration
   2. Chemical precipitation (aluminum sulfate)
   3. Chemical disinfection (chlorination)
   4. Boiling
   5. Distillation
   6. Ion exchange; resin filtration

Hard versus soft water

A. Dissolved calcium or magnesium bicarbonates form "temporary" hard water; boiling or use of chemicals (washing soda) precipitates salts, leaving water "soft"
B. Dissolved calcium or magnesium sulfates form "permanently" hard water; chemical agents needed to precipitate the salts
C. If unprecipitated, the dissolved salts react with soaps (but usually not with the newer detergents) and little lather can be obtained

Body regulation of water content

A. The osmoreceptors of the hypothalamus influence the neurohypophysis in its release of ADH (antidiuretic hormone or vasopressin); working through the kidney tubules, this hormone regulates water reabsorption from urine
B. The thirst center of the hypothalamus detects body dehydration and gives us the sensation of thirst

SOLUTIONS
Substances that dissolve in other substances form solutions

A. A solution can be classified as a homogeneous mixture
B. Solids, liquids, and gases can be dissolved in other solids, liquids, and gases
   1. Substance dissolved is called the solute
   2. Substance in which the solute is dissolved is called the solvent
   3. Common solution is one where a solid, liquid, or gas is dissolved in a liquid

Solubility is affected by various factors

A. Chemical and physical nature of the solvent

B. Chemical and physical nature of the solute
C. Amount of solvent versus amount of solute
D. Temperature—warming aids some solutes (solids) to dissolve; cooling aids others (gases) to dissolve
E. Presence or absence of mixing; mixing usually speeds solution reaction
F. Pressure—especially when one of the components is a gas

Types of solutions

A. Dilute—a small amount of solute in a relatively large amount of solvent
B. Concentrated—a large amount of solute in a relatively small amount of solvent
C. Unsaturated—a solution holding less solute than is possible for it to dissolve at a certain temperature and pressure
D. Saturated—a solution holding all the solute that it can dissolve at a certain temperature and pressure
E. Supersaturated solution—unique case of a solution holding more solute than it normally should for a particular temperature and pressure
 1. Very unstable condition
 2. Excess solute easily precipitates from solution
F. Percent solution—grams of solute per gram of solution
G. Molar solution (M)—the number of gram-molecular weights of solute per liter of solution
H. Normal solution (N)—the number of gram-equivalent weights of solute per liter of solution
I. Method of obtaining normal solutions
 1. Compute gram-molecular weight (sum of atomic weights of atoms in molecule) of substance
 2. Divide the computed gram-molecular weight by the atomic weight of hydrogen in the molecule
 3. The result of this division produces the gram-equivalent weight
 4. The gram-equivalent weight in a liter of solution is a "normal" solution
J. Molal solution—a gram-molecular weight of solute in 1000 g. of solvent

Nonvolatile substances put into solution

These tend to raise the boiling point and lower the freezing point of the solvent in which they are dissolved; e.g., water and ethylene glycol (commercial antifreeze) freezes at a lower temperature and boils at a higher temperature than pure water

Osmosis

A. Process of selective diffusion
B. More concentrated solution is separated from a less concentrated solution by a membrane that is permeable only to the solvent—a semipermeable membrane
C. Solvent moves more rapidly from the dilute solution into the concentrated solution than in the reverse direction
D. Pressure forcing the solvent across the membrane is called osmotic pressure
E. Isotonic solutions—when the osmotic pressures of 2 liquids are equal, the flow of solvent is equalized and the 2 solutions are said to be isotonic to each other
 1. Physiologic saline—0.89% NaCl in distilled water—is isotonic to blood and body tissues
 2. Five percent dextrose in water is isotonic to blood and body tissues
 3. When isotonic solutions are administered intravenously, the blood cells remain intact
F. Hypertonic solutions—when one solution has less osmotic pressure (is more concentrated) than another, it draws fluid from the other and is said to be hypertonic to it
G. Hypotonic solutions—when one solution has more osmotic pressure (is more dilute) than another, it forces fluid into the other and is said to be hypotonic to it
H. Both hypertonic and hypotonic types of solution are destructive to body cells and should not be used in intravenous injections
I. Osmosis constantly occurs as part of the normal physiology of human beings
 1. Capillary membrane—the colloid osmotic pressure of the plasma draws fluid from the tissue spaces back into the capillaries; edema results when disease states upset the normal colloid osmotic pressure (starvation, kidney disease)
 2. Plasma membranes—water freely flows from interstitial fluid into intracellular fluid and vice versa depending on the relative concentration of water in these 2 fluid compartments
 3. Kidney tubules—the reabsorption of

water from glomerular filtrate involves the osmosis of water from the lumen of the collecting tubules into the surrounding tubule cells

4. Mucous membrane of the gastrointestinal tract—absorption of ingested water involves osmosis across the membranes of the tract

Size of the particle of solute determines type of solution

A. Atomic, ionic, and most molecular-sized particles are extremely small particles—submicroscopic
   1. Particles are freely dispersed by solvent
   2. Particles are kept in solution by movement and attraction of solvent molecules
   3. Substances of this class are called *crystalloids*
   4. Crystalloids form true solutions
      a. Clear in appearance—particles cannot be seen
      b. Solute stays in solution as long as the solvent is not removed by evaporation or other means
      c. Solute accompanies solvent as it passes through filters and most membranes
B. Large particles of matter do not form solutions in the real sense of the term
   1. Solute particles easily settle out of solvent
   2. Solute particles can be seen by naked eye or with microscope when suspended in solvent
   3. Solute can be removed by ordinary filtration
   4. Substances of this class are called coarse suspensions
C. The colloid particle
   1. Intermediate in size between the crystalloid and the coarse suspensoid
   2. Particle size much larger than that of crystalloid although smaller than particle of coarse suspensoid; diameter size of colloid around 0.0000001 to 0.00001 mm.
   3. Solutions of colloids
      a. Solute particles dispersed by solvent
      b. Solution—clear, cloudy, or opalescent
      c. Show bright path of reflected light when a beam of light is passed through solution—the Tyndall effect
      d. More stable than coarse suspensoids, less stable than true solutions
      e. With time, the colloid particles will settle out
      f. Affect osmotic pressure less than crystalloids
   4. Colloid particles will pass through ordinary filters but will be held back by most membranes
   5. Colloid particles carry electric charges on their surfaces—not to be confused with ionic charges
      a. Charges sometimes help keep particles in solution
      b. Colloid particles having charges that attract the solvent are called lyophilic (solvent-loving) colloids
      c. Colloid particles having charges that repel the solvent are called lyophobic (solvent-hating) colloids
      d. Lyophilic colloids form more stable solutions than do lyophobic colloids
      e. Lyophobic colloids easily separate out of solution
      f. Lyophobic colloids can be made to stay in solution by coating their particles with a layer of lyophilic colloid
      g. The stabilizing lyophilic colloid is called an emulsifying agent; the stabilized lyophobic colloid is said to have been emulsified; for example:
         (1) Oil and water make a lyophobic colloid solution (separate easily)
         (2) Oil, water, and soap make an emulsified solution, with the soap (lyophilic colloid) coating the oil (lyophobic colloid) and holding it in solution
   6. Importance of colloid suspensions
      a. Proteins, fats, and many carbohydrates form molecules in the colloid range in size
      b. These form colloid solutions in the cells and body fluids
      c. Protoplasm of cell itself is a colloid
      d. Colloid chemistry is the chemistry of life
   7. Sol-gel equilibrium

a. Most colloids can exist in 2 forms, a sol and a gel
b. Sol—a solution where the solid particles are suspended in a liquid
c. Gel—a solution where the liquid particles are suspended in the solid medium
d. Most of the physical and chemical characteristics of protoplasm can be explained by the equilibrium that exists between the sol and gel states

BASES, ACIDS, AND SALTS
Bases

A. Definition—a base is a substance that usually adds an OH^- (hydroxyl) ion to any solution in which it is placed; e.g.,

$$NaOH \xrightarrow{\text{in water}} Na^+ + OH^-$$

B. Properties of a base
1. Bitter taste
2. Slippery feeling to touch
3. Electrolyte in water
4. Reacts with indicators, giving a base color
   a. Methyl orange—yellow
   b. Litmus—blue
   c. Phenolphthalein—red
5. Reacts with acids to form water and a salt (neutralization)
6. Reacts with certain metals to release hydrogen gas
7. Combines with organic acids (fatty acids) to form soaps
8. In high concentration destroys organic material; corrosive

C. Names and formulas of common bases
1. Calcium hydroxide ($Ca[OH]_2$)—water solution, called lime water
2. Sodium hydroxide ($NaOH$)—caustic soda
3. Potassium hydroxide (KOH)—soap making
4. Ammonium hydroxide (NH_4OH)—household cleaner
5. Magnesium hydroxide ($Mg[OH]_2$)—water solution marketed under trade name Milk of Magnesia—antacid, mild laxative
6. Aluminum hydroxide ($Al[OH]_3$)—component of antacid pills

Acids

A. Definition—an acid is ordinarily thought of as a substance that liberates an H^+ (hydrogen ion) to a solution in which it is placed; e.g.,

$$H_2CO_3 \xrightarrow{\text{in water}} H^+ + HCO_3^-$$

B. Properties of an acid
1. Sour taste
2. Reacts with indicators, giving an acid color
   a. Methyl orange—red
   b. Litmus—red
   c. Phenolphthalein—colorless
3. Combines with certain metals, releasing hydrogen gas
4. Reacts with bases to form water and a salt (neutralization)
5. Reacts with carbonates to give carbon dioxide gas
6. Acts as an electrolyte in water
7. In high concentration destroys organic materials—corrosive

C. Names and formulas of common acids
1. Hydrochloric acid (HCl)—secreted by the parietal cells of the stomach; transforms pepsinogen into pepsin, which is a protein-digesting enzyme of gastric juice
2. Nitric acid (NHO_3)—used in test for proteins
3. Sulfuric acid (H_2SO_4)—in storage batteries
4. Carbonic acid (H_2CO_3)
   a. One form in which CO_2 is transported in the blood
   b. Part of the bicarbonate buffer system, which is the most important buffer system regulating the pH of body fluids
5. Boric acid (H_3BO_3)—mild antiseptic
6. Acetic acid ($C_2H_3O_2H$)—vinegar
7. Lactic acid ($CH_3CHOHCOOH$)—builds up in muscle tissue during exercise; most lactic acid is then transported to the liver via the circulatory system where it is completely oxidized into CO_2, water, and energy (as ATP)

General considerations concerning acids and bases

A. Weak acids produce few hydrogen ions in solution while strong acids produce many
B. Weak bases produce 10 hydroxyl ions in solution while strong bases produce many

C. Strong acids and bases can cause serious damage to human tissue
D. Acids and bases can be used to neutralize each other—therefore, in the event of acid or base burn, flood with water and add the opposite chemical in weak, diluted form

Salts

A. Definition—the compound (besides water) formed when an acid is neutralized by a base is a salt; e.g.,

HCl + KOH → H_2O + KCl
Acid   **Base**   **Water**   **Salt**

B. Properties of a salt
 1. Crystalline in nature
 2. Ionic even in the dry crystal
 3. Electrolyte in solution
 4. "Salty" taste
C. Names and formulas of common salts
 1. Sodium chloride (NaCl)—salt of intercellular and extracellular spaces
 2. Calcium phosphate ($CaPO_4$)—bone and tooth formation
 3. Potassium chloride (KCl)—salt of intracellular spaces
 4. Calcium carbonate ($CaCO_3$)—limestone
 5. Barium sulfate ($BaSO_4$)—when taken internally, outlines internal structures for x-ray studies
 6. Silver nitrate ($AgNO_3$)—antiseptic, photographic work
 7. Iron (II) sulfate ($FeSO_4$)—treatment of anemia
 8. Sodium bicarbonate ($NaHCO_3$)—antacid
 9. Calcium sulfate ($CaSO_4$)—hydrated form is plaster of Paris (casts for broken bones)
 10. Magnesium sulfate ($MgSO_4$)—Epsom salt

Hydrogen ion concentration—pH

A. The *p* in pH comes from the French word *puissance* meaning power
B. The *H* in pH stands for *hydrogen*
C. Thus pH denotes the power or strength of hydrogen (ions) in a solution
D. A neutral solution has the same amount of acid reacting ions, H$^+$ (actually H_3O^+), as basic reacting ions, OH$^-$
E. An acid reacting solution has more H$^+$ than OH$^-$

F. A basic reacting solution has more OH$^-$ than H$^+$
G. pH is used to represent these conditions
 1. The pH of a solution is defined as the logarithm of 1 divided by the concentration of H$^+$—$\log \dfrac{1}{(H^+)}$
 2. A neutral solution has a pH of 7.00
 3. An acid solution would have a pH in the range from 0 to 6.99; the lower the pH, the more acid the solution
 4. A basic solution would have a pH in the range from 7.01 to 14.00; the higher the pH, the more basic the solution
 5. The pH of the extracellular fluid (vascular and interstitial fluid) is in the narrow range of 7.35 to 7.45; fluctuations in pH of 0.4 unit above or below this range can result in body distress; a prolonged blood pH of 7 or less or 7.8 or more can result in death
 6. Certain body fluids have a pH different than 7.4; gastric juice has a pH of 1 or 2 caused by the presence of hydrochloric acid; bile is basic; urine may be acidic or basic

Buffers

A. A poorly ionized acid or base, plus a salt formed from that acid or base, acts as a buffer in solution
B. A buffer allows the addition of acid ions (H_3O^+) and basic ions (OH$^-$) without a change occurring in the pH of the solution to which the addition is made
C. A typical buffer of the blood is carbonic acid (H_2CO_3) plus its salt, sodium bicarbonate ($NaHCO_3$)
D. Many medications are buffered before administration; e.g., protamine zinc insulin
E. The body regulates its pH through buffer systems
 1. During normal metabolism, the body builds up CO_2, which forms carbonic acid with water; the subsequent ionization of carbonic acid would tend to lower the body fluid pH; but through increased rate and depth of breathing, the excess CO_2 is expelled from the body; thus the respiratory system interacting with buffer systems helps to regulate the body's pH
 2. During disease conditions such as pneumonia or emphysema, when the

respiratory system cannot adequately expel CO_2 from the body, the kidneys secrete an acid urine and conserve bicarbonate ions; the effect of this is to raise the body's pH back to normal; thus under disease conditions, as well as normal conditions, the kidneys interact with buffer systems to regulate the pH of the body fluids

RADIOACTIVITY
Radioactive elements

A. Certain elements (such as radium) have atoms whose nuclei are naturally unstable and are constantly breaking down at a set rate
B. In the breakdown process these elements emit high-energy particles and rays that can penetrate other materials—radioactive rays
  1. Alpha particle—fast-moving helium nucleus
    a. Weight—4 atomic weight unit (a.w.u.)
    b. Charge—2$^+$
    c. Penetration—slight
  2. Beta particle—fast-moving electrons
    a. Weight—practically 0 a.w.u.
    b. Charge—1$^-$
    c. Penetration—moderate
  3. Gamma ray—penetrating ray, similar to light ray
    a. Weight—none
    b. Charge—none
    c. Penetration—high
C. Use of radioactive elements—radium treatment of cancer, radioactive bomb for defense
D. Measurement of radioactivity
  1. The roentgen—1.6×10^{12} ion pairs/g. of air (radioactive rays ionize gases)
  2. The curie—37,000,000,000 nuclear disintegrations/second
  3. The millicurie—0.001 curie
  4. The microcurie—0.000001 curie
E. Certain radioactive materials take a long time to disintegrate; others take less than a second
  1. The time during which one half of a certain radioactive material disintegrates is called its *half-life*
  2. Short half-life elements are used on humans in medicine to cut down on the amount of exposure to radiation
  3. Determining the half-life of a radio-

active element is used in dating fossils and telling the age of antiques

Radioactive isotopes

A. In a certain element, one isotope may be nonradioactive and others be radioactive; e.g., the cobalt isotope ^{59}Co, atomic weight 59 a.w.u., is nonradioactive but the cobalt isotope ^{60}Co, atomic weight 60 a.w.u., is radioactive
B. Stable nuclei of nonradioactive elements can be made radioactive through bombardment by subatomic particles

Uses of radioactivity in medicine

A. Radium treatments for malignancy
B. ^{60}Co—total body radiation for malignancy; also, wires made of ^{60}Co can be placed directly in malignant tissue
C. Studies on body fluids, using radioactive isotope of sodium (^{24}Na)
D. Leukemia, polycythemia, and bone cancer treatments with radioactive phosphorus (^{32}P); radiophosphorus has also been useful in localizing breast tumors because of the uptake of the ^{32}P into the rapidly growing, cancerous tissue
E. Tracing metabolic pathways of food and drugs by means of radioactive carbon (^{14}C)
F. Studies on red cells (erythrocytes) and hemoglobin formation with radioactive iron (^{59}Fe) and radioactive chromium (^{51}Cr)
G. Radioiodine (^{131}I) is helpful in studying the functioning of the thyroid gland since iodine is selectively taken up by the gland; radioiodine is also useful in detecting and localizing brain tumors since serum albumin tagged with ^{131}I is absorbed by a growing tumor
H. Radiogold (^{198}Au) has been used in the treatment of carcinomas that have metastasized to the pleural and peritoneal cavities
I. Radioactive tantalum (^{82}Ta), a gamma emitter, has been shaped into a wire and used in the treatment of retinoblastoma

Protection from radiation

A. Radiation danger decreases as distance from radioactive material increases
B. Heavy materials can shield from radioactive rays; e.g., lead, concrete
C. Radiation hazard increases with increase in time of exposure

ORGANIC CHEMISTRY—THE STUDY OF CARBON COMPOUNDS
General information

A. Compounds thought at one time to be formed only by living organisms—thus "organic"
B. Carbon combines covalently with many other elements and with itself to form a vast array of compounds
C. Carbon compounds exist as isomers—compounds containing the same number and kinds of atoms but differing in structure and in physical and chemical properties
D. Organic compounds form families of compounds called "homologous" series

Hydrocarbons

A. Compounds containing only carbon and hydrogen
B. Saturated hydrocarbons
  1. If all of the carbon bonds are attached to other carbon or hydrogen atoms, compound is called saturated
  2. Saturated hydrocarbons are relatively unreactive and chemically stable
C. Unsaturated hydrocarbons
  1. When a hydrocarbon does not have all of its carbon bonds attached to other carbon or hydrogen atoms, the compound is called unsaturated
  2. Bonds that are unattached tend to combine with each other and form double or triple bonds
  3. Unsaturated hydrocarbons are less stable and more chemically reactive than the saturated hydrocarbons; double and triple bonds tend to break and add in other atoms, becoming saturated
  4. Hydrocarbons can be treated with halogens to replace one or more of the hydrogen atoms (a process called substitution); these substitution reactions produce such medically important compounds as
    a. Methyl chloride (CH_3Cl)—local anesthetic
    b. Chloroform ($CHCl_3$)—general anesthetic
    c. Carbon tetrachloride (CCl_4)—fat solvent
    d. Ethyl chloride (C_2H_5Cl)—local anesthetic
    e. Iodoform (CHI_3)—antiseptic

Alcohols

A. All alcohols contain an OH (hydroxyl) group
B. Reactions of alcohols
  1. Neutral in solution—neither acid nor base
  2. Intense oxidation causes alcohol to burn, as in alcohol lamps
C. Important alcohols
  1. Methyl alcohol—wood alcohol (CH_3OH)—used as a solvent; poisonous if taken internally
  2. Ethyl alcohol—grain alcohol (CH_3CH_2OH)—used as a solvent for medications, as an antiseptic and rubbing compound; not poisonous; used as a beverage in social situations; large quantities taken internally cause the depression and confusion classified as drunkenness
  3. Propyl alcohol (C_3H_7OH)—used as a rubbing compound, industrial solvent, antiseptic
  4. Benzyl alcohol—local anesthetic; basis for the synthesis of ephedrine and the hormone epinephrine
  5. Glycerol—trihydric alcohol used in skin creams and as a solvent; nitrated form used in explosives; basis for synthesis of fats

Phenols

A. All phenols contain an OH (hydroxyl) group like alcohol, but in phenols this group is attached directly to a benzene ring
B. A phenol reacts as an acid producing hydrogen ions in solution
C. Phenol will react with bases to form an organic salt
D. Phenols will undergo oxidation, reduction, and substitution
E. Phenols can react with other compounds to form esters and ethers
F. Important phenols
  1. Phenol (carbolic acid)—used as disinfectant, antiseptic, poison
  2. Cresol (Lysol)—disinfectant
  3. Resorcinol—antiseptic

Aldehydes

A. All aldehydes contain a $\overset{\displaystyle O}{\overset{\|}{C}}$—H group
B. Reactions of aldehydes

1. Mild oxidation of aldehyde forms organic acid
2. Alkaline copper reagents cause this oxidation to occur—the basis of Benedict's (Fehling's, Clinitest) tests for aldehyde sugars
3. Condensation (polymerization)—aldehydes will join with themselves and other aldehydes to form large aggregates
4. Reduction forms a primary alcohol

C. Important aldehydes
   1. Formaldehyde—acrid-smelling gas; water solution of formaldehyde is called formalin; useful as an insecticide, fumigating agent, antiseptic, disinfectant, and fixative for tissues for histologic examination
   2. Acetaldehyde—liquid with a sharp odor; polymerizes to paraldehyde; fumigation; forms chloral hydrate, a sedative and hypnotic; used in manufacture of DDT, an insecticide
   3. Benzaldehyde—used for manufacture of drugs, dyes, perfumes
   4. Cinnamic aldehyde—active ingredient of oil of cinnamon
   5. Vanillin—active ingredient in vanilla extract

Ketones

A. All ketones contain a C=O group
B. Reactions of ketones
   1. Ketones are formed by the mild oxidation of secondary alcohols
   2. Reduction of ketones forms secondary alcohols
   3. Ketones are relatively unreactive
C. Important ketones
   1. Acetone—one end product of fat metabolism; solvent for paints and varnish
   2. Dihydroxyacetone—intermediate product of carbohydrate metabolism
   3. Methyl ethyl ketone—solvent
   4. Benzophenone—perfumes, soaps, cosmetics
   5. Acetophenone—perfumes, soaps, cosmetics

Organic acids

A. All organic acids contain the $\overset{\overset{\textstyle O}{\textstyle \|}}{C}$—OH (carboxyl) group

B. Organic acids form organic salts by reacting with a base
C. Important organic salts
   1. Lead acetate—making lead pigments, treating poison ivy dermatitis
   2. Sodium acetate—component of a well-known buffer
   3. Copper acetate—insecticide (Paris green)
   4. Aluminum acetate—dye making
   5. Calcium propionate—mold inhibitor in baked goods
   6. Calcium lactate—calcium therapy
   7. Ferric ammonium citrate—iron therapy
   8. Sodium citrate—anticoagulant in blood for transfusions
   9. Sodium oxalate—anticoagulant in blood for laboratory examinations
   10. Sodium benzoate—mold inhibitor for food
   11. Sodium salicylate—antipyretic, analgesic agent
D. Important organic acids
   1. Formic acid—found in insect sting venom
   2. Acetic acid—acid of vinegar, used in manufacture of cellulose acetate
   3. Lactic acid—acid of sour milk, intermediate in metabolism of carbohydrates
   4. Oxalic acid—bleach
   5. Citric acid—acid in citrus fruits, intermediate in metabolism of carbohydrates, fats, and proteins (citric acid cycle)
   6. Pyruvic acid—intermediate in carbohydrate metabolism
   7. Benzoic acid—synthesis of other products like the benzoate salts
   8. Chaulmoogric acid—has been used in the treatment of Hansen's disease
   9. Salicylic acid—synthesis of aspirin and sodium salicylate
   10. Picric acid—treatment of burns, precipitant of proteins in clinical tests
E. Certain organic acids are produced from hydrolysis of fats and are called fatty acids; e.g., butyric acid, stearic acid, palmitic acid, oleic acid

Esters

A. Reactions of esters
   1. Esters formed in reaction between an acid and an alcohol
   2. Esters easily hydrolyzed by acids

(acid hydrolysis) and bases (saponification)

3. When the ester contains the acid residue of a fatty acid, the hydrolysis of the ester by a base results in the formation of a soap—the basic salt of a fatty acid

4. When fatty acids react with glycerol, they form esters that are called fats or oils

B. Important esters
   1. Ethyl acetate—solvent, stimulant, and antispasmodic
   2. Butyl acetate—solvent
   3. Ethyl nitrite—diuretic and antispasmodic
   4. Amyl nitrite—lowers blood pressure, aids in asthma and angina pectoris
   5. Glycerol trinitrate (nitroglycerin)—vasodilator, explosive
   6. Methyl benzoate—perfumes and flavoring agents
   7. Methyl salicylate—flavoring (oil of wintergreen), liniments
   8. Acetylsalicylic acid—aspirin
   9. Phenolsulfonphthalein—an indicator for acid-base reactions
   10. Many flavors and odors in foods, fruits, flowers, and perfumes are the result of volatile esters (amyl acetate, banana, ethyl butyrate, pineapple, etc.)

Ethers

A. Reactions of ethers
   1. Ethers are formed from condensation of alcohol molecules with H_2SO_4 (sulfuric acid) acting as a catalyst
   2. Use of ether and oxygen in operating rooms makes for explosive conditions; care must be exercised preventing sparks
   3. Ethers can cause nausea and irritation of tissues; cause much postoperative discomfort

B. Important ethers
   1. Diethyl ether—general anesthetic, solvent for fats
   2. Dimethyl ether—solvent
   3. Divinyl ether—anesthetic
   4. Methyl propyl ether—anesthetic

Amines

A. Organic compounds containing an NH_2 group that can be considered as derivatives of ammonia

B. Reactions of the amines
   1. Amines give a basic reaction in water solution
   2. Amines react like a base with acids, forming complex ions

C. Important amines
   1. Dimethyl amine—used in processing of leathers, in production of liquid fuel for rocket propulsion, and in making ion exchange resins
   2. Trimethyl amine—preparation of ion exchange resins
   3. Para-amino phenol—used in photographic developers and for making analgesic drugs
   4. Aniline—used in the manufacture of dyes, rubber, drugs, antioxidants
   5. Acetanilid—antipyretic and analgesic drug
   6. Sulfanilamide—an important sulfa drug
   7. Sulfathiazole and sulfadiazine—important sulfa drugs
   8. In general, amines are used in dyes, drugs, soaps, disinfectants, insecticides

Amino acids

A. Amino acids possess 2 functional groups; an amine group and an acid or carboxyl group

B. Amino acids are amphoteric—act as both acids or bases; therefore, proteins act as buffers in body fluids

C. Reactions of amino acids
   1. Amino acids are able to act as an acid and as a base (amphoteric character)
   2. Condense via peptide bond to form proteins

D. Essential amino acids cannot be synthesized well enough in the body to maintain health and growth and must be supplied in the food

Heterocyclic compounds

A. Cyclic compounds containing atoms other than carbon

B. Important heterocyclic compounds
   1. Furfural—an aldehyde derivative of furan; used as a solvent, in manufacture of nylon, and in clinical test for sugars
   2. Pyrrole—constituent of porphyrins that make up hemoglobin, chlorophyll, cytochromes, and the amino acid tryptophan

3. Imidazole—found in the purines of nucleic acids and in the amino acid histidine
4. Thiazole—found in penicillin and in the structure of the vitamin thiamin
5. Pyridine—important to formation of members of the B complex of vitamins
6. Purine—found in nucleic acids, uric acid, stimulants such as tea and coffee, and in Dramamine (motion sickness-relieving drug)
7. Pyrimidine—used to synthesize nucleic acids, the vitamin thiamin (B_1), and barbiturates (phenobarbital, Amytal, Seconal, etc.)

Alkaloids

A. Nitrogen-containing organic materials extracted from plants
B. Important alkaloids
1. Nicotine—alkaloid in tobacco; used in manufacture of insecticides
2. Atropine—derived from belladonna plant; dilates pupil of eye, used to dry secretions of respiratory tract
3. Cocaine—found in cocoa plant; local anesthetic and nerve stimulant
4. Quinine—from cinchona bark; antimalaria drug
5. Atabrine—synthetic drug; similar in action to quinine
6. Morphine—derived from a type of poppy (raw material opium); central nervous system depressant
7. Codeine—opium derivative; central nervous system depressant
8. Demerol—synthetic compound; similar in action to morphine

BIOCHEMISTRY

See sections on anatomy and physiology and nutritional science

Carbohydrates

A. Aldehyde or ketone derivatives of single oxidation of polyhydric alcohols, or compounds yielding aldehyde or ketone derivatives upon hydrolysis
B. Include simple sugars, starches, celluloses, gums, and resins
C. Widespread in plant and animal tissue
D. Contain carbon, hydrogen, and oxygen with the hydrogen and oxygen present in approximately the ratio of 2 to 1

E. Synthesis—plants synthesize carbohydrates from carbon dioxide and water with the aid of the green pigment chlorophyll (which acts as an enzyme) and the solar energy of the sun
F. Classification
1. By functional group
a. Carbohydrates having the aldehyde group are called aldoses
b. Carbohydrates having the ketone group are called ketoses
2. By complexity of the molecule
a. Carbohydrate having a single ketose or aldose molecule is called a monosaccharide—a simple sugar
b. Carbohydrate formed by combining 2 aldose molecules or an aldose and a ketose molecule is called a disaccharide
c. Carbohydrate having more than 2 simple sugars joined in a molecule is called a polysaccharide
G. Tests for glucose in urine
1. Benedict's test and Clinitest tablets use copper ions in basic medium—show presence of sugar in urine by change in color
2. Positive reaction gives colors from green (very little sugar) to brick red (more than 2 g. of sugar per 100 ml. of urine)
3. Iron ions and silver ions can be used instead of copper to give a test for sugar
4. Most monosaccharides and disaccharides except sucrose are reducing sugars; therefore, sucrose put into urine will not produce a reaction
H. Important carbohydrates
1. Glycerose and dihydroxyacetone—triose intermediates in cellular metabolism of carbohydrates
2. Ribose and deoxyribose—pentose constituents in nucleic acids
3. Glucose (dextrose)—hexose monosaccharide; a sugar found abundantly in body fluids, fruits, and vegetables; the pancreatic hormones, insulin and glucagon, regulate the blood glucose concentration in the normal range of 70 to 105 mg. per 100 ml. of blood; glucose is the basic food molecule that is broken down first in glycolysis (in the cytoplasm of cells) and then in the Krebs' cycle (in mitochondria); the breakdown of each molecule of

glucose results in the release of 38 molecules of ATP, which can be used in almost all cellular energy requiring functions

4. Fructose (levulose)—ketose monosaccharide; found in fruits and honey, sweetest sugar known; important intermediate in cellular metabolism of carbohydrates

5. Galactose—hexose monosaccharide; present in brain and nervous tissue

6. Lactose (milk sugar)—disaccharide of glucose and galactose molecules; bacterial fermentation of lactose to lactic acid causes milk to sour

7. Sucrose (cane sugar)—disaccharide of glucose and fructose molecules; nonreducing sugar, common table sugar used in sweetening and baking

8. Maltose—disaccharide of 2 glucose molecules; found in grains and malt

9. Starch—mixed polysaccharide of glucose molecules found in plants
   a. Amylose—straight-chained glucose polymer
   b. Amylopectin—branched-chain glucose polymer
   c. Chief food carbohydrate in human nutrition
   d. Starch polymers react with iodine to form a blue colored complex; used as a test for starch
      (1) Test becomes colorless as starch is hydrolyzed
      (2) Starch (blue) → amylodextrin (purple) → erythrodextrin (red) → achroodextrin (colorless) → maltose (colorless) → glucose (colorless)

10. Glycogen—polysaccharide polymer of glucose molecules found in human and animal tissue; storage compound in body; hydrolyzes to glucose, maintaining blood glucose levels

11. Cellulose—polysaccharide polymer of glucose found in plants; not digestible by humans; important in manufacture of cotton cloth, paper, and cellulose acetate synthetics

12. Inulin—polysaccharide polymer of fructose, used in kidney function test (inulin clearance test)

13. Agar-agar—polysaccharide polymer of galactose used as a solid medium for bacteriologic studies

Lipids

A. Organic substances essentially insoluble in water but soluble in organic solvents (ether, chloroform, acetone, etc.)

B. Fatty acids—important constituents of all lipids (except sterols)
   1. Usually straight-chained carboxylic acids
   2. Naturally occurring fatty acids contain even numbers of carbon atoms
   3. Saturated fatty acids—have no double bonds (points of unsaturation) between their carbon atoms
   4. Unsaturated fatty acids—have 1 or more points of unsaturation between their carbon atoms
   5. Essential fatty acids—cannot be synthesized by body; must be taken in by diet

C. Classification of lipids
   1. Simple lipids—esters of fatty acids and alcohols
      a. Fats—the alcohol of fats is the trihydric alcohol glycerol
         (1) Solid fats—fats that are solid at room temperature contain long-chained, saturated fatty acids
         (2) Liquid fats (oils)—fats that are liquid at room temperature contain short-chained, unsaturated fatty acids
      b. Waxes—esters of long-chained fatty acids and an alcohol other than gylcerol; lanolin, a mixed wax from wool, is used in creams and salves
      c. Reactions of simple lipids
         (1) Hydrolysis—splitting into fatty acid(s) and alcohol by breaking ester bond, is effected by acid, base, or enzymatic action
         (2) Saponification—basic hydrolysis; soap is formed from organic salts of fatty acid and metal ion of base
         (3) Addition—fats containing unsaturated fatty acids will form addition products at points of unsaturation
            (a) Addition of oxygen will cause fat to become rancid; antioxidants slow this reaction in packaged foods

(b) Unsaturated oils used in paints add oxygen and oils become hard and glossy

(c) Hydrogenation—liquid fats can form solid fats by adding in hydrogen at double bonds

2. Compound lipids—fats containing chemical substances other than fatty acids and alcohols

a. Phospholipids—contain alcohol, fatty acids, phosphoric acid, and a nitrogenous base (or inositol)

(1) Lecithins—contain the alcohol glycerol, fatty acids, phosphoric acid, and the nitrogenous base choline; are found in brain and nervous tissue; in blood, lecithin serves to render fats soluble in plasma (a lipotropic agent)

(2) Cephalins—similar in structure to lecithin except base is ethanolamine; important in brain and nerve tissue; help blood-clotting mechanism

(3) Sphingomyelins—made from amino alcohol (sphingosinol), a fatty acid, phosphoric acid, and choline; important in brain and nerve tissue

b. Cardiolipids—made from unsaturated fatty acids, glycerol, and phosphoric acid; found in heart tissue

c. Glycolipids (cerebrosides)—structure contains the monosaccharide galactose, amino alcohol (sphingosinol), and a fatty acid; found in brain tissue and the myelin sheaths of nerves

3. Steroids—complex monohydroxy alcohols found in plant and animal tissues —basic structure, the phenanthrine structure plus a cyclo-pentane ring; characteristic side chains determine specific steroids

a. Cholesterol—a sterol found in human and animal tissue, chiefly in brain and nerve tissue; an important, normal component of membranes; found in blood within a normal range of 150 to 300 mg. per 100 ml.; high blood cholesterol seems associated with coronary thrombosis

b. Ergosterol—a plant sterol that can be converted to vitamin D by ultraviolet light

c. Bile acids—sterols that aid in digestion and absorption of fats

d. Steroid hormones—sex and adrenal gland hormones

e. Vitamin D—steroid helping to control calcium metabolism by regulating calcium uptake from the gastrointestinal tract

Proteins

A. Polymers of alpha amino acids connected by peptide bonds

B. Characteristics of proteins

1. Protein molecules are very large

2. Proteins form colloid particles in solution

3. Synthesis of proteins is in ribosomes of cell, according to specific genetic patterns under direction of the nucleic acids DNA and RNA

4. Structure patterns of proteins are extremely specific; proteins differ from species to species, individual to individual, organ to organ; present problems for transplant operations

5. Proteins are the tissue builders of the body

C. Classification of proteins

1. Simple proteins—give amino acids on hydrolysis

a. Albumins—water soluble, coagulated by heat; e.g., lactalbumin (milk), serum albumin (blood), egg white; albumin is most important in the development of the plasma colloid osmotic pressure, which helps control (through osmosis) the flow of water between the plasma and interstitial fluid; during a condition such as starvation, a fall in the albumin level of the blood results in a fall in the plasma colloid osmotic pressure; this results in edema caused by less fluid being drawn by osmosis into the capillaries from the interstitial spaces

b. Globulins—insoluble in water, soluble in dilute salt solutions, coagulated by heat; e.g., lactoglobulin (milk), serum globulin (blood), gamma serum globulin—forms antibodies of blood

c. Glutelins—soluble in dilute bases

or acids, insoluble in neutral solutions; coagulated by heat; e.g., glutenin (wheat)

d. Albuminoids—soluble in water; e.g., collagen (connective tissue), elastin (ligaments)

e. Histone—water-soluble; e.g., globin (hemoglobin)

f. Prolamines—insoluble in water, soluble in 70% to 80% alcohol; e.g., gliadin (wheat), zein (corn)

g. Protamines—water-soluble; e.g., protamine (fish spermatozoa)

2. Compound proteins—contain molecules other than amino acids

a. Chromoproteins—proteins containing a colored molecule; e.g., hemoglobin, flavoproteins

b. Glycoproteins—proteins containing carbohydrate molecule(s); e.g., mucopolysaccharide of synovial fluid

c. Lipoproteins—simple proteins combined with lipid substances; e.g., lipovitellin in egg yolk

d. Nucleoproteins—proteins complexed with nucleic acids; e.g., the DNA (genetic material) found in chromosomes is complexed with proteins; chromosomes are sometimes referred to as nucleoprotein structures

e. Metalloproteins—proteins containing metal ions; e.g., ferritin (iron transport compound of plasma)

f. Phosphoproteins—proteins containing phosphoric acid radical; e.g., casein of milk

3. Derived proteins—also called *denatured* proteins; treatment with acids, bases, heat, x-ray films, ultraviolet rays, and many other agents causes proteins to alter their molecular arrangements

D. Reactions of proteins

1. Amphoteric properties—like the amino acids forming them, proteins can act as acid or base in solutions; can act as buffers

2. Hydrolysis—acid, base, or enzyme hydrolysis splits peptide bond; yields proteose → peptones → peptides → amino acids

3. Denaturation—change in structure renders the protein less soluble, leads to coagulation of protein

a. Heat—protein and heat → coagu-

lated protein; e.g., cooked egg white, cooked meat, etc.

b. Salts of heavy metals—silver, lead, mercury, etc.; taken internally, poison because they denature the enzymes of the cells, which are protein in nature

c. Acetone and alcohol—both harden skin proteins

d. Inorganic acids and bases—coagulate and hydrolyze proteins

e. Alkaloids and organic acids—tanning of hides, precipitation of blood proteins for clinical tests

f. Rays—x-ray films, infrared rays, ultraviolet rays—long exposure can cause cataracts (precipitation of lens protein in eye)

4. Salting out—concentrated salt solutions render soluble proteins insoluble

5. Color reactions

a. Xanthoproteic test—protein having benzene ring (as found in the amino acids tyrosine and phenylalanine) will turn yellow on addition of concentrated nitric acid; heat and a second addition of sodium hydroxide will turn the yellow to orange

b. Millon's test—protein having a phenolic ring (as found in the amino acid tyrosine) will form red precipitate on addition of a mixture of mercuric and mercurous nitrates

c. Biuret test—test for the peptide bond; violet color appears on addition of a hydroxide and dilute copper sulfate solution; negative for free amino acids (no peptide bond)

d. Hopkins-Cole test—protein that contains the indole structure (amino acid tryptophan) shows a violet color on addition of glyoxylic acid and concentrated sulfuric acid

e. Ninhydrin test—test for free amino acids, ninhydrin reagent gives blue color

Nucleoproteins

A. Specific proteins found in cells, made of large and complex molecules having important functions

B. Composition of nucleoproteins

1. Hydrolysis of nucleoproteins results in nucleic acids and protein

2. Hydrolysis of nucleic acid yields
   a. Phosphoric acid—H_3PO_4
   b. Pentose sugars—ribose or deoxyribose
   c. Purine or pyrimidine bases
      (1) Purine bases—adenine, guanine
      (2) Pyrimidine bases—cytosine, uracil, thymine
3. Combination of a purine or pyrimidine base with either ribose or deoxyribose forms a nucleoside
4. Addition of phosphoric acid to a nucleoside forms a nucleotide
5. Polymerization of nucleotide molecules via ester bonds yields a nucleic acid—the shape of DNA is that of a double helix

C. Two main forms of nucleic acid—RNA and DNA (ribonucleic acid and deoxyribonucleic acid)
   1. RNA yields the following on hydrolysis: adenine, guanine, cytosine, uracil, ribose, phosphoric acid
   2. DNA yields the following on hydrolysis: adenine, guanine, cytosine, thymine, deoxyribose, phosphoric acid

D. Role of DNA and RNA in protein synthesis
   1. DNA is found chiefly in the chromatin material of interphase cells and in the chromosomes of cells in mitosis
      a. Portions of DNA molecules are the genes of classic genetics; the genetic code consists of sequences of bases (adenine, guanine, cytosine, and thymine) linearly arranged along the DNA molecule; every 3 bases represent a code for 1 amino acid (a triplet code)
      b. One enormous DNA molecule represents thousands of genes separated from each other by specific triplets (codons) representing periods or commas; i.e., the linear triplet code is punctuated so that it can be eventually translated correctly on the ribosome
      c. DNA is also found in mitochondria, chloroplasts, and certain other cellular organelles (like centrioles) and is thought to play some role in their replication and metabolism
   2. RNA is found both inside the nucleus and in the cytoplasm of cells
   3. RNA occurs in three forms: messenger RNA (mRNA), transfer RNA (tRNA), and ribosomal RNA (rRNA)
      a. DNA transcribes its coded message of how to make proteins into messenger RNA (mRNA); the function of mRNA is to carry this coded genetic information from the DNA in the nucleus to the ribosome in the cytoplasm where proteins can be synthesized
      b. The transcribed genetic code being carried by mRNA is translated into the synthesis of proteins on the ribosomes; these proteins then serve both structurally and enzymatically in the cell
      c. Transfer RNA (tRNA) molecules each carry an amino acid to the ribosome where protein synthesis is occurring; there is a specific tRNA molecule for each amino acid
      d. Ribosomal RNA (rRNA) is part of the structure of the ribosome
   4. The protein difference between individuals is ultimately determined by differences in the genetic code carried by DNA; the DNA and RNA molecules are presently the only known molecules that store information and can result in the accurate transmission of genetic information from one generation of cell or organism to the next; the cellular mitotic and meiotic processes are elaborate and precise mechanisms for partitioning the genetic material appropriately between daughter cells

E. Other important related compounds
   1. ATP and ADP (adenosine triphosphate and adenosine diphosphate) are energy-storing compounds in cells
   2. NAD (nicotinamide adenine dinucleotide) and NADP (nicotinamide adenine dinucleotide phosphate) are important in hydrogen transport in the metabolism of foods

Enzymes

A. Organic catalysts that enter into reactions and are reformed at end of reaction
B. Needed in minute amounts
C. Protein in nature and inactivated by all things denaturing proteins; e.g., high temperature, changes in pH

D. Substrate is the substance acted upon by an enzyme
E. Enzymes usually have ending "ase" added on to name of substrate or to action of enzyme; e.g., sucrase—enzyme hydrolyzing sucrose; lactic acid dehydrogenase—enzyme removing hydrogen from lactic acid
F. Enzymes, being proteins, are usually quite specific in action
  1. One enzyme will usually catalyze only 1 reaction—substrate specificity
  2. Enzyme activity will be high at temperature specific for the enzyme and low at other temperatures—temperature specificity
  3. Enzyme activity will be high at the pH specific for the enzyme and low at the other pH values—pH specificity
G. Certain inorganic ions act to speed up or slow down enzyme activity—enzyme activators and enzyme inhibitors
H. Enzymes acting within cells are called intracellular enzymes; e.g., the enzymes bringing about the breakdown of glucose and other sugars, the synthesis of carbohydrates, proteins, and nucleic acids all function within cells and are intracellular enzymes
I. Enzymes acting outside cells are called extracellular enzymes; e.g., the digestive enzymes found in the mouth, stomach, and small intestine all function outside of cells and are extracellular enzymes
J. Some enzymes exist in 2 parts
  1. Apoenzyme—protein part of enzyme
  2. Coenzyme—nonprotein part of enzyme
  3. Holoenzyme—the apoenzyme and the coenzyme together

Chemistry of digestion

A. Digestion is carried on by a series of hydrolytic reactions
B. The catalysts in digestion are enzymes
C. Function of digestion is to render food small enough to be absorbed into body
D. The digestive process is summarized in Table 2-2

Vitamins

A. Materials needed in minute quantities in the diet that the body cannot synthesize
B. Many have coenzyme roles in metabolism
C. Classification
  1. Fat-soluble
    a. Vitamin A—maintains cells and tissue in healthy state; needed for vision in dim light
    b. Vitamin D—regulates calcium metabolism
    c. Vitamin E—antioxidant
    d. Vitamin K—essential for prothrombin synthesis for proper blood clotting
  2. Water-soluble
    a. Vitamin B complex—many act as coenzymes in metabolism
    b. Vitamin B_{12}—extrinsic factor necessary to prevent pernicious anemia
    c. Folic acid—needed for normal maturation of erythrocytes
    d. Ascorbic acid (vitamin C)—maintains connective tissue in normal state
D. Other essential food factors not strictly vitamins that appear to be needed in small amounts in diet for health
  1. Choline—used in synthesis of lecithin; widely distributed in foods so human deficiency is rare; seems to prevent fatty livers
  2. Inositol—importance in human nutrition still under investigation; possible role in carbohydrate metabolism suggested; widely distributed in foods
  3. Bioflavonoids—lack in diet causes increased capillary permeability and fragility; exact role in human nutrition under investigation; found in citrus fruits, other fruits, and vegetables
  4. Lipoic acid—role in human nutrition under investigation; possible enzymatic role in carbohydrate and protein metabolism indicated; found in yeast and liver

Chemistry of blood, urine, and hormones
Blood

A. Liquid tissue circulating in body composed of fluid (plasma) and cells (erythrocytes, leukocytes, and platelets)
B. Chemical nature
  1. Water
  2. Proteins
  3. Amino acids
  4. Glucose
  5. Inorganic salts
  6. Vitamins
  7. Waste products—urea, uric acids, etc.
  8. Hormones
  9. Enzymes

Table 2-2. Chemistry of digestion

Secretion	Gland of secretion	Enzyme	Optimum reaction	Substrate	Example	End product
Saliva	Sublingual Submaxillary Parotid	Ptyalin (salivary amylase)	pH 6.7-7.2	Carbohydrates	Bread Potatoes	Maltose Dextrin
Bile	Liver	Action due to salts	pH 7.5-8.2	Fats	Butter	Emulsified fats
Pancreatic juice	Pancreas	Trypsin	pH 6.0-9.0	Protein	Meat, beans	Proteoses, peptones, polypeptides
		Chymotrypsin	pH 6.0-10.0	Protein		
		Amylopsin (amylase)	pH 7.5-8.2	Carbohydrates	Bread, starch, flour	Maltose
		Steapsin	pH 7.5-8.2	Fats	Fat meat, ham, butter	Fatty acids and glycerol
Succus entericus (intestinal juice)	Glands of intestinal wall	Maltase	pH 7.5-8.2	Maltose		Glucose
		Carboxypeptidase	pH 7.5-8.2	Peptides		Amino acids
	Brunner's glands Lieberkühn's glands	Aminopeptidase	pH 7.0-9.0	Peptides		Amino acids
		Dipeptidase (erepsin)	pH 7.0-9.0	Dipeptides		Amino acids
		Maltase	pH 7.0-9.0	Maltose		Glucose
		Lactase	pH 7.0-9.0	Lactose		Glucose and galactose
		Sucrase (invertase)	pH 7.0-9.0	Sucrose		Glucose and fructose
		Nuclease	pH 7.0-9.0	Nucleic acid		Mononucleotides
		Phosphatase	pH 7.0-9.0	Mononucleotides		Nucleosides, phosphates
		Nucleosidase	pH 7.0-9.0	Nucleosides		Pentoses, purines, and pyrimidines
Gastric juice	Glands of stomach mucosa (chief cells)	Pepsin	pH 1.5-1.8	Protein	Meat, beans, legumes	Proteoses, peptones, peptides
		Rennin (infants)	pH 5.0	Milk casein	Milk	Paracasein + Ca^{++}
		Lipase		Fats, oils	Butter, cocoa oil, olive oil	Fatty acids and glycerols

C. Function
1. Transport of food materials
   a. From intestinal tract to tissues
   b. From storage tissues to metabolizing cells
2. Transport of gases
   a. Oxygen from lungs to cells
   b. Carbon dioxide from cells to lungs
3. Transport of waste materials from cells to organs of excretion
4. Distribution of hormones, antibodies, and certain enzymes
5. Defense against infection, by action of antibodies and leukocytes
6. Wound healing through clot formation
7. Regulation and distribution of body temperature
8. Regulation of body acid-base balance through blood buffers
D. Coagulation
1. Function—prevention of blood loss and promotion of wound healing
2. Mechanism
   a. Blood contains prothrombin, calcium salts, fibrinogen
   b. Blood platelets and tissues contain thromboplastin
   c. Injury causes blood platelets and tissue to break and blood vessels to rupture, mixing blood and thromboplastin
   d. Calcium ions necessary for clotting, chemicals that bind up calcium act as anticoagulants outside of body; e.g., potassium oxalate
   e. Heparin blocks the conversion of prothrombin to thrombin; is used in and out of body to prevent clotting
   f. Antithrombin in blood dissolves clots, helps prevent clots in the body
   g. Vitamin K necessary for synthesis of prothrombin in liver
E. Blood buffers
1. Proteins, amino acids, bicarbonates, phosphates all act to prevent changes in the pH of the blood
2. Blood buffers are necessary to prevent changes in the pH of the blood that are incompatible with life
F. Blood gases
1. Oxygen transported by blood chiefly through combination with hemoglobin of red blood cells

2. Carbon dioxide transported by blood as bicarbonates and dissolved in plasma
3. Carbonic anhydrase, an enzyme in the red blood cells, aids in converting carbon dioxide to bicarbonates
G. Changes in the body are often reflected by changes in the components of the blood; e.g., pH, cell content, blood gases, waste products

Urine

A. Water solution of inorganic salts and organic compounds
B. Important in excretion of wastes
C. Analysis yields information of physical condition in health and disease
D. Normal urine
1. Amount—800 to 1800 ml. per 24 hours
2. Color—light yellow to dark brown, resulting from pigments (urobilin, urochrome, etc.)
3. Odor—aromatic (fresh); food and drugs alter odor
4. Sediment—varies; caused by diet and other normal changes
   a. Few blood cells
   b. Few epithelial cells
   c. Phosphates
   d. Urates
   e. Uric acid crystals
   f. Calcium oxalate
5. Specific gravity (1.005 to 1.025) varies greatly, depending on fluid intake and the quantity of solutes dissolved in the urine; the individual having diabetes insipidus may excrete 5 to 15 L. of urine daily; this urine has a very low specific gravity (very close to that of pure water); an individual having diabetes mellitus may excrete urine of high specific gravity caused by excessive quantities of glucose dissolved in the urine
6. Reaction—usually acid (pH 4.5 to 7.5 is the normal range); alkaline immediately after a meal
7. Proteins—negative; protein in urine is usually associated with pathology although albumin traces may occasionally appear after heavy exercise or cold showers (these traces being of no consequence)
8. Sugar—trace to negative; presence of urinary carbohydrate usually pathologic

9. Ketone bodies—negative; ketone bodies in urine appear in metabolic disorders
10. Indican—negative; positive results indicate intestinal obstruction
11. Bile—negative; positive results indicate liver or gallbladder dysfunction
12. Blood—trace to negative; positive results indicate bleeding in organs of urinary system

Hormones

A. Produced by glands of internal secretion —endocrine glands (ductless glands)
B. Discharged into blood
C. Carried by blood to site of activity
D. Regulate functioning of body
E. Some important hormones
   1. Thyroid hormone (thyroxine)—regulates metabolism
   2. Parathyroid hormone—regulates calcium metabolism
   3. Pancreatic hormones (insulin and glucagon)—regulate carbohydrate metabolism
   4. Anterior pituitary hormones
      a. Growth hormone—influences growth, maintains tissues and bones
      b. Gonadotropic hormone—regulates sexual growth and function
      c. Thyrotropic hormone—regulates thyroid gland
      d. Adrenocorticotropic hormone (ACTH)—maintains adrenal gland function
   5. Posterior pituitary gland hormone
      a. Oxytocin—stimulates smooth muscle
      b. Vasopressin (antidiuretic hormone, ADH)—increases water absorption in the kidneys
   6. Cortical adrenal gland hormones
      a. Mineralocorticoids; e.g., aldosterone —regulate salt balance
      b. Glucocorticoids; e.g., cortisone— regulate carbohydrate and protein metabolism
   7. Medullary adrenal gland hormones
      a. Epinephrine—regulates
         (1) Heart rate and cardiac output
         (2) Blood pressure; acts as a vasoconstrictor
         (3) Muscle constriction
         (4) Conversion of glycogen to glucose; thereby affects blood sugar

      b. Norepinephrine
         (1) Acts as vasoconstrictor
         (2) Regulates and raises blood pressure
   8. Sex hormones
      a. Male and female hormones are produced by gonad tissues
      b. Chemically related to cholesterol
      c. Determine primary and secondary sex characteristics, regulate sexual function, and in the female maintain pregnancy and lactation
      d. Chief female sex hormones are estrogens and progesterone
      e. Chief male sex hormone is testosterone
      f. Chorionic gonadotropic hormone present in urine in early pregnancy is the basis of pregnancy tests
   9. Gastrointestinal hormones function to regulate digestion
      a. Gastrin—stimulates flow of gastric juices
      b. Enterogastrone—inhibits flow of gastric juices
      c. Secretin—stimulates flow of sodium bicarbonate from the pancreas to the duodenum
      d. Pancreozymin—stimulates the flow of pancreatic enzymes from the pancreas to the duodenum
      e. Cholecystokinin—stimulates contraction of gallbladder
      f. Enterocrinin—stimulates flow of intestinal juice

Metabolism of carbohydrates, fats, and proteins

A. Breakdown products of digestion utilized for energy and tissue synthesis in body
B. Glycolysis
   1. Enzymatic anaerobic process occurring in cytoplasm of cells; no oxygen necessary
   2. Produces 2 ATP molecules per glucose molecule metabolized (quickly converts simple sugars to energy)
   3. End products, pyruvic and lactic acids
C. Citric acid cycle (Krebs' cycle)
   1. Main oxidative, metabolic pathway; pyruvic acid enters the mitochondrion where it is completely oxidized to carbon dioxide and water
   2. When a glucose molecule is completely oxidized through glycolysis

and the citric acid cycle, 38 ATP molecules are obtained; thus the aerobic oxidation of glucose involving the citric acid cycle in the mitochondria is considerably more efficient in yielding energy (as ATP) than the anaerobic oxidation of glucose (glycolysis)

3. Enzymes catalyze each step of the process

PHYSICS

MEASUREMENT

The metric system

A. Used universally in medicine and nursing
B. Based on units of 10 and the use of certain prefixes such as "kilo," "centi," and "milli"
C. Standard unit of length—meter (m.)
   1. Kilometer (km.) = 1000 meters
   2. Centimeter (cm.) = $\frac{1}{100}$ meter
   3. Millimeter (mm.) = $\frac{1}{1000}$ meter
D. Standard unit of weight—gram (g.)
   1. Kilogram (kg.) = 1000 grams
   2. Milligram (mg.) = $\frac{1}{1000}$ gram
E. Standard unit of volume—liter (L.)
   1. Milliliter (ml.) = $\frac{1}{1000}$ liter
   2. Cubic centimeter = 1 milliliter
F. Conversions
   1. One meter = 39.37 inches; 2.54 centimeters = 1 inch
   2. One kilogram = 2.2 pounds; 453 grams = 1 pound
   3. One liter = 1.06 quarts

Temperature

A. The 3 common measures of temperature are
   1. Celsius or centigrade
   2. Fahrenheit
   3. Absolute or Kelvin
B. Conversions
   1. If
      T_f = temperature in Fahrenheit degrees,
      T_c = temperature in Celsius degrees, and
      T_k = temperature in absolute (Kelvin) degrees,
      then
   2. $T_f = (\frac{9}{5}T_c) + 32$
   3. $T_c = (T_f - 32) \times \frac{5}{9}$
   4. $T_k = T_c + 273°$
   5. In practice, tables are generally available for these interconversions

Sources of error in measurement

A. Errors in calibration of instruments; e.g., the markings on a ruler or a thermometer may be incorrectly placed or spaced
B. Errors caused by parallax; e.g., the temperature on a thermometer may be read incorrectly as a result of varying the relative position of the eye and the thermometer
C. Random, accidental errors in taking readings; can be minimized by taking more than one reading

MECHANICS

The study of motion and the action of forces on bodies

Three basic laws of motion developed by Isaac Newton

A. First law: A body remains at rest or in uniform motion in a straight line unless forces act on the body making it change its state of rest or uniform motion; in other words, bodies continue to do whatever they are doing unless some force acts on them
   EXAMPLE: If a nurse is rapidly pushing a patient in a wheelchair and the wheelchair is suddenly stopped, the patient (a body) continues in motion straight ahead and may fall forward out of the chair; to prevent this from happening, the nurse would have to apply a force to stop the forward motion
B. Second law: If a body is accelerated, the greater the force applied to the body, the greater the acceleration; the greater the mass of the body, the more force needed to produce a desired acceleration
   EXAMPLE: All other bodily factors being the same, a runner with more powerful muscles will accelerate faster than a runner with less powerful muscles; if a 150 lb. weight were placed on the runner's shoulders, those same powerful muscles would produce less acceleration because of the increased mass
C. Third law: For every action there is an equal and opposite reaction
   EXAMPLES:
   1. While walking, the soles exert an action force backward on the floor; the floor exerts a reaction force on the soles propelling the body forward
   2. As blood flows through an artery it exerts an action force on the walls of the artery; the walls of the artery ex-

ert a reaction force on the blood, which helps to provide the pressure to keep the blood flowing

D. The three laws of motion imply an understanding of the difference between mass and weight
   1. Mass—quantity of matter in a body; does not change with the location of the body; measured in grams, kilograms, or milligrams
   2. Weight—the force of gravitational attraction upon a body (see Law of gravitation below); commonly measured in pounds or kilograms
   3. Weight will change as gravitational attraction changes; mass however will remain the same

E. Technology based on Newton's laws of motion
   1. Centrifuge—a motor-driven device used in research laboratories and blood banks that rapidly spins mixtures of particles of different mass (or weight); the heavier particles are sedimented (move to the bottom of the centrifuge tube) faster than the lighter particles; the particles are sedimented because of their own inertia (proportional to their mass) and Newton's first law (the particles tend to follow a straight line path to the bottom of the tube since there is no force to oppose such a motion); similarly the spin cycle of a washing machine utilizes the principle of Newton's first law
   2. Ballistocardiograph—a device that measures and records the movement of the body as a whole in response to the pumping action of the heart; the forces caused by the surge of blood into the aorta produce reaction forces that move the rest of the body; measurements from this machine provide information that can be used along with electrocardiograph information to determine the condition of the heart

Law of gravitation

A. Any 2 objects in the universe are attracted to each other with a force equal to the product of the masses of the 2 objects divided by the square of the distance between them; i.e., the greater the mass of the bodies, the greater the gravi-

tational force; the closer they are together, the greater the gravitational force

B. Applications
   1. Postural drainage—positioning of individual so that the throat is below level of lungs to help drain fluid from the lungs
   2. Rocking beds—abdominal viscera alternately push against and then away from the diaphragm, thus aiding in respiration
   3. Position of head postoperatively—head is placed on one side; thus, the force of gravity pulls the tongue down, breathing remains unobstructed and allows for drainage in case of vomiting
   4. Semi-Fowler's position—fluid in peritoneal cavity flows toward the pelvis where it is more easily drained

Center of gravity

A. Position in a body where all the weight may be considered to be located; sphere, such as a rubber ball, has its center of gravity in its center

B. An object is stable (will not topple over) as long as a line dropped from its center of gravity to the ground is within the base of the object; in a human, the center of gravity is in the pelvic cavity and for upright balance the line drawn from this point to the ground must fall somewhere between the legs
   1. When lifting a patient, the back should be kept straight to keep torque at a minimum (see material on levers, p. 104); in addition, when bending over, the body's center of gravity shifts from a stable position between the legs to an unstable position outside the legs; the back muscles must then work even harder to prevent the body from toppling over
   2. When walking and carrying a load, the load should be carried as close to the body (center of gravity) as possible to maintain balance and to avoid strain

Momentum

A. Basic concept—an object's momentum is dependent on its mass and the velocity at which it is moving; a 250 lb. person in a heavy motorized wheelchair moving down a corridor at 3 miles per hour has greater momentum than a 100 lb. person in a light wheelchair rolling along at 5 miles per hour

B. Changes in momentum—an object's momentum can be changed by applying a force to an object for a certain length of time; the greater the force applied and/or the longer the time that the force is applied, the greater is the change in momentum of the object

1. During exercise, the contracting heart imparts great momentum to the blood because the force of contraction of the myocardium is great, and the duration of contraction of the myocardium is relatively long compared with skeletal muscle, which has a shorter duration of contraction

2. During micturition, the walls of the urinary bladder exert a force of prolonged duration that imparts great momentum to the urine being expelled from the body

3. During a cough or a sneeze, the abdominal and intercostal muscles apply a large force on the air in the lungs; the sudden opening of the vocal cords and epiglottis results in the explosive propulsion of air from the lungs; in this case momentum of the air stream is great, not because of the mass of the particles (since the molecules of gasses in air are light), but because of their high velocity

4. When a person speaks, the vocal cords vibrate and in turn produce vibrations in the air molecules surrounding them; the momentum in these vibrating molecules is transferred from air molecule to air molecule all the way to the ear of the listener, where the vibrations are converted into nerve impulses that the brain interprets as sound

Energy

A property that enables a body to perform work

A. Examples

1. A wound-up spring has energy because it can do the work of running a clock

2. Muscles possess energy because they are capable of doing the work of moving the body

3. Epithelial cells of the human respiratory tract possess energy because their cilia beat back and forth and thus do the work of pushing mucus and foreign matter up toward the throat

4. Every living cell in the body possesses energy because it does work to maintain certain water and electrolyte concentrations within itself

B. Work—the product of the force exerted and the distance through which the force moves; using the examples above

1. The spring exerts a force that moves gears in the clock through a certain distance

2. The muscles exert a force that moves the bones of the body through a certain distance

3. The cilia exert a force that moves them through a certain distance in the fluid surrounding them

4. The cell membranes exert a force that moves ions a certain distance through the membrane

C. Types of energy

1. Potential energy—energy stored in an object because of its position

a. A coiled spring has potential energy because it could do work if it were allowed to uncoil

b. An ATP molecule has potential energy because it could do work when chemical changes occur; during chemical changes the positions of electric charges within and between molecules are altered

c. A glucose molecule has potential energy that can be released to accomplish work during chemical changes; enzyme systems in the cytoplasm of cells and in the mitochondria of cells chemically change the glucose molecule releasing the energy stored in the bonds holding the molecule together

2. Kinetic energy—the energy of motion; the basis for many other forms of energy

a. Heat

(1) Measured through temperature

(2) Based on the energy of movement (kinetic energy) of the molecules composing matter

b. Sound, as interpreted by the brain, is caused by the energy of motion (kinetic energy) of air molecules stimulating the ear to send nerve impulses to the brain

c. Electricity—caused by the energy of motion (kinetic energy) of electrons

D. Laws concerning energy

1. First law of thermodynamics (law of conservation of energy)—energy cannot be created or destroyed but may be transformed from one form into another

    a. Sunlight or radiant energy is transformed into chemical bond energy by green plants in the process of photosynthesis

    b. The potential energy of an ATP molecule is transformed into the kinetic energy of muscles, cilia, and flagella in motion

    c. The potential energy in an intravenous bottle hanging above a patient's bed is transformed into kinetic energy when the bottle's contents are allowed to flow by gravity into the patient

2. Second law of thermodynamics—all systems in the universe have a natural tendency to become disorderly or randomized; the energy of the system continually becomes more spread out and dilute

    a. Molecules tend to move from areas where they are in high concentration to areas where they are in low concentration; this is usually stated as the law of diffusion

        (1) The diffusion of oxygen and carbon dioxide between the air sacs and capillaries of the lungs

        (2) The diffusion of water through the membrane systems of cells (osmosis)

    b. Heat always flows from a hot body into a colder one

        (1) Some of the chemical energy stored in muscles is transformed into heat when muscles contract; this heat flows from the hot body (the muscles) into cooler bodies (the surrounding tissues, including blood) and helps to maintain the human body temperature of 37°C. (98.6°F.)

        (2) When the human body is

too hot, vasodilation occurs in the skin and heat radiates from the body into the cooler surrounding air

    c. The human body is highly organized; this organization is achieved during embryonic development and maintained throughout life by expending energy; this energy must be expended because the human body, obeying the second law of thermodynamics, would radiate its heat out to the surrounding air until the body temperature was the same as the temperature of the surrounding air; ions would flow into and out of the cells until they were in equal concentration on either side of the cell membrane and no new cells would be formed to replace the hundreds of thousands that die in each second of existence; this expenditure of energy offsets the natural tendency for disorganization and disorder in the body; the body dies when, for a variety of reasons, it can no longer work to maintain the particular order associated with human life

3. Applications of the energy laws—machines

    a. Apart from friction, the work output of a machine is equal to the work input to the machine; the first law of thermodynamics indicates that energy cannot be created or destroyed; a machine can multiply force, that is, provide a mechanical advantage, but at the expense of distance

        (1) Lever—a rigid bar that moves about a fixed point known as the fulcrum; a small force is applied through a large distance and the other end of the lever exerts a large force over a small distance

            (a) Automobile jack—a small force applied over a large distance exerts a force large enough to lift the end of the automobile a small distance; overall the automobile has been lifted a few inches but the arm has moved up and down through 20 or more feet

(b) Types of levers

(1) First-class lever— fulcrum between resistance and effort; e.g., scissors, hemostat

(2) Second-class levers —resistance between fulcrum and effort; e.g., wheelbarrow, oxygen tank carrier

(3) Third-class lever— effort between resistance and fulcrum; e.g., forceps, bending over and using your back muscles to lift an object with your hips acting as the fulcrum

(2) Pulleys—this machine can also multiply force at the expense of distance; the use of a number of pulleys together, as in a block and tackle, provides a mechanical advantage equal to the number of ropes excluding the pull rope; thus a block and tackle with two ropes gives a mechanical advantage of two; a 100 lb. weight can be lifted by application of a force of 50 lb.; e.g., traction, lifting heavy objects like engines

(3) Wedge—inclined plane; e.g., ramps in place of stairs, bevelled shape of hypodermic needles

(4) Wheel and axle—steering wheel of car, doorknob

b. Efficiency—never total, as friction that occurs when two surfaces rub together produces resistance and heat; the greater the efficiency, the less heat produced; friction causes mechanical devices to eventually wear out by wearing away

(1) Human digestive system offsets friction by producing mucus—lubrication helps food to slide along the digestive tract

(2) Synovial fluid in the joints of the skeletal system along with smooth articular cartilage helps to prevent friction in joints

(3) Use of lubricants when inserting rectal thermometers or catheters

(4) Friction allows for walking by producing the action force on the floor

c. Use of body lever systems in lifting

(1) In lifting, hips are the fulcrum and the effort is made by the back muscles to lift the load (third-class lever system)

(2) Torque (force × length of lever arm) increases as the distance between the fulcrum (hips) and the resistance (shoulder joints) increases

(3) To minimize the torque and to avoid back strain, objects should be lifted with the back straight; this keeps the length of the lever arm (the back) as short as possible and also utilizes the relatively powerful leg muscles to lift

E. Common units used in discussions of energy concepts

1. Foot-pound (ft.-lb.)—a unit of work in the English system; in carrying a 55 lb. load up a flight of stairs 10 ft. high, a nurse has done 550 ft.-lb. of work on the 10 lb. load (work = force × distance)

2. Joule and erg—units of work in the metric system; conversions

1 joule = 10,000,000 ergs (10^7 ergs)
1 joule or 10^7 ergs = 0.7376 ft.-lb.

3. Calorie—amount of heat required to raise the temperature of 1 g. of water 1°C.

4. Horsepower (hp.)—a unit of power; power is the rate at which work is done; if some mechanical device could lift a 55 lb. load up the 10 ft. flight of stairs in 1 second, the power output of the device would be 1 hp.

5. Watt—a unit of power usually associated with electricity; conversions

1 watt = 1 joule/second = 10^7 ergs/second
1 hp. = 745.7 watts

EXAMPLE: If all the light bulbs in your house added together have a power output of 750 watts, then their power output could also be expressed as slightly greater than 1 hp.

MATTER AND ITS PHYSICAL PROPERTIES
Solids
Composed of atoms or molecules bonded together in a rigid framework
A. Important physical properties of solids
1. Density and specific gravity—the amount of mass found in a particular volume of a solid; commonly expressed as grams per cubic centimeter (g./cc.) with water, as the standard, arbitrarily given a density of 1 g./cc.; density of iron is 7.8 g./cc. so iron is 7.8 times as dense as water; this number is called specific gravity, which is numerically equal to density
   a. Compact bone is more dense and stronger than cancellous bone
   b. In most humans, the body as a whole (with lungs inflated with air) is less dense than fresh or salt water and thus floats
2. Elasticity—because of external or internal stresses, solids may change their shape or size
   a. Skin stretches when pulled because elastic connective tissue fibers loosely bind the skin to the underlying body tissues; e.g., pregnancy, obesity
   b. During mitosis, the plasma membrane exhibits great elasticity resulting in division of the cytoplasm and production of daughter cells
3. Size of solids
   a. A small body has proportionately more surface area when compared with its volume; a large body has proportionately less surface area compared with its volume
      (1) The cells composing the human body are small and therefore have a large surface to volume ratio; since foods and wastes must exchange through these surface membranes, size is critically important; a large cell having a small surface to volume ratio will not have enough surface area to provide for the needs of its huge interior volume, but a small cell, having a large surface to volume ratio, will have enough space because of its relatively huge surface area
      (2) The mucous membrane of the intestinal tract is thrown into tiny folds called villi; the small size of the villi provides them with a great surface area compared to their volume and results in increased surface area for both digestion and absorption of foods
      (3) The proximal convoluted tubules of the nephron have a brush border consisting of numerous microvilli that have very high surface to volume ratio; these tiny cellular extensions greatly increase the surface area of the tubule for reabsorption of materials from the glomerular filtrate
      (4) Infants have a higher metabolic rate than adults partly because they must generate more body heat to make up for the heat they lose by radiation from the comparatively large surface area of their bodies
   b. As the size of a body is increased, its weight increases in proportion to its volume
B. Atoms or molecules in a solid are most commonly found in the crystalline state—the atoms or molecules are in a three dimensional, orderly arrangement
1. Enzymes—the chemical reactions that maintain life are the result of the catalytic action of enzymes; the enzyme and its substrate act in a key-lock manner; while enzymes may be found dissolved in body fluids, their crystalline nature still accounts for their biologic activity
2. Structural proteins
   a. Proteins that are constituents of cell membranes include membranes of mitochondria, lysosomes, endoplasmic reticulum, Golgi apparatus, and plasma
   b. The major protein in connective tissue, which helps to bind all the

tissues and cells of the human body together, is collagen

3. Hemoglobin and myoglobin—hemoglobin transports respiratory gases in the blood while myoglobin binds oxygen in muscle tissue and is similar to although simpler than hemoglobin

4. Actin and myosin—the contractile proteins of muscle

5. Lipids—the lipids composing cell membranes are believed in some cases to be arranged in a repeating, crystalline pattern called a "bimolecular leaflet"

6. The inorganic calcium salts of bone have a crystalline structure and impart great hardness to bone substance

Liquids

Composed of molecules that are not as rigidly bound to each other as in solids, assume the shape of the container in which they are placed and are practically incompressible

A. Pressure

1. Hydrostatic—in a liquid, pressure is caused by the weight of the fluid above a submerged object; therefore, pressure on an object is dependent on how far the object is below the surface of the liquid not on the overall volume of the liquid

   a. Rate of intravenous infusion—depends, in part, on the height of the reservoir of fluid above the site of entry into the body; rate can be increased by raising the reservoir and decreased by lowering it

   b. Bladder irrigation and tidal drainage—hydrostatic pressure (which depends on gravity) forces fluid from the reservoir container above the bladder; then hydrostatic pressure again drains the fluid from the bladder to another container below the level of the bladder

   c. Wangensteen suction—depends on hydrostatic pressure; as a reservoir is slowly emptied of its water content, a mild vacuum is created, which, through various connections, produces a gentle suction often used for gastrointestinal drainage

2. Buoyant force—pressure caused by a liquid is exerted on a submerged object in all directions with the lower part of an object (like the undersurface of a swimmer) submerged deeper in the liquid than the upper part; therefore, since pressure increases with depth, there is a greater pressure pushing up on the most submerged part of the object; the net upward force is called the buoyant force; individuals rehabilitating from certain diseases or maintaining muscles or joints may exercise with the limbs under water to use this force; less effort is needed to exercise, and atrophy of muscles and deformity of joints are minimized

3. Archimedes' principle—as an object is submerged in water the water molecules must move out of the way since the object itself takes up space; the volume of water displaced by the object always equals the volume of the object itself; this displaced volume of water has weight; this principle states that the weight of this displaced water equals the buoyant force; an object will float in water if the weight of water displaced by the object is greater than the weight of the object; conversely, an object will sink in water if the weight of water displaced by the object is less than the weight of the object

   a. Life jackets increase the volume and thus the weight of water displaced by the person, therefore the buoyant force increases and the person floats; by strapping on a life jacket, very little weight and a great volume is added to the body, which then bobs on the surface of the more dense material, the water

   b. Hydrometer (urinometer)—measures density (sp. gr.) of urine or other liquids; the sealed, weighted, glass tube sinks or rises in the liquid depending on the weight of fluid displaced; a liquid of low density can not buoy up the tube very much and it floats low whereas a liquid of high density can and it floats high

4. Pascal's principle—when pressure is applied to a fluid in a closed, nonflexible container, that pressure is transmitted undiminished throughout

all parts of the fluid and the pressure acts in all directions

a. Cerebrospinal fluid—an abnormal increase of pressure on this fluid is transmitted to all parts of the central nervous system containing the fluid

   (1) Brain tumor—a mass of tissue displaces fluid and increases the pressure of the cerebrospinal fluid

   (2) Hydrocephalus—blockage in the canal of Sylvius or overactivity of the choroid plexuses results in a tremendous collection of fluid and increased pressure

b. Urination—in conditions resulting in the lack of a micturition reflex, manual pressure over the bladder region will be transmitted to the urine, which results in the opening of the sphincters and the expulsion of urine from the bladder

c. Circulatory system—the pressure exerted as a result of the contracting ventricles is transmitted throughout the blood vessels of the circulatory system; this pressure is responsible for blood flow

   (1) Pressure—fluid always flows from regions of higher pressure to those of lower pressure; the pressure in the human circulatory system is highest in the ventricles during systole, decreases throughout the length of the circulatory system, and is lowest in the atria; the normal pressure of blood in the circulatory system varies with age and disease

   (2) Lumen of the tube—the flow of fluid through a tube is directly proportional to the radius of the tube; e.g., the degree of constriction of the arterioles for the most part determines the quantity of blood entering the capillary beds and returning to the heart

   (3) Length of the tube—the longer the tube, the less fluid flow there is through the tube in a unit of time; when blood circulation to the skin is greatly increased the heart must increase its output to maintain normal circulation, since many more miles of tubing (capillaries) have been added to the system

   (4) Viscosity—the molecular components of a fluid exert forces of attraction on each other; as the fluid flows along, an internal friction, caused by the molecular attractions of the fluid's components, tends to impede fluid flow; this internal resistance to fluid flow is viscosity

      (a) Anemia—because of a reduced number of red blood cells, the viscosity of the blood is decreased; therefore blood returns to the heart more rapidly, increasing cardiac output, which may overwork the heart during periods of increased exercise

      (b) Polycythemia—an increased number of red blood cells in the blood increases its viscosity; blood flows more sluggishly and the blood pressure will increase to compensate

B. Surface tension—the molecules of a liquid exert forces of attraction on one another; at the surface of the liquid the molecules are attracted by other molecules at the bottom and sides, but not at the top since air is there; this results in a force of contraction at the liquid surface called surface tension

1. A thin razor blade will float on the surface of water unless the surface of the water is pierced and then the razor sinks

2. Soaps and detergents lower the surface tension of water by reducing the degree of the interaction of the water molecules with each other

a. Detergents reduce water surface tension by allowing the water molecules on the surface to interact

with detergent molecules, which then interact with the material to be cleaned; thus the detergent is a molecular bridge between the water and the dirt
  b. Detergents in bile (bile salts) lower the surface tension of fat globules and water in the intestinal tract, allowing greater surface contact between the fat molecules and the lipases
  c. Hot water has a lower surface tension than cold water and is consequently a better cleaning agent
  d. The alveoli and respiratory passages of the human lungs have a mixture of surface tension-reducing substances collectively called surfactant that reduce surface tension and the pull that the water molecules would ordinarily have on each other if these surface active agents were absent; breathing is therefore much easier because of this agent
  e. Surface tension principles are thought to be involved in both the ameboid motion of red blood cells and in their phagocytic action
C. Capillarity—when a small diameter tube is dipped into water or other fluid, the water will rise in the tube because of adhesion of the water molecules to the components of the glass; surface tension then causes the film of water to contract and pull itself up the tube; the water continues to rise until the weight of the water balances the adhesive force; this rise of the fluid level in a tube is called capillarity or capillary action
  1. Capillarity draws blood into a capillary tube when a technician takes a small blood sample for various analyses
  2. Water rising between the cotton fibers of a washcloth, a ball of absorbent cotton, gauze acting as a surgical drain, or a paper towel drying one's hands

Gases

The molecules composing gases are so far apart that they do not exert any cohesive forces on each other; consequently, the gas will expand to fill any container and will exert pressure on the container because of

elastic rebound of the gas molecules with the walls of the container
A. The atmosphere is an ocean of air surrounding the earth whose moving molecules of gas are kept from diffusing away from the earth by gravity while exerting a pressure upon the earth known as atmospheric pressure, which can be measured by barometers
B. Boyle's law—at constant temperature, the pressure exerted by a gas is inversely proportional to its volume; as the volume of a gas is decreased, its pressure increases and as the volume is increased, the pressure decreases
  1. Respiration—the contraction and downward movements of the dome-shaped diaphragm increase the volume of the thoracic cavity containing the lungs; since the volume of air in the lungs is increased, the pressure exerted by the air is decreased; air now flows from the area of higher pressure outside the body to the area of lower pressure inside the lungs; conversely, during expiration, the upward movement of the diaphragm and the elastic recoil of the lungs themselves decrease the volume of air in the thoracic cavity and lungs as air flows out
  2. Pneumothorax—an opening connecting the outside air with the intrapleural space results in air flowing into the intrapleural space; this eliminates the pressure gradient between the thoracic cavity and the atmosphere, and the lungs cannot inflate
  3. Intermittent positive pressure breathing apparatus (IPPB)—a special valve is operated by the individual's own respirations; on inspiration, one part of the valve opens and oxygen or a mixture of gases is forcefully pushed under greater than atmospheric pressure (positive pressure) into the lungs through a special mouthpiece or face mask
C. Laws concerning gases and absolute temperature
  1. Charles' law—the volume of a gas is proportional to the absolute temperature; i.e., gases expand and contract in proportion to temperature
  2. Gay-Lussac's law—the pressure of a gas is proportional to the absolute temperature; the higher the tempera-

ture the greater the pressure exerted by the gas

3. Examples
   a. Autoclave—by keeping the volume of a gas (steam) constant and raising the pressure, the temperature of the gas rises; the high temperatures of the steam reached in an autoclave kill microorganisms
   b. Aerosol sprays of any type must not be stored in excessively hot places since the rise in temperature increases the pressure in the can and may cause it to explosively burst open

D. Laws concerning gases and partial pressure
   1. Dalton's law—the pressure exerted (in millimeters of mercury—mm. Hg) by a gas in a mixture of gases is proportional to its percentage in the mixture; e.g., partial pressure of O_2 in alveoli is 104 mm. Hg; partial pressure of O_2 in pulmonary artery and alveolar capillaries is 40 mm. Hg; therefore, O_2 diffuses from alveoli air sacs into capillaries
   2. Henry's law—the quantity of gas dissolving in a liquid is proportional to the partial pressure of the gas at a given temperature; i.e., a person overcome by smoke inhalation or who has some obstruction to normal breathing can benefit from inhalation of either pure O_2 or a mixture of gases having a higher partial pressure of O_2 than is found in air

E. Effects of atmospheric pressure changes on the human body
   1. Descent below the earth, in scuba diving or in watertight enclosures, *caissons,* for tunnel construction, causes the gases normally found in the human body to occupy a smaller volume; when the person rapidly ascends to sea level the pressure decreases suddenly and the body gases begin occupying larger volumes, which can result in nitrogen bubbling out of the blood; these bubbles can stimulate and damage nerves causing great pain and paralysis; the bubbles can also form emboli that can block normal functioning in the circulatory system (the bends or decompression sickness)
   2. Ascent above the earth, as in high-altitude jet airplanes or spaceflights, causes the gases normally found in the human body to occupy a larger volume because of the decreased pressure at high altitudes; thus as one ascends:
      a. Gases in the gastrointestinal tract expand bringing about abdominal distention and pain
      b. Gases in the paranasal sinuses expand and, if the sinus exits are clogged, can result in sinus headache
      c. Gases in the middle ear expand and, if the eustachian tubes are collapsed, can cause middle ear discomfort
      d. Bubbles of O_2 form in the blood if ascent is extremely rapid
      Airliners are pressurized to avoid these discomforts

F. Bernoulli's principle—the pressure in a fluid decreases with increased velocity of the fluid; i.e., the energy in a fluid (liquid or gas) can be considered to exist in 2 forms: kinetic energy expressed as the velocity at which the fluid is moving, and potential energy expressed as the lateral pressure exerted by the fluid; if one component increases, then the law of conservation of energy demands that the other component decrease, so that the total amount of energy remains constant
   1. The ability of an airplane to fly—the wings of the airplane are constructed so that air rushes over the top of the wing faster than it does under the bottom; therefore the air pressure is less at the top of the wing than underneath and the plane rises
   2. Atomizer (sprayer)—as air rushes across the top of the tube connected to the fluid below, the pressure at the top of the tube decreases and atmospheric pressure pushes the fluid up the tube where it mixes with the air and exits from the device as a fine mist
   3. Other applications producing suction that operate on Bernoulli's principle include
      a. Gravity suction apparatus
      b. Siphon suction apparatus
      c. Water seal or closed drainage system or drainage of the thorax
      d. Thoracic thermotic pump

Plasma

Hot gas molecules have been stripped of their electrons producing a mass of ions and electrons
A. Most of the matter in the universe is in the form of plasma (in the interior of suns)
B. Fluorescent lighting—mercury vapor is ionized by high voltage between the ends of the long tube; the vapor conducts an electric current and radiates energy that causes the phosphor coating on the inner surface of the tube to glow
C. Neon signs and vapor lamps in street lighting operate as in fluorescent lighting

HEAT

Atomic movement

A. All atoms and molecules constantly vibrate and move
B. The rate of these vibrations determines whether the molecules will be in the solid, liquid, gaseous, or plasma state
C. The more rapidly the atoms and molecules vibrate, the hotter the substance

Temperature

A. The quantity that measures how hot or cold a body is, as compared with some standard
B. Temperature is a measure of the average kinetic energy of the molecules composing a substance; when a hot and cold body touch, thermal energy in the form of heat always passes from the hot to the cold body
C. Measurement
　1. Thermometers—measure temperature through expansion and contraction of the liquids—mercury or colored alcohol
　2. The scale of the thermometer exists between certain arbitrarily fixed points
　　a. On the centigrade or Celsius scale the freezing point of water is 0; the boiling point of water is 100; the space between 0 and 100 is divided into 100 equal units called degrees
　　b. On the Fahrenheit scale the freezing point of water is 32; the boiling point of water is 212
　3. Mercury is used in thermometers because it is opaque and easily read through glass; it conducts heat rapidly and responds by expanding or con-

tracting; it has a low freezing point and a high boiling point; it has a relatively large degree of expansion or contraction in response to heat; and its expansion between 35°C. and 43°C. is uniform, making it ideal for carefully measuring the human body temperature
　4. Clinical thermometers are maximum reading thermometers since the mercury level stays at the highest reading attained

Intensity and quantity of heat

A. Temperature measures the intensity of heat
B. The unit that expresses the quantity of thermal energy or the amount of heat that could be produced in a body is the calorie
C. The British Thermal Unit (BTU) is defined as the quantity of heat required to change the temperature of 1 lb. of water 1°F.

Specific heat

A. The quantity of heat required to raise the temperature of a substance 1°C.
B. Some substances heat faster than others and some substances cool faster than others
C. Water has a high specific heat, which means that a relatively large quantity of energy must be added to water to bring about small temperature changes
　1. A hot water bottle stays hot for a long time because water possesses a great deal of thermal energy
　2. Water is ideal for baseboard heating systems since water carries a lot of heat
　3. Water is excellent for cooling automobiles or other large engines since a relatively small reservoir of water is sufficient to carry away a great deal of heat from the engine
　4. If it were not for the vast amounts of water on the earth, both in the oceans and in the air as vapor, the earth's temperature would be extremely inhospitable for life

Expansion and contraction caused by heat

A. Matter expands when heated because of increased vibrations of the component molecules

B. Matter contracts when cooled because of decreased molecular vibrations
  1. Metal covers on glass jars can be loosened by heating under hot water
  2. Pyrex glassware is used extensively in laboratories because of its very slight expansion when heated; it is less likely to crack during experimental procedures requiring heat
  3. Dental fillings must expand and contract to the same degree as tooth substance; if this were not the case, fillings might easily fall out or teeth might crack

Transmission of heat

A. Conduction—the transmission of heat from one part of a substance to another
  1. Good heat (and electric) conductors in order of effectiveness are silver, copper, aluminum, iron, and water; the body fluids conduct heat efficiently to all cells
  2. Poor heat (and electric) conductors are called insulators and include wool, wood, styrofoam, paper, cork, straw, and air; in the human body fat is the best insulator and helps to reduce heat loss
  3. Applications
    a. Hot moist compresses are excellent transmitters of heat and must be carefully applied
    b. Thermal blankets contain air spaces that trap body heat and serve as insulators
    c. Rubber is a good insulator for hot water bottles but the skin must still be protected
B. Convection—the heating or cooling of liquids or gases by means of currents
  1. When air or water is heated, the hot molecules are moving more rapidly than the cooler molecules; as they spread outward they encounter the least opposition to their movement when they move upward; therefore warmer fluid and air rise
  2. As the hot fluid and air rise and spread out they cool because of a slowing down of their molecules; once the heat is dissipated, the cooler molecules descend to take the place of warmer molecules that are rising
  3. Application
    a. Radiators and baseboard heating devices are placed under windows so that a "curtain" of rising warm air will bring about descent of colder air coming from the window toward the radiator where it can be warmed
    b. Clothing decreases convection of air currents tending to cool the body
C. Radiation—a hot object emits radiant energy that is transformed into heat when it strikes some object
  1. When radiant energy strikes an object, the object absorbs some of that energy and the object heats up
  2. Radiation is the transmission of radiant energy *not* the transmission of heat
  3. Application
    a. Radiant heat lamps (infrared lamps) are sometimes used therapeutically for warming parts of the body; the heat transfer via radiation is more penetrating than through conduction or convection
    b. Cryosurgery is surgery performed at low temperature so tissue needs for oxygen are diminished and the surgeon can spend more time repairing or replacing the damaged tissues or organs; body temperature can be artificially lowered through immersion in cold water, packing in ice, cold water enemas, or irrigating the stomach with ice water
    c. The normal metabolism in each of the cells of the human body produces heat; in addition, heat is a by-product of muscular contraction; the body maintains its temperature at 37°C. by emission of radiant energy from the surface of the body, evaporation of water from the lungs and skin, defecation, and urination

Change of state

A. Evaporation—molecules of a liquid become molecules of gas; since the most energetic molecules leave the surface of a liquid during evaporation, the average kinetic energy and temperature of the remaining liquid molecules is lower; thus evaporation causes cooling
  1. Rubbing alcohol applied to the skin will rapidly evaporate, cooling the body

2. Sweating is an important physiologic process because its evaporation helps to control body temperature
B. Condensation—molecules of a gas become molecules of a liquid; to become a liquid, gaseous molecules must give up some of their energy; since the liquid's temperature rises, condensation causes heat
   1. Steam burns can be severe since the heat of condensation is transferred to the tissues, causing extensive damage
   2. If an individual is to have steam inhalation, the face must be protected from the direct steam
C. Boiling—the evaporation occurring beneath the surface of a liquid; the gas bubbles so formed are buoyed to the liquid's surface and escape into the atmosphere; this evaporation can be speeded up by (1) adding heat to the liquid molecules so that they possess enough energy to burst out from the surface of the liquid, and (2) reducing the atmospheric pressure above the liquid
   1. Autoclave—by increasing the pressure inside the autoclave (which is like a giant pressure cooker) higher water temperatures can be reached and bacteria and their spores can be readily destroyed by the steam generated; thus the autoclave sterilizes materials placed in it for specified lengths of time
   2. Distillation (all chemical and drug solutions are made in distilled water) —purifying water by boiling and collecting the vapor; impurities are left behind during water evaporation
D. Melting—when a solid melts into a liquid, it must absorb energy to break the chemical bonds holding the molecules rigidly together; as the molecules absorb the energy they vibrate more and more violently until they are relatively free to move about as they please; putting an ice cube in the mouth or on the skin cools because each gram of melting ice absorbs calories from the surfaces of the mouth or skin
E. Freezing—when a liquid freezes, it must give up some of its energy so that the molecules of the substance will be held to each other (cohesion) in the rigid framework of a solid; frostbite is a freezing of a part of the surface of the body,

generally the ear lobes, tip of the nose, or ends of the digits of hands and feet; unless the process can be reversed, destruction of tissue occurs
F. Sublimation—change of state from a solid directly to a gas with no intervening liquid state
   1. Camphor or naphthalene (mothballs or flakes) sublimate
   2. Solid CO_2 (dry ice) also sublimates and is useful as a cooling agent; the solid CO_2 molecules absorb large quantities of heat to change directly to the gaseous state

Sterilization

Heat is used to kill all living organisms on medical instruments and other materials; dry heat at a temperature of 170°C. (338°F.) for 30 minutes is considered sufficient for sterilization; dry heat sterilization has an advantage over steam sterilization in that no damage is done to the fine cutting edges of surgical instruments or to ground glass surfaces

Humidity

The amount of water vapor in the air; if air is saturated with water, it contains all the water vapor it can at that temperature
A. Absolute humidity—the actual percentage of water vapor that is in a sample of air
B. Relative humidity—the amount of water vapor in the air compared to the amount of vapor present in saturated air at the same temperature; if the relative humidity is 25%, the air is holding one fourth of the total amount of water it could hold at that temperature
   1. When the relative humidity as well as the temperature is high, discomfort occurs because the high humidity, or vapor pressure in the air, counteracts evaporation of sweat from the body surface; i.e., as much or nearly as much water condenses on the body from the atmosphere as evaporates from it
   2. Air conditioners remove moisture from the air (dehumidify the air) as well as cool it; this is important because a temperature of 80°F. with low relative humidity can be comfortable whereas 70°F. with high relative humidity can be uncomfortable

SOUND
Basic concept
A. Sound is a mechanical vibration that cannot occur in a vacuum; it is propagated best through solids and through liquids better than gases; sound travels in waves from a vibrating source such as human vocal cords, a loud speaker, or a dropped object
  1. A very faint heartbeat might be heard by placing the ear on the chest; even strong heartbeats cannot be heard distinctly with just the ears
  2. The sound vibrations (waves) pass readily through the tissue of the human body to the surface of the skin where a stethoscope can pick them up

Properties of waves
A. Transverse waves—if the particles of the medium vibrate at right angles to the direction of the wave, the wave is transverse; waves upon the surface of liquids and all electromagnetic waves (light, infrared, and ultraviolet) are transverse waves
B. Longitudinal waves—the particles of the medium vibrate back and forth along the same direction as the wave; sound waves are longitudinal waves
C. Frequency—the number of complete vibrations (or waves) generated or moving along per second; referred to as cycles per second or as a hertz (Hz.)
D. The passage of a wave through a medium (either gas, liquid, solid, or plasma) is actually the passage of a disturbance in the medium, not a flowing of the medium itself; the wave represents sequential vibration or swinging of the molecules of the medium from the vibrating source to the ears
E. Refraction of sound waves—sound travels faster in warm air than cool air; in warm air the average kinetic energy of the air molecules is higher than in cooler air and the wave can be propagated more quickly
F. Reflection of sound waves—many solid objects reflect sound waves from their surfaces resulting in an echo; a reverberation is a series of echoes
G. The energy of sound waves—all waves possess energy but to differing degrees; ultraviolet waves and gamma radiation possess high energy while sound waves possess little energy; the structure of the ear reflects the need to amplify the relatively weak energy of sound waves into more energetic waves capable of stimulating the liquid-filled organ of hearing, the cochlea in the inner ear
H. The velocity of sound—the frequency of the wave × the length of the wave; the velocity of sound waves varies with the nature and temperature of the medium; since light travels much faster than sound, lightning is seen before thunder is heard

The interpretation of sounds
A. Loudness—a neurologic or psychologic interpretation of intensity; while the exact relationship is complex, one could say that the greater the intensity of the sound waves stimulating the organ of Corti, the greater the frequency of nerve impulses reaching the auditory centers of the brain and the louder the sound seems to be
  1. Noise level is measured in decibels (db.); a normal conversation is about 65 db., amplified rock music about 120 db., and the sound of a nearby jet airplane about 140 db.; the decibel scale is logarithmic so that 120 db. is 1 million times more intense than 60 db.
  2. Excessive noise can result in hearing loss at certain frequencies of sound; noise levels of about 85 db. and over can damage the organ of Corti; damage increases with the length and intensity of noise and is irreversible
  3. The Doppler effect—when a vibrating source or a receiver of sound move toward each other, the pitch or frequency of the sound produced by the source becomes higher; as the vibrating source and the receiver move away from each other, the frequency of the sound becomes lower
  4. Speech audiometry—this technique detects the threshold of hearing of actual speech for individuals by presenting groups of two-syllable words at successively lower levels until the person fails to hear; this data is presented as a speech reception threshold (SRT) in db.; phonetically balanced single-syllable words can also be presented; these words represent a fre-

quency of sounds of speech that approximate a typical conversation; the percentage of words repeated correctly is the Davis' Social Adequacy Index (SAI); a score of 94% to 100% is considered normal

B. Pitch—corresponds to frequency; the higher the frequency, the higher the pitch of the sound
  1. The human ear can potentially hear sounds whose frequencies range from 16 Hz. to 20,000 Hz.; with increasing age, the upper range decreases slightly, which presents no problem in hearing speech since speech falls in the range of 85 Hz. to 1050 Hz.
  2. The audiometer electronically produces sounds at a variety of frequencies as well as intensities and is used to measure hearing loss

C. Quality—people have different and distinct qualities or timbres to their voices; similarly, the sounds of different musical instruments are easily recognized; a musical sound or a voice rarely represents a pure tone but usually many frequencies are occurring simultaneously

D. Ultrasonic sound—vibrational frequencies exceeding the upper level of human hearing (20,000 Hz.)
  1. Can be used in cleaning metal parts; the high-frequency vibrations shake the solution and produce bubbles that help in the cleaning process; ultrasonic cleaners are available for hospital use in cleaning syringes and needles
  2. Low-intensity ultrasonic waves have been used to treat arthritis and bursitis, to break kidney stones, and to help dissolve scars
  3. Ultrasonic dental drills can quickly drill into teeth without the pain associated with tooth vibrations, which stimulate the nerve of the tooth
  4. Sonograms are pictures of the body derived through differential reflection or transmission of sound waves
  5. Ultrasonic fetal heart monitors can detect the fetal heart beat in as early as the twelfth week of gestation

E. Deafness—the condition where sound vibrations are not transmitted to the brain for interpretation
  1. Perforation or tear of the tympanic membrane

  2. Inflexibility of the 3 middle ear bones or ossicles; vibrations are now only poorly transmitted to the oval window
  3. Otosclerosis—abnormal bone formation over the oval window immobilizes the stapes
    a. Surgery can remove the abnormal bony tissue in the early stages of the disease
    b. In later stages, the stapes can be removed and a prosthesis can be implanted
    c. If the oval window is ossified, a new opening in the cochlea is made to replace the oval window (fenestration)
    d. Bone conduction hearing aids as described below can essentially bypass the middle ear
  4. Deafness caused by auditory nerve damage; the nerve cannot be regenerated nor can hearing be helped by hearing aids

F. Hearing aids—electronic devices that amplify sounds and assist partially deaf persons to hear; a miniature microphone picks up the sound, sends it to an amplifier and then to a miniature loudspeaker fitted in or behind the ear
  1. Air conduction type sends an amplified sound wave into the ear, thus utilizing the person's own middle ear
  2. Bone conduction type bypasses the middle ear and transmits amplified vibrations to the skull bones, which in turn produce vibrations in the inner ear

ELECTRICITY
Electric force

A. The atoms composing all matter represent an almost perfect balance of protons and electrons; the attraction of a positive proton for a negative electron (opposite charges attracting) is the electric force that also results in like charges repelling

B. Coulomb's law—the greater the magnitude of the charges and the shorter the distance between the charges, the greater the magnitude of the electric force

C. Advantages of electricity—convenient, quiet, and easily transformed into other forms such as light or mechanical energy

D. Fields—the electric forces can be thought of as a force field existing and acting in the space between the charged particles; an electric field travels only through a conductor like a copper wire

E. Shielding—any material placed between the charged particles will reduce the magnitude of the electric force and have a shielding effect; if an automobile is struck by lightning, the energy from the lightning travels along the surface of the metal of the car and arcs to the ground; thus, passengers inside will not be electrocuted since the metal conducts electric energy while shielding objects within the car

F. Electric forces hold atoms and molecules together and thus hold solid matter together; electric forces also provide the source for all chemical energy; the molecular rearrangements associated with cellular metabolism derive their energy from electric forces between enzymes, substrates, and cofactors

Conductors and insulators

A. Conductors are good transferrers of electric fields and the energy they contain
 1. Metals such as silver, copper, aluminum, and iron and in fact most metals are good electric conductors
 2. Copper and aluminum are commonly used for all electric wiring

B. Insulators are poor transferrers of electric fields and the energy they contain
 1. Rubber, many plastics, and most nonmetals are good insulators
 2. Copper wires are almost always insulated with a thin outer layer of rubber

C. Water as a conductor—distilled water is a poor conductor while tap water contains enough charged particles (ions) to make it a fairly good electric conductor
 1. Frayed and wet electric cords can give serious shocks; infants with wet diapers sitting on frayed electric cords can be electrocuted
 2. Electrocution can occur by touching ungrounded electric fixtures such as switches and pull chains with wet hands, since the ions (electrolytes) of body fluids make them excellent conductors of electric energy

D. Semiconductors—substances such as pure germanium and pure silicon are poor electric conductors, but when impurities are added they suddenly are capable of

carrying electric energy; transistors, solid state circuits, and many copying machines use semiconductors

Static electricity

A. Substances can be charged by friction whereby a negatively charged object picks up positive charges, which it discharges via a spark when touching an object that is a good conductor

B. Applications
 1. Removing blankets and sheets from a bed will build up electric charge through the hands that should be discharged by touching a grounded object before touching others
 2. Wool, silk, nylon, and dacron may set off sparks caused by static electric charges and should not be used around combustible gases or monitoring equipment
 3. Electric equipment and operating room tables should be grounded to allow static charges to drain off, thus preventing sparks

Current electricity

A. Direct current (DC)—the flow of electric charge is in only one direction; e.g., the electric system of an automobile

B. Alternating current (AC)—electric charge in the circuit moves first in one direction and then in the opposite direction with the voltages and currents alternating back and forth; e.g., the outlets in homes and hospitals

C. Concept of electric energy and work
 1. By attaching conductors from an electric socket, battery, or generator to various devices such as motors, lamps, etc., an energy-filled electric field is conducted to these devices and is converted to other useful forms of energy such as mechanical energy, light energy, or heat energy
 2. The potential energy of the electric field is called electric potential and is measured in volts
 3. The rate of flow of electric current is measured in amperes or amps; 1 amp is a current flow of 1 coulomb/second; a coulomb is 6.25 billion electrons
 4. The resistance to flow of electricity depends on the properties of the material and on the size and length of the conductor

a. The greater the diameter of a conductor and the shorter a conductor, the less resistance the conductor offers to the flow of electricity

b. The smaller the diameter of a conductor and the longer a conductor, the greater the resistance to flow of electricity

5. Ohm's law—electric potential (volts), rate of flow of electric charge (amps), and resistance are related; the rate of flow of electricity between two points is directly proportional to the impressed voltage and inversely proportional to the resistance between the two points; thus the rate of flow of electricity can be increased by either increasing the voltage or decreasing the resistance

a. Dry fingers or hands touching an ungrounded or faulty electric source can result in a definite shock; the source touched with wet fingers or while standing in water can result in enough electric energy to be fatal

b. As little as 0.05 amp can be fatal and 0.1 amp is practically always fatal since the electric currents upset the natural electric rhythms of the heart and can result in fibrillation and also stop the breathing center from working

c. The shock obtained via alternating current is not caused by electrons pouring from the socket into the body but by the powerful vibrations of electrons and ions already inside the body that are energized via the electric field that is flowing from the outlet

Power

A. Power represents the quantity of energy used per unit of time and is expressed in watts

B. The kilowatt is 1000 watts; power companies compute the number of kilowatt hours of power used for billing purposes; a kilowatt hour is the quantity of electric power consumed in 1 hour at a rate of 1 kw. per hour

C. Types of electric circuits

1. Series circuits—current must flow through each electric device in the circuit in turn to make a complete circuit; there is only one electric pathway in the circuit; if any switches are turned off, if any fuse blows, or if any single light burns out, flow of current in the entire circuit ceases

2. Parallel circuits—current flows independently through each electric device in the circuit; there are many electric pathways in the circuit; a break in any single pathway has no effect on the flow of current in the other pathways

3. Microelectronic circuits—utilize blocks or chips of semiconducting materials like silicon or germanium since these materials allow for incredible miniaturization of electric circuits; tiny pocket electronic calculators utilize microelectronic circuits

Application of electricity

A. Electronic devices used in health care

1. Electronic cardiac pacemakers—battery-operated devices supplement or replace defective electric stimulation in the human heart and thus help to maintain the individual's heartbeat at a selected rate

2. Electrosurgery—an extremely high-frequency device called an oscillator is utilized to generate high temperatures in a small area to coagulate or desiccate tissue thus preventing bleeding during surgery; electric cutting (using the oscillator) vibrates the tissues apart and simultaneously cauterizes the small blood vessels, thus preventing bleeding

3. High frequency diathermy—utilizes an oscillator to produce a high frequency electromagnetic field that vibrates the molecules of the tissue, thus heating it up; the heat may be produced deep below the skin's surface making it useful in treating such conditions as muscular strain, arthritis, and other types of inflammation

4. Electronic thermometers—in this device, temperature change in a crystal alters the resistance of the crystal to electric flow; an individual's temperature changes the resistance of the crystal, allowing a certain amount of current to flow through and the amount read on a scale calibrated for temperature readings; these thermom-

eters give readings more accurate than mercury thermometers in about 5 to 7 seconds

B. Applications to the human body
1. The nerve impulses involving depolarization and repolarization of axons and dendrites involve the flow of a charge (carried by ions) down the length of the axon or dendrite
2. The contraction of all types of muscle is preceded by depolarization of the muscle fibers; ions carry the electric charges
   a. Electrocardiograms measure and record the electric activity of the heart as this activity is carried to the surface of the body by the ions of the body fluids; this information provides an electric picture of the heart's activity
   b. Electromyography—measures and records the electric activity of skeletal muscles of the body

MAGNETISM
Basic concepts

A. Stationary electrically charged particles exert electric forces on each other according to Coulomb's law; in addition, when electrically charged particles are in motion, the particles exert a magnetic force on each other
B. Magnetic fields contain energy; the greater the degree of movement of the electrically charged particle, the stronger the magnetic field
C. Most substances are not magnetic because for every electron spinning in a given direction, there is another electron nearby spinning in the opposite direction and their magnetic fields cancel each other
1. A common, iron horseshoe magnet possesses its magnetic properties because of the movement of negatively charged electrons in the iron atoms composing the magnet; as the electrons spin, magnetic fields are created
2. In iron, nickel, and cobalt, all the magnetic fields are not cancelled and the substance as a whole possesses magnetic properties
D. Domains—the magnetic field around a single iron atom induces adjacent iron atoms to line up with it; each cluster of aligned atoms is called a magnetic domain
1. A magnetized piece of iron has its domains aligned so that their magnetic fields add to each other, thus building up a powerful magnetic field
2. If a magnet is dropped or heated, some of the domains shift out of alignment and partially cancel the magnetic field of the magnet and the magnet becomes weaker
3. An unmagnetized piece of iron such as a nail or paper clip has a random arrangement of domains that cancel each other's magnetic effects
4. If an unmagnetized piece of iron is stroked with or brought near a powerful magnet, some of the domains are induced to align with each other, making the formerly unmagnetized iron weakly magnetic
E. Magnets have north and south poles; like poles repel and opposite poles attract
1. Since a freely suspended magnet will line up with the magnetic field of the earth itself, which acts as if it were a giant magnet, magnets are useful as compasses for determining direction
2. Since a moving beam of electrons has its own associated magnetic field, the beam can be deflected in different directions by an impressed magnetic field
   a. Television—the electron beam ultimately producing the image on the screen can be adjusted by altering the strength of the magnetic fields surrounding it
   b. Cathode ray oscilloscope—monitors heart electricity or muscle and nerve action potentials since the incoming electric signal modifies the magnetic fields surrounding the electron beam of the oscilloscope deflecting the beam up or down
3. Tremendous amounts of potentially dangerous radiation are deflected from hitting the earth's surface because of the Van Allen radiation belts that surround the earth; the magnetic field of Van Allen belts interacts with the magnetic field of the incoming radiations and the radiations are

either deflected away or drawn into the Van Allen belts

Generators

A. Generators produce the electric power used to run all of the electric devices in a technologic society
B. Generators operate on the basic principle that an electric current will flow in a wire that is moved through a magnetic field
C. By increasing the number of coils in the wire and the rate at which the coils move through the magnetic field, current can be increased
D. Generators can use hydroelectric power, wood, coal, oil, or nuclear fuel as sources of energy

Motors

A. A motor has the same 2 basic elements as a generator: a coil of wire called the armature and a magnetic field
B. By allowing current to flow through the armature, which is in the magnetic field, the electrons are deflected at right angles to the long axis of the wire; the wire as a whole begins rotating and mechanical energy is produced

LIGHT
Basic concepts

A. Visible light is a type of electromagnetic radiation; all electromagnetic radiation consists of moving electric and magnetic energy fields that come into existence because of the vibrations of electrically charged particles
B. All types of electromagnetic radiation have the same electric and magnetic nature and travel at the same constant velocity: 186,000 miles per second (speed of light)
C. The electromagnetic spectrum varies from extremely long AM and FM radio waves measured in miles to very short gamma and cosmic rays measured in millimeters
D. The product of the frequency of vibration and the wavelength is constant (the velocity of light); the lower the frequency of vibration of the wave, the longer the wavelength, and the higher the frequency, the shorter the wavelength
E. The higher the frequency (or the shorter the wavelength) of electromagnetic radi-

ation, the greater the energy content of the radiation

Wavelengths of electromagnetic radiations

A. Wavelengths are measured in either millimicra or Angstrom units
   1. A millimicron is one thousandth of a micron; a micron is one millionth of a meter (39 inches)
   2. An Angstrom unit is one tenth of a millimicron
B. The wavelength of visible light possesses just the right amount of vibrational energy to excite the photoreceptor cells (rods and cones) of the retina
C. Different wavelengths of light are bent or refracted to slightly different degrees and appear to the eyes and brain as different colors; this principle of dispersion is responsible for a rainbow
D. Emission of light—atoms can be excited by absorbing energy that causes orbiting electrons to jump to higher energy levels within the atom; as the electrons fall back to their lower, more stable energy levels (de-excitation) the energy of excitation is released and may appear as visible light; e.g., advertising signs and mercury vapor street lamps
   1. A characteristic pattern of wavelengths of light (a discontinuous spectrum) is emitted from every element in the vapor state; this pattern is best seen using a spectroscope
   2. Fluorescence—the property of absorbing radiation of one frequency and re-emitting radiation of a lower frequency and energy; a substance is said to be fluorescent if it emits visible light when energized or bombarded with ultraviolet (UV) light; high-intensity fluorescent light bulbs have been used to treat jaundice in newborn infants; the excess bilirubin in the blood, which is responsible for the jaundice, is oxidized by exposure to the bright light as blood passes through the vessels of the thin skin
   3. Phosphorescence—the atoms of a phosphorescent substance become de-excited a relatively long period of time after being excited; the phosphorescent atoms in the dial of a luminous clock are excited during the day by the visible light striking it; it glows

throughout the night as billions of excited atoms gradually become de-excited, releasing their energy as visible light

Lasers

A. Laser stands for light amplification by stimulated emission of radiation; a laser produces coherent light, which means that the light waves are all of the same frequency, are all in phase with each other (peak with peak, trough with trough), and are all travelling in the same direction; in coherent light, millions of light waves become additive and form a single, concentrated beam of light that travels in a straight line without spreading out and that can be precisely focused on minute areas

B. As coherent light leaves the laser (ruby crystal) it can be utilized for a variety of purposes
   1. Eye surgery—the energy in the coherent light produced by a laser is used to fuse minute areas of the retina to the surrounding choroid coat; an ophthalmoscope is used to precisely focus the coherent light on specific, tiny areas of the retina; a detached retina can in this way be re-attached and the fusion points are so tiny that there is no apparent loss of light sensitive retinal tissue; the machine used in this type of surgery is called a photocoagulator and uses a ruby laser
   2. Cancer therapy—the laser has been used to selectively treat pigmented skin cancers, which apparently absorb the light more readily than the surrounding, less pigmented normal tissue

Color

A. The perception of color is the result of the translation and interpretation of certain nerve impulses in the brain that come from the retina; the frequency of light determines the color that is seen; the lowest frequency stimulating the retina is red, the highest is violet, in between are all of the colors of nature

B. An object may appear to be colored because it emits electromagnetic radiation that falls within the visible range; an object may also appear colored not because it emits light, but because of selective reflection

C. Color mixing
   1. Red, green, and blue are the additive primaries; any color in the spectrum can be obtained with the proper blend of these three colors; equal amounts of the three of them produce white light
   2. Magenta, yellow, and cyan (turquoise) are the subtractive primaries; any color in the spectrum can be obtained using the proper blend of these three colors; they are sometimes loosely called respectively, red, yellow, and blue
   3. Complementary colors are any two colors that when added together produce white; red and cyan, magenta and green, and yellow and blue

D. Perception of color is believed to depend on the cones of the retina that are located most densely at the part of the retina called the fovea centralis; one type of cone detects red, another detects green, and another detects blue; it is generally believed that the brain blends nerve impulses from these three types of cones to produce all the colors of nature
   1. Faulty color vision is thought to be caused by cones that are either missing or not functioning properly; red-green colorblindness is the most common type and is a genetically inherited trait resulting in individuals seeing red and green objects as shades of gray; more men are affected than women since the trait appears to be sex-linked
   2. Color and emotion—even though red light has a lower frequency and therefore less energy than a quantum of blue light, the human mind generally associates red with warmth, excitement, and mental stimulation, and blue with coolness and calmness; for many individuals, the color of an object or a room determines to a great extent whether or not they will keep and use the object or stay in the room; thus, color has a physical basis in electromagnetic radiation but involves complex interpretation by the human mind

Reflection and refraction

A. General principles
1. Source of light—the sun is the primary outdoor source; incandescent and fluorescent bulbs are indoor light sources
2. Most objects are visible because they reflect light emitted from various sources
3. An object such as a pane of glass is transparent if it allows light to pass through it in straight lines
4. An object such as a thin, cloth window shade or a piece of paper is translucent if it allows light to pass through it in a diffused manner so that objects cannot be seen; in hospitals, use of shades or blinds diffuses light and cuts down on harsh glare
5. An object such as a heavy pair of drapes is opaque if light cannot pass through it
6. Light travelling in any single, given medium travels in straight lines; each straight line is called a ray

B. Reflection
1. When light strikes a surface off which it can reflect, the angle of incidence equals the angle of reflection as measured from the normal (a line perpendicular to the plane of the reflecting surface)
   a. When successive elevations of any surface are less than about one fourth the wavelength of the incident light, the light reflected from the surface travels mainly in one direction and the surface is polished
   b. Light reflected from rougher surfaces travels in many directions and is diffusely reflected; it is easier to read a page of text that is printed on paper that provides more diffuse than polished reflection as glare is eliminated
   c. The word *ambulance* is often printed backwards on the front of small ambulances so that motorists seeing the lettering via reflected light through their rearview mirrors will read the lettering correctly
2. Virtual images—as light reflects off a mirror the angles of incidence and reflection are equal; the reflected rays of light appear to come from a point behind the mirror; because the light rays do not actually come from this point, the image is referred to as a virtual image as opposed to a real image; the virtual image of a mirror is as far behind the mirror as the object is in front of the mirror

C. Refraction
1. Refraction—the bending of an oblique ray of light as it travels from one transparent medium into another; refraction is caused by the change in average velocity of light as it passes through the medium
2. Index of refraction—the average speed of light varies in different, transparent media; the average speed of light in water is only 75% of its average speed in a vacuum; the average speed of light in a diamond is 41% of its average speed in a vacuum; the index of refraction is a measure of how much the average speed of light differs from the speed of light in a vacuum; index of refraction = speed of light in vacuum ÷ speed of light in medium; the higher the index of refraction, the slower the average speed of light through the medium
   EXAMPLES
   a. A thermometer or syringe half immersed in a beaker of water appears to be bent at the point of immersion in the water
   b. An object in water appears to be nearer to the surface than it actually is; thus the object seems larger because it is magnified
   c. A mirage—the average speed of of light is slightly greater in hot air than cool air; on a hot paved road or a desert, the light reflected from an object is refracted upward, away from the hot surface and may then produce an upside-down virtual image to an individual some distance away; the wet shimmering look of a hot road is refracted light from the sky reaching a motorist's eye after passing through hot air layers
   d. Total internal reflection—at a certain critical angle, light between two media is not refracted (or

bent) through the two media, but reflected back into the first medium
(1) This phenomenon permits viewing of the interior walls of the stomach, intestines, and blood vessels
(2) A dentist's flashlight will "curve" the light (via total internal reflection) to the appropriate part of an individual's mouth
(3) Total internal reflection via the paired prisms in a pair of binoculars permits higher magnifications in a short optic tube

Light scattering

A. When light strikes some tiny particles in the air like dust or molecules of water vapor, the tiny particles absorb and re-emit the light in all directions
B. As white light from the sun passes through the atmosphere, the blue light waves are scattered by nitrogen and oxygen atoms and the sky appears blue
C. At sunset, light from the sun must travel through a longer path in the atmosphere before reaching the eyes; since most of the blue light waves have been scattered and the red wavelengths are more readily transmitted through the atmosphere, the sunsets are reddish and orange

Diffraction

A. The bending of light or any type of electromagnetic wave around corners is called diffraction; the longer the wavelength of electromagnetic radiation, the larger the object that it can be bent around
EXAMPLES
1. AM radio waves, some of which are over 3 miles long, easily bend around objects, thereby allowing AM radio broadcasts to come in clearly even in cities having many tall buildings and mountainous regions
2. FM radio waves, which are from 9 to 12 feet long, cannot easily bend around large objects; consequently, a specific location in a city or suburban area with large obstructing objects can determine the quality of the reception of FM broadcasts
3. Some spectrophotometers used in cer-

tain laboratory analysis of blood and urine rely on diffraction gradings to disperse white light into its component wavelengths and to utilize these specific wavelengths in the analytic procedure
4. X-ray diffraction—because of their very short wavelengths, x-rays diffract around the atoms in large molecules and produce diffraction patterns on photographic plates; analyses of these patterns can reveal the details of the arrangement of the atoms in a molecule; used in DNA analysis

Interference

A. When waves of any type are superimposed upon one another, a resulting wave different from the 2 original waves is produced; i.e., crests meet crests in some places and the resulting wave is augmented; in other areas, crests meet troughs and the waves cancel; the waves are said to interfere with each other; many superimposed waves produce patterns of interference
B. The interference of longitudinal sound waves produces beats; the interference of transverse light waves produces colors
C. When observing the top surface of a stack of microscope slides a pattern of colored rings is noted; this is caused by the interference of light as it reflects to the eyes from the many reflective surfaces of the stacked glass slides
D. Iridescence—when light reflects off 2 surfaces of a thin film, a spectrum of colors resulting from interference is observed
1. A film of gasoline on water is iridescent because of interference of light waves reflected from the top and bottom of the gasoline layer; the thickness of the gasoline film determines which wavelengths of visible light will interfere constructively or destructively; different colors result because of destructive interference (cancelling) of a particular wavelength (color) of visible light and the complementary color then appears; thus, the color pattern is a contour map indicating different thicknesses of the gasoline layer
2. A soap film left on poorly rinsed dishes will reflect light from both its top and bottom surfaces; the resulting in-

terference of light waves produces a spectrum of colors; as the dish is turned the colors at any particular point will change since different angles of light result in cancellation of different wavelengths

E. Holography—coherent light from a laser illuminates an object; before the light reflected from the object strikes a photographic plate, it is made to interfere with coherent light that does not strike the object but which is derived from the same light that illuminates the object; the photographic plate called a hologram is thus a photograph of the interference pattern of light reflected from the object; when coherent light is directed through a hologram, diffraction of the light occurs at each of the thousands of interference patterns present on the hologram; the diffracted light waves so produced form a virtual image that reforms the three dimensional shape of the object on a surface

Polarization

A. Certain naturally occurring crystals, like tourmaline and herapathite, absorb light waves striking them in all planes but one; the light transmitted through and emerging from the crystal vibrates in only one plane; this light is called plane polarized light

EXAMPLES

1. Polaroid filters contain a material, like herapathite or certain man-made molecules, that will only permit light vibrating in a single plane to pass through; when used in sunglasses, they cut down on glare and eye strain; much of the light reflected from non-metallic surfaces, such as water, glass, or roadways, is already polarized because these surfaces tend to absorb light waves perpendicular to their surfaces and to reflect light waves parallel to their surfaces; when this polarized light strikes the Polaroid filters in the sunglasses, many of the light waves are absorbed; thus fewer waves are transmitted and the harsh glare is reduced

2. Polarizing filters for cameras cut down on glare in photographs and also have the effect of deepening the blue color of the sky

3. Polarizing microscopes are used in research laboratories to analyze the molecular structure of many substances

Lenses

A. The refraction of light through transparent, glass (or quartz or fluorite) lenses is of great practical importance; magnification of objects is possible using simple lenses as well as groups of lenses arranged in telescopes and microscopes; the principal axis of a lens is the line joining the two points that represent the centers of curvature of the curved surfaces of a given lens

B. Convex lenses (converging or positive lenses) converge light rays passing through them; concave lenses (diverging or negative lenses) diverge light rays passing through them

C. When light rays parallel to the principal axis pass through a converging lens, they converge on a point called the focal point; light rays not parallel to the principal axis converge in a series of points above and below the focal point making up the focal plane

1. A converging lens will magnify an object (acting as a simple magnifying glass) if it is held inside the focal point of the lens; the image is enlarged, right side up and virtual; this means that the image only appears to exist but has no physical reality

2. When an object is placed outside the focal point of a converging lens, a real, inverted image is obtained that can be focused on a screen; whenever a real image is formed, the object and image are on opposite sides of the lens

EXAMPLES

a. Motion pictures utilize converging lenses, and the movie screen is the plane where light rays are converged; slide projectors also operate via the same principle

b. In cameras, the film is flattened out and placed in the focal plane of the camera's lens; in popular single lens reflex (SLR) cameras, a mirror diverts the light to a prism, which erects the image allowing the viewer to see exactly what will be focused on the film; when the shutter button is pushed and the mirror flips out of the way, light is focused on and exposes the photographic film

D. Diverging lenses used alone produce smaller, virtual images; they are used on some cameras (not SLR cameras) as "finders" since the virtual image seen approximates the proportions of the photograph; whenever a virtual image is formed, the object and the image are on the same side of the lens

E. Lens defects—the distortions in an image produced by a given lens are called aberrations; combining a number of lenses as a system can usually minimize aberrations; this is the reason that microscopes and telescopes employ compound lenses in their construction

1. Spherical aberration—an unsharp (uncrisp) image is formed because light refracted from the outer edges of the lens is focused at a slightly different point than light refracted from more central areas of the lens

   a. In cameras and microscopes, this is corrected by using more than one lens and also by using diaphragms to cover the outer regions of the lens

   b. In the human eye, the iris is generally contracted to varying degrees and acts, in effect, like a diaphragm to block light from being refracted through the outer regions of the lens

2. Chromatic aberration—each wavelength of visible light refracts through lenses at different angles; thus each wavelength (color) of white light is brought to focus at a slightly different point; the result of this is that objects take on colors that they do not possess; this is corrected in cameras, microscopes, and telescopes by using combinations of simple lenses made of different types of glass called achromatic lenses; in the human eye, vision is sharpest when the pupil is the smallest; cutting down on light moving through the periphery of the lens minimizes chromatic as well as spherical aberration

3. Astigmatism—in the human eye, astigmatism is a type of aberration caused by the surface of the cornea possessing irregular curves; since the cornea in addition to the lens is important in refracting (focusing) light on the retina, the result of astigmatism is blurred vision, which can be corrected by using glasses whose lenses have variable curvature to compensate for the irregular curvature of the cornea

F. Focusing—the camera focuses on objects at varying distances by changing the distance between the lens and the film; the human eye focuses on objects at varying distances by changing the degree of curvature of the lens; this ability of the human eye to change the focal length of the lens is called accommodation; while the cornea, aqueous humor, and vitreous humor all help to focus light on the retina, only the crystalline lens can be accommodated; the muscle responsible for accommodation is the ciliary body; when the ciliary body contracts, the suspensory ligaments loosen and the lens rounds out and is in position for focusing on near objects; when the ciliary body relaxes, the suspensory ligaments pull the lens into a flattened position, which allows for focusing on distant objects; the limit for accommodation is represented by the near point; objects closer to the eye than the near point (about 6 inches from the surface of a normal eye) cannot be clearly focused on the retina

1. Emmetropia—the normal refractive state of the eye

2. Ametropia—any abnormality in refractive ability of the eye

   a. Myopia—the eye focuses light anterior to the retina (somewhere in the vitreous humor): from this abnormal focal point, light rays diverge and produce a blurred image on the retina; however, if objects are held about 1 inch from the eye, they will focus on the retina; for this reason, myopia is also called near-sightedness; glasses containing diverting lenses correct this condition

   b. Hyperopia—the eye focuses light posterior to the retina; thus a circle of not-yet-conveyed light strikes the retina producing a blurred image; hyperopia is also called far-sightedness and can be corrected using glasses containing converging lenses

3. Contact lenses—thin lenses that are molded to the shape of the outer surface of the cornea; this can correct near-sightedness, far-sightedness, and astigmatism; the lens is applied to the surface of the eye using a saline solution that helps adhere the lens to the eye's surface

G. Eye examination with the ophthalmoscope and the retinoscope
 1. Ophthalmoscope—the interior of the eye as well as the vision can be studied with this instrument; light is shined into the eye and if the eye has normal refractive ability, the light will be focused on the retina and will be reflected back to the observer's eye; persons with myopia or hyperopia will not converge the light on the retina and the observer will not clearly see the eye's interior; then by using lenses of varying refractive abilities the observer can compensate for the person's abnormal refraction and study the interior of the eye and determine the state of vision
 2. Retinoscope—permits diagnosis and evaluation of the refractive state of the eye; a beam of light is shined into the eye and the observer watches the red glow of reflected light from the retina as it leaves the pupil; by observing the distribution of the light as it leaves the pupil, the observer can determine the refractive error in the eye

H. Binocular vision—the visual fields of the 2 human eyes overlap; while each eye sees some areas of the environment that the other eye cannot see, both eyes see large areas in common; the human brain interprets these overlapping fields in terms of depth; the environment appears in three dimensions as opposed to the visual effect of a movie projected on a flat screen; the blind spot of the right eye can be seen by the left eye and vice versa, therefore, there are no visual gaps in the field of vision

Other types of medically important electromagnetic radiation

A. X-ray—high-frequency electromagnetic waves emitted as a result of the excitation of the innermost orbital electrons of atoms; to excite the innermost orbital electron considerable energy must be expended
 1. X-rays have great penetrating power—soft body tissues are easily passed through and expose a photographic plate; hard tissue like bone stops the x-rays and appears as lighter areas on the x-ray photograph
 2. Hard x-rays (higher frequency and more energy) have great penetrating power and can be used for deep (cancer) therapy
 3. Soft x-rays (lower frequency and less energy) are used for more superficial therapy
 4. Pneumoencephalogram—the ventricles of the brain can be x-rayed if the cerebrospinal fluid of the ventricles is temporarily replaced by air; as x-rays pass through the brain, the ventricles are outlined; the picture obtained is called a pneumoencephalogram
 5. GI series and barium enemas—allow visualization of the soft tissues of the upper and lower gastrointestinal tract; the barium salts coat the inner walls of the alimentary tube and absorb the x-rays striking them; as a result, the organ surfaces are outlined
 6. Fluoroscopy—can be considered the observation of "live" x-ray images; after the x-rays pass through the individual, they strike a fluorescent screen that absorbs the x-rays and emits visible light; by using x-ray opaque chemicals the intestinal, renal, and biliary tracts can be observed; fluoroscopy can also be used in the placement of catheters in the heart or the large blood vessels connected to the heart
 7. Radiation hazards—individuals working with x-rays should leave the room, stand behind a lead shield, or wear a lead apron when activating the x-ray machine since there is some scattering of radiation in all directions even though the x-ray beam is aimed at a particular area; film badges (photographic film) should be worn when working near sources of radiation to provide a record of the individual's overall exposure to the radiation

B. Gamma rays—electromagnetic radiation having frequencies and energy content even higher than x-rays; cobalt therapy involves exposure of cancerous tissue to a source of radioactive cobalt; the gamma rays emitted from the disintegrating cobalt atoms pass through the tissues and ionize molecules that they strike along their path; damage through ionization to vital cellular molecules (such as the nucleic acids, DNA and RNA) can result in cell death; it is believed that the greater destruction of cancerous tissue by high-energy radiation (compared with normal tissue) is caused by the higher mitotic rate of the cancer tissue; in any population of cancer cells, a greater proportion will be in some state of mitosis compared with slower dividing noncancerous tissue; supposedly, the shortened and thickened chromosomes in mitosis present better targets for the radiation than the chromatin material of interphase cells; the normally rapidly dividing body tissues (bone marrow, germinal layers of the skin, and gastrointestinal tract) are also selectively damaged by radiation resulting in the side effects that commonly occur as a result of this therapy

REVIEW QUESTIONS FOR PHYSICAL SCIENCE
Chemistry

1. Radioactive iodine (^{131}I) has a half-life of 8 days. If, then, we have 200 mg. of this isotope at a given instant, how much will we have at the end of 24 days?
   1. 25
   2. 50
   3. 12.5
   4. 75
2. Which combination of electrolytes is normally present in highest concentrations inside the cell?
   1. K^+, HPO_4^-
   2. Na^+, Cl^-
   3. K^+, Cl^-
   4. Na^+, HPO_4^-
3. Like carbohydrate and fat, protein is composed of C, H, and O. Protein differs, however, in that it also contains
   1. Phosphorus
   2. Nitrogen
   3. Potassium
   4. Sodium
4. The breakdown of triglyceride molecules can be expected to produce
   1. Urea nitrogen
   2. Amino acids
   3. Simple sugars
   4. Fatty acids

5. Chemical substances important to life that contain phosphate paired nitrogenous bases and deoxyribose sugar would be
   1. Fats
   2. Polysaccharides
   3. ATP
   4. DNA
6. Charles, a young teenager, is hospitalized with a severe asthma attack. The acid-base imbalance complicating his condition is
   1. Respiratory alkalosis caused by his accelerated respirations and loss of CO_2
   2. Respiratory acidosis caused by his impaired respirations and increased formation of H_2CO_3
   3. Metabolic acidosis caused by excessive production of acid metabolites
   4. Metabolic acidosis caused by his kidney's inability to help compensate for the increased H_2CO_3 formed
7. The most effective agent creating the osmotic pressure (osmotic forces) of the water *outside* the cell membrane is
   1. Sodium
   2. Potassium
   3. Glucose
   4. Calcium
8. An aqueous solution containing free ions that permits the passage of an electric current is called
   1. A salt
   2. An acid
   3. A base
   4. An electrolyte
9. The sharing of electrons between two atoms forms
   1. An ionic bond
   2. A buffer
   3. A covalent bond
   4. A system
10. A solution with more OH^- ions than H^+ ions is
    1. An acid
    2. An alkaline
    3. Neutral
    4. Salty
11. The taste, color, and texture of substances in our environment are the result of
    1. The arrangement of electrons in the outer orbitals of atoms
    2. The number of protons in the nucleus of atoms
    3. The number of neutrons in the nucleus of atoms
    4. The total number of electrons possessed by an atom
12. The ability of an organic molecule to dissolve in water depends on its ability to form which type of bond with water molecules?
    1. Van der Waals bonds
    2. Ionic bonds
    3. Hydrogen bonds
    4. Covalent bonds
13. Sodium ions are most important and directly involved in the human body fluids for
    1. Blood clotting

2. Generation of action potentials in nervous and muscular tissue
3. Transport of respiratory gases
4. Bone formation

14. The average adult human body has what percentage of water?
    1. 80
    2. 60
    3. 40
    4. 20

15. Phosphorus (or phosphate ions) is important in the human body for
    1. Membrane potentials
    2. Osmotic regulation of cell size
    3. Cellular energy metabolism
    4. Blood clotting

16. The receptors for the regulation of body water (through detection of osmotic pressure) are located in the
    1. Hypothalamus
    2. Neurohypophysis
    3. Kidney tubules
    4. Blood

17. The reabsorption of water from glomerular filtrate (in the kidney tubules), the flow of water between the intracellular and interstitial compartments, and the exchange of fluid between plasma and interstitial fluid spaces is caused by what important physical process?
    1. Dialysis
    2. Active transport
    3. Osmosis
    4. Diffusion

18. Two body systems that interact with the bicarbonate buffer system to preserve the normal body fluid pH of 7.4 are the
    1. Respiratory and urinary systems
    2. Muscular and endocrine systems
    3. Skeletal and nervous systems
    4. Circulatory and urinary systems

19. The capillary endothelium is a selectively permeable membrane. Which of the following molecules cannot easily pass through it?
    1. O_2 and CO_2
    2. Plasma proteins
    3. Glucose, O_2, and CO_2
    4. Ions, amino acids, and water

20. Substances that establish the pH of an aqueous solution and also resist changes in the pH of the solution are called
    1. Foods
    2. Electrolytes
    3. Enzymes
    4. Buffers

21. An important function of the albumin of the blood is
    1. Red blood cell formation
    2. The activation of white blood cells
    3. Blood clotting
    4. The development of the colloid osmotic pressure

22. The glucose concentration of the blood is regulated primarily through hormones secreted by the
    1. Liver
    2. Pancreas

3. Kidneys
4. Spleen

23. Chromosomes are sometimes referred to as
    1. Nucleoprotein structures
    2. Glycoprotein structures
    3. Lipoprotein structures
    4. Mucopolysaccharide structures

24. Cholesterol is important in the human body for
    1. Bone formation
    2. Blood clotting
    3. Cellular membrane structure and function
    4. Muscle contraction

25. Functional portions of double-helix DNA molecules are known as
    1. Chromosomes
    2. Genes
    3. Nuclei
    4. Nucleoli

26. Transfer RNA molecules
    1. Carry amino acids to the ribosome
    2. Carry the transcribed genetic code to the ribosome
    3. Are part of the structure of ribosomes
    4. Store genetic information as part of genes

27. Messenger RNA molecules
    1. Carry amino acids to the ribosome
    2. Store genetic information as part of genes
    3. Are part of the structure of ribosomes
    4. Carry the transcribed genetic code to the ribosome

28. Genetic information can be stored in
    1. Protein and DNA only
    2. DNA and RNA only
    3. RNA and protein only
    4. DNA, RNA, and proteins

29. Glucocorticoids and mineralocorticoids are secreted by the
    1. Pancreas
    2. Hypophysis
    3. Adrenal glands
    4. Gonads

30. DNA is found
    1. Only in the nucleus
    2. Only in the cytoplasm
    3. In nuclei, mitochondria, and chloroplasts
    4. In mitochondria and centrioles only

31. Secretin and pancreozymin are hormones secreted by the
    1. Duodenum
    2. Pancreas
    3. Adrenals
    4. Liver

32. An individual with untreated diabetes mellitus might be expected to have urine with a
    1. High pH
    2. High specific gravity
    3. Low pH
    4. Low specific gravity

33. The constant source of glucose for maintaining blood glucose at normal levels at all times is
    1. Ingested food
    2. Intestinal hydrolysis
    3. Liver glycogen
    4. Gluconeogenesis

34. The chemical name for aspirin is
    1. Salicylic acid

2. Sal soda
3. Acetylsalicylic acid
4. Sodium salicylic acid

35. A calorie is a unit of
    1. Heat
    2. Weight
    3. Mass
    4. Light
36. The crossroad of metabolism where all metabolic paths meet in a common oxidation pathway is called
    1. Citric acid cycle
    2. Glycolysis
    3. Ornithene cycle
    4. Positive nitrogen balance
37. An example of a chemical change is
    1. Shattering of glass
    2. Freezing of water
    3. Fermentation of fruit
    4. Hardening of gelatin
38. Two solutions having the same osmotic pressure are said to be
    1. Isotonic
    2. Hemolyzed
    3. Hypotonic
    4. Hypertonic
39. The best first-aid treatment for acid burns on the skin is to wash them with water and then apply a solution of
    1. Sodium hydroxide
    2. Sodium chloride
    3. Sodium bicarbonate
    4. Sodium sulfate
40. The process by which oxygen is being constantly returned to the air is
    1. Hydrogenation
    2. Photosynthesis
    3. Hydration
    4. Saponification
41. An increase in positive valance or a loss of electrons by an element is called
    1. Combustion
    2. Photosynthesis
    3. Reduction
    4. Oxidation
42. A solution of sodium hydroxide would be expected to have a pH of
    1. 3
    2. 7
    3. 6
    4. 10
43. A solution containing 1 gram-equivalent weight of solute in 1 liter of solution is called
    1. An isotonic solution
    2. A normal solution
    3. A molar solution
    4. A saturated solution
44. Water can be made chemically pure by
    1. Boiling
    2. Filtration
    3. Distillation
    4. Sublimation
45. Acetic acid is classed as a weak acid because it
    1. Lacks hydrogen
    2. Is poorly ionized
    3. Contains oxygen
    4. Contains carbon
46. A good first-aid treatment for an alkali (base)

burn is to wash it with water and then flood it with
    1. A weak acid
    2. A weak base
    3. A solution of salt
    4. Alcohol
47. A substance that acts as a coenzyme is
    1. Ascorbic acid
    2. Vitamin B_1
    3. Vitamin K
    4. Vitamin D
48. An enzyme important in carbon dioxide transport is
    1. Phosphatase
    2. Zymase
    3. Trypsin
    4. Carbonic anhydrase
49. Fats in the body are rendered easy to digest because of the emulsifying action of
    1. Hydrolysis
    2. Bile salts
    3. Enzymes
    4. Proteins
50. Urea is formed from the breakdown of
    1. Purines
    2. Proteins
    3. Carbohydrates
    4. Fats
51. Excessive loss of gastric juice caused by gastric lavage or pernicious vomiting can lead to
    1. Acidosis
    2. Alkalosis
    3. Loss of osmotic pressure of the blood
    4. Loss of oxygen from the blood
52. Many hormones of the body have a chemical structure similar to
    1. Fats
    2. Amino acids
    3. Sterols
    4. Glucose
53. A substance that acts as a poison because it unites with the iron of hemoglobin and prevents it from combining with oxygen is
    1. H_2CO_3
    2. CO
    3. CO_2
    4. N_2HCO_3
54. A homogenous mixture of 2 or more substances is a
    1. Suspension
    2. Solvent
    3. Hydrate
    4. Solution
55. The name for an organic catalyst in the body is
    1. Polypeptide
    2. Enzyme
    3. Phospholipid
    4. Emulsifier
56. An example of a buffer system is a mixture of
    1. Acetic acid and carbonic acid
    2. HCl and NaOH
    3. Carbonic acid and sodium bicarbonate
    4. Carbonic acid and KOH
57. Radium is stored in lead containers because
    1. Considerable heat is produced when radium disintegrates
    2. The lead absorbs the harmful radiations

3. Radium is a heavy substance
4. Lead prevents disintegration of the radium
58. An overexercised muscle that has too little oxygen supply may become sore from a buildup of
   1. Butyric acid
   2. Lactic acid
   3. Aceto-acetic acid
   4. Acetone
59. A weak base is
   1. $CaCO_3$
   2. $Ca(OH)_2$
   3. KOH
   4. NH_4OH
60. Ammonia is excreted by the kidney to help maintain
   1. Blood clotting
   2. Osmotic pressure of the blood
   3. Acid-base balance of the body
   4. Normal red blood cell production

Physics

1. One meter is equal to
   1. 3 ft.
   2. 39.37 in.
   3. 1000 cm.
   4. 100 cm.
2. A weight of 154 pounds is equal to
   1. 7 kg.
   2. 77 kg.
   3. 70 kg.
   4. 308 kg.
3. On the Celsius scale, normal body temperature (98.6°F.) reads
   1. 68°
   2. 37°
   3. 72°
   4. 20°
4. The apparent resistance that a body offers to changes in its state of motion is called
   1. Inertia
   2. Friction
   3. Momentum
   4. Deceleration
5. The rate at which the velocity of a body changes with time is called
   1. Momentum
   2. Acceleration
   3. Speed
   4. Inertia
6. The quantity of matter in a body is its
   1. Volume
   2. Weight
   3. Mass
   4. Force
7. The force of gravitational attraction on a body is its
   1. Mass
   2. Volume
   3. Position
   4. Weight
8. Placing unconscious persons on the side or with the head turned to the side may save their life by preventing suffocation (from vomiting or breathing obstruction by the tongue). The major physical principle behind this position is
   1. The law of gravity

2. Newton's first law
   3. Newton's second law
   4. Newton's third law
9. The amount of space occupied by a body is its
   1. Volume
   2. Mass
   3. Weight
   4. Density
10. The property possessed by an object that enables it to do work is
    1. Mass
    2. Energy
    3. Power
    4. Efficiency
11. A collision of a heavy person in a heavy wheelchair might be more damaging to the person and the chair than the collision of a light person in a light wheelchair. This is explained by the concept of
    1. Gravity
    2. Acceleration
    3. Momentum
    4. Speed
12. The product of a force and the distance through which it moves is
    1. Power
    2. Efficiency
    3. Work
    4. Energy
13. The momentum possessed by the airstream leaving the lungs during a cough or sneeze is caused mainly by the
    1. Mass of the particles in the airstream
    2. Weight of the particles in the airstream
    3. Diameter of the particles in the airstream
    4. Velocity of the airstream
14. Work accomplished in a unit of time is
    1. Energy
    2. Momentum
    3. Efficiency
    4. Power
15. The energy of motion is
    1. Kinetic
    2. Potential
    3. Thermal
    4. Electromagnetic
16. When the fluid in a bottle is allowed to flow into a person intravenously
    1. Chemical energy is converted to kinetic energy
    2. Potential energy is converted to kinetic energy
    3. Potential energy is converted to chemical energy
    4. Kinetic energy is converted to potential energy
17. The diffusion of water through the various cellular membrane systems is described by the
    1. First law of thermodynamics
    2. Law of universal gravitation
    3. Second law of thermodynamics
    4. Newton's third law of motion
18. The product of the mass of a body and its velocity is called its
    1. Energy
    2. Speed
    3. Momentum
    4. Force

19. Gravity can be considered to act on a body at a point known as the
    1. Gravitational point
    2. Center of inertia
    3. Center of momentum
    4. Center of gravity
20. A pair of scissors or a hemostat are examples of a
    1. First-class lever system
    2. Second-class lever system
    3. Third-class lever system
    4. Fourth-class lever system
21. The rotational force equal to the product of force and lever arm distance is
    1. Torque
    2. Centrifugal force
    3. Centripetal force
    4. Rotational inertia
22. The synovial fluid of the joints minimizes
    1. Velocity of movement
    2. Friction in the joints
    3. Efficiency
    4. Work output
23. An object following a circular path experiences a force tending to draw it toward the center of the circular path called
    1. Centrifugal force
    2. Centripetal force
    3. Torque
    4. Inertia
24. If the density of iron is 7.8 g./cc. and the density of water is 1 g./cc. the specific gravity of iron is
    1. 7.8 g./cc.
    2. 15.6
    3. 7.8
    4. 1 g./cc.
25. The reaction force to centripetal force is
    1. Torque
    2. Momentum
    3. Centrifugal force
    4. Inertia
26. Compact bone is stronger than cancellous bone because of its greater
    1. Volume
    2. Size
    3. Weight
    4. Density
27. The mass of a substance per unit volume is its
    1. Weight
    2. Specific gravity
    3. Structure
    4. Density
28. Human body cells are necessarily small so that
    1. Their surface to volume ratio is large
    2. Their nutritional requirements will be small
    3. Their surface to volume ratio is small
    4. More cells can be packed into a given area
29. Force per unit area is referred to as
    1. Pressure
    2. Surface
    3. Density
    4. Specific gravity
30. The tendency of a liquid's surface to contract an area is called
    1. Capillarity
    2. Surface tension

---

    3. The principle of flotation
    4. Pascal's principle
31. Rehabilitating exercises carried out under water use
    1. Water pressure
    2. Water vapor
    3. Water's buoyant force
    4. Water temperature
32. The physical principle that explains the ability of a person to float in water is
    1. Pascal's principle
    2. Bernoulli's principle
    3. The principle of gravitation
    4. Archimedes' principle
33. The nurse irrigates the front of the eye under low pressure to avoid damaging the retina (in the back of the eye). The nurse's actions indicate a knowledge of
    1. Pascal's principle
    2. Archimedes' principle
    3. Surface tension
    4. The second law of thermodynamics
34. Most of the matter in the universe is in a physical state known as
    1. Plasma
    2. Solid
    3. Liquid
    4. Gas
35. Providing an air-conditioned environment (in hot, humid weather) for persons with heart disease is important because
    1. The internal body temperature drops below 37°C.
    2. The heart is relieved of the strain of pumping blood through many miles of blood vessels in the skin
    3. The increased circulation in the skin causes excess body heat to radiate away
    4. The increased circulation in the skin gives the heart the exercise it needs
36. Persons having prolonged anemia or polycythemia may eventually place a strain on their heart. The concept underlying this strain is
    1. Pressure
    2. Surface tension
    3. Viscosity
    4. Temperature
37. The transfer and distribution of thermal energy from molecule to molecule within a body is called
    1. Convection
    2. Radiation
    3. Conduction
    4. Circulation
38. Hot water and detergents are useful cleaning aids primarily because
    1. They melt the dirt away
    2. Greater pressure develops
    3. Dirt is less soluble in hot water having detergents
    4. The surface tension of water becomes lower
39. The transfer of heat in a gas or liquid via currents in the fluid is called
    1. Conduction
    2. Circulation
    3. Radiation
    4. Convection

40. The lack of surfactant in newborn infants results in hyaline membrane disease. The principle underlying the respiratory distress of these infants is
    1. Surface tension
    2. Pascal's principle
    3. Second law of thermodynamics
    4. Archimedes' principle
41. The transfer of energy through electromagnetic waves is called
    1. Radiation
    2. Convection
    3. Circulation
    4. Conduction
42. The pressure volume relationships accounting for the movement of air into and out of the lungs is described by
    1. Charles' law
    2. Boyle's law
    3. Dalton's law
    4. Gay-Lussac's law
43. Steam produces a more damaging burn than water at the same temperature because
    1. Steam contains fewer calories of energy than water at the same temperature
    2. Steam contains more calories of energy than water at the same temperature
    3. Steam absorbs a great deal of energy on condensation
    4. The hot water absorbs a great deal of energy on cooling
44. An autoclave kills microorganisms directly because of
    1. Low volume
    2. High pressure
    3. High temperature
    4. High density
45. The change in state of liquid to a gas is called
    1. Sublimation
    2. Condensation
    3. Evaporation
    4. Regulation
46. Breathing pure oxygen can benefit a person overcome by smoke inhalation since the high partial pressure of oxygen results in greater dissolving of oxygen in the tissues. This is described by
    1. Charles' law
    2. Gay-Lussac's law
    3. Boyle's law
    4. Henry's law
47. The change in state from a vapor to a liquid is called
    1. Evaporation
    2. Sublimation
    3. Regulation
    4. Condensation
48. The unit used to express the quantity of thermal energy in a body is the
    1. Newton
    2. Degree (Celsius or Fahrenheit)
    3. Calorie
    4. Erg
49. The material composing a dental filling should respond to temperature changes by expanding and contracting
    1. To a greater degree than tooth substances
    2. To the same degree as tooth substances
    3. To a lesser degree than tooth substances
    4. As slightly as possible
50. Water is a useful liquid to use in a hot water bottle because water possesses a
    1. High specific heat
    2. High specific gravity
    3. Low specific gravity
    4. Low specific heat
51. The outside surface of many refrigerators is white or silver-metallic because
    1. Radiant energy can be efficiently absorbed
    2. Convection is kept to a minimum
    3. Conduction is maximized
    4. Radiant energy is efficiently reflected
52. Infrared lamps (heat lamps) transfer heat via
    1. Radiation
    2. Diffusion
    3. Convection
    4. Conduction
53. A very faint heartbeat might be detected by placing your ear to someone's chest because sound propagates better through
    1. Solids than through liquids or gases
    2. Liquids than through solids
    3. Gases than through liquids
    4. Gases than through solids
54. If the bell of a stethoscope does not have a diaphragm built into it, then
    1. The stethoscope is broken
    2. No sounds can be heard
    3. The stethoscope is of poor quality
    4. The skin surface acts as the diaphragm
55. Physiologically, the middle ear (containing the 3 ossicles) serves primarily to
    1. Communicate with the throat via the eustachian tube
    2. Amplify the energy of sound waves entering the ear
    3. Translate sound waves into nerve impulses
    4. Maintain one's balance
56. Air conduction type hearing aids would increase hearing sensitivity in cases of
    1. Diminished sensitivity of the cochlea
    2. Perforation of the tympanic membrane
    3. Immobilization of the auditory ossicles
    4. Destruction of the auditory nerve
57. The body fluids are good conductors of electricity because of
    1. Their water content
    2. Their content of ions such as Na^+ and Cl^-
    3. Their content of nonionized molecules such as glucose
    4. Their high concentration of copper and silver atoms
58. Silk or nylon nursing uniforms, rubber soled shoes, and low relative humidity should be avoided in operating rooms because of the hazard of
    1. Electrocution
    2. Magnetism
    3. Static electricity
    4. Current electricity
59. An improperly grounded 110 volt, 60 cycle AC electric fixture may kill you if you are shocked because
    1. The cells of the body die instantly
    2. The brain cells are electrocuted

3. Normal electric patterns in the heart are disrupted
4. Violent muscle spasms destroy the body

60. Thermistor thermometers, high-frequency diathermy, electrocardiography, and electron microscopy are all related in that they require which of the following types of energy to function?
    1. Thermal energy
    2. Sound energy
    3. Electric energy
    4. Light energy

61. The word "ambulance" is oftened printed backward on the front of small ambulances because
    1. A motorist will read the word correctly (and move aside) because of reflection of light through the rearview mirror
    2. The printing of the word backward catches your attention and makes you read it
    3. The printer made a mistake
    4. Federal law requires the word to be printed backward

62. Window shades or venetian blinds reduce harsh "glare." The shades or blinds work because of

1. Interference
2. Polarization of light
3. Refraction of light
4. Scattering and diffusion of light

63. Barium salts in GI series and barium enemas serve to
    1. Give off visible light and illuminate the alimentary tract
    2. Fluoresce and thus illuminate the alimentary tract
    3. Dye the alimentary tract and thus give it color contrast
    4. Absorb x-rays and thus give contrast to the soft tissues of the alimentary tract

64. An individual having thyroid difficulties is being given radioactive iodine internally. Thus the individual is
    1. Not radioactive and can be handled as any other individual
    2. Highly radioactive and should be isolated as much as possible
    3. Mildly radioactive and should be treated with standard precautions
    4. Not radioactive but may still transmit some dangerous radiations and must be treated with precautions

CHAPTER 3

Microbiology

During the past 100 years the science of microbiology has placed valuable tools in the hands of the modern nurse. This material presents the characteristics of microorganisms, their ability to produce disease, and the nature and spread of infection. In a practical sense, it provides the basis for aseptic clinical methods and immunization.

At the end of this review is a list of diseases and their causative agents. Many of these diseases are rather common, while others are exotic; however, today's nurses have had to respond to the mobility of society, which requires a more comprehensive knowledge of all diseases.

DEFINITIONS

A. Microbiology—the branch of biology dealing with microorganisms (microbes)
B. Microorganism—an organism seen or studied only through the microscope; may be unicellular or multicellular
C. Pathogen—any microorganism that can produce disease
D. Parasite—an organism that lives in or on the body of another species (the host) and benefits at the expense of the host
E. Saprophyte—any organism that lives on dead or decaying organic matter; includes some fungi and bacteria

MICROBIAL DISTRIBUTION

A. Normal flora—found within body cells, on glaciers, in hot springs, and wherever life is possible, even in areas devoid of free oxygen
B. Normal flora distribution in the body—microbes normally present on body surfaces and in the oropharynx, nasopharynx, ileum, colon, male urethra, and female vaginal area

MICROBIAL CLASSIFICATION

Modern classification places microbes in the kingdom Protista—the other kingdoms being Plants and Animals
A. Protista—the Kingdom of Microbes
  1. Eucaryota—the subkingdom to which the higher protists belong; higher protists, like all higher forms of life, have cells possessing a nuclear membrane and organelles (those of medical concern are protozoa and fungi)
  2. Procaryota—the subkingdom to which the lower protists belong; the cells of lower protists lack a nuclear membrane and organelles (those of medical concern include bacteria, rickettsiae, chlamydiae, and viruses)
B. Phyla—the major division of a kingdom or subkingdom; in turn, phyla are divided into classes, classes into orders, orders into families, families into genera, and genera into species
C. Nomenclature—every living thing has a 2-part scientific name (binomial nomenclature); the first is the genus, which is capitalized, and the second is the species, which is not capitalized; both names are italicized; e.g., *Clostridium tetani*—the organism causing tetanus

MICROSCOPY

Investigation employing the microscope
A. Compound (light) microscope—consists of a tube, which holds an ocular lens (eye piece) at the top and an objective lens at the other end; a gear mechanism adjusts the tube to proper focus, and

magnification equals the ocular power (usually 10×) × the objective power
B. Darkfield microscope—a compound microscope equipped in such a way that objects and particles with a refractive index different from that of their suspending medium will scatter light and appear bright against the dark background (useful in demonstrating *Treponema pallidum*, the causative organism of syphilis)
C. Fluorescent microscope—utilizes invisible ultraviolet light in conjunction with fluorescent dyes such as auramine
   1. When the dye is combined with bacteria, the bacteria appear as luminous objects
   2. Combining fluorescent dyes with specific antibodies provides rapid identification of certain antigens
D. Phase contrast microscope—a special microscope that alters the phase relationships of the light passing through and around an object
   1. Permits visualization of details beyond the resolution of conventional microscopy
   2. Permits visualization of cell structures without staining, which usually kills the cells and alters cell structures
E. Electron microscope—a class of microscopes using electrons rather than visible light to produce magnified images, especially of objects having dimensions smaller than the wavelengths of visible light, with linear magnifications up to or exceeding 1 million
   1. Transmission electron microscope (TEM)—electron beam is passed through specimen as in light microscopy and is visualized on a fluorescent screen
   2. Scanning electron microscope (SEM)—electron beam made to strike specimen at an angle and the reflected rays visualized as in TEM; image is three-dimensional, with a depth of field well beyond TEM

BACTERIA

A. Definition—bacteria are lower protists, the vast majority of which are unicellular and without chlorophyll
B. Classification—according to *Bergey's Manual of Determinative Bacteria*, ed. 8, the bacteria are divided into 10 major orders (a forthcoming major revision of bacterial taxonomy will place bacteria into 17 parts plus rickettsia and mycoplasmas)
C. Some examples of medically important orders
   1. Eubacteriales ("true bacteria")—typically unicellular microbes having a rigid cell wall; the morphologic types are
      a. Rod-shaped bacilli—variations of the rod shape may be curved or clubbed (some of the gram-positive rods form endospores)
      b. Spherical cocci
      c. Eubacteriales are divided into 5 families based on shape, gram stain, and endospore formation
         (1) Gram-positive cocci include
            (a) Diplococci—occurring predominantly in pairs; e.g., *Diplococcus pneumoniae*
            (b) Streptococci—occurring predominantly in chains; e.g., *Streptococcus pyogenes*
            (c) Staphylococci—occurring predominantly in grapelike bunches; e.g., *Staphylococcus aureus*
         (2) Gram-negative cocci include *Neisseria gonorrhea* and *Neisseria meningitidis*
         (3) Gram-negative rods include enterobacteria such as *Escherichia, Salmonella,* and *Shigella*
         (4) Gram-positive rods that do not produce endospores include *Corynebacterium diphtheriae*
         (5) Gram-positive rods producing endospores include *Bacillus anthracis, Clostridium botulinum, Clostridium tetani*
   2. Actinomycetales (actinomycetes)—moldlike microbes with elongated cells, frequently filamentous; e.g., *Mycobacterium tuberculosis* and *Mycobacterium leprae*
   3. Spirochaetales (spirochetes)—flexuous, spiral organisms; e.g., *Treponema pallidum*
   4. Mycoplasmatales (mycoplasmas)—

delicate, nonmotile microbes displaying a variety of sizes and shapes
  a. Commonly referred to as pleuro-pneumonia-like organisms (PPLO)
  b. Mycoplasmas are the smallest organisms known that are capable of growth and reproduction outside living cells

D. Bacterial cell
  1. Size—from 0.5 mm. to 15 mm.
  2. Cell wall—gram-positive species are rich in muramic acid and low in lipids; the opposite is true of the gram-negative species
  3. Capsule—a thickened protective material (generally a polysaccharide) that is secreted by the cell, thereby protecting it from being phagocytized and increasing its virulence; e.g., *Diplococcus pneumoniae*
  4. Spores—the inactive resistant structures into which bacterial protoplasm can transform under adverse conditions (under favorable conditions a spore germinates into an active and growing vegetative cell)
    a. The endospores are resistant to heat and desiccation
    b. Spore formers *Clostridium tetani* and *Clostridium botulinum* are difficult to destroy; therefore, their destruction is used to set the standards of sterilization for the hospital and food industries
  5. Flagella—organelles of locomotion possessed by all motile bacteria; some species have 1 flagellum (monotrichous) whereas others have flagella over their entire surface (peritrichous)
  6. Reproduction—bacteria reproduce by binary fission, an asexual process dividing the cell into new daughter cells; bacteria are also able to conjugate and exchange genetic material

E. Growth needs
  1. Nutrition
    a. Autotrophic organisms—may do well on simple diet of carbon dioxide, inorganic salts, and water
    b. Heterotrophic organisms—demand organic nutrients
      (1) Saprophytes—derive nourishment from dead or decaying organic matter
      (2) Parasites—derive nourishment from living tissue; obligate parasites cannot be cultured except in living tissue

  2. Culturing
    a. Definitions
      (1) Culture—growth of large numbers of microbes on suitable food media; e.g., broth, agar, milk, etc.
      (2) Culture media—food substances in or on which cultures are grown
      (3) Colony—cluster of millions of microbes, presumably all descendants from single bacterium, visible to naked eye
    b. Types of culture media commonly used
      (1) Liquid—beef broth in tubes or flasks, peptone water
      (2) Solid—beef broth with agar added to cause it to solidify
        (a) Agar broth poured into test tube and allowed to solidify on slant, called agar slant
        (b) Broth poured into Petri dish, called agar plate
        (c) Beef agar inoculated with bacteria before it solidifies, called pour plate
        (d) Beef agar inoculated by streaking after hardened, called streak plate
      (3) Various other substances such as blood, gelatin, and sugars (dextrose, lactose, maltose, etc.) may be added to either liquid or solid culture media
      (4) Living tissue cultures—used to grow rickettsiae and viruses
    c. Special kinds of culture media used
      (1) Selective media—promote growth of one kind of microbe, inhibit growth of others in the same culture; e.g., bile salts added to media permits the growth of enteric organisms while inhibiting other organisms
      (2) Differential media—differentiate certain organisms from others growing in the same culture; e.g., eosin-methylene blue (EMB), an agar differential medium especially valu-

able for helping diagnose intestinal infections (*Escherichia coli* produces a green metallic sheen on EMB agar)

d. Types of cultures
  (1) Classified according to the number of kinds of bacteria
    (a) Pure cultures—contain only one kind of bacteria
    (b) Mixed cultures—contain two or more kinds of bacteria
  (2) Classified according to the species of bacteria; e.g., *Staphylococcus epidermidis* culture, *Bacillus subtilis* culture

e. Ways in which cultures are studied
  (1) Smears made and organisms studied microscopically either with or without staining
  (2) Cultural characteristics observed
    (a) Media most favorable to growth
    (b) Appearance of colonies—the color, shape, and texture, whether large or small, smooth or rough, opaque or translucent
    (c) Molecular oxygen requirement (anaerobic, aerobic, or facultative)

F. Biochemical reactions
  1. Fermentation—anaerobic oxidation reactions by which some organisms use carbohydrates to generate energy-rich adenosine triphosphate (ATP) molecules; various kinds of fermentation reactions are useful for identifying different groups of microorganisms
    a. Nonfermenters
    b. Fermenters that produce only acid
    c. Fermenters that produce acid and gas; e.g., *Escherichia coli*, a normal inhabitant of intestinal tract
    d. Lactose fermenters; e.g., *Escherichia coli* and other nonpathogens in intestinal tract
    e. Nonlactose fermenters; e.g., *Shigella* and *Salmonella* pathogens in intestinal tract
  2. Urea-splitting reaction—identifies organisms as
    a. Urease-positive organisms (contain enzyme urease, which catalyzes conversion of urea to ammonia); e.g., *Proteus bacilli* (gram negative, normal inhabitants of intestinal tract)
    b. Urease-negative organisms—do not contain urease so cannot convert urea to ammonia; e.g., *Salmonella* and *Shigella*, pathogens in intestinal tract

G. Hydrogen ion concentration (pH)—majority of bacteria grow and culture best at a pH of about 7.5; most fungi (molds and yeasts) culture best at a pH of about 5

H. Oxygen utilization
  1. Obligate aerobes—organisms that cannot grow without free (molecular) oxygen
  2. Obligate anaerobes—organisms that cannot grow in the presence of free (molecular) oxygen
  3. Facultative—organisms that can grow with or without free oxygen

I. Temperature
  1. Psychrophiles—organisms growing best at low temperatures (10° to 20° C.; 50° to 68°F.)
  2. Mesophiles—organisms growing best at "middle temperatures" (20° to 45° C.; 68° to 113°F.); this range includes human pathogens that have an optimum temperature of 37°C. or 98.6° F.
  3. Thermophiles—organisms growing best at high temperatures (45° to 65° C.; 113° to 149°F.)

J. Staining—artificial coloration to facilitate visualization and identification of tissues and microorganisms
  1. Gram stain—gram-positive organisms retain the crystal violet color when treated with ethyl alcohol; gram-negative organisms are decolorized with ethyl alcohol
  2. Acid-fast stain—after being stained with carbolfuchsin, acid-fast organisms resist decolorization with dilute acid alcohol and do not take counterstain (usually methylene blue); non-acid-fast organisms decolorize and take counterstain

K. Pathogenicity—some 2000 species of bacteria most of which are harmless; those causing disease (pathogens) are usually heterotrophic mesophiles

RICKETTSIAE

A. Definition—obligate intracellular parasites closely related to gram-negative bacteria; culture only in living tissue
B. Characteristics—rod-shaped microbes with average dimensions of 0.5 mm. by 2 mm.; simpler than bacterial cell; reproduce by binary fission
C. Pathogenicity—with the exception of Q fever can only be transmitted to humans by the bite of an infected louse, flea, tick, or mite

CHLAMYDIAE (BEDSONIAE)

A. Definition—obligate intracellular parasites thought to be distantly related to gram-negative bacteria; culture only in living tissue
B. Characteristics—about 0.3 mm. in diameter; reproduces by a rather complex form of binary fission, and is unable to produce adenosine triphosphate (ATP)
C. Pathogenicity—unlike rickettsiae, chlamydiae are transmitted from one host to another without the intervention of a vector; cause trachoma, psittacosis, lymphogranuloma venerum, as well as other diseases

VIRUSES

Here considered a microbe or protist merely for convenience
A. Definition—obligate intracellular parasite of unknown relationship to other forms of life
B. Characteristics—virions (virus particles)—range in size from 1.0 to 350 nanometers (nm.), which is equal to one billionth of a meter or $\frac{1}{1000}$ of a millimeter; some cuboidal and others rod-shaped; unlike rickettsiae and chlamydiae, composed of either ribonucleic acid (RNA) or deoxyribonucleic acid (DNA), not both
C. Classification
   1. Animal viruses—some contain RNA and others DNA; divided into 14 categories on the basis of particle size, symmetry, and nucleic acid content
   2. Plant viruses—contain RNA
   3. Bacterial viruses—most contain DNA; those that destroy bacterial cells called bacteriophages
D. Culturing—being obligate parasites, viruses demand living tissues such as embryonated hen's eggs, tissue cultures, and animal inoculation
E. Pathogenicity—viruses cause cancer in animals and Burkitt's lymphoma, mumps, rubeola, rubella, smallpox, chickenpox, herpes simplex, encephalitis, yellow fever, and many other infections in humans

FUNGI

A. Definition—higher protists; include morels, truffles, cup fungi, mildews, mushrooms, puffballs, smuts, rusts, molds, and yeasts (molds and yeasts are of medical concern)
B. Molds—fuzzy growths of interlacing filaments called hyphae
   1. Hyphae—filaments of a mold; in some species hyphae divided by partial septa and appear to be multicellular, whereas in others they are nonseptate
   2. Mycelium—a tuft of interwoven hyphae
   3. Spores—means by which molds reproduce; a single spore in the proper environment gives rise to new mycelium; spores produced sexually and asexually
C. Yeasts—organisms that usually are single-celled and usually reproduce by budding
   1. Yeast cell—round or ovoid in shape and much larger and more complex than bacterial cell
   2. Reproduction—usually by the asexual process of budding, but many species also reproduce sexually by means of ascospores
   3. True yeasts—reproduce sexually as well as asexually (by budding); many species, such as *Saccharomyces cerevisiae* (baker's yeast) convert glucose into alcohol and carbon dioxide (alcoholic fermentation); *Candida albicans,* another type of yeast, causes "thrush" in humans (this yeast is part of the normal flora but may become an opportunistic pathogen in persons with low resistance)
   4. Pathogenicity—certain species of molds cause infection, particularly those belonging to the class Fungi Imperfecti (Deuteromycetes), which account for diseases such as athlete's foot, ringworm of the scalp and axillary regions, and systemic mycosis

PROTOZOA

A. Definition—unicellular animals or animal-like microbes (higher protists) comprising phylum Protozoa; most are free living but other species may be parasitic to animals and humans

B. Characteristics—typically large, mobile, and of various shapes; complex internal structure and said to be the most advanced form of the one-celled state; certain species exist in either active (trophozoite) stage or resistant (cyst) stage, depending on conditions

C. Reproduction—sexual (by conjugation) and asexual (by binary fission)

D. Classification
   1. Sarcodina (Rhizopoda)—movement by means of pseudopodia (*Entamoeba histolytica*)
   2. Flagellata (Mastigophora)—movement by means of flagella (*Trypanosoma, Trichomonas vaginalis, Giardia intestinalis*)
   3. Ciliatia (Infusoria)—movement by means of cilia (*Balantidium coli*)
   4. Sporozoa—all parasitic; reproduce by sporulation (*Plasmodium,* causative agent of malaria)

METAZOANS

A. Definition—multicellular animals (helminths and ectoparasites are of medical concern)

B. Helminths—parasitic worms that fall into three categories: nematodes, cestodes, and trematodes
   1. Nematodes (roundworms)—animal phylum Aschelminthes
      a. Characteristics—elongated cylindrical body, usually pointed at both ends; vary in length from less than 1 inch to several inches; includes trichinella, pinworms, and hookworms
      b. Life cycle—example: the roundworm (*Ascaris lumbricoides*) lives in the intestine of humans (the host); female lays eggs (ova), which escape in the feces and gain entrance into new host via food or water; ova liberate larvae, the latter entering the blood and in turn the lungs; from lungs larvae travel up the trachea, down the esophagus, and back into the intestine where they develop into adult worms
   2. Cestodes (tapeworms)—animal phylum Platyhelminthes
      a. Characteristics—ribbonlike intestinal worms ranging from 6 to 30 feet in length in humans; head (scolex) equipped with suckers and/or hooklets; body divided into segments (proglottids); each structurally and functionally autonomous
      b. Life cycle—example: beef tapeworm (*Taenia saginata*); adult worm (in intestine) releases fertile eggs that contaminate soil and water; cattle (intermediate host) ingest eggs, which then develop and enter muscle and other tissue forming cysticerci; the tissue is ingested by humans (definitive host); scolices are set free and hook into intestinal lining where they produce an adult tapeworm generation; pigs and fish may also serve as intermediate hosts for tapeworms
   3. Trematodes (flukes)—unsegmented flatworms
      a. Characteristics—have suckers or hooklets for anchoring themselves to host
      b. Life cycle—complex with sexual and asexual generations; generally 2 or more hosts are involved; typical cycle: fertile eggs passed by host (in feces or urine) and develop into ciliated miracidia, which, in presence of water, swim about and enter a certain species of snail; in the snail, miracidia eventually develop into cercariae, which are released into the water and eventually enter the definitive host; important Trematode parasites of humans are the blood flukes (*Schistosoma*) and the liver fluke (*Clonorchis*)

C. Ectoparasites—parasites living on the exterior surface of another organism such as lice, mites, fleas, and ticks
   1. Mites—members of the order Acarina (phylum Arachnida); parasitic on humans and domestic animals; cause scabies and transmit rickettsial diseases
   2. Lice—insects of the suborder Anoplura (phylum Insecta); parasitic on humans and animals; certain species serve as vectors of disease such as

epidemic typhus; eggs of lice are recognized as "nits," which are attached to hairs

3. Fleas—insects of the order Siphonaptera; many parasitic and may serve as vectors of disease such as endemic typhus and bubonic plague

4. Ticks—members of the order Acarina; parasites on wild and domestic animals; responsible for the transmission of the various forms of spotted fever

MICROBIAL CONTROL

A. Definitions
   1. Disinfection—the removal of or destruction of pathogenic microbes
   2. Sterilization—the removal or destruction of all microbes
B. Physical methods
   1. Heat sterilization
      a. Moist heat
         (1) Steam under pressure (autoclave)—usually operated at 121°C. (250°F.) (15 lb. pressure per square inch); time needed for procedure depends on material(s) being sterilized
         (2) Boiling water—object(s) to be sterilized immersed in water and boiled for 15 minutes; because some spores resist boiling, procedure not suitable for surgical instruments
      b. Dry heat (hot-air oven)
         (1) Operating temperature—160° to 170°C. (310° to 338°F.) (usually for 2 hours)
         (2) Items sterilized—petrolatum gauze dressings and other items that might be damaged by steam or water
      c. Pasteurization—the disinfection of milk and other substances by use of moderate heat; pathogenic organisms killed and microbial development considerably delayed (thus retarding spoilage)
         (1) Holding method—heating to 63°C. (145°F.) for 30 minutes, followed by rapid cooling
         (2) Flash method—heating to 71.7°C. (161°F.) for not less than 15 seconds, followed by rapid cooling
   2. Radiation—all types of radiation injurious to microbes

      a. Gamma rays—used to sterilize food and drugs
      b. Ultraviolet light—used to inhibit microbial population of air in operating rooms, nurseries, laboratories, school rooms, and food establishments (the disadvantage of ultraviolet light is that it has little penetration power)
   3. Filtration—removal of microbes from liquids by means of porous materials (diatomaceous earth, asbestos, porcelain); used to sterilize drugs, culture media, and certain other heat-sensitive substances
   4. Refrigeration—low temperature inhibits microbial multiplication; used for food preservation
   5. Hypertonicity—by their osmotic effects hypertonic solutions inhibit microbial multiplication; e.g., brine and syrups
   6. Desiccation (drying)—removal of water; bacterial spores and certain vegetable cells resistant to such treatment; commonly used in food preservation
C. Chemical agents (for body surfaces and inanimate objects)
   1. Definitions—many terms used to describe action of chemical agents on microorganisms; in actual practice such terms often have little meaning because of variables
      a. Antiseptic—inhibits microbial growth
      b. Disinfectant—destroys pathogenic microbes
      c. Germicide—destroys pathogenic microbes
      d. Bactericide—destroys bacteria
      e. Fungicide—destroys fungi
      f. Virucide—destroys viruses
   2. Conditions (variables) affecting action of chemical agents
      a. Types and number of microbes—microbes respond differently to different agents; spores are resistant to most agents
      b. Concentration—typically the greater the concentration of chemical, the greater the effect
      c. Time—a certain time needed for maximum effect
      d. Temperature—a rise usually hastens action
      e. Organic matter—presence inhibits action

3. Evaluation—various tests used to evaluate antiseptics and disinfectants; all have limitations
   a. Phenol coefficient—bactericidal activity of a chemical agent in relation to the bactericidal action of phenol
   b. Culture inhibition—filter paper disks impregnated or saturated with chemical agent placed on agar plates previously inoculated with test organism; clear zone observed around disk (following incubation) if agent is inhibitory to organism (this is the same procedure used in determining the sensitivity of a culture to chemotherapeutic agents)
4. Commonly used chemical agents
   a. Ethyl alcohol (70%)
   b. Isopropyl alcohol (80%)
   c. Zephiran (1:1000)
   d. Hydrogen peroxide (3%)
   e. Silver nitrate (1%)
   f. Iodine and iodine-releasing compounds
   g. Chlorine and chlorine-releasing compounds
   h. Substituted phenols
   i. Cresols
   j. Ethylene oxide
D. Chemotherapy—the systemic use of chemical agents (anti-infectives) in the treatment of infection
   1. Anti-infectives (major classes) (see Pharmacology, p. 243)
      a. Antibiotics (p. 243)
      b. Sulfonamides (p. 245)
      c. Anthelmintics (p. 250)
      d. Antiprotozoals (p. 248)
      e. Tuberculostatics (p. 247)
   2. Antibiotic sensitivity—determined by 2 general techniques
      a. Paper disks—multilobed disk impregnated with different antibiotics placed on surface of inoculated plate; zones of inhibition (following incubation) surround lobes containing antibiotics to which microbe is sensitive
      b. Tube dilution—antibiotic in question diluted out in growth broth and tubes then inoculated with the organisms in question; minimal inhibitory concentration (MIC) determined (following incubation) by

noting minimal concentration preventing growth

INFECTION

A. Definitions
   1. Infection (or infectious disease)—invasion of the body by pathogenic microorganisms (pathogens) and the reaction of the tissues to their presence and to the toxins generated by them
   2. Communicable disease—an infectious disease caused by a pathogen that may pass from one person to another directly or indirectly
   3. Contagious disease—a term usually used to indicate an infectious disease that is spread easily and directly from one person to another
   4. Incubation period—the period of time between the infection of a susceptible person or animal and the moment of entrance of the infecting microbe into the body to the first appearance of signs or symptoms of the disease in question
B. Occurrence
   1. Endemic—disease constantly present in a given locality
   2. Epidemic—the occurrence of a disease clearly in excess of normal expectancy in a community or region
   3. Pandemic—a widespread or worldwide epidemic
   4. Sporadic—an occasional occurrence of a disease
C. Types
   1. Local, focal, or systemic
      a. Local infection—one in which etiologic agent is limited to one locality of the body such as a boil; often a local infection may have systemic repercussions such as fever and malaise
      b. Focal infection—a local infection such as an abscess from which the organisms themselves spread to other parts of body; e.g., a tooth abscess that continues to seed organisms into blood
      c. Systemic infection—one in which the infectious agent is spread throughout the body; e.g., typhoid fever
   2. Acute or chronic
      a. Acute infection—one that develops

rapidly, usually resulting in a high fever and severe sickness
   b. Chronic infection—one that develops slowly, with mild but longer-lasting symptoms; sometimes an acute infection may become chronic and vice versa
3. Primary or secondary
   a. Primary infection—the initial infection unrelated to other health problems
   b. Secondary infection—an infection occasioned when invaders (or opportunists) take advantage of the weakened defenses resulting from the primary infection; e.g., staphylococcal pneumonia as a sequela of measles or pneumonia
4. Bacteremia—the presence of nonmultiplying bacteria in the blood
5. Septicemia—bacterial cells actively multiplying in the blood
6. Toxemia—the presence of microbial toxins in the blood
7. Viremia—the presence of viruses in the blood
D. Proof of etiology (Koch's postulates)—4 requirements must be fulfilled to establish a given microbe as the etiologic agent of a given disease
   1. Particular microbe must be found in every case of the particular disease
   2. Particular microbe must be isolated and grown in pure culture
   3. Particular microbe must cause particular disease when inoculated into susceptible animal
   4. Particular microbe must be recovered from inoculated animal and its identity established
E. Source and transmission of pathogens
   1. Source—ultimate source (or reservoir) of almost all pathogens are humans or animals; human sources include:
   a. Persons exhibiting symptoms of disease
   b. Carriers—persons who harbor a pathogen in the absence of a discernible clinical disease
      (1) Types of carriers
         (a) Healthy carriers—those who never had the disease in question
         (b) Incubatory carriers—those in the incubation period of a disease

(c) Chronic carriers—those who have recovered from a disease but continue to harbor pathogen
      (2) Diseases commonly spread by carriers
         (a) Typhoid fever
         (b) Diphtheria
         (c) Meningitis
         (d) Pneumonia
         (e) Dysentery
   2. Transmission
   a. Direct
      (1) Body contact
      (2) Droplets (droplet infection)
   b. Indirect
      (1) Food
      (2) Water
      (3) Air
      (4) Soil
      (5) Fomites
      (6) Vectors (insects)
         (a) Mechanical transfer—insects' feet
         (b) Biologic transfer—microbe undergoes part of its life cycle in insect's body
   3. Portals of entry and exit
   a. Portal of entry—where microbe enters body
      (1) Nose
      (2) Mouth
      (3) Urogenital tract
      (4) Skin: wounds, abrasions, and insect bites
   b. Portal of exit—where microbe leaves body
      (1) Nose
      (2) Mouth
      (3) Feces
      (4) Urine
      (5) Vaginal discharges
      (6) Pus and exudates
      (7) Vomitus
      (8) Blood
F. Development
   1. Definitions
   a. Pathogenicity—the ability of a microbe to cause disease
   b. Virulence—the degree of pathogenicity
   2. Determinants of pathogenicity
   a. Chemical products
      (1) Exotoxins—heat-labile proteins readily released from

bacterial cell; most deadly of all biologic poisons; e.g., botulism, tetanus, and diphtheria

(2) Endotoxins—heat-stable lipo-polysaccharide-protein complexes released from gram-negative bacteria; less deadly than exotoxins; e.g., typhoid fever and dysentery

(3) Other toxic products
    (a) Hemolysins—destroy red cells
    (b) Leukocidins—destroy white cells
    (c) Coagulase—clots blood plasma
    (d) Hyaluronidase—dissolves intercellular cement
    (e) Kinases—dissolve clots or inhibit their formation
    (f) Collagenase—disintegrates collagen

b. Cellular destruction—some microbes damage tissues and cause disease by direct mechanical injury to the cells, particularly intracellular parasites; e.g., viruses and rickettsiae

c. Capsules—increase virulence apparently by making microbes possessing them less vulnerable to destruction by phagocytosis

G. Resistance
  1. Nonspecific—resistance directed against all invading microbes; varies considerably from one species to another and even among individuals of same species
    a. Body surface barriers
      (1) Intact skin and mucosa
      (2) Cilia and secretion of mucus
    b. Antimicrobial secretions
      (1) Oil of skin—contains fatty acids effective against many bacteria and fungi
      (2) Tears—contain lysozyme, a bactericidal (gram-positive) enzyme
      (3) Gastric juice—contains highly bactericidal hydrochloric acid
      (4) Vaginal secretions—low pH acts to inhibit microbial growth
    c. Internal antimicrobial agents

(1) Interferon—an antiviral substance produced within the cells in response to a viral attack; it inhibits viral growth and multiplication

(2) Properdin—a protein agent in blood that destroys certain gram-negative bacteria and viruses

(3) Lysozyme—ubiquitous; destroys mainly gram-positive bacteria

d. Phagocytosis—part of the role of the reticuloendothelial system
  (1) Phagocytes—cells that ingest and destroy microbes
    (a) Microphages—the polymorphonuclear leukocytes of the blood, of which the neutrophils are the most active; in the inflammatory response they pass through the intact capillary wall (diapedesis) into the intercellular area
    (b) Macrophages
      (1) Fixed (or sessile) macrophages— phagocytes lining the capillary endothelium and sinuses of liver (Kupffer's cells), spleen, bone marrow, lymph nodes, and other organs where they remove microbes from the blood
      (2) Wandering macrophages (histiocytes) —blood monocytes that enter the tissues (via diapedesis) and devour intercellular debris, including debilitated microphages

2. Specific resistance—resistance directed against a specific pathogen (foreign protein) or its toxin
  a. Antigen—any substance, including allergens, that stimulates the production of antibodies when introduced into the body; typically antigens are foreign proteins, the

most potent being microbial cells and their products

(1) Plasma cells—the antibody-producing cells that arise from B lymphocytes in the presence of antigens; a specific antigen provokes the production of a specific antibody (homologous antibody), which is considered to be ineffective against any other antigen

(2) Memory cells—a large population of antibodies that develop upon first encounter with an antigen; they become somewhat dormant until stimulated by subsequent encounters with the antigen; this phenomenon explains the dramatic rise in antibody titer following a booster shot of a vaccine (anamnestic reaction)

b. Antibody—an immune substance produced by plasma cells; antibodies are gamma globulin molecules and are commonly referred to as immunoglobulin (Ig)

(1) Chemical structure—the antibody molecule is made up of 4 polypeptide chains in 2 pairs

(2) Classification—there are 5 major classes of antibodies

(a) Immunoglobulin G (IgG) antibodies—most important class making up more than 80% of the total immunoglobulins; only immunoglobulin that passes the placental barrier providing natural passive immunity to the newborn

(b) Immunoglobulin A (IgA) antibodies—present in blood, mucus, and human milk secretions; play an important role against respiratory pathogens

(c) Immunoglobulin M (IgM) antibodies—the first antibodies to be detected after an injection of antigen; bactericidal for gram-negative bacteria under specific conditions

(d) Immunoglobulin D (IgD) antibodies—present in small numbers in normal individuals; specific immunologic role presently under investigation

(e) Immunoglobulin E (IgE) antibodies—responsible for hypersensitivity and allergies; these antibodies exist tightly bound to the surface of mast cells (large basophilic connective tissue cells)

(1) Upon introduction of their homologous antigens (allergens), they cause the mast cells to release histamine and other pharmacologic agents

(2) The release of histamine and other pharmacologic agents causes the symptoms of hypersensitive reactions

(3) This process explains the relief of symptoms by the administration of antihistamines

c. Antigen-antibody reactions

(1) Agglutination—the clumping together of cells and specific antigens by homologous antibodies called agglutinins

(2) Cytolysis—the disruption or dissolution of cells (lysis) by homologous antibodies called cytolysins or lysins

(3) Opsonification—the rendering of bacteria and other cells susceptible to phagocytosis by homologous antibodies called opsonins

(4) Neutralization (viral)—the rendering of viruses noninfective by homologous antibodies called neutralizing antibodies

(5) Neutralization (toxin)—the chemical neutralization of a toxin by homologous antibodies called antitoxins

(6) Precipitation—the formation of an insoluble complex (precipitate) in the reaction between a soluble antigen and its homologous antibodies called precipitins

d. Complement-fixation—a group of blood serum proteins needed in certain antigen-antibody reactions; both the complement and the antibody must be present for a reaction to occur

H. Immunity
1. Species immunity—certain species are naturally immune to specific microorganisms; e.g., humans are immune to distemper, dogs are immune to measles
2. Active immunity—antibodies formed in the body
   a. Natural active immunity—antibodies formed by the individual during the course of the disease; in some instances the antibodies provide lifelong immunity; e.g., measles, chickenpox, yellow fever, smallpox
   b. Artificial active immunity—the use of a vaccine or toxoid to stimulate the formation of homologous antibodies; revaccination (booster shots) are often needed to sustain antibody titer (anamnestic effect)
      (1) Killed vaccines—antigenic preparations containing microbes grown in the laboratory separated from growth medium and killed by heat or a chemical agent; usually injected subcutaneously; less often given by intramuscular or oral routes; e.g., pertussis vaccine, typhoid vaccine
      (2) Live vaccines—antigenic preparations containing microbes weakened (attenuated) by drying, continued and prolonged passage through culture media or animals (to induce mutations), or by other means; typically such vaccines are more antigenic than killed preparations; e.g., oral (Sabin) poliomyelitis vaccine, measles vaccine
      (3) Toxoids—antigenic preparations composed of inactivated bacterial toxins (generally an exotoxin treated with formaldehyde); e.g., tetanus, diphtheria toxoids

3. Passive immunity—antibodies acquired from an outside source
   a. Natural passive immunity—the passage of preformed antibodies from mother through the placenta or colostrum to the baby; therefore, during the first few weeks of life the newborn is immune to certain diseases to which the mother has active immunity
   b. Artificial passive immunity—the injection of antisera derived from immunized animals or humans; antisera (antiserums) provide immediate and often complete protection in susceptible exposed persons and also are of value in treatment; e.g., diphtheria antitoxin, tetanus antitoxin (individuals may be hypersensitive to certain sera such as horse serum and pretesting for hypersensitivity must be carried out before administration)

I. Diagnosis—made on the basis of signs and symptoms, skin tests, and/or laboratory findings
1. Signs and symptoms—certain infections, especially those of childhood, made almost exclusively on the basis of signs and symptoms; e.g., measles, mumps, chickenpox
2. Skin tests—in certain infections the individual becomes hypersensitive to the microbe or its toxin and develops an area of redness (positive reaction) at the site of its injection; e.g., persons showing a positive reaction to tuberculin either currently have tuberculosis or have been infected in the past
3. Laboratory findings
   a. Isolation or demonstration of pathogen in a suitable specimen such as pus or blood
   b. Serology—the demonstration of tell-tale antibodies in blood serum

via antigen-antibody reactions; the presence of antibody indicates either infection or previous contact with pathogen

(1) Specific agglutination tests—known antigen (agglutinogen) is used to demonstrate the presence of homologous antibody (agglutinin); the reciprocal of the highest dilution of the serum sample showing agglutination is referred to as the titer, a rising titer indicating infection; e.g., diagnosis of typhoid fever using the pathogen *Salmonella typhosa* as the test antigen (Widal test)

(2) Nonspecific agglutination tests (heterophil tests)—in some infections antibodies arise that cause the agglutination of unrelated (heterophil) antigens; e.g., antibodies associated with rickettsial infections agglutinate *Proteus* group bacteria (Weil-Felix reaction) and the antibody of infectious mononucleosis agglutinates the red blood cells of sheep (Paul-Bunnell test)

(3) Precipitation tests—known soluble antigen (precipitinogen) is used to demonstrate the presence of antibody (precipitin), a rising titer indicating infection

(4) Flocculation tests—the use of appropriate antigen (in the colloidal state) to demonstrate presence of antibody by means of flocculation (the coalescence of colloidal particles); e.g., the VDRL test for syphilis

(5) Complement-fixation tests—known antigen and a known amount of complement demonstrate the presence of homologous antibody in a number of infections; e.g., syphilis, pertussis, histoplasmosis; the test is based on the fact that complement becomes "fixed" or used up in the presence of homologous antibody

(6) Fluorescent antibody tests—antihuman antibody, obtained from animals that have been injected with human immunoglobulin, is made fluorescent by reaction with a fluorescent dye and used as a "tag" to identify the presence of antibodies under fluorescent light

(7) Neutralization tests—known viruses used to demonstrate the presence of neutralizing antibodies

(a) Hemagglutination inhibition tests—red blood cells and known hemagglutinating viruses (those causing red cells to agglutinate) are used to demonstrate presence of antibody against the test virus

(b) Pathogenic inhibition tests—known viruses are treated with patient's blood serum and then inoculated into appropriate animal or tissue culture

MAJOR PATHOGENS

A. Bacterial pathogens

1. *Actinomyces*—*Actinomyces bovis* and *Actinomyces israelii* (considered by some to be identical) are anaerobic, gram-positive actinomycetes; they cause actinomycosis (lumpy jaw)

2. *Bacillus anthracis*—large, aerobic, gram-positive, spore-forming bacillus; causes anthrax, primarily a disease of sheep and cattle; humans become infected through the skin by contact with hides of infected animals

3. *Brucella*—*Brucella abortus*, *Brucella suis*, and *Brucella melitensis* are small, gram-negative bacilli that are somewhat pleomorphic (variable in shape); they cause brucellosis, an infection primarily of domestic animals (cattle, goats, swine, sheep), which humans acquire by drinking infected milk

4. *Bordetella pertussis*—small, gram-negative coccobacillus; causes pertussis or whooping cough

5. *Borrelia vincentii*—an actively motile, anaerobic spirochete believed to func-

tion in consort with *Fusobacterium fusiforme* (and perhaps other bacteria) to produce fusospirochetal disease commonly referred to as Vincent's angina or trenchmouth

6. *Clostridium tetani*—large, gram-positive, motile bacillus forming large terminal spores; like all clostridia, it is an obligate anaerobe; causes tetanus (lockjaw)

7. *Clostridium perfringens*—gram-positive, anaerobic, motile, spore-forming bacillus; the most common cause of gas gangrene

8. *Clostridium botulinum*—a large, gram-positive bacillus; an obligate anaerobe; its exotoxin, the most powerful biologic toxin known, is responsible for botulism (the most serious, often fatal, form of food poisoning)

9. *Corynebacterium diphtheriae* (Klebs-Löffler bacillus)—gram-positive, non-spore-forming, nonmotile, pleomorphic bacillus; causes diphtheria

10. *Diplococcus pneumoniae*—gram-positive, encapsulated diplococcus; on the basis of the antigenic nature of the capsule there are about 100 types, the most important being Types I, II, and III; causes pneumococcal pneumonia (most commonly lobar) and often responsible for sinusitis, otitis media, and meningitis

11. *Escherichia coli*—small, gram-negative bacillus composing the major portion of the normal flora of the large intestine; certain strains are the most common cause of urinary tract infections and infantile diarrhea

12. *Enterobacter aerogenes*—small, gram-negative bacillus (morphologically indistinguishable from *Escherichia coli*); causes urinary tract infections

13. *Hemophilus influenzae*—small, gram-negative, highly pleomorphic bacillus; causes acute meningitis and upper respiratory infections

14. *Hemophilus aegyptius* (Koch-Weeks bacillus)—indistinguishable morphologically from *Hemophilus influenzae*; causes a common conjunctivitis called pinkeye

15. *Hemophilus ducreyi*—morphologically indistinguishable from *H. influenzae* and *H. aegyptius;* causes the venereal ulcer called chancroid (soft chancre)

16. *Klebsiella pneumoniae (Friedländer's bacillus)*—gram-negative, encapsulated, nonspore-forming bacillus; causes pneumonia and urinary tract infections

17. *Leptospira icterohaemorrhagiae*—long, tightly-coiled spirochete similar in appearance to *Treponema pallidum;* causes infectious jaundice (Weil's disease)

18. *Mima polymorpha*—short, gram-negative rod with bipolar staining resembling the *Neisseria;* infections of polymorpha may be confused with *Neisseria* infections; causes many (nosocomial) infections

19. *Mycobacterium tuberculosis* (tubercle bacillus)—acid-fast actinomycete (thin, waxy rods, often bent, nonmotile, nonspore forming) causes tuberculosis

20. *Mycobacterium leprae* (Hansen's bacillus)—acid-fast actinomycete very similar to *M. tuberculosis;* causes leprosy

21. *Neisseria gonorrhoeae*—gram-negative diplococcus; causes gonorrhea

22. *Neisseria meningitidis*—gram-negative diplococcus; causes epidemic (meningococcic) meningitis

23. *Pasteurella pestis*—a small gram-negative pleomorphic coccobacillus; causes bubonic plague

24. *Pasteurella tularensis (Francisella tularensis)*—a short, gram-negative, highly pleomorphic bacillus; causes tularemia (rabbit fever)

25. *Pseudomonas aeruginosa*—gram-negative, motile bacillus; a common secondary invader of wounds, burns, outer ear, and urinary tract; the infection characterized by blue-green pus; may be transmitted by catheters and other hospital instruments

26. *Salmonella typhosa*—gram-negative, motile bacillus, morphologically indistinguishable from the normal flora of large intestine; causes typhoid fever

27. *Salmonella paratyphi* A, B, and C—gram-negative bacilli morphologically indistinguishable from *S. typhosa;* causes paratyphoid fever

28. *Salmonella*—a great many species of *Salmonella* cause a local gastrointestinal infection in which organisms do

not enter blood (unlike S. *typhosa* and S. *paratyphi*); such infections are referred to as salmonellosis or salmonella food poisoning

29. *Shigella*—gram-negative bacilli, similar to *Salmonella; Shigella dysenteriae* and a number of other species cause an illness known as bacillary dysentery, dysentery, or shigellosis

30. *Staphylococcus aureus*—gram-positive staphylococcus strain, which clots plasma (coagulase positive), is the most virulent; causes a variety of infections; e.g., boils, carbuncles, impetigo, osteomyelitis, staphylococcus pneumonia, and staphylococcus food poisoning

31. *Streptococcus pyogenes*—a gram-positive streptococcus; the most virulent strain (Group A beta hemolytic streptococci) causes scarlet fever, septic sore throat, tonsillitis, cellulitis, puerperal fever, erysipelas, rheumatic fever, and glomerulonephritis

32. *Streptococcus viridans*—gram-positive streptococcus; distinguishable from S. *pyogenes* by its alpha hemolysis (rather than beta) of red blood cells; the most common cause of subacute bacterial endocarditis

33. *Spirillum minus*—gram-negative, highly motile spirillum; causative agent of sodoku rat-bite fever

34. *Streptobacillus moniliformis*—gram-negative, highly pleomorphic bacillus; a common parasite of rats and mice; causes a rat-bite fever (Haverhill fever)

35. *Treponema pallidum*—a long, slender, highly motile spirochete; causes syphilis

36. *Treponema pertenue*—very similar to T. *pallidum;* causes yaws

37. *Vibrio cholerae* (formerly V. *comma*) —curved, gram-negative bacillus with a single polar flagellum; causes Asiatic cholera

B. Rickettsial pathogens
  1. *Coxiella burnetii*—the only species of rickettsiae not associated with a vector; causes Q fever, an infection clinically similar to primary atypical pneumonia
  2. *Rickettsia prowazekii*—causes epidemic typhus fever; human louse serves as vector
  3. *Rickettsia quintana*—causes trench fever; louse serves as vector
  4. *Rickettsia rickettsii*—causes Rocky Mountain spotted fever; in the western part of the country the wood tick serves as vector and in the eastern part, the dog tick
  5. *Rickettsia tsutsugamushi*—causes scrub typhus; mite serves as vector
  6. *Rickettsia typhi (mooseri)*—causes endemic (or murine) typhus; rat serves as primary reservoir and rat flea serves as vector

C. Chlamydial pathogens (now considered distinct from rickettsiae and viruses) infect the eye (trachoma and inclusion conjunctivitis), the genitals (lymphogranuloma venereum), and the lung (psittacosis, ornithosis)

D. Viral pathogens
  1. DNA viruses
     a. Adenoviruses—spherical in shape and 70 to 80 nm. in diameter; cause acute respiratory disease, adenoidal-pharyngeal conjunctivitis, and other respiratory infections
     b. Herpesviruses—spherical in shape and 150 to 200 nm. in diameter; cause herpes simplex, varicella (chickenpox), herpes zoster (shingles), infectious mononucleosis, and cytomegalic inclusion disease
     c. Papovaviruses—spherical and 45 to 55 nm. in diameter; cause warts in humans and various tumors in animals
     d. Poxviruses—brick-shaped virions (100 × 200 × 300 nm.); cause smallpox (variola) and molluscum contagiosum in humans and various infections in animals
  2. RNA viruses
     a. Coronaviruses—enveloped pleomorphic viruses; frequently associated with a mild upper respiratory infection
     b. Myxoviruses—spherical or filamentous and 80 to 120 nm. in greatest dimension; causes influenza in humans and animals
     c. Paramyxoviruses—spherical or filamentous and 100 to 300 nm. in greatest dimension; cause mumps and rubeola (measles) and a number of infections in animals
     d. Picornaviruses—spherical in shape

and 20 to 30 nm. in diameter; cause poliomyelitis, Coxsackie disease, common cold, and various diseases of animals

e. Reoviruses—double stranded RNA virus involved in mild respiratory infections of humans

f. Rhabdoviruses—large bullet-shaped viruses; rabies virus is a member of this group

g. Togaviruses—spherical in shape and 40 to 60 nm. in diameter; mostly borne by mosquitoes and ticks; cause eastern equine encephalomyelitis, western equine encephalomyelitis, Venezuelan equine encephalomyelitis, and a number of other infections

E. Fungal pathogens

1. Dermatophytes—fungi infecting the skin, hair, and nails; such infections are collectively referred to as dermatomycoses or dermatophytoses

   a. *Epidermophyton*—cause tinea pedis (athlete's foot) and tinea unguium (ringworm of nails)

   b. *Malassezia furfur*—causes ringworm of the neck, trunk, and arms

   c. *Microsporum*—causes tinea capitis (ringworm of scalp)

   d. *Trichophyton*—causes tinea pedis (athlete's foot), tinea unguium (ringworm of nails), and tinea capitis (ringworm of scalp)

2. Systemic fungi—pathogenic fungi involving deeper structures of the body

   a. *Blastomyces dermatitidis*—dimorphic yeastlike fungus; causes North American blastomycosis (an infection marked by ulceration of the skin and abscesses throughout the body)

   b. *Candida albicans* (formerly *Monilia albicans*)—pathogenic yeast; may infect various body areas, including the skin, mouth, vagina, and lungs; such infections generally referred to as candidiasis, moniliasis

   c. *Coccidioides immitis*—dimorphic fungus, growing as a yeast in tissues and as a mold on artificial media; causes acute coccidioidomycosis (a respiratory disease) and chronic coccidioidomycosis (a progressive disease involving any organ of the body)

   d. *Cryptococcus neoformans*—pathogenic yeast with a characteristic large capsule around the cell; causes cryptococcosis (torulosis, European blastomycosis), a serious infection involving the lungs and central nervous system

   e. *Histoplasma capsulatum*—dimorphic fungus producing characteristic spores (chlamydospores) in infected tissue; causes histoplasmosis (a primary lung infection)

   f. *Sporotrichum schenckii*—dimorphic fungus, appearing in infected tissues as cigar-shaped yeast cells that reproduce by budding; causes sporotrichosis (usually marked by necrotic ulceration of the skin)

F. Protozoal pathogens

1. *Balantidium coli*—ciliated protozoan; causes enteritis

2. *Entamoeba histolytica*—an ameba; causes amebiasis (amebic dysentery)

3. *Giardia lamblia*—flagellated protozoan; causes enteritis

4. *Leishmania donovani*—flagellated protozoan; causes kala azar; transmitted by sand flies

5. *Plasmodium*—sporozoans (motile in immature forms and nonmotile in mature forms); *P. vivax, P. ovale, P. malariae,* and *P. falciparum* cause malaria; transmitted by female anopheles mosquito

6. *Toxoplasma gondii*—sporozoan; causes toxoplasmosis

7. *Trichomonas vaginalis*—flagellated protozoan; causes trichomonas vaginitis (a venereal disease)

8. *Trypanosoma*—flagellated ribbonlike protozoa; *T. gambienese* and *T. rhodesiense* cause African sleeping sickness (transmitted by tsetse flies) and *T. cruzi* causes South American trypanosomiasis or Chagas' disease (transmitted by reduviid bugs)

G. Parasitic pathogens

1. Nematodes (roundworms)

   a. *Ancylostoma duodenale* (hookworm)—intestinal parasite very similar to *Necator americanus*

   b. *Ascaris lumbricoides* (roundworm)—intestinal parasite very much resembling the earthworm

   c. *Enterobius vermicularis* (pinworm, seatworm)—small, white parasitic worm found in the upper part of the large intestine; the female lays eggs in perianal area causing irritation

d. *Loa loa*—a threadlike worm; infests subcutaneous tissues, especially about the eye

e. *Necator americanus* (American hookworm)—intestinal parasite about ½ inch in length

f. *Onchocerca volvulus*—a type of filarial worm; causes onchocerciasis (subcutaneous nodules on the head)

g. *Trichinella spiralis*—one of smallest parasitic nematodes (about 1.5 mm. in length), causes trichinosis (muscle infestation with trichina)

h. *Trichuris trichiura* (whipworm)—intestinal parasite about 2 inches in length

i. *Wuchereria bancrofti*—a white threadlike worm; causes filariasis (elephantiasis)

2. Cestodes (tapeworm)

a. *Diphyllobothrium latum* (fish tapeworm)—large tapeworm (about 20 feet in length) found in adult form in the intestine of cats, dogs, and humans (vertebrate and aquatic hosts in sequence)

b. *Echinococcus granulosa* (dog tapeworm)—small tapeworm of dogs; larval stage (hydatid) may develop in humans forming hydatid tumors or cysts in the liver, lungs, kidneys, and other organs

c. *Hymenolepsis nana* (dwarf tapeworm)—a species about 1 inch in length; found in the adult form in the intestine

d. *Taenia marginata* (beef tapeworm)—the common tapeworm of humans, a species from 12 to 25 feet in length, found in the adult form in the human intestine

e. *Taenia solium* (pork tapeworm)—a species 3 to 6 feet in length, found in the adult form in the intestine of humans

3. Trematodes (flukes)

a. *Clonorchis sinensis*—one of the most common liver flukes, especially in China and Japan

b. *Fasciola hepatica*—the common liver fluke of herbivorous animals; occasionally found in the human liver

c. *Fasciolopsis buski*—the largest of the intestinal flukes

d. *Paragonimus westermani*—the lung fluke; found in cysts in the lungs, liver, abdominal cavity, and elsewhere

e. *Schistosoma*—blood flukes; e.g., S. *mansoni*, S. *haematobium*, and S. *japonicum;* cause schistosomiasis

REVIEW QUESTIONS FOR MICROBIOLOGY

1. A gram-negative microbe
   1. Cannot be stained by Gram's method
   2. Retains the original stain when stained by Gram's method
   3. Takes the counterstain when stained by Gram's method
   4. Weighs less than a gram
2. An acid-fast microbe
   1. Cannot be destroyed by acids
   2. Retains the original stain even though treated with acid-alcohol and counterstained
   3. Is destroyed quickly by acids
   4. Takes a counterstain after treatment with acid-alcohol
3. The body cannot readily destroy pneumococci by phagocytosis because they have which of the following structures?
   1. Nuclei
   2. Capsules
   3. Spores
   4. Flagella
4. A mechanical defense having stratified epithelium and sebaceous glands is the
   1. Alimentary tract lining
   2. Skin
   3. Respiratory tract lining
   4. Kidney
5. A mechanical defense having ciliated epithelium and goblet cells is the
   1. Alimentary tract lining
   2. Skin
   3. Respiratory tract lining
   4. Mouth cavity
6. A substance found in granular leukocytes that acts against gram-negative organisms is
   1. Phagocytin
   2. Properdin
   3. Lysozyme
   4. Interferon
7. Organisms that live on dead or decayed organic matter are
   1. Parasites
   2. Opportunists
   3. Saprophytes
   4. Commensals
8. An organism that lives in or on the body of the host at the expense of the host is a
   1. Saprophyte
   2. Opportunist
   3. Commensal
   4. Parasite

9. Autoclaving is used for sterilizing surgical supplies more often than boiling because
   1. More articles can be sterilized at one time
   2. Pressurized steam is surer to penetrate all parts of the material
   3. Steam is less injurious to materials
   4. A higher temperature can be attained, assuring the destruction of spores

10. Immunity by injecting serum from an immune animal into an individual is
    1. Active natural immunity
    2. Active artificial immunity
    3. Passive natural immunity
    4. Passive artificial immunity

11. A child has come into the hospital after exposure to diphtheria and is given antitoxin. This is what type of immunity?
    1. Active natural immunity
    2. Active artificial immunity
    3. Passive natural immunity
    4. Passive artificial immunity

12. An injection consisting of bacterial cells that have been modified is
    1. A vaccine
    2. An antitoxin
    3. A toxoid
    4. A toxin

13. Immunity transferred to young from an immune mother through the placenta is
    1. Active natural immunity
    2. Active artificial immunity
    3. Passive natural immunity
    4. Passive artificial immunity

14. Immunity by antibody formation during the course of a disease is
    1. Active natural immunity
    2. Active artificial immunity
    3. Passive natural immunity
    4. Passive artificial immunity

15. A substance that dissolves connective tissue cement is
    1. Hemolysin
    2. Collagenase
    3. Coagulase
    4. Hyaluronidase

16. A term used to indicate the degree of pathogenicity is
    1. Susceptibility
    2. Infestation
    3. Virulence
    4. Commensalism

17. An organism capable of producing disease is referred to as a
    1. Saprophyte
    2. Pathogen
    3. Infection
    4. Mutualism

18. An interaction between a parasite and host in which microorganisms are in or on the body of the host is
    1. Infection
    2. Susceptibility
    3. Mutualism
    4. Saprophyte

19. The lack of resistance to disease is called
    1. Infection
    2. Susceptibility
    3. Parasitism
    4. Virulence

20. A substance that destroys red blood cells is
    1. Hemolysin
    2. Collagenase
    3. Hyaluronidase
    4. Leukocidin

21. A substance that dissolves fibrin is
    1. Hemolysin
    2. Fibrinolysin
    3. Collagenase
    4. Coagulase

22. An antibiotic is
    1. An agent that interferes with the growth and activities of microbes
    2. A substance of microbial origin that has antimicrobial properties
    3. Prevents growth of bacteria
    4. Reduces the number of organisms to safe levels prescribed by law

23. A germicide
    1. Prevents growth of bacteria
    2. Destroys all forms of life
    3. Kills all kinds of microbes
    4. Prevents growth or action of microorganisms

24. An antimicrobial
    1. Kills all kinds of microbes
    2. Reduces the number of organisms to safe levels prescribed by law
    3. Is an agent that interferes with the growth and activities of microbes
    4. Prevents growth of bacteria

25. An antiseptic
    1. Prevents growth of bacteria
    2. Destroys all forms of life
    3. Kills all kinds of microbes
    4. Prevents growth or action of microorganisms

26. Pasteurization means
    1. Treating material at 62.5°C. for 30 minutes
    2. Treating material with intermittent periods of steam and incubation
    3. Reducing the number of organisms to safe levels prescribed by law
    4. The lowest temperature at which a suspension of bacteria is killed in 10 minutes

27. Sterilization means to
    1. Prevent growth of bacteria
    2. Destroy all forms of life
    3. Kill all kinds of microbes
    4. Prevent growth or action of microorganisms

28. The complete destruction of all microscopic forms of life including bacterial endospores can be brought about and assured through
    1. Disinfection
    2. Sterilization
    3. Application of antiseptics
    4. Boiling at 100°C. for 10 minutes

29. The ability of a microorganism to overcome the normal defense mechanism of the human body, survive, and grow within the body by establishing a position of superiority is recognized as
    1. Pathogenicity
    2. Passive resistance
    3. Virulence
    4. Motility

30. The administration of corticosteroids to con-

trol the symptoms of one disease can cause infections because it
1. Interferes with the inflammatory response of the body
2. Prevents the production of leukocytes
3. Promotes the growth and spread of enteric viruses
4. Stops antibody production in lymphatic tissue

31. Parasitic microorganisms such as bacteria, protozoa, rickettsia, and viruses can be maintained and studied in the laboratory if consideration is given to
1. Cultivation in suitable host cell media
2. Maintaining strict anaerobic conditions
3. Adding beef extract to nutrient agar media
4. Growth in nutrient broth at body temperature only

32. The most persistent structures that can survive harsh environmental conditions such as high temperature are
1. Viruses
2. Spirochetes
3. Bacterial endospores
4. Protozoa

33. Any disease caused by microbes may properly be called
1. A communicable disease
2. A contagious disease
3. An infectious disease
4. A viral disease

34. Antibodies are produced by
1. Plasma cells
2. Eosinophils
3. Lymphocytes
4. Erythrocytes

35. The vegetative cells of a spore former produce spores when
1. Oxygen is present
2. Conditions are unfavorable
3. Air is absent
4. pH is neutral

36. Which statement relates to active immunity?
1. Blood antigens are aided by phagocytes in defending the body against pathogens
2. Protein antigens are formed in the blood to fight invading antibodies
3. Protein substances are formed by the body to destroy or neutralize antigens
4. Lipid agents are formed by the body against antigens

37. Which of the following is a rickettsial disease?
1. Diphtheria
2. Scarlet fever
3. Gonorrhea
4. Spotted fever

38. A disease produced by a gram-negative diplococcus that generally invades the urogenital tract is
1. Cholera
2. Syphilis
3. Gonorrhea
4. Chancroid

39. An infection caused by the yeast *Candida albicans* often occurring in infants and debilitated individuals is
1. Typhoid fever
2. Thrush

3. Malta fever
4. Dysentery

40. An anaerobic spore-forming rod that produces an exotoxin in canned food is
1. *Salmonella typhosa*
2. *Clostridium botulinum*
3. *Clostridium tetani*
4. *E. coli*

41. A disease characterized by producing a "pseudomembrane" in the throat and producing general toxemia by excreted toxins is
1. Diphtheria
2. Malaria
3. Smallpox
4. Anthrax

42. A viral disease caused by one of the smallest human viruses that infects the motor cells of the anterior horn of the nerve cord is
1. Rubeola
2. Rubella
3. Poliomyelitis
4. Chickenpox

43. A dermatophytic fungus that infects skin, hair, and nails causes a disease commonly known as
1. Ringworm
2. Carbuncle
3. Boil
4. Anthrax

44. A disease produced by the acid-fast organism *Mycobacterium leprae* is
1. Scarlet fever
2. Hansen's disease
3. Bubonic plague
4. Anthrax

45. Streptococcus infection characterized by swollen joints, fever, and the possibility of endocarditis and death is
1. Whooping cough
2. Measles
3. Tetanus
4. Rheumatic fever

46. A disease produced by *Treponema pallidum* that usually invades the urogenital tract is
1. Gonorrhea
2. Chancroid
3. Syphilis
4. Measles

47. A disease usually produced by a gram-positive diplococcus that invades the respiratory tract is
1. Tuberculosis
2. Diphtheria
3. Scarlet fever
4. Lobar pneumonia

48. A disease produced when a clostridium enters wounds and produces a toxin causing muscle contraction is
1. Tetanus
2. Gas gangrene
3. Botulism
4. Anthrax

49. Which of the following is caused by protozoa?
1. Gonorrhea
2. Malaria
3. Diphtheria
4. Typhoid

50. The presence of *Escherichia coli* in water is
1. Important as a pathogen

2. An index of fecal pollution
3. Important in production of toxin
4. A harmless finding

51. The protozoan *Entamoeba histolytica* invades the intestinal mucosa and produces
    1. Typhoid
    2. Cholera
    3. Amebic dysentery
    4. Tuberculosis

52. A disease produced by a small bacterium and transmitted by the rat flea is
    1. Typhoid
    2. Cholera
    3. Tuberculosis
    4. Bubonic plague

53. A viral infection characterized by red blotchy rash and Koplick's spots in the mouth is
    1. Rubeola
    2. Rubella
    3. Chickenpox
    4. Mumps

54. A viral infection of the parotid gland is
    1. Rubeola
    2. Rubella
    3. Mumps
    4. Thrush

55. A viral infection characterized by brain inflammation and usually transmitted by insect vectors is
    1. Epidemic viral encephalitis
    2. Smallpox
    3. Infectious hepatitis
    4. Poliomyelitis

56. A viral disease with grave complications producing respiratory inflammation and skin rash is
    1. Rubeola
    2. Rubella
    3. Yellow fever
    4. Chickenpox

57. A viral infection characterized by vesicular rash on the trunk, usually of children, is
    1. Smallpox
    2. Chickenpox
    3. Measles
    4. Yellow fever

58. What kind of organism causes infectious hepatitis?
    1. Bacteria
    2. Molds
    3. Rickettsiae
    4. Viruses

59. What kind of organism causes measles?
    1. Bacteria
    2. Protozoa
    3. Rickettsiae
    4. Viruses

60. Gram-negative diplococci found in a vaginal smear are presumed to be
    1. Gonococci
    2. Meningococci
    3. Pneumococci
    4. *Treponema pallidum*

61. Acid-fast rods found in sputum are presumed to be
    1. Influenza virus
    2. *Bordetella pertussis*
    3. Diphtheria bacillus
    4. *Mycobacterium tuberculosis*

62. Bubonic plague is transmitted by the
    1. Tsetse fly
    2. Rat flea
    3. Body louse
    4. Aedes mosquito

63. Epidemic typhus is transmitted by the
    1. Anopheles mosquito
    2. Body louse
    3. Aedes mosquito
    4. Rat flea

64. The most important method of preventing Rocky Mountain spotted fever is
    1. Kill the Anopheles mosquito
    2. Kill the bloodsucking bug
    3. Proper sewage disposal
    4. Tick control

65. The most important method of preventing epidemic typhus fever is
    1. Kill body lice
    2. Tick control
    3. Kill rat fleas
    4. Kill biting gnats

66. The most important method of preventing malaria is
    1. Kill the Anopheles mosquito
    2. Kill the bloodsucking bug
    3. Kill the tsetse fly
    4. Kill biting gnats

67. The most important method of preventing amebic dysentery is
    1. Proper pasteurization of milk
    2. Kill biting gnats
    3. Proper sewage disposal
    4. Tick control

68. The most important method of preventing endemic typhus fever is
    1. Kill body lice
    2. Tick control
    3. Kill rat fleas
    4. Proper sewage disposal

69. An example of a disease caused by protozoa is
    1. African sleeping sickness
    2. Plague
    3. Syphilis
    4. Yellow fever

70. What kind of organism causes mumps?
    1. Bacteria
    2. Molds
    3. Rickettsiae
    4. Viruses

71. Tularemia is transmitted by the
    1. Body louse
    2. Aedes mosquito
    3. Animal skins and the bite of insects
    4. Rat flea

72. Malaria is transmitted by the
    1. Anopheles mosquito
    2. Tsetse fly
    3. Body louse
    4. Aedes mosquito

73. African sleeping sickness is transmitted by the
    1. Anopheles mosquito
    2. Tsetse fly
    3. Body louse
    4. Aedes mosquito

74. Dermatomycoses are infections of the body that can best be controlled and treated with
    1. Fungicides
    2. Bacteriostats

   3. Viricides
   4. Bacteriocides

75. The major benefit in using tetanus antitoxin is that it
   1. Stimulates plasma cells directly
   2. Provides high titer of antibodies
   3. Provides immediate active immunity
   4. Provides long-lasting passive immunity

76. Antitoxins are used to treat
   1. Whooping cough and septic sore throat
   2. Typhoid fever and dysentery
   3. Diphtheria and botulism
   4. Scarlet fever and tetanus

77. Rickettsial diseases are spread primarily by
   1. Food and water
   2. Body contact
   3. Fomites
   4. Vectors

78. A very common type of food poisoning in the United States is
   1. Salmonellosis
   2. Botulism
   3. Paratyphoid toxicity
   4. Bacillary dysentery

79. Under certain circumstances the virus that causes chickenpox can also cause
   1. Athlete's feet
   2. Infectious hepatitis
   3. Herpes zoster
   4. German measles

80. The mosquito is the vector of
   1. Encephalitis
   2. Typhus
   3. Rocky Mountain spotted fever
   4. Cholera

81. Johnny has been in the hospital for a month. He has just completed a course of penicillin therapy and blood cultures are negative. The throat culture report shows *Candida albicans*, and the physician's comment is "It's a super-infection." This means that it is
   1. Easier to treat than some of the resistant organisms the physician thought would be present
   2. Limited to the superior aspect of the respiratory tract
   3. New organisms that grew rapidly because natural flora were absent
   4. Overwhelming and will require potent antibiotic therapy

82. Typhus fever, which is transmitted to humans by the bite of an infected arthropod, is caused by a
   1. Virus
   2. Micrococcus
   3. Saprophyte
   4. Rickettsia

83. A fungal disease of the lungs normally transmitted by soil and dust contaminated with droppings from birds or bats is caused by the microorganism

   1. *Mycobacterium leprae*
   2. *Histoplasma capsulatum*
   3. *Hemophilus influenzae*
   4. *Mycoplasma pneumoniae*

84. A disease that may arise from a normal microbial flora organism, especially after prolonged antibiotic therapy, is
   1. Moniliasis or candidiasis
   2. Scarlet fever
   3. Q fever
   4. Herpes zoster

85. The common factor of the following diseases—puerperal sepsis, scarlet fever, otitis media, bacterial endocarditis, rheumatic fever, and glomerulonephritis—is that all
   1. Can be easily controlled through childhood vaccination
   2. Result from streptococcal infections that enter via the upper respiratory tract
   3. Are noncontagious, self-limiting infections by spirilla
   4. Are caused by parasitic bacteria that normally live outside the body

86. The common microorganism that is part of the normal flora of the upper respiratory tract and skin surfaces of healthy persons, but necessitates preoperative scrubbing and the use of surgical masks, gowns, and gloves during surgery is
   1. *Mycobacterium tuberculosis*
   2. *Clostridium tetani*
   3. *Staphylococcus aureus*
   4. *Streptococcus pyogenes*

87. An obligate, intracellular parasite, capable of causing diseases such as smallpox, meningitis, hepatitis, and yellow fever, is a
   1. Virus
   2. Saprophyte
   3. Rickettsia
   4. Protozoa

88. The syphilis organism can best be seen by
   1. A gram stain
   2. Darkfield illumination
   3. Acid fast stain
   4. Nutrient agar

89. A slide flocculation test for syphilis is the
   1. Wassermann test
   2. Dick test
   3. Kahn test
   4. VDRL

90. A stool specimen for determining if amebiasis is the cause of clinical symptoms is generally maintained by which of the following methods?
   1. Refrigerated for 24 hours or longer
   2. Frozen in transit or storage
   3. Desiccated if held at room temperature
   4. At or near body temperature for fresh examination

CHAPTER 4

Nutritional science: community and clinical nutrition

Human health and well-being are based on the interaction of numerous factors. Fundamental among these factors is nutrition, both from a biologic standpoint of maintaining physical health and from a cultural and psychosocial standpoint of maintaining emotional health. Thus, food and feeding practices are by no means simple events in human life but are filled with great meaning for all persons.

Several objectives become apparent in applying nutritional science to nursing care. First is the recognition of the role of nutrition in sustaining optimum health and integrity of tissue, and thus preventing disease and illness. Second is the concern for adapting food patterns of individuals to their nutritional needs within the framework of their particular cultural, economic, and psychologic life situation and style. Third is the awareness of the need in specific disease states to modify nutritional factors for therapeutic purposes.

Certain basic nutritional knowledge is required by nurses to meet these objectives. This knowledge should include a general understanding of the nutrients, their sources, functions, and utilization in the body. It should also include an awareness of key interrelationships among these nutrients in body function, as well as knowledge of the needed amounts of each.

Some basic definitions for the review of nutrition include the following.

nutrition the science that deals with the physiologic needs of the body in health and disease; the combination of processes by which a living organism receives and uses materials necessary for maintenance of its functions and growth

dietetics the science and art of applying principles of nutrition in the feeding of groups or individuals

food culturally acceptable substances that will supply heat and energy, build and repair tissue, and regulate body processes

nutrients basic chemical constituents of food, such as proteins, fats, carbohydrates, vitamins, minerals, and water

metabolism overall chemical changes (reactions) occurring in the body to sustain life, including activities that build tissue and substances (anabolism) and activities that break down tissue and substances (catabolism); frequently used to refer to chemical actions following absorption

NUTRITIONAL SCIENCE

NUTRIENTS SUPPLYING ENERGY
Carbohydrates

Primary source of fuel for quick energy

Definition

Organic compounds (saccharides— starches and sugars) composed of carbon, hydrogen, and oxygen; hydrogen to oxygen usually occurs in ratio of 2 to 1, as in water

Classification of carbohydrates

A. Monosaccharides—simple sugars
1. Glucose (dextrose)
   a. Principle form in which carbohydrate is used by the body; blood sugar
   b. Found in this form in few foods; mainly derived from starch digestion and conversion of other sugars
2. Fructose (levulose)
   a. Sweetest of simple sugars
   b. Found in honey, fruits, some vegetables
   c. Converted to glucose in the body
3. Galactose
   a. Not found free in foods
   b. Produced from lactose (milk sugar) by digestion
   c. Converted to glucose in the body
B. Disaccharides—double sugars
1. Sucrose (ordinary table sugar)
   a. Processed from cane and beet sugar
   b. Found in fruits, vegetables, syrups, sweet food products
   c. Converted to glucose and fructose in digestion
2. Lactose (milk sugar)
   a. Only source is milk and milk products with the exception of cheese
   b. Converted to glucose and galactose in digestion
3. Maltose
   a. Not found free in foods
   b. Produced by hydrolysis of starch
   c. Converted to glucose in digestion
C. Polysaccharides—complex carbohydrates of many saccharide units
1. Starch
   a. Most significant polysaccharide in human nutrition
   b. Major food sources include cereal grains, potatoes and other root vegetables, legumes
   c. Converted entirely to glucose upon digestion
2. Dextrins
   a. Not found free in foods
   b. Formed as intermediate products in the breakdown of starch
3. Cellulose
   a. Framework of plants found in unrefined grains, vegetables, fruits
   b. Nondigestible by humans; no specific enzyme is present
   c. Provides important bulk in the diet
4. Pectins
   a. Nondigestible, colloidal polysaccharides having a gel quality
   b. Found mostly in fruits
5. Glycogen—"animal starch"
   a. Formed from glucose and stored in liver and muscle tissue
   b. Food sources mainly meats and seafoods
   c. Converted entirely to glucose upon digestion

Digestion of carbohydrates

A. Mouth
1. Enzyme—ptyalin
2. Action—begins breakdown of starch to dextrins and maltose; food usually does not remain in the mouth long enough for much of this action to occur
B. Stomach
1. Enzyme—none for carbohydrates
2. Action—none; above action by ptyalin may continue to a minor degree
C. Small intestine
1. Pancreatic enzyme—amylopsin—converts starch to dextrins and maltose
2. Intestinal enzymes (disaccharidases)
   a. Sucrase—converts sucrose to glucose and fructose
   b. Lactase—converts lactose to glucose and galactose
   c. Maltase—converts maltose to glucose

Absorption of carbohydrates

A. Factors influencing absorption
1. Rate of entry into small intestine; rate depends upon motility and control of pyloric valve
2. Type of food mixture present will affect competition for absorbing sites and available carrier transport systems

3. Condition of intestinal membranes and time food mass is held in contact with absorbing surfaces
4. Normal endocrine activity and effect of certain hormones
B. Sugars absorbed at different rates through specific selectivity
1. Galactose most rapid
2. Glucose almost as rapid
3. Fructose absorbed most slowly
C. Mechanism of absorption
1. Diffusion when osmotic gradient provides positive pressure; e.g., after a meal
2. Active transport with aid of sodium carrier
D. Route of absorption
1. Water-soluble, so absorbed directly into villi capillaries of blood
2. Carried through portal blood system to liver and other tissues

Metabolism of carbohydrates

A. Sources of blood glucose
1. Carbohydrate sources
   a. Dietary carbohydrates
   b. Liver glycogen
   c. Products of intermediary cell metabolism; e.g., lactic acid and pyruvic acid
2. Noncarbohydrate sources
   a. Protein—glucogenic amino acids, deaminized
   b. Fat—small portion, glycerol
3. Production of glucose from protein, fat, and various intermediate carbohydrate metabolites—gluconeogenesis
B. Uses of blood glucose
1. Burned for energy—glycolysis
2. Stored for reserve use
   a. Converted to liver glycogen—glycogenesis
   b. Converted to adipose fat—lipogenesis
3. Converted to other forms of nutrient metabolites
   a. Other carbohydrate compounds necessary for total body metabolism
   b. Certain amino acids required for protein synthesis
C. Hormonal influences
1. Hormone that lowers blood sugar level—insulin
   a. Affects cell wall permeability to glucose, hence increases cell entry

b. Fosters conversion of glucose to glycogen—glycogenesis
   c. Fosters conversion of glucose to fat—lipogenesis
2. Hormones that raise blood sugar
   a. Glucagon—stimulates breakdown of liver glycogen to glucose—glycogenolysis
   b. Steroid hormones (adrenal cortex) —act as insulin antagonists; stimulate breakdown of protein to form glucose—gluconeogenesis
   c. Epinephrine (adrenal medulla)—stimulates breakdown of stored glycogen to glucose—glycogenolysis
   d. Growth hormone (GH) and adrenocorticotropic hormone (ACTH) from anterior pituitary—act as insulin antagonists
   e. Thyroid hormone (thyroxine)—influences rate of insulin breakdown; stimulates glucose absorption from intestine; liberates epinephrine
D. Energy production
1. First stage: production of common molecule (active acetate or acetyl CoA)—2 carbon fragments that are the cell's ultimate fuel for energy via the final common energy cycle (Krebs' cycle)
2. Second stage: burning of common molecule (active acetate) in mitochondria via specific reactions of the Krebs' cycle
3. Third stage: trapping energy in high energy compounds (ATP) via respiratory chains (hydrogen ion transfer) attached to Krebs' cycle at various points, thus enabling energy to be available and released as needed for cell work; final products of glucose oxidation—carbon dioxide and water

Functions of carbohydrates

A. Supply major energy source
B. Spare protein
C. Supply bulk
D. Provide essential metabolites for tissue function and metabolism
E. Aid in utilization of fat through balance of Krebs' cycle
F. Protect liver against toxins through deposits of glycogen
G. Promote growth of desirable intestinal flora

Role of carbohydrates

A. Supply 40% to 50% of total calories in average American diet
B. Inexpensive; used in greater amounts by people in lower income groups, providing up to 80% of total calories
C. Provide important sources of B vitamins and minerals through enrichment of bread and cereal products
D. Foods high in carbohydrates; e.g., sugar and sweets, breads, cereal and cereal products, dried fruits, bananas, grapes, potatoes, milk
E. Foods low in carbohydrates; e.g., most fresh fruits and vegetables

Modification of intake to meet therapeutic needs

A. Decrease for obesity, hypoglycemia, dumping syndrome; adequate but not excessive for balance of nutrients required in diabetes control
B. Elimination of gummy-textured sweets (caramels) to protect teeth against dental caries
C. Increase for liver disease (hepatitis), fever, malnutrition or underweight, to increase calories
D. Low cellulose or fiber content in gastrointestinal diseases and surgery
E. Increased fiber intake recommended for lower gastrointestinal problems such as diverticulosis
F. Decrease, especially of sucrose, in certain lipid disorders

Fats

Most concentrated source of fuel for stored energy

Definition

Organic compounds composed of carbon, hydrogen, and oxygen, chiefly as triglycerides (glycerol esters of fatty acids); belong to class of fats and fat-related compounds called lipids

Classification of fats

A. Simple lipids
1. Triglycerides (neutral fats) esters of fatty acids with glycerol base, in ratio of 3 fatty acids to each glycerol base
2. Waxes
B. Compound lipids (combinations of triglyceride with other components)
1. Phospholipids—lecithin
2. Glycolipids—cerebrosides
3. Lipoproteins—important transport form of fat in blood
C. Derived lipids (simple derivatives from fat digestion or other more complex products)
1. Fatty acids—structural components of fats
2. Glycerol—water-soluble base for fat
3. Steroids—cholesterol, ergosterol, bile salts, certain provitamins, and adrenal and gonadotropic hormones

Chemical structure of fatty acids, relation to food fats

A. Saturated fatty acids—all possible valence bonds in carbon chain filled with hydrogen, producing a harder more dense fat; found in animal fats
B. Unsaturated fatty acids—some carbon valence bonds unfilled (double bonds), producing a softer, less dense fat; found in vegetable oils
C. Food fats highest in saturated fat found mostly in meat and dairy fats; food fats highest in unsaturated fat found mostly in vegetable oils
D. Essential fatty acid—linoleic acid

Digestion of fats

A. Mouth
1. Enzyme—none
2. Action—only mechanical, mastication
B. Stomach
1. Enzyme—none
2. Action—mechanical separation of fats as protein and starch are digested out
C. Small intestine
1. Gallbladder—bile salts emulsify fats in preparation for digestion
2. Pancreas
   a. Pancreatic lipase (steapsin)—converts triglycerides to diglycerides and monoglycerides in turn, then to fatty acids and glycerol
   b. Cholesterol esterase—combines free cholesterol and fatty acids to form cholesterol esters
3. Intestinal wall—lecithinase converts lecithin to glycerol, fatty acids, phosphoric acid, and choline

Absorption of fats

A. Stage I: transport into intestinal wall mucosa
1. Short and medium chain fatty acids,

being more water-soluble, may be absorbed directly into bloodstream through portal system
2. Remaining insoluble products require bile as a carrier
B. Stage II: preparation for final transport
   1. Bile separated out and recirculated for same task again
   2. Completion of breakdown of triglycerides, diglycerides, and monoglycerides with enzyme enteric lipase
   3. Synthesis of new triglycerides and formation of lipoprotein compounds (chylomicrons) to serve as carriers into lacteals (lymphatic system), hence to portal blood

Metabolism of fats

Two main sites, liver and adipose tissue
A. Adipose tissue
   1. Fat synthesis and deposit—most active site of lipogenesis in body
   2. Fat mobilization and oxidation—fat tissue constantly being broken down and mobilized to body tissues for fuel as fatty acids
B. Liver tissue
   1. Converts fat to transport form (lipoproteins) for immediate removal from liver to body cells, thus preventing a fatty liver
   2. In addition to the lipoproteins (chylomicrons), the liver synthesizes 3 other lipoproteins continuously from body fat or circulating endogenous fat to transport fat to cells
      a. Pre-beta lipoproteins
      b. Beta lipoproteins
      c. Alpha lipoproteins
C. Hormonal influences
   1. Close relation with carbohydrate metabolism so the same hormones are operative
   2. Growth hormone (GH), adrenocorticotropic hormone (ACTH), and thyroid-stimulating hormone (TSH) increase release of fatty acids from adipose tissue by imposing energy demands on the body
   3. Cortisone causes release of fatty acids
   4. Epinephrine stimulates breakdown of tissue fat
   5. Insulin stimulates lipogenesis
   6. Thyroxine stimulates adipose tissue release of fatty acids and also lowers cholesterol in blood

Functions of fats

A. Provide most concentrated source of energy
B. Aid in digestion, absorption, and utilization of other nutrients
C. Provide fat-soluble vitamins and aid in their absorption and use
D. Provide essential fatty acid—linoleic acid
E. Assist in regulation of body temperature
F. Provide structural protective tissue for vital organs

Role of fats

A. Supply 40% to 60% of total calories in average American diet, an amount in excess of needs for best health
B. Provide flavor and satiety to foods
C. A higher ratio of unsaturated to saturated fats is beneficial to health

Modification of intake to meet therapeutic needs

A. Increase in polyunsaturated fats and decrease in saturated fats recommended to reduce risks of atherosclerosis; reduction of calories, sucrose, and cholesterol may also be indicated
B. Decrease in fat may be indicated in gallbladder disease and surgery, diarrhea, other malabsorption conditions
C. Increase in fat recommended in dumping syndrome, underweight

ENERGY METABOLISM
Definitions

A. Energy—force or power enabling the body to do its work
B. Metabolism—total of chemical processes in the body by which substances are changed into other substances to sustain life; thus, the dynamic concept underlying all life is change

Measurement of energy

A. Kilocalorie (commonly called calorie)—measure of heat energy given off when fuel substances in food are used by the body; 1 calorie is the amount of heat required to raise 1 kg. of water 1°C.
   1. Fuel factor of carbohydrate—4 calories per gram
   2. Fuel factor of fat—9 calories per gram
   3. Fuel factor of protein—4 calories per gram
B. Joule—energy measure in the metric sys-

tem; 1 calorie (kilocalorie) equals 4.184 joules (kilojoules)

Human energy system

A. Energy transformation and cycle
 1. Ultimate energy source is the sun
 2. Body transforms stored energy in plants and animals to different forms of energy—chemical, mechanical, electrical, thermal
 3. Metabolism converts potential energy bound in chemical compounds to free energy to do body work
B. Control agents in human energy system
 1. Enzymes—a specific cell enzyme governs each specific reaction process that changes one compound to another
 2. Coenzymes—necessary partners for many reactions to proceed; a function performed by many vitamins
 3. Hormones—substances that act as chemical messengers to control or trigger an enzyme action
C. Overall system control—chemical bonding
 1. Covalent bonds—carbon bonds
 2. Hydrogen bonds
 3. High-energy phosphate bonds—adenosine triphosphate (ATP) is the main energy compound in the body
D. Types of metabolic reactions in human energy balance system
 1. Anabolism—reactions that synthesize more complex compounds
 2. Catabolism—reactions that break down compounds to simpler ones

Energy metabolism—calorie requirements

A. Basal metabolism—measure of energy needed by body at rest for all its internal chemical activities; approximately 1 calorie per kilogram body weight per hour for an adult
 1. Basal metabolic rate (BMR)—rate of basal metabolism in a given person at a given time and situation
 2. Factors influencing BMR—growth, surface area, sex, pregnancy and lactation, fever, climate, diseases, malnutrition and starvation, thyroxine
B. Physical activities—calorie requirements depend on type and amount of exercise
C. Total energy metabolism—total calorie requirement for both basal and physical activity needs combined

THE NUTRIENT SUPPLYING BUILDING MATERIAL—PROTEIN

Definition

A. Contains nitrogen in addition to the basic carbon, hydrogen, and oxygen
B. More complex compounds of high molecular weights, structured in specific arrangements and numbers of their simpler building units, amino acids

Classification of proteins

A. Simple proteins—contain only amino acids and their derivatives; e.g., albumin, globulin, collagen
B. Compound proteins (conjugated)—compounds of simple protein with some nonprotein group; e.g., nucleoproteins such as purines; metalloproteins such as hemoglobin; phosphoproteins such as casein in milk; lipoproteins such as pre-beta lipoprotein carriers of triglycerides in the blood
C. Derived proteins—fragments of various sizes produced in the process of protein digestion; e.g., proteoses, peptones, and polypeptides

Chemical structure of proteins

A. Basic structure has dual nature with both acid and base (amino) radicals
 1. Gives buffering capacity
 2. Provides ability to form peptide chains and hence proteins
B. Essential and nonessential amino acids
 1. Essential ones cannot be synthesized by body and are necessary in diet
  a. Tryptophan
  b. Lysine
  c. Valine
  d. Threonine
  e. Leucine
  f. Isoleucine
  g. Methionine
  h. Phenylalanine
 2. The remaining 12 or 14 amino acids are nonessential since they can be synthesized by the body so they are not dietary essentials
 3. Both essential and nonessential amino acids are necessary to body metabolism
C. Complete and incomplete proteins
 1. Complete proteins contain sufficient amounts of all the essential amino acids; these foods are of animal origin; e.g., meat, milk, egg, cheese

2. Incomplete proteins lack one or more of the essential amino acids in sufficient amount to meet needs; these foods are of plant origin; e.g., grains, legumes, nuts, seeds
3. A mixed diet provides a balanced mix of all the amino acids
4. A vegetarian diet may be planned so as to include all the essential amino acids in a complementary fashion

Digestion of proteins

A. Mouth
1. Enzyme—none
2. Action—only mechanical mastication
B. Stomach (acid)
1. Enzyme—pepsin, produced first as inactive precursor pepsinogen then activated by the hydrochloric acid
2. Action—converts protein to proteoses and peptones
3. In infants, enzyme rennin converts casein to coagulated curd
C. Small intestine (alkaline)
1. Pancreas
a. Trypsin (produced first as inactive precursor trypsinogen and then activated by enterokinase) converts proteins, proteoses, and peptones to polypeptides and dipeptides
b. Chymotrypsin (produced first as inactive precursor chymotrypsinogen and then activated by active trypsin) converts proteoses and peptones to polypeptides and dipeptides; also coagulates milk
c. Carboxypeptidase converts polypeptides to simpler peptides, dipeptides, and amino acids
2. Intestine
a. Aminopeptidase converts polypeptides to peptides and amino acids
b. Dipeptidase converts dipeptides to amino acids

Absorption of proteins

A. Water-soluble amino acids do not require a wetting agent as fats do
B. Absorbed by active transport with aid of vitamin B_6 (pyridoxine) as a carrier
C. A few whole proteins may be absorbed intact and are not used in protein synthesis; e.g., antibodies

Metabolism of proteins

A. Balance among body activities—dynamic system

1. Protein turnover between tissue protein and plasma protein is constant in health
2. Metabolic amino acid pool maintained by liver as reserve for specific needs in tissue synthesis
3. Nitrogen balance—the balance between nitrogen intake (food protein) and nitrogen output (urine, etc.)
a. Positive nitrogen balance occurs when nitrogen intake exceeds output as in growth during childhood and pregnancy, or in tissue building with large protein input for healing after injury
b. Negative nitrogen balance occurs when nitrogen output (loss) exceeds nitrogen input (food protein) as in postsurgery and initial stages of traumatic injuries before build-up to positive balance with treatment (high-protein formula food); debilitating disease and immobilized states such as paralysis also require such protein therapy (remember that sufficient calories for energy are always needed in such protein therapy to spare protein for tissue synthesis purposes)
B. Anabolism—building tissue
1. Substances governing protein synthesis
a. Deoxyribonucleic acid (DNA)—genetic design in nucleus for a specific protein pattern
b. Ribonucleic acid (messenger RNA)—receives specific imprint of protein pattern from DNA in the cell nucleus and moves out into the cell to ribosome granules to form a working site for the specific protein synthesis
2. Stages in process of protein synthesis
a. All activated amino acids needed for the specific protein pattern must be present—law of "all or none"
b. Transfer RNA—segments of the RNA pattern chain fitted to respective amino acids carry each acid into correct sequence in the pattern
c. Peptide linkage forms polypeptide chain that comprises that specific protein; the protein chain then breaks free of the mold of RNA,

leaving the mold free to reproduce the same protein as needed
C. Catabolism—breaking down tissue for resynthesis of needed materials or for energy
 1. Nitrogenous radical (NH_2) is split off—deamination
 2. Remaining nonnitrogen residues (Keto-acids) may be used as a base for making other amino acids for tissue synthesis or for synthesizing carbohydrate or fat for energy
 3. Common metabolic (dynamic turnover) pool of metabolites from protein, carbohydrate, and fat maintained in balance with amino acid pool
D. Hormonal influences
 1. Anabolic effect—growth hormone (GH), androgens, insulin, thyroid hormone
 2. Catabolic effect—adrenal steroids, large amounts of thyroid hormone

Functions of proteins

A. Build, maintain, and repair tissue
B. Secondary energy source
C. Perform specific functions as component part of tissue and substances
 1. Hormones (insulin)
 2. Enzymes (all enzymes are proteins)
 3. Antibodies
 4. Blood components
  a. Bind and transport nutrients; e.g., iron-binding protein
  b. Regulate water balance by supplying albumin to maintain necessary colloidal osmotic pressure for operation of the capillary fluid shift mechanism
  c. Help regulate acid-base balance
 5. Form vitamins; e.g., niacin and folic acid

Role of proteins

A. Supplies 10% to 15% of total calories in average diet
B. About one third of dietary protein should be supplied by complete protein
C. Each meal should supply a complete protein food or food combinations (grains, legumes) to supply all 8 essential amino acids
D. Essential amino acids may be supplied by a complementary mix of plant proteins or by supplementing plant protein with animal protein

E. Protein foods tend to be relatively expensive, hence there is a concern in planning adequate diets on low incomes

Requirements for human nutrition

A. Quality of protein fundamental to life and health
B. General daily recommendations of Food and Nutrition Board of the National Research Council
 1. Adult—0.9 g. per kg. body weight
 2. Children—growth needs vary according to age and growth patterns
 3. Pregnancy—rapid growth demands require an increase of 30 g. or about two thirds increase over that of the nonpregnant woman
 4. Lactation—requires an increase of 20 g.

Modifications of intake to meet therapeutic needs

A. Restriction indicated in advanced renal disease that impairs nephron capacity to excrete nitrogen and maintain nitrogen balance and in liver disease such as advanced cirrhosis involving hepatic coma that lowers liver capacity to detoxify nitrogenous substances; e.g., ammonia
B. Increase indicated in any degenerative or debilitating disease where tissue regeneration and healing are needed; any wound healing situation following injury or surgery; general body tissue rebuilding as in malnutrition

NUTRIENTS CONTROLLING BODY PROCESSES
Fat-soluble vitamins
Vitamin A (retinol)

A. Chemical and physical nature
 1. Preformed vitamin A—animal sources
 2. Provitamin A—precursor carotene; pigment found in green and yellow plants; body converts to vitamin A
B. Absorption and storage
 1. Absorption aided by bile salts, pancreatic lipase, and dietary fat
 2. Carotene converted to vitamin A in intestinal wall
 3. Absorbed through lymphatic system and portal blood to liver (same route as fat)
 4. Large storage capacity in liver, hence,

potential toxicity levels with large intakes
C. Physiologic functions
1. Vision cycle—necessary component of visual purple (rhodopsin), light-sensitive pigment in the retina enabling it to make adjustments to light and dark
2. Epithelial tissue—necessary material for proper synthesis and maintenance of epithelial tissue, hence, integrity of skin and internal mucosa, growth and formation of tooth buds
D. Food sources—animal (preformed vitamin); e.g., liver, butterfat, egg yolk; plant (carotene); e.g., yellow and green vegetables and fruits

Vitamin D (calciferol)

A. Chemical and physical nature
1. Sterols, more hormonelike in source and action
2. Formed in skin by irradiation of cholesterol by sunlight
B. Absorption and storage
1. Absorption accompanies that of calcium and phosphorus in the small intestine
2. Formed by sunlight in skin absorbed into systemic circulation as are hormones
3. Storage in liver, but not as great as that of vitamin A
C. Physiologic functions
1. Absorption of calcium and phosphorus
2. Calcification—bone formation
D. Food sources
1. Very few—mainly in those foods to which it has been added in enrichment process; e.g., milk
2. Main source—sunlight's irradiation of body cholesterol

Vitamin E (tocopherol)

A. Chemical and physical nature
1. Resistant to oxidation (valuable as an antioxidant)
2. Fat-soluble, stable to heat and acids
B. Absorption and storage
1. Absorbed with other fat-soluble vitamins, aided by bile and fats
2. Stored especially in adipose tissue
C. Physiologic functions
1. Antioxidant properties, especially in protection of polyunsaturated lipids
2. Helps sustain tissue integrity, especially structural parts containing unsaturated lipids; e.g., cell wall

D. Food sources—vegetable oils, leafy vegetables, cereals

Vitamin K (phylloquinone, menadione)

A. Chemical and physical nature
1. Fat soluble
2. Synthesized by normal intestinal bacteria
B. Absorption and storage
1. Absorbed by usual route for fats—lacteals, portal blood to liver
2. Stored in liver in small amounts
C. Physiologic function—necessary for the synthesis of prothrombin in the liver, hence, vital component in blood clotting mechanism
D. Food sources—only small amounts in foods such as leafy vegetables, liver, egg yolk; major source—synthesized by the normal intestinal bacteria; see Table 4-1 for summary of fat-soluble vitamins

Water-soluble vitamins
Vitamin C (ascorbic acid)

A. Chemical and physical nature
1. Water-soluble acid, easily oxidized, unstable
2. Other animals can synthesize vitamin C from glucose but humans lack the necessary specific enzyme
B. Absorption and storage
1. Easily absorbed from small intestine
2. Not stored in tissue depots; distributed to tissue saturation levels in general circulation, remainder being excreted; large amounts present in adrenal tissue
C. Physiologic functions
1. Intercellular cement substance, hence, vital in tissue synthesis and maintenance, wound healing, reaction to stress
2. Supports general body metabolism
D. Food sources
1. Main source—citrus fruits
2. Other sources include tomatoes, cabbage, potatoes, berries, melons, chili peppers, broccoli, leafy vegetables

B complex vitamins

A. Group I: classic disease factors
1. Thiamin (B$_1$)—antiberiberi factors; essential in carbohydrate metabolism, energy systems, and integrity of nerve tissue
2. Riboflavin (B$_2$)—essential in tissue respiration and energy metabolism,

Table 4-1. Summary of fat-soluble vitamins

Vitamin	Physiologic functions	Results of deficiency	Requirements	Food sources
A (retinol) Provitamin A (carotene)	Production of rhodopsin (visual purple) Formation and maintenance of epithelial tissue Toxic in large amounts	Xerophthalmia Night blindness Keratinization of epithelium Follicular hyperkeratosis Skin and mucous membrane infections Faulty tooth formation	Adult: 5000 I.U. Pregnancy: 6000 I.U. Lactation: 8000 I.U. Children: 1500 to 5000 I.U. depending on age	Liver Butterfat (cream, butter, whole milk) Egg yolk Green and yellow vegetables and fruits Fortified margarine
D (calciferol)	Absorption of calcium and phosphorus Calcification of bones Renal phosphate clearance Toxic in large amounts	Rickets in children Faulty bone growth Osteomalacia in adults	400 I.U.—children, pregnancy, lactation	Fish oils Fortified or irradiated milk
E (tocopherol)	Related to action of selenium Antioxidant with vitamin A and polyunsaturated fats Hemopoiesis Reproduction in animals	Hemolysis of red blood cells, anemia Weakening of integrity of cell wall structure Sterility in rats	Adult: 25 to 30 mg.	Vegetable oils
K (menadione)	Blood clotting, necessary for synthesis of prothrombin Toxic in large amounts	Hemorrhagic disease of newborn Bleeding tendencies in biliary disease or cholecystectomy Deficiency in intestinal malabsorption or prolonged antibiotic therapy Slowed clotting time and possible internal bleeding with anticoagulant therapy (Dicumarol counteracts vitamin K)	Unknown	Main source synthesized by intestinal bacteria Green leafy vegetables Liver Egg yolk Cheese

growth and prevention of skin disorders

3. Niacin (nicotinic acid)—pellagra prevention factor; essential to tissue oxidation and cell metabolism

B. Group II: more recently discovered coenzyme factors

  1. Pyridoxine (B$_6$)—essential coenzyme in protein metabolism and absorption

  2. Pantothenic acid—essential component of coenzyme A or acetyl CoA (active acetate); a vital factor in overall body metabolism

  3. Lipoic acid—coenzyme associated with thiamin in glucose metabolism; a fatty acid, not a true vitamin

  4. Biotin—coenzyme in CO$_2$ fixation reactions in energy metabolism

C. Group III: cell-growth and blood-forming factors

  1. Folic acid—essential to growth and reproduction of cells; associated with

Table 4-2. Summary of water-soluble vitamins

Vitamin	Physiologic functions	Clinical applications	Requirement	Food sources
C (ascorbic acid)	Intercellular cementlike substance Collagen formation Firm capillary walls General metabolism Makes iron available for hemoglobin and maturation of red blood cells Influences conversion of folic acid to folinic acid	Scurvy (deficiency) Megaloblastic anemia Wound healing, tissue formation Fevers and infections Stress reactions Growth periods	Adults: 60 mg. Children: varies with age	Citrus fruits Tomatoes Cabbage Potatoes Strawberries Melon Broccoli Green peppers Chili peppers
B_1 (thiamin)	Coenzyme in carbohydrate metabolism TPP—decarboxylation TDP—transketolation	Beriberi (deficiency) GI: anorexia, gastric atony, indigestion, deficient hydrochloric acid CNS: fatigue, apathy, neuritis, paralysis CV: cardiac failure, peripheral vasodilation, and edema of extremities	0.5 mg. per 1000 calories	Pork Beef Liver Whole or enriched grains Legumes
B_2 (riboflavin)	Coenzyme in protein of energy metabolism (flavoproteins) FMN (flavin mononucleotide) FAD (flavin adenine dinucleotide)	Wound aggravation Cheilosis (cracks at corners of mouth) Glossitis Eye irritation; photophobia Seborrheic dermatitis	0.6 mg. per 1000 calories (0.07 mg./kg. 0.75)	Milk Liver Enriched cereals
Niacin (nicotinic acid: precursor—tryptophan)	Coenzyme in tissue oxidation to produce energy (ATP) NAD (nicotinamide adenine dinucleotide) NADP (nicotinamide adenine dinucleotide phosphate)	Pellagra (deficiency) Weakness, lassitude, anorexia Skin: scaly dermatitis CNS: neuritis, confusion	14 to 19 mg. (niacin equivalent)	Meat Peanuts Enriched grains
B_6 (pyridoxine)	Coenzyme in amino acid metabolism Decarboxylation Deamination Transamination Transsulfuration Niacin formation from tryptophan Heme formation Amino acid absorption	Anemia (hypochromic microcytic) CNS: hyperirritability, convulsions, neuritis Isoniazid therapy requires supplemental B_6 Pregnancy: anemia	2 mg.	Wheat Corn Meat Liver

Table 4-2. Summary of water-soluble vitamins—cont'd

Vitamin	Physiologic functions	Clinical applications	Requirement	Food sources
Pantothenic acid	Coenzyme in formation of active acetate (CoA)—acetylation	Contributes to Lipogenesis Amino acid activation Formation of cholesterol, steroid hormones, and heme Excretion of drugs		Liver Egg Skimmed milk
Lipoic acid (sulfur-containing fatty acid)	Coenzyme (with thiamine) in carbohydrate metabolism to reduce pyruvate to active acetate Oxidative decarboxylation	Undetermined (see Thiamin)		Liver Yeast
Biotin	Coenzyme in decarboxylation (synthesis of fatty acids, amino acids, purines); deamination	Undetermined		Egg yolk Liver
Folic acid	Coenzyme for single carbon transfer—purines, thymine, hemoglobin Transmethylation	Blood cell regeneration in pernicious anemia but not control of its neurologic problems Megaloblastic anemia Macrocytic anemia of pregnancy Sprue treatment Aminopterin is folic acid antagonist	Adults: 0.4 mg. Pregnancy: 0.8 mg. Lactation: 0.5 mg.	Liver Green leafy vegetables, asparagus
PABA (part of folic acid)		Treatment of rickettsial diseases Anemias (see Folic acid)		Same as folic acid
B$_{12}$ (cobalamin)	Coenzyme in protein synthesis Formation of nucleic acid and cell proteins —red blood cells Transmethylation	Extrinsic factor in pernicious anemia—combines with intrinsic factor of gastric secretions for absorption; forms red blood cells (with folic acid) Sprue treatment (with folic acid)	5 μg.	Liver Meat Milk Egg Cheese
Inositol	Lipotropic agent (?)	Undetermined		Citrus fruit Grains Meat Milk
Choline	Lipotropic agent Forms nerve mediator —acetylcholine	Fatty liver—hepatitis, cirrhosis (undetermined in human nutrition)		Meat Cereals Egg yolk

Table 4-3. Summary of minerals

Mineral	Metabolism	Physiologic functions	Clinical application	Requirement	Food sources
Calcium (Ca)	Absorption according to body need, aided by vitamin D; favored by protein, lactose, acidity; hindered by excess fats and binding agents (phosphates, oxylates, phytate) Excretion chiefly in feces, 70% to 90% of amount ingested Deposition—mobilization in bone compartment constant; deposition aided by vitamin D Parathyroid hormone controls absorption and mobilization	Bone formation Teeth Blood clotting Muscle contraction and relaxation Heart action Nerve transmission Cell wall permeability Enzyme activation (ATPase)	Tetany-decrease in ionized serum calcium Rickets Renal calculi Hyperparathyroidism Hypoparathyroidism	Adults: 0.8 g. Pregnancy and lactation: 1.3 g. Infants: 0.7 g. Children: 0.8 to 1.4 g.	Milk Cheese Green leafy vegetables Whole grains Egg yolk Legumes Nuts
Phosphorus (P)	Absorption with calcium aided by vitamin D; hindered by excess binding agents (calcium, aluminum, and iron) Excretion chiefly by kidney according to renal threshold blood level Parathyroid hormone controls renal excretion balance with blood level Deposition—mobilization in bone compartment constant	Bone formation Overall metabolism: Absorption of glucose and glycerol (phosphorylation) Transport of fatty acids Energy metabolism (enzymes, ATP) Buffer system	Growth Hypophosphatemia: Recovery state from diabetic acidosis Sprue, celiac disease (malabsorption) Bone diseases (upset Ca:P balance) Hyperphosphatemia: Renal insufficiency Hypoparathyroidism Tetany	Adults: 1½ times calcium intake Pregnancy and lactation: 1.3 g. Infants: 0.2 to 0.5 mg. Children: 0.8 to 1.4 g.	Milk Cheese Meat Egg yolk Whole grains Legumes Nuts
Magnesium (Mg)	Absorption increased by parathyroid hormone; hindered by excess fat, phosphate, calcium Excretion regulated by kidney	Constituent of bones and teeth Activator and coenzyme in carbohydrate and protein metabolism Essential intracellular fluid (ICF) cation Muscle and nerve irritability	Tremor, spasm; low serum level following gastrointestinal losses	300 to 350 mg. Deficiency in humans unlikely	Whole grains Nuts Meat Milk Legumes
Sodium (Na)	Readily absorbed Excretion chiefly by kidney, controlled by aldosterone, acid-base balance	Major extracellular fluid (ECF) cation Water balance; osmotic pressure	Fluid shifts and control Buffer system Losses in gastrointestinal disorders	About 0.5 g. Diet usually has more: 2 to 6 g.	Table salt (NaCl) Milk Meat Egg

Mineral	Metabolism	Physiological functions	Clinical application	Daily requirement	Food sources
		Acid-base balance Cell permeability; absorption of glucose Muscle irritability; transmission of electrochemical impulse and resulting contraction			Baking soda Baking powder Carrots, beets, spinach, celery
Potassium (K)	Secreted and reabsorbed in digestive juices Excretion guarded by kidney according to blood levels; increased by aldosterone	Major ICF cation Acid-base balance Regulates neuromuscular excitability and muscle contraction Glycogen formation Protein synthesis	Fluid shifts Losses in: Starvation Diabetic acidosis Adrenal tumors Heart action—low serum potassium (tachycardia, cardiac arrest) Treatment of diabetic acidosis (rapid glycogen production reduces serum potassium) Tissue catabolism—potassium loss	About 2 to 4 g. Diet adequate in protein, calcium, and iron contains adequate potassium	Whole grains Meat Legumes Fruits Vegetables
Chlorine (Cl)	Absorbed readily Excretion controlled by kidney	Major ECF anion Acid-base balance—chloride-bicarbonate shift Water balance Gastric hydrochloric acid—digestion	Hypochloremic alkalosis in prolonged vomiting, diarrhea, tube drainage	About 0.5 g. Diet usually has more: 2 to 6 g.	Table salt
Sulfur (S)	Absorbed as such and as constituent of sulfur-containing amino acid, methionine Excreted by kidney in relation to protein intake and tissue catabolism	Essential constituent of cell protein Activates enzymes High-energy sulfur bonds in energy metabolism Detoxification reactions	Cystine renal calculi Cystinuria	Diet adequate in protein contains adequate sulfur	Meat Egg Cheese Milk Nuts Legumes
Iron (Fe)	Absorption according to body need controlled by mucosal block–ferritin mechanism; aided by vitamin C, gastric hydrochloric acid Transport—transferrin Storage—ferritin, hemosiderin Excretion from tissue in minute quantities; body conserves and re-uses	Hemoglobin formation Cellular oxidation (cytochrome system producing ATP)	Growth (milk anemia) Pregnancy demands Deficiency—anemia Excess—hemosiderosis; hemochromatosis	Men: 10 mg. Women: 18 mg. Pregnancy: 18 mg. Lactation: 18 mg. Children: 10 to 18 mg.	Liver Meat Egg yolk Whole grains Enriched bread and cereal Dark green vegetables Legumes Nuts

Continued.

Table 4-3. Summary of minerals—cont'd

Mineral	Metabolism	Physiologic functions	Clinical application	Requirement	Food sources
Copper (Cu)	Transported bound to an α-globulin as ceruloplasmin Stored in muscle, bone, liver, heart, kidney, and central nervous system	Associated with iron in: Enzyme systems Hemoglobin synthesis Absorption and transport of iron Involved in bone formation and maintenance of brain tissue and myelin sheath in nervous system	Hypocupremia: Nephrosis Malabsorption Wilson's disease—excess copper storage	2 to 2.5 mg. Diet provides 2 to 5 mg.	Liver Meat Seafood Whole grains Legumes Nuts
Iodine (I)	Absorbed as iodides, taken up by thyroid gland under control of thyroid-stimulating hormone (TSH) Excretion by kidney	Synthesis of thyroxine, the thyroid hormone, which regulates cell oxidation	Deficiency—endemic colloid goiter; cretinism	Men: 140 μg. Women: 100 μg. Infants: 25 to 45 μg. Children: 55 to 140 μg.	Iodized salt Seafoods
Manganese (Mn)	Absorption limited Excretion mainly by intestine	Activates reactions in: Urea formation Protein metabolism Glucose oxidation Lipoprotein clearance and synthesis of fatty acids	No clinical deficiency observed in humans Inhalation toxicity in miners	Unknown Diet provides 3 to 9 μg.	Cereals Soybeans Legumes Tea, coffee Nuts
Cobalt (Co)	Absorbed chiefly as constituent of vitamin B_{12}	Constituent of vitamin B_{12}; essential factor in red blood cell formation	Deficiency associated with deficiency of vitamin B_{12}—pernicious anemia	Unknown	Supplied by preformed vitamin B_{12}
Zinc (Zn)	Transported with plasma proteins Excretion largely intestinal Stored in liver, muscle, bone, and organs	Essential enzyme constituent: Carbonic anhydrase Carboxypeptidase Lactic dehydrogenase Combines with insulin for storage of the hormone	Possible relation to liver disease	Unknown Average diet supplies 10 to 15 mg.	Widely distributed Liver Seafood
Molybdenum (Mo)	Minute traces in the body	Constituent of specific enzymes involved in: Purine conversion to uric acid Aldehyde oxidation		Unknown	Organ meats Milk Whole grains Leafy vegetables Legumes

	Function			Excreted in urine
(Fl)		...dental caries	Excess causes endemic dental fluorosis	Excreted in urine
Selenium (Se)	Associated with fat metabolism	Constituent of "factor 3," which acts with vitamin E to prevent fatty liver		
Chromium (Cr)	Associated with glucose metabolism	Infants unable to metabolize sugar and adult diabetics showed definite improvement when small amounts of chromium added to diet	Possible link with cardiovascular disorders and diabetes	

anemias because of vital role in formation of red blood cells

2. Para-aminobenzoic acid (PABA)—part of the folic acid molecule; not a true vitamin alone
3. Cobalamin (B_{12})—cobalt-containing vitamin essential to hemoglobin formation; failure to absorb the vitamin because of lack of intrinsic factor in gastric secretions produces pernicious anemia

D. Group IV: other related factors (pseudovitamins)
   1. Inositol—lipotropic agent in animal nutrition
   2. Choline—essential metabolite, nerve mediator, lipotropic agent

See Table 4-2 for summary of water-soluble vitamins

Minerals

A. Group I: major minerals
   1. Calcium (Ca)
   2. Magnesium (Mg)
   3. Sodium (Na)
   4. Potassium (K)
   5. Phosphorus (P)
   6. Sulfur (S)
   7. Chlorine (Cl)
B. Group II: trace minerals
   1. Iron (Fe)
   2. Copper (Cu)
   3. Iodine (I)
   4. Manganese (Mn)
   5. Cobalt (Co)
   6. Zinc (Zn)
   7. Molybdenum (Mo)
C. Group III: other trace minerals (functions undetermined)
   1. Fluorine (Fl)
   2. Aluminum (Al)
   3. Boron (Br)
   4. Selenium (Se)
   5. Cadmium (Cd)
   6. Chromium (Cr)
   7. Vanadium (V)

See Table 4-3 for summary of minerals

COMMUNITY AND CLINICAL NUTRITION

The objective of community and clinical nutrition is to help promote, restore, and maintain health for all persons through nutrition.

EXAMPLES OF COMMUNITY RESOURCES RELATED TO NUTRITION

A. International nutrition
  1. World Health Organization (WHO) —administers programs in community and clinical nutrition in many parts of the world
  2. Food and Agriculture Organization (FAO)—provides technical assistance in agricultural development, food production and distribution
  3. United Nations International Children's Fund (UNICEF)—distributes food, equipment, and materials for child and maternal health
B. Federal government
  1. Department of Health, Education and Welfare
     a. Food and Drug Administration (FDA)—responsibility for safety of food; administers programs in public education, food labeling, monitoring, testing
     b. Public Health Service—research, materials, and services on nutrition and chronic diseases, community problems, nutrition surveys
  2. Department of Agriculture
     a. Agricultural Research Service
     b. Agricultural Extension Service
     c. Food assistance programs such as Food Stamps, Commodities
     d. School Lunch Program
C. Provincial, state, and local governments
  1. Public Health Services
  2. Public Health Nursing Services
D. Private foundations—promote research and publish recommended nutrient standards
  1. National Academy of Sciences
  2. National Research Council
  3. Food and Nutrition Board
E. Professional organizations (national and regional groups)
  1. American Dietetic Association
  2. Society for Nutrition Education
  3. American Home Economics Association
  4. American Public Health Association, Food and Nutrition Section
  5. American Medical Association
  6. American Dental Association
  7. American Nurses Association
  8. The Nutrition Today Society
F. Volunteer health organizations
  1. American Heart Association
  2. American Diabetes Association
  3. American Red Cross

SITUATIONS INVOLVING NUTRITIONAL NEEDS

A. Care of individuals throughout the life cycle
B. Care of patients with chronic diseases; e.g., diabetes, heart disease, allergies, arthritis
C. Care of persons with obesity or undernutrition
D. Nutrition education and care to prevent problems from
  1. Disease
  2. Lack of knowledge
  3. Food faddism
  4. Food habits
  5. Inadequate economic means
  6. Cultural and social situations

NUTRITIONAL NEEDS DURING LIFE CYCLE
Pregnancy and lactation

A. Nutritional objectives
  1. Ensure optimum nutrition before, during, and after pregnancy and during lactation
  2. Provide adequate nutrition to meet increased maternal and fetal nutrient demands
B. Observed nutritional influences
  1. Higher prematurity rate, low birth weight babies, and complications such as toxemia are frequently associated with malnutrition and underweight in the mother
  2. Higher risk pregnancies in teenagers
C. Nutritional needs
  1. Increased calories to meet increased basal metabolic needs and spare protein for growth, to promote weight gain to support pregnancy (averages 11.4 kg. or 25 lb. but is individual according to need), and for lactation
  2. Increased protein to provide for growth demands
  3. Increased vitamins, especially folic acid supplement to prevent anemia
  4. Increased minerals with supplement of iron to prevent anemia
  5. Iodized salt to provide needed sodium and iodine
D. Food guide may be based on basic 4 food groups with
  1. Increased protein foods—1 qt. milk,

2 eggs, 2 servings of meat, added cheese
2. Additional servings from each of the remaining food groups—grains, vegetables, fruits
3. Additional calories, protein, and fluids during lactation
See Table 4-4 for listing of food groups
E. Complications of pregnancy and possible dietary modifications
1. Underweight—careful monitoring of diet intake to ensure adequate amount of increased nutrients and desirable weight gain
2. Nausea and vomiting—limited fluids with meals, small frequent feedings, restricted fats, high carbohydrate
3. Constipation—increased fluids and residue or fiber
4. Toxemia—increased protein and calories

Infancy

A. Nutritional objectives
1. Provide nutritional base for rapid growth and development of the child during the first year of life
2. Establish the foundation for good food habits and attitudes
B. Emphasis on all nutrients to meet high energy needs and rapid growth demands
C. Diet
1. Breast-feeding
   a. Has physiologic and psychologic value for mother and infant
   b. Meets nutrient needs of early months (see comparison with cow's milk)
      (1) Calories: 110 to 120 per kg. body weight from birth to 6 months of age; 100 per kg. body weight from 6 to 12 months of age
      (2) Protein: 2.2 to 2.0 g. per kg. body weight from birth to 6 months of age; 1.8 g. per kg. body weight from 6 to 12 months of age
   c. Provides immunity factor
   d. Reduces chances for infection
2. Bottle-feeding
   a. Formula designed to match nutrient ratio of breast milk composition: water dilution to reduce protein and mineral concentration,

added carbohydrate to increase energy value
   b. Comparison of breast milk and cow's milk

	Human milk	Cow's milk (whole)
Water	88%	88%
Protein	1.0 to 1.5%	3.5 to 4.0%
Sugar (lactose)	6.5 to 7.5%	4.5 to 5.0%
Fat	3.5 to 4.0%	3.5 to 5.0%
Minerals	0.15 to 0.25%	0.7 to 0.75%
Calories (per fluid oz.)	20	20

   c. May meet needs of working mother
   d. Must be prepared under clean conditions and sterilized to prevent contamination
3. Supplement of vitamins A, C, and D usually given
   a. Requirement of vitamin A—1500 I.U.; needed for rapid growth of epithelial tissue and vision adaption
   b. Requirement of vitamin C—35 mg.; needed for rapid tissue growth
   c. Requirement of vitamin D—400 I.U.; needed for absorption and use of calcium and phosphorus for growth of bones and teeth
4. Solid food additions
   a. Introduce gradually beginning about 6 weeks of age, one at a time, in small amounts (a teaspoon or so at first increasing to servings of about 2 to 3 tablespoons by latter part of first year)
   b. Iron source, such as enriched cereal and egg yolk, among first solid food additions because milk does not contain iron and fetal storage supply lasts only about 3 to 6 months
   c. Gradual additions of a variety of strained, then soft, fruits and vegetables to supply needed vitamins, especially A and C
   d. Continuing additions include meat, potatoes, other grain forms, whole egg, puddings, toast, crackers as energy needs increase
   e. Emphasis is on variety of foods as child grows so that food tastes and habits may expand with interest
   f. Some iron and calcium absorption

may be hindered by certain binders in foods such as phytic acid in cereal hulls (especially wheat) or oxalic acid in spinach; however, absorption mechanisms usually assure adequate supply if diet contains a variety of foods

D. Diseases or conditions during infancy with possible diet modifications
1. Diarrhea—sterile feedings, decreased fat and carbohydrate
2. Constipation—increased fluids, added prune juice or strained fruit, change in type of carbohydrate
3. Celiac disease (malabsorption syndrome)—sometimes due to gluten sensitivity; diet is low in gluten, which is found in wheat, rye, and oat grains, so these grains are eliminated and rice and corn are substituted
4. Allergy—individual diet modification according to specific food sensitivity; e.g., if milk allergy exists, substitute forms of soybean or meat formula preparations are used
5. Lactose intolerance—found in non-Caucasian races; lactose-free diet used with Nutramigen as a milk substitute
6. Other examples of inborn errors of metabolism
   a. Galactosemia—missing enzyme to convert galactose to glucose, so galactose builds up in blood leading to mental retardation, liver failure, cataracts; diet is galactose-free with Nutramigen as milk substitute
   b. Phenylketonuria (PKU)—missing enzyme to convert essential amino acid phenylalanine to another amino acid, tyrosine; increase of phenylalanine and abnormal metabolites in blood leads to mental retardation, central nervous system disturbances; diet is low in phenylalanine with milk substitute Lofenalac and calculated food selections from those foods low in phenylalanine

Childhood

A. Nutritional objectives
1. Provide adequate nutrient intake to meet continuing growth and development needs
2. Provide basis for support of psychosocial development in relation to food patterns, eating behavior, and attitudes
3. Provide sufficient calories for increasing physical activities and energy needs
B. Diet—calorie and nutrient requirements increase with age
1. Increased variety in types and textures of foods
2. Increased involvement in feeding process, stimulation of curiosity about food environment, language learning
3. Consideration for child's appetite, choices, motor skills
C. Possible nutritional problem areas
1. Anemia—increase foods containing iron; e.g., enriched cereals, meat, egg, green vegetables
2. Obesity or underweight—increase or decrease calories; maintain core foods
3. Low intake of calcium, iron, vitamins A and C—usually caused by dietary fads
4. Often omitting breakfast before school

Adolescence

A. Nutritional objectives
1. Provide optimum nutritional support for demands of rapid growth and high energy expenditure
2. Support development of good eating habits through variety of foods, regular pattern, good quality snacks
B. Nutrient needs increased in all respects so adequate intakes of all nutrients should form basis of diet
C. Possible nutritional problems
1. Low intakes of calcium, vitamins A and C, iron in girls
2. Anemia—increase foods containing iron
3. Obesity or underweight—decrease or increase calories as needed
4. Skin problems—use well-balanced diet, high in protein, vitamins, minerals
5. Nutritional deficiencies related to
   a. Psychologic factors—food aversions, emotional problems
   b. Fear of overweight or crash diets—mainly in girls; cultural pressure
   c. Fad diets—caused by misinformation; need for sound counseling
   d. Poor choice of snack foods—usually high in sugar; use more fruit and protein forms
   e. Irregular eating pattern

6. Additional stress of pregnancy—need high protein, calorie intake
D. Nutrition education may be made through association with teenagers' concerns about physical appearance, figure control, complexion, physical fitness, athletic ability

Adulthood

A. Young adults
　1. Nutrition as basis of health and fitness
　2. Economic problems related to education or early careers
　3. Beginning of family, concern for welfare of young children's health and eating habits

B. Middle adults
　1. Pressures of increased family and job responsibilities
　2. Adjustments as children grow and leave home
　3. Beginnings of aging process
C. Older adults
　1. Nutritional objective—provide adequate nutrition to ensure and promote health
　2. Nutritional needs require
　　a. Calories in relation to ideal weight and activity
　　b. Consistency of diet in relation to physical, physiologic, or mechanical capacity

Table 4-4. Daily food guide: the basic four food groups

Food group	Main nutrients	Daily amounts°
Milk 　Milk, cheese, ice cream, or other products made with whole or skimmed milk	Calcium Protein Riboflavin	1 cup = 8 oz. fluid milk or designated milk equivalent† Children under 9 years of age: 2 to 3 cups Children 9 to 12 years of age: 3 or more cups Teenagers: 4 or more cups Adults: 2 or more cups Pregnant women: 3 or more cups Nursing mothers: 4 or more cups
Meats 　Beef, veal, lamb, pork, poultry, fish, eggs 　Alternates—dry beans, dry peas, nuts, peanut butter	Protein Iron Thiamin Niacin Riboflavin	2 or more servings Count as 1 serving: 　2 to 3 oz. of lean, boneless, cooked meat, poultry, or fish 　2 eggs 　1 cup cooked dry beans or peas 　4 tablespoons peanut butter
Vegetables and fruits	 Vitamin A Vitamin C (ascorbic acid) Smaller amounts of other vitamins and minerals	4 or more servings Count as 1 serving: 　½ cup vegetable or fruit, or a portion such as 1 medium apple, banana, orange, potato, or ½ medium grapefruit, melon Include: 　A dark-green or deep-yellow vegetable or fruit rich in vitamin A, at least every other day 　A citrus fruit or other fruit or vegetable rich in vitamin C daily 　Other vegetables and fruits including potatoes
Breads and cereals	 Thiamin Niacin Riboflavin Iron Protein	4 or more servings of whole grain, enriched or restored Count as one serving: 　1 slice of bread 　1 oz. (1 cup) ready to eat cereal, flake or puff varieties 　½ to ¾ cup cooked cereal 　½ to ¾ cup cooked pasta (macaroni, spaghetti, noodles) 　Crackers: 5 saltines, 2 squares graham crackers, etc.

°Use additional amounts of these foods or added butter, margarine, oils, sugars, etc., as desired or needed.
†Milk equivalents: 1 oz. cheddar cheese, 3 servings cottage cheese, 1 cup fluid skimmed milk, 1 cup buttermilk, ¼ cup dry skimmed milk powder, 1 cup ice milk, 1⅔ cups ice cream, ½ cup evaporated milk.

c. Adequate intake of all nutrients to meet adult needs
3. Diet based on Daily Food Guide (Table 4-4)
4. Possible nutritional problems
   a. Low intake of calcium and vitamins A and C
   b. Obesity or underweight
   c. Faulty eating patterns resulting from
      (1) Poor lifelong eating habits
      (2) Psychologic factors
      (3) Economic factors
      (4) Health status
      (5) Physical and physiologic capacity
      (6) Food fads

FAMILY NUTRITIONAL NEEDS AND COSTS

A. Nurse's role in nutrition counseling
   1. Establish rapport
   2. Identify nutrition problems
   3. Collect pertinent information concerning influences on food habits and patterns
      a. Age, weight, height, sex, and activity of family members
      b. General appearance and health status
      c. Cultural and religious customs
      d. Social and psychologic meanings of food
      e. Financial status
      f. Physical and mental capacity
      g. Good storage, preparation, and serving facilities
      h. Food marketing and preparation methods
      i. Knowledge of nutrition
      j. General interest and concern
   4. Take nutritional history
      a. Kind and amounts of food in usual pattern on daily or weekly basis, including weekend variances
      b. Distribution and time of meals and snacks
      c. Personal preferences
      d. Time and number of meals
      e. Place meals eaten
   5. Evaluate nutritional intake based on standards of nutrition
   6. Set goals and work out a practical food plan with the family, within their life situation and style, for meeting identified nutritional needs
   7. Plan follow-up visits for continued support, education, and encouragement
   8. Use available resource persons and materials
      a. Nutritionist, dietitian, physician, social worker
      b. Community agencies, associations, clinics, hospitals
      c. Textbooks, booklets, visual materials
B. Economic considerations in food planning
   1. Plan menus and market lists in advance
   2. Select most economic market
   3. Take advantage of sales
   4. Purchase foods in season
   5. Purchase food sizes, amounts, and grades most suitable
   6. Compare prices according to method of preserving, freshness, edible portion, processed versus regular plain form
   7. Compare nutritive return in relation to cost

CLINICAL NUTRITION

A. Objectives of nutritional care in disease
   1. Supply optimum nutrition
   2. Heal tissue, cure disease
   3. Support recovery from disease
   4. Improve function of involved tissue or organ system
   5. Reduce work of affected organ to promote healing
B. Factors in planning modified diets
   1. Disease state, its nature, duration, intensity
   2. Food form or nutrient modification required by the disease
   3. Patient's individual food tolerances and food habits
   4. Nutritional adequacy of modified diet
   5. Patient's physical ability and home situation
C. Modifications of normal diet to meet clinical needs
   1. Texture, residue
   2. Specific nutrients—modifications in one or more of the basic nutrients (protein, carbohydrate, fat, minerals, vitamins)
   3. Energy—calorie increase or decrease
   4. Meal pattern, food distribution

D. Diet management tools—food exchange groups (Table 4-5)
1. Calorie and nutrient control
2. Flexible food choices
E. Standard hospital diets—liquid, soft, light, full
1. Liquid diets
   a. Clear liquid—clear broth, bouillon, juices, plain gelatin, fruit-flavored water ices, ginger ale, coffee, tea
   b. Full liquid—may add milk and items made with milk, such as cream soups, milk drinks, sherbet, ice cream, puddings, custard
2. Soft diet—may add all soft cooked foods, such as refined cereals, pasta, rice, white bread and crackers, eggs, cheese, meat, potatoes, cooked whole vegetables, cooked fruits, few soft ripe plain fruits without membranes or skins, simple desserts
3. Light diet—same as soft with few additional whole cooked foods, light raw foods as fruit; mainly avoids heavily seasoned or fried foods
4. Full diet (or general diet)—full, well-balanced diet of all foods as desired and tolerated, including a wide variety for interest and flavor
F. Therapeutic diets
1. Obesity and weight control
   a. Considerations—individual decision and support, individual diet plan with calorie and situational adaptations, a planned follow-up program
   b. Characteristics of diet
      (1) Realistic goals of total loss and rate of loss
      (2) Calories lowered according to individual nutritional need, to effect a gradual loss of 1 or 2 pounds a week
      (3) Nutritional adequacy of all nutrients; ratio of about 12% to 15% of calories as protein, no more than 35% as fat with reduced intake of saturated fats, with rest of calories as carbohydrate, using little or no sucrose and including a variety of foods
      (4) Culturally desirable—to form the basis for permanent re-education of eating habits
      (5) Calorie adjustment to maintain weight when desired weight goal is reached
   c. Basic tools for planning diet—food exchange groups, using the exchange system of dietary control
2. Diabetes mellitus
   a. Considerations—individual nutritional needs, maintenance of ideal weight, calories, and situational adaptations, a planned follow-up program according to need
   b. Characteristics of diet
      (1) Calories as needed to maintain ideal weight
      (2) Protein—optimum, normal age group needs; usually 65 to 85 g. for average adult
      (3) Carbohydrate—adequate for need but not excessive; usually about 100 to 250 g. for an adult
      (4) Fat—moderation is the guideline; substitution of vegetable fats for some of the animal fats; usually about 70 to 100 g. for adult
      (5) Dietary ratio—carbohydrate to protein to fat usually about 2:1:1
      (6) Distribution—fairly even distribution of food throughout the day in 3 meals, with snacks added between as needed from the day's total food allowances according to need and therapy with insulin or oral hypoglycemics
   c. Basic tools for planning diet—food exchange groups, using the exchange system of dietary control
3. Gastrointestinal diseases
   a. Peptic ulcer
      (1) Traditional conservative management used by some physicians
         (a) Acid neutralizing—milk, soft bland foods such as refined grains, egg, mild cheeses, a few cooked or or pureed vegetables and fruits, tender meat; may be initially limited to Sippy diet
         (b) Nonirritating chemically (avoid strong flavors and seasonings)

(c) Nonirritating mechanically (avoid raw foods, plant fiber, "gas-formers")

(d) Nonirritating thermally (avoid hot or cold foods)

(2) Liberal individualized approach (more widely used in current practice)

(a) Treated individually, with detailed initial diet history, attitudes, living situation, food reactions, tolerances, then dietary program that can be followed is planned

(b) Activity of ulcer from time to time influences dietary management to control acid and promote healing; however, a variety of foods as tolerated is the guideline, with regular unhurried meals

b. Diverticulosis and diverticulitis

(1) Well-balanced diet with variety of foods, adequate protein

(2) Acute episodes may require liquids and low residue foods, excluding roughage; however, some clinicians are increasingly favoring increased fiber in the diet rather than less, with more use of bran, whole grains, and cellulose foods as a means of reducing muscle contractions of the colon and facilitating normal muscle tone

c. Malabsorption syndrome (celiac, sprue)

(1) Fat poorly absorbed, so fat foods limited

(2) Gluten a factor in the etiology of nontropical sprue; gluten foods (wheat, rye, oat) eliminated with all other foods used according to individual tolerance

d. Ulcerative colitis

(1) Treatment—rest, nutritional therapy, sulfonamides

(2) Diet therapy

(a) High protein—extensive colon lesions require healing; protein supple-ments used with food sources to supply 120 to 150 g. of protein per day; milk causes some difficulty for some patients at first, so is omitted and added later in cooked form; use egg, cheese, meat

(b) High calorie—about 3000 calories a day needed to spare protein for healing and restore nutrient deficits from daily loss in stools and consequent weight loss

(c) Increased minerals and vitamins—supplements of vitamins and minerals, as well as food sources as tolerated (grains, fruits, vegetables, protein foods)

(d) Low residue—diet fairly low in residue in acute stages with gradual increases as tolerated, avoiding only heavy roughage to prevent irritation

4. Diseases of the liver and gallbladder

a. Hepatitis

(1) Treatment—rest, optimum nutritional therapy

(2) Diet therapy

(a) High protein—healing of liver tissue vital; daily intake should include 1 qt. milk, 2 eggs, 8 oz. lean meat, fish, or cheese; total should approximate 75 to 100 g. protein

(b) High carbohydrate—energy needs, restore glycogen reserves; use daily 4 servings vegetables including potato, 4 servings fruit with frequent juices, 6 to 8 servings bread or cereal; total carbohydrate should be 300 to 400 g.

(c) Moderate fat—2 to 4 tablespoons butter or fortified margarine, sufficient for making food palatable; a moderate amount of easily usable foods such as whole milk, cream, butter, margarine, or vegetable oil is beneficial; total fat should be 100 to 150 g. daily

    (d) High calorie—increased energy needs for disease process and tissue regeneration and to spare protein for healing; these food amounts should provide about 2500 to 3000 calories daily

b. Cirrhosis

    (1) Treatment—rest, supportive care, nutritional therapy

    (2) Diet therapy

        (a) Protein according to tolerance—with increasing liver damage protein metabolism is hindered; hold to 80 to 100 g. as long as tolerated, reduce as necessary

        (b) Continue high carbohydrate, moderate fat as in hepatitis to supply energy; vitamin supplements especially B complex

        (c) Low sodium—usually restricted to 500 to 1000 mg. daily by eliminating salt and controlling foods processed with salt or sodium-based preservatives; sodium restriction helps to control the increasing ascites

        (d) Soft foods—if esophageal varices develop to prevent danger of rupture and bleeding

        (e) Alcohol strictly forbidden to avoid continued irritation and malnutrition

c. Hepatic coma

    (1) Treatment—rest, removal of sources of ammonia as advanced liver damage brings failure of liver to detoxify ammonia through its urea cycle, hence ammonia intoxication and coma follow ingestion of protein

    (2) Diet therapy

        (a) Low protein—reduced according to tolerance, 15 to 30 g.

        (b) High calories and vitamins according to need —about 1500 to 2000 calories sufficient to prevent tissue catabolism and the liberation of additional nitrogen

        (c) Fluid carefully controlled according to output

d. Gallbladder

    (1) Cholecystitis—diet low in fat to avoid stimulus to gallbladder, which constricts to excrete bile with subsequent pain; calories principally from carbohydrate foods in acute phases; if weight loss indicated, as is often the case, calories reduced to 1000 to 1200

    (2) Cholecystectomy—removal of the gallbladder, usually for stones, may require a low fat diet after surgery, with resumption of moderate fat diet intake on a maintenance basis

5. Cardiovascular diseases

a. Atherosclerosis, coronary heart disease

    (1) Etiology—relation to general lipid metabolism, fatty deposits in artery walls; cholesterol and serum lipids elevated

    (2) Types of lipid disorders

        (a) Type I—elevation of chylomicrons (lipoprotein formed in intestinal wall from dietary fats) with normal levels of other lipoproteins (beta, pre-beta); genetic type, rare, in children with missing enzyme lipoprotein lipase to clear chylomicrons with dietary load of triglycerides from blood following intestinal absorption; diet very low in fat, about 25 to 35 g. daily, since fat cannot be handled, with major energy source coming from carbohydrate; may use special short and medium chain fatty acid product MCT (medium chain triglycerides) as a commercially prepared oil since it can be absorbed directly into the blood and go to the liver for metabolism

(b) Type II—cholesterol is elevated as well as beta lipoproteins; hence diet is low in cholesterol, less than 300 mg. per day, and decreasing saturated fats; this eliminates foods high in cholesterol such as egg (yolk only involved), organ meats, shellfish, and animal fats such as butter, cream, whole milk, fatty meat, cheeses; this is a common disorder and may occur at either younger or older ages

(c) Type III—relatively uncommon, elevation of an abnormal form of beta lipoprotein, also increase in plasma cholesterol and triglycerides; patients display characteristic orange streaks in palmar creases of hands; apparently genetic; diet designed for weight loss if obese, with low cholesterol and high unsaturated fatty acid foods (vegetable oils)

(d) Type IV—common pattern, associated with glucose intolerance and diabetic tendency; plasma triglycerides high but cholesterol may be normal; usually compounded by obesity; after weight loss, diet is maintained

on low carbohydrate level, low in cholesterol, low saturated fats (animals), and high unsaturated fatty acids are substituted for animal fats

(e) Type V—rare form, elevation of chylomicrons and pre-beta lipoproteins, also cholesterol and triglycerides; the diet is designed to reduce weight to normal, then maintain patient on low fats and carbohydrates, with main calories coming from proteins

(3) Fat control in diets

(a) Amount of fat—no more than 35% of diet calories or lower if weight reduction is needed

(b) Kind of fat—reduction of animal fats (saturated) and increased substitution of plant fats (unsaturated)

b. Congestive heart failure

(1) Edema—imbalance in capillary fluid shift mechanism caused by increased venous pressure from failing heart, compounded by aldosterone mechanism, which causes more sodium retention and by ADH mechanism, which causes more water retention

(2) Diet therapy

(a) Low sodium—helps control edema

(1) Mild restriction—2 to 3 g. sodium: no added table salt (light use in cooking) and no obviously salty foods; all other foods as desired

(2) Moderate restriction —1000 mg. sodium: same as above plus elimination of salt in cooking and canned vegetables; basic

foods as desired, un-
processed with salt
(3) Strict restriction—
500 mg. sodium:
same as above plus
increased control of
foods with higher
amounts of natural
sodium (smaller
amounts of meat,
egg, milk limited to
2 cups) also limiting
of vegetables such as
leafy greens, beets,
carrots, celery
(4) Severe restriction—
250 mg. sodium: all
of above restrictions
plus tighter control
of natural food
sources; e.g., no regu-
lar milk (use low so-
dium milk only),
meat limit 2 to 3 oz.
daily and 2 to 3 eggs
per week
(b) Calorie control—reduced
for cardiac rest in acute
stages or continuing for
weight reduction
(c) Texture control—soft
foods in acute stages to
reduce work of eating
c. Hypertension
(1) Etiology—unclear but studies
have linked it to a sensitivity
to salt use; probably associated with imbalance in renin-
angiotensin-aldosterone mechanism for conserving body
sodium
(2) Diet therapy—low sodium,
moderate restriction to 1000
mg. if needed; usually with
diuretic therapy milk restriction to 2 to 3 g. is sufficient—
no added salt after light use
in cooking
6. Renal disease
a. Acute glomerulonephritis—usually
short-term problem so overall nutrition is of greater concern with
adequate rather than restricted
protein and no sodium restriction
b. Nephrotic syndrome—nephron lesions with massive albuminuria as

well as other protein losses in urine;
general malnutrition ensues; diet is
high in protein to help replace
losses, 100 to 150 g. daily; calories
also high to spare protein for tissue
synthesis and to provide energy;
edema is severe so sodium is restricted to 500 mg.
c. Chronic renal failure (uremia)
(1) Diet
(a) Protein low to moderate
according to tolerance,
30 to 50 g.
(b) Carbohydrate relatively
high for energy, 300 to
400 g.
(c) Fat relatively moderate,
70 to 90 g.
(d) Calories adequate for
maintenance to prevent
tissue breakdown, 2000
to 2500 daily
(e) Sodium controlled ac-
cording to serum levels
and excretion tolerance,
varying from 400 to 2000
mg.
(f) Potassium controlled according to serum levels
and excretion capacities,
varying from 1300 to
1900 mg.
(g) Water controlled according to excretion, about
800 to 1000 ml.; careful
intake-output records
vital
(2) General diet management
(a) General protein and electrolyte control
(b) The low protein–essential
amino acid diet (modi-
fied Giordano-Giovan-
netti regimen) to sus-
tain patients with uremia
and alleviate their difficult symptoms
(1) Very low protein—
20 g., minimal essen-
tial amino acids
(2) Controlled potassium
—1500 mg., fed only
essential amino acids,
causing the body to
use its own excess
urea nitrogen to syn-

thesize the nonessential amino acids needed for tissue protein production; foods used include 1 egg, 6 oz. milk, low protein bread, 2 to 4 fruits, and 2 to 4 vegetables from special lists to control protein and potassium

d. Renal calculi
  (1) Treatment
    (a) Fluid intake—large fluid intake to produce a dilute urine and help prevent concentration of stone constituents
    (b) Urinary pH—an attempt to control the solubility factor by increased acidity or alkalinity, depending upon the composition of the stones formed; e.g., for an alkaline stone, an acid urine
    (c) Stone composition—reduction of material composing the stone
  (2) Diet according to type of stone
    (a) Calcium stone—low calcium, low phosphate or oxalate according to calcium compound, acid ash; calcium foods, mainly dairy products, are eliminated; acid ash foods such as meat, egg, grains are emphasized; alkaline foods such as milk, vegetables, fruits are controlled
    (b) Uric acid stones—low purine (uric acid is a metabolic product of purines in the body), controlling purine foods such as meat, especially organ meats, meat extractives, and to a lesser extent plant sources such as whole grains and legumes; alkaline ash since the stone composition is acid
    (c) Cystine stones—rare genetic type; diet is low methionine, since methionine is the essential amino acid from which the nonessential amino acid cystine is formed, controlling such protein foods as meat, milk, egg, cheese; alkaline ash since the stone is an acid composition

7. Surgery
  a. Postoperative nutritional needs
    (1) Protein—increased protein caused by protein losses and catabolic period of recovery and tissue healing; a period of negative nitrogen balance initially
    (2) Calories—adequate amount to supply energy and spare protein for tissue building
    (3) Water—adequate fluid therapy to avoid dehydration caused by large fluid losses
    (4) Minerals—replacement of deficiencies and insurance of continued adequacy essential to maintain electrolyte balance
    (5) Vitamins—vitamin C especially needed for tissue synthesis and wound healing; B complex essential in energy production and tissue building
  b. Dietary management
    (1) Initial IV therapy for water and electrolytes, but oral intake needed as soon as possible for adequate nutrition
    (2) Hyperalimentation—parenteral nutrition of high nutrient density; solutions of amino acids, glucose, electrolytes, minerals, vitamins; usually inserted into larger veins (inferior or superior vena cava) to avoid thrombosis in peripheral veins; used in cases of major tissue trauma or injury, extensive surgery
    (3) Postoperative diet—liquid, soft, to full diet as soon as

possible to supply nutritive demands

c. Special gastrointestinal surgery
  (1) Mouth, throat, or neck surgery —oral liquid feedings or tube feedings, either blenderized food mixtures or special formula preparations such as Sustagen to achieve a high protein, high calorie intake
  (2) Gastric resection
      (a) Immediate postoperative period—gradual buildup of foods a few at a time until tolerance established
      (b) Later—"dumping syndrome" may develop; rapid food passage draws water from surrounding blood volume causing shock symptoms; relief achieved by diet— 5 or 6 small meals low in carbohydrate, mainly protein and fat, with liquids only between meals
  (3) Cholecystectomy—low fat following surgery to avoid pain from constriction at wound site; general avoidance of heavy fat intake on a continuing basis
  (4) Ileostomy and colostomy— initial period of reduced residue diet may be indicated, but return to regular full diet as soon as possible for both nutritional and psychologic reasons
  (5) Rectal surgery—nonresidue immediately, then low residue diet as needed with return to full diet as soon as possible
d. Burns
  (1) Immediate shock period— days 1 to 3
      (a) Initial fluid and electrolyte problems, massive flooding edema at burn site pulling water from other parts of the body, as well as protein loss and electrolyte loss (sodium); potassium drawn from cells to replace sodium loss with rising serum levels of potassium
      (b) Immediate parenteral— protein through blood or plasma expander (Dextran), sodium and chloride replacement through lactated Ringer's solution, water (dextrose solution) to cover losses
  (2) Recovery period—days 3 to 5
      (a) As fluid and electrolytes are reabsorbed, pattern shifts and a sudden diuresis follows
      (b) Oral liquid solutions, such as Holdrane's solution (water, salt, baking soda), may now be tolerated
  (3) Secondary feeding period— days 6 to 15
      (a) Critical nutrition stage of tissue regeneration, turning from initial catabolic period of negative nitrogen balance to an active tissue rebuilding stage
      (b) Diet therapy—high protein (150 to 400 g.) with protein supplements, high calorie (3500 to 5000), high vitamins, especially C for wound healing and B complex for energy and protein metabolism; record keeping of intake vital to ensure meeting high nutrient requirements
  (4) Follow-up reconstruction period—from second week on
      (a) Grafting and plastic surgery—continued optimum nutrition essential
      (b) Rehabilitation period— rebuilding both physically and emotionally requires much support

THE EXCHANGE SYSTEM OF DIETARY CONTROL

The exchange system, set up by professional organizations including the American

Dietetic Association, is based on a simple grouping of common foods according to generally equivalent nutritional values. This system may be used for any situation requiring calorie and food value control.

The foods are divided into 6 basic groups, called the exchange groups. Each food within a group contains approximately the same food value as any other food item in that same group, allowing for free exchange within any given group; hence the term food exchange is used throughout. The total number of exchanges per day depends on individual nutritional needs, based always on normal nutritional recommendations of the Food and Nutrition Board, National Research Council.

Although there is some variation in the composition of foods within the exchange groups, for simplicity the following values for carbohydrate, protein, and fat are used.

Food	Approximate measure	Carbohydrate (g.)	Protein (g.)	Fat (g.)	Calories
Fruit exchange	Varies	10	—	—	40
Bread exchange	1 slice	15	2	—	70
Meat exchange	1 oz.	—	7	5	75
Vegetable B exchange	½ cup	7	2	—	40
Milk exchange	1 cup	12	8	10	170 (skimmed = 80)
Fat exchange	1 tsp.	—	—	5	45

Table 4-5. Food exchange groups

Food group	Unit of exchange	Composition Carbohydrate (g.)	Protein (g.)	Fat (g.)	Calories	Characteristic items
Milk						
Whole	1 cup	12	8	10	170	Equivalents to 1 cup whole milk listed; 1 cup skimmed and 2 fat exchanges = whole milk
Skimmed	1 cup	12	8	—	80	
Vegetables A	As desired	—	—	—	—	Free use: 3% carbohydrates and below (tomatoes, green beans, leafy vegetables)
B	½ cup	7	2	—	35	Medium carbohydrate: pod and root varieties (green peas, carrots)
Fruit	Varies	10	—	—	40	Fresh or canned without sugar Portion size varies with carbohydrate value of item; all portions equated at 10% carbohydrate
Bread	Varies; 1 slice bread	15	2	—	70	Variety of starch items, breads, cereals, vegetables; portions equal in carbohydrate value to 1 slice bread
Meat	1 oz.	—	7	5	75	Protein foods, exchange units equal to protein value of 1 oz. lean meat (cheese, egg, seafood)
Fat	1 tsp.	—	—	5	45	Fat food items equal to 1 tsp. butter or margarine (bacon, oil, mayonnaise, olives, avocado)

Table 4-6. Food exchanges

Milk exchanges

Whole milk	1 cup	(Cream portion of whole milk equals 2 fat
Skim milk	1 cup	exchanges; 1 cup of whole milk equals 1 cup
Buttermilk	1 cup	of skim milk plus 2 fat exchanges)
Evaporated milk	½ cup	
Powdered skim milk	¼ cup	
Yogurt, plain	1 cup	

Vegetable exchanges—served plain, without fat, seasoning, or dressing (any fat used is taken from fat exchange allowance)

GROUP A (Use as desired; negligible carbohydrate, protein, and fat in amounts commonly eaten)

Asparagus	Greens	Mushrooms
Bak choi, Gai choi	Beet greens	Okra
Bamboo shoots	Chard	Peppers (bell, chili, etc.)
Broccoli	Collards	Radishes
Brussels sprouts	Kale	Sauerkraut
Cabbage	Mustard	String beans, young
Cauliflower	Salad greens	Summer squash
Celery	Lettuces	Tomatoes
Chicory	Spinach	Watercress
Chinese cabbage	Turnip greens	Parsley
Cucumbers		Pimientos
Escarole, endive		
Eggplant		

GROUP B (½ cup equals 1 serving)

Artichoke (1 medium)	Onions	Rutabaga
Beets	Peas, green	Squash, winter
Carrots	Pumpkin	Turnip

Fruit exchanges—unsweetened, fresh, frozen, canned, cooked (1 exchange is portion indicated by each fruit)

Berries		Others	
Blackberries	1 cup	Apple	1 small
Blueberries	⅔ cup	Apple juice	⅓ cup
Raspberries	¾ cup	Applesauce	½ cup
Strawberries	1 cup	Apricots (fresh)	2 medium
Citrus fruits		Banana	½ small
Grapefruit	½ small	Cherries	10 large
Grapefruit juice	½ cup	Figs (fresh)	1
Orange	1 small	Grapes	12 medium
Orange juice	½ cup	Grape juice	¼ cup
Tangerine	1 large	Peach	1 medium
Dried fruits		Pear	1 small
Apricots	4 halves	Pineapple	½ cup, 1 slice
Dates	2	Pineapple juice	⅓ cup
Figs	1 small	Plums	2 medium
Prunes	2 medium	Prunes (fresh)	2
Raisins	2 tablespoons	Prune juice	¼ cup
Melons			
Cantaloupe	¼ medium		
Honeydew	⅛ medium		
Watermelon	½ center slice		

Bread exchanges (equivalent portions indicated by each item)

Bread		Graham (2½ in. square)	2
Bagel	½	Oyster	½ cup
Biscuit, roll (2 in. diam.)	1	Round, thin (½ in. diam.)	6-8
Bread (white or dark)	1 slice	Saltines (2 in. square)	5
Cornbread (1½ in. cube)	1	Soda (2½ in. square)	3
Frankfurter roll	1 small	Matzos (6 in. diam.)	1 piece
Hamburger roll	½ large	Muffin (2 in. diam.)	1
Tortilla	1 medium	Melba thins	4
Crackers		Pretzels (22 per lb.)	1 medium
Animal	8	Pretzel sticks (avg. thin)	14

Continued.

Table 4-6. Food exchanges—cont'd

Bread exchanges—cont'd

Cereal		Corn on the cob	½ large ear, 1 small ear
Cereal, cooked	½ cup		
Cereal, dry (flakes, puffed)	¾ cup	Popcorn (popped)	1 cup
Flour	2½ tbs.	Parsnips	⅔ cup
Rice, grits (cooked)	½ cup	Potatoes, white	1 small
Corn	⅓ cup	Potatoes, mashed white	½ cup
Spaghetti, macaroni, noodles (cooked)	½ cup	Potatoes, sweet or yams	¼ cup
Vegetables and others		Sponge cake, plain	1½ in. cube
Baked beans, no pork	¼ cup	Ice cream, vanilla (omit 2 fat exch.)	½ cup
Beans, peas, dried, cooked	½ cup	Ice milk, vanilla	½ cup

Meat exchanges (all items refer to cooked weight)

Lean meat, poultry	1 oz.	Fish	
Cold cuts (4½ in. × ⅛ in.)	1 slice	Cod, halibut	1 oz.
Frankfurter (8 or 9 per lb.)	1	Salmon, tuna, crab, lobster	¼ cup
Egg	1	Shrimp, clams, oysters, etc.	5 small
Cheese, cheddar	1 oz.	Sardines	3 medium
Cheese, cottage	¼ cup	Scallops (12 pieces per lb.)	1 large
Sausage (3 in. × ½ in.)	2	Peanut butter (limit 1 exch. per day)	2 tbs.

Fat exchanges

Avocado (4 in. diam.)	⅛	French dressing	1 tbs.
Bacon, crisp	1 slice	Half and half (10% cream and milk)	4 tbs.
Butter or margarine	1 tsp.	Mayonnaise	1 tsp.
Cream, light (20%)	2 tbs.	Nuts	6 small
Cream, heavy (40%)	1 tbs.	Oil or cooking fat	1 tsp.
Cream cheese	1 tbs.	Olives	5 small
Cheese spreads	1 tbs.	Sour cream	2 tbs.

Miscellaneous foods allowed as desired (negligible carbohydrate, protein, fat)

Artificial sweeteners	Gelatin, plain	Rennet tablets, plain
Bouillon, fat-free	Lemon	Rhubarb
Broth, clear	Mustard	Spices
Coffee	Pepper	Tea
Cranberries, unsweetened	Pickles, dill and sour	Vinegar
Catsup		

Table 4-7. Weight reduction diets using the exchange system

Food exchange group	Approximate measure	Total number of exchanges per day			
		800 calories	1000 calories	1200 calories	1500 calories
Milk (nonfat)	1 cup	2	2	2	2
Vegetable group A	As desired	Free	Free	Free	Free
Vegetable group B	½ cup	1	1	1	1
Fruit	Varies	3	3	3	4
Bread	1 slice	1	3	4	4
Meat	1 oz.	6	6	7	9
Fat	1 tsp.	1	1	2	4
		Distribution of food exchanges			
Breakfast					
Fruit		1	1	1	1
Meat		1	1	1	1
Bread		1	1	1	1
Fat		1	1	1	1
Lunch and dinner					
Meat		2 to 3	2 to 3	3	4
Vegetable A		Any	Any	Any	Any
Vegetable B (either meal)		1	1	1	1
Bread		0	1	1 to 2	1 to 2
Fat		0	0	0 to 1	1 to 2
Fruit		1	1	1	1 to 2
Milk		1	1	1	1

Table 4-8. American dietetic association meal plan for diabetics

	Diet plan number								
	1	*2*	*3*	*4*	*5**	*6**	*7**	*8*	*9*
Calories	1200	1500	1800	2200	1800	2600	3500	2600	3000
Carbohydrate (g.)	125	150	180	220	180	250	370	250	300
Protein (g.)	60	70	80	90	80	100	140	115	120
Fat (g.)	50	70	80	100	80	130	165	130	145
Total food exchanges									
Milk	2	2	2	2	4	4	4	2	2
Vegetable group A	†	†	†	†	†	†	†	†	†
Vegetable group B	1	1	1	1	1	1	1	1	1
Fruit	3	3	3	4	3	4	6	4	4
Bread	4	6	8	10	6	10	17	12	15
Meat	5	6	7	8	5	7	10	10	10
Fat	1	4	5	8	3	11	15	12	15

*These diets contain more milk and are planned for children.
†As desired.

REVIEW QUESTIONS FOR NUTRITIONAL SCIENCE: COMMUNITY AND CLINICAL NUTRITION

1. The government agency charged with the responsibility of food safety is the
   1. U.S. Department of Agriculture
   2. U.S. Department of Commerce
   3. Food and Drug Administration
   4. U.S. Public Health Service
2. Our food environment is rapidly changing as advances in food technology make possible a wide variety of new food items with the use of food additives. These materials are
   1. Chemicals used with foods during processing to achieve a particular purpose or product
   2. Naturally occurring chemicals in plants and animals
   3. Incidental chemicals unintentionally getting into foods during growing or processing for market
   4. Pesticides used in agriculture to increase crop yields
3. The Government Regulated Additives and Substitution (GRAS) list is
   1. A listing of food additives proved to be harmful and subsequently banned
   2. A group of additives used for nutrient enrichment of food products
   3. A record of all the food additives that have been fully tested and therefore declared safe for use
   4. A listing of several hundred food additives in general use that have been declared safe but lack comprehensive testing
4. The unique chemical compound produced in the human energy system in the cell, which traps and stores energy in its high-energy bonds, is
   1. DNA—deoxyribonucleic acid
   2. ATP—adenosine triphosphate
   3. RNA—ribonucleic acid
   4. AMP—adenosine monophosphate

5. The weight of extracellular body fluid is approximately 20% of the total body weight of an average individual. Which component of the extracellular fluid contributes the greatest portion to this amount?
   1. Interstitial fluid
   2. Plasma fluid
   3. Fluid in body secretions
   4. Fluid in dense tissue
6. The building units of protein, which are amino acids, have a unique fundamental structure—a *dual nature*. This refers to the
   1. Acid and base parts of their structure
   2. Balanced amino groups
   3. Two different modes of absorption
   4. Two different pathways to produce energy
7. A complete protein, a food protein of high biologic value, is one that contains
   1. All 22 of the amino acids in sufficient quantity to meet human requirements
   2. All 8 of the essential amino acids in correct proportion to meet human needs
   3. The 8 essential amino acids in any proportion, since the body can always fill in the difference needed
   4. Most of the 22 amino acids from which the body will make additional amounts of the 8 essential amino acids needed
8. Twenty-two amino acids are involved in total body metabolism, building and rebuilding various tissues. Of these, 8 are termed *essential* amino acids. This means that
   1. The body cannot synthesize these 8 amino acids and hence must obtain them in the diet
   2. These 8 amino acids are essential in body processes and the remaining 14 are not
   3. These 8 amino acids can be made by the body because they are essential to life
   4. After synthesizing these 8 amino acids the body uses them in key processes essential for growth
9. The end products of protein digestion, the

"building blocks"—amino acids, are absorbed from the small intestine by
1. Simple diffusion because of their small size
2. Active transport with aid of vitamin B$_6$ (pyridoxine)
3. Osmosis caused by their greater concentration in the intestinal lumen
4. Filtration according to the osmotic pressure direction

10. Proteins whose biologic activity has been altered by heat, ultraviolet light, or other physical means are
    1. Denatured
    2. Deactivated
    3. Attenuated
    4. Neutralized

11. In the body's blood transport system, lipoproteins function as carriers of
    1. Glucose to cells for energy supply and conversion to fat for storage
    2. Triglycerides and some fatty acids as a major fuel source for cell metabolism
    3. Fat-soluble vitamins to regulate specific cell functions
    4. Amino acids to supply structural units for cell synthesis of protein for adipose fat tissue

12. The terms *saturated* and *unsaturated,* when used in reference to fats, indicate degrees of
    1. Color
    2. Taste
    3. Hardness
    4. Digestibility

13. The main function of adipose tissue in fat metabolism is synthesizing
    1. Lipoproteins for fat transport
    2. And storing triglycerides for energy reserves
    3. Cholesterol as needed
    4. And releasing glucose for energy

14. Cholesterol is frequently discussed in relation to atherosclerosis. It is a substance that
    1. All persons would be better off without because it causes the disease process
    2. Circulates in the blood, the level of which responds usually to dietary substitutions of unsaturated fats for saturated fats
    3. Is found in many foods, both plant and animal sources
    4. May be controlled entirely by eliminating food sources

15. When the transport fat compounds accumulate in abnormal levels in the blood, the diet may be modified as one effort to control them. The foods most affected by such diet therapy would be
    1. Vegetable oils
    2. Fruits
    3. Grains
    4. Animal fats

16. The two main sites for handling fat metabolism are the liver and adipose tissue. Of its several functions concerning fat, the *main* role of the liver is
    1. The production of phospholipids
    2. Oxidizing fatty acids to produce energy
    3. Converting fat to lipoproteins for rapid transport out into the body
    4. Storing fat for energy reserves

17. Because fat is insoluble in water it cannot travel free in the blood. The main type of compound formed, therefore, to serve as a vehicle of transport is
    1. Triglyceride
    2. Plasma protein
    3. Phospholipid
    4. Lipoprotein

18. An important material produced in the liver and stored in the gallbladder is needed to prepare food fats for change to usable fuel forms. This material is
    1. Lipase
    2. Amylase
    3. Bile
    4. Cholesterol

19. The major digestive changes in fat are accomplished in the small intestine by a lipase from the pancreas. This enzymatic activity
    1. Easily breaks down all the dietary fat to fatty acids and glycerol
    2. Splits off all the fatty acids in only about 25% of the total dietary fat consumed
    3. Synthesizes new triglycerides from the dietary fat consumed
    4. Emulsifies the fat globules and reduces their surface tension

20. The fuel glucose is delivered to the cells by the blood for "production" of energy. The hormone controlling the use of glucose by the cell is
    1. Thyroxine
    2. Growth hormone
    3. Adrenal steroids
    4. Insulin

21. Carbohydrates provide one of our main fuel sources for energy. Which of the following carbohydrate foods provides the *quickest* source of energy?
    1. A slice of bread
    2. A glass of orange juice
    3. A glass of milk
    4. Chocolate candy bar

22. A readily available form of energy, though limited in amount, is stored in the liver by conversion of glucose to
    1. Glycogen
    2. Glycerol
    3. Tissue fat
    4. Amino acids

23. Most of the work of changing raw fuel forms of carbohydrates to the refined usable fuel glucose is accomplished by enzymes located in the
    1. Mouth
    2. Stomach mucosa
    3. Small intestine
    4. Large intestine

24. After the raw fuel forms of carbohydrate are changed to the refined usable fuel monosaccharides, these simple sugars, mainly glucose, are absorbed from the intestine directly into the portal blood system by
    1. Pinocytosis
    2. Active transport

3. Simple diffusion
4. Osmosis

25. Vitamin C has been advocated in megadoses to prevent infections such as the common cold. Which of the following chemical characteristic of the vitamin would seem to refute these claims?
    1. Vitamin C is a complex compound of high molecular weight and hence unavailable metabolically in such large amounts
    2. The liver and adipose tissue already accumulate large storage reserves of this vitamin and release it as needed
    3. When general tissue saturation levels are reached, the rest of the vitamin is excreted in the urine
    4. Vitamin C is fat soluble and hence excess becomes bound in fat compounds and is unavailable to the body

26. The food group lowest in natural sodium is
    1. Meat
    2. Milk
    3. Vegetables
    4. Fruits

27. Many vitamins and minerals regulate the many chemical changes of cell metabolism by acting in a coenzyme role. This means that the vitamin or mineral
    1. May become a structural part of the enzyme controlling a particular reaction
    2. May be a necessary catalyst present for the reaction to proceed
    3. Forms a new compound by a series of complex changes
    4. Prevents unnecessary reactions by neutralizing the controlling enzyme

28. Vitamin A is a fat-soluble vitamin produced by humans and other animals from its precursor carotene—provitamin A. One of the main sources of this vitamin is
    1. Skim milk
    2. Leafy greens
    3. Oranges
    4. Tomatoes

29. Because vitamin A is fat soluble, it requires a helping agent for absorption. This agent is
    1. Lipase
    2. Amylase
    3. Hydrochloric acid
    4. Bile

30. The vision cycle in the eye requires vitamin A. Here the vitamin functions as
    1. A necessary component of rhodopsin (visual purple), which controls light-dark adaptations
    2. A part of the rods and cones that control color blindness
    3. The material in the cornea that prevents cataract formation
    4. An integral part of the retina's pigment melanin

31. Which of the following statements are true about the sources of vitamin K?
    1. Vitamin K is found in a wide variety of foods so there is no danger of a deficiency
    2. Vitamin K can easily be absorbed without assistance so that all that is consumed is absorbed

3. Vitamin K is rarely found in dietary food sources so a natural deficiency can easily occur
4. Almost all vitamin K sufficient for metabolic needs is produced by intestinal bacteria

32. Overall calcium balance in the body is maintained between two sets of balances: (1) absorption-excretion, regulating the amount that will be absorbed; and (2) deposition-mobilization as bone tissue, regulating the amount for building of bone and withdrawing from bone. This dynamic homeostasis is controlled by two interbalanced regulatory agents
    1. Vitamin A and thyroid hormone
    2. Ascorbic acid and growth hormone
    3. Phosphorus and ACTH
    4. Vitamin D and parathyroid hormone

33. Advocating megadoses of vitamin A must be questioned because
    1. The vitamin cannot be stored and the excess amount would saturate the general body tissues
    2. The vitamin is highly toxic even in small amounts
    3. The liver has a great storage capacity for the vitamin even to toxic amounts
    4. Although the body's requirement for the vitamin is very large, the cells can synthesize more as needed

34. Vitamin C in human nutrition is related to tissue integrity and hemorrhagic disease. It controls such disorders by
    1. Preserving the structural integrity of tissue by protecting the lipid matrix of cell walls from peroxidation
    2. Preventing tissue hemorrhage by providing essential blood clotting materials
    3. Facilitating adequate absorption of Ca and P for bone formation to prevent bleeding in the joints
    4. Strengthening capillary walls and structural tissue by depositing cementing material to build collagen from ground substance and hence prevent tissue hemorrhage

35. Many factors involving agent, host, and environment work together to produce malnutrition. This basic interrelationship of external and internal factors "housed" in a person's life system that causes disease is called the
    1. Biology of malnutrition
    2. Ecology of malnutrition
    3. Geography of malnutrition
    4. Psychology of malnutrition

36. In starvation, the imbalance of which *primary* homeostatic mechanism causes nutritional edema?
    1. The capillary fluid shift mechanism
    2. The aldosterone mechanism
    3. The ADH mechanism
    4. Nitrogen balance

37. The nurse should be aware that a potassium deficit would demonstrate itself by
    1. Extreme muscle weakness, tachycardia, and possible cardiac arrest
    2. Development of tetany with muscle spasm
    3. Nausea, vomiting, and leg and stomach cramps
    4. Skin rash, diarrhea, and diplopia

38. Following surgery, major concern centers on the depletion of which of the following electrolytes?
    1. Sodium
    2. Calcium
    3. Chloride
    4. Potassium
39. A night feeding planned for a juvenile diabetic includes milk, crackers, and cheese. This will provide
    1. High carbohydrate nourishment for immediate utilization
    2. Nourishment with latent effect to counteract late insulin activity
    3. Encouragement for the child to stay on a diet
    4. Added calories to help the child gain weight
40. An adult intolerance to milk, found mostly in black populations, is caused by a genetic deficiency of the enzyme
    1. Sucrase
    2. Lactase
    3. Maltase
    4. Amylase
41. The most prevalent nutritional disorder among children in this country is iron deficiency anemia. A major reason for this in young children is
    1. Overfeeding of milk
    2. Lack of adequate iron reserves from mother
    3. Blood disorders
    4. Introduction of solid foods too early for proper absorption
42. Anemia, a nutritional problem encountered in children and adults, involves several different nutrients. The nutrients include proteins, iron, vitamin B$_{12}$, and
    1. Carbohydrates
    2. Thiamin
    3. Calcium
    4. Folic acid
43. Mrs. White, a hospitalized patient with essential hypertension, is on a 1 g. Na diet that she does not like and tells you her sister is bringing in some "good old home-cooked food." Your initial *most* effective nursing action would be to
    1. Call in the dietitian for patient teaching
    2. Tell Mrs. White that she cannot have salt as it will raise her blood pressure
    3. Wait for Mrs. White's sister and discuss the diet with both of them
    4. Catch Mrs. White's sister before she goes into the room and tell her about the diet
44. Since sodium is the major cation controlling fluid outside the cells, diet therapy in congestive heart failure with subsequent cardiac edema is aimed at reducing the sodium intake. The foods most affected by such restriction would be
    1. Fruits
    2. Vegetables
    3. Grains
    4. Processed foods
45. Sodium reduction is an effective therapeutic tool in the treatment of congestive heart failure primarily because

1. It helps to prevent potassium accumulation that occurs when sodium intake is higher
2. It helps to control food intake and thus weight
3. It causes excess tissue fluid to be withdrawn and excreted
4. It aids the weakened heart muscle to contract and improves cardiac output
46. On a sodium restricted diet it is difficult to maintain the
    1. Protein and vitamin B intake
    2. Carbohydrate and vitamin D intake
    3. Fat and vitamin C intake
    4. Protein, fat, and carbohydrate intake
47. The posterior pituitary gland secretes antidiuretic hormone (ADH), which influences normal kidney function by stimulating the
    1. Glomerulus to control the quantity of fluid passing through it
    2. Glomerulus to withhold the proteins from the urine
    3. Nephron tubules to reabsorb water
    4. Nephron tubules to reabsorb glucose
48. A patient with acute renal failure complains of nausea, pain in the abdomen, diarrhea, and muscular weakness. You note an irregularity in pulse and signs of pulmonary edema. These are probably manifestations of
    1. Calcium deficiency
    2. Calcium excess
    3. Sodium deficiency
    4. Potassium excess
49. Diet therapy for renal calculi of calcium phosphate composition would probably be
    1. High calcium and phosphorus, alkaline ash
    2. High calcium and phosphorus, acid ash
    3. Low purine
    4. Low calcium and phosphorus, acid ash
50. Metabolic acidosis develops in renal failure as a result of
    1. Depression of respiratory rate by metabolic wastes causing carbon dioxide retention
    2. Inability of renal tubules to secrete hydrogen ions and conserve bicarbonate
    3. Inability of renal tubules to reabsorb water to achieve dilution of the acid contents of the blood
    4. Impaired glomerular filtration causing retention of sodium and metabolic waste products
51. Patients having renal failure may develop tetany. This is caused by
    1. Acidosis
    2. Potassium retention
    3. Calcium depletion
    4. Sodium chloride depletion
52. The modified Giordano-Giovannetti dietary regimen for patients with uremia is based on which of the following principles?
    1. A high protein intake ensures an adequate daily supply of all amino acids to compensate for losses
    2. Essential and nonessential amino acids are necessary in the diet to supply materials for tissue protein synthesis
    3. Urea nitrogen cannot be used to synthesize amino acids in the body, hence all the

nitrogen for amino acid synthesis must come from the dietary protein
4. If the diet is low in protein and supplies only essential amino acids, the body will use the excess urea nitrogen to synthesize the nonessential amino acids needed for tissue protein production

53. A patient with renal stones of calcium oxalate composition would need a diet
    1. Low in calcium and oxalate, acid ash
    2. Low in calcium and oxalate, alkaline ash
    3. Low in methionine, acid ash
    4. Low in purines, alkaline ash

54. If you were instructing a cardiac patient on a high unsaturated fatty acid diet, which of the following foods would you increase in the diet?
    1. Liver and other glandular organ meats
    2. Enriched whole milk
    3. Red meats, such as beef
    4. Vegetable oils, such as corn oil

55. A therapeutic diet frequently used in the treatment of heart disease is the low saturated fat diet. Which of the following foods should be avoided by the patient on this diet?
    1. Whole milk
    2. Corn oil
    3. Special soft margarine
    4. Whole grains

Mrs. Simon, in congestive heart failure, is having difficulty breathing as a result of pulmonary edema. She is being treated with digitalis and diuretic therapy and also with a 1 g. sodium diet. Questions 56 and 57 refer to this situation.

56. At 9:00 P.M. Mrs. Simon asks for a glass of juice and you know that the only kinds on the ward are pear nectar, apple, and tomato. You would
    1. Explain to her that she should not have juice between meals, but you will give her a glass of water
    2. Ask her which she prefers, the apple juice or the pear nectar
    3. Explain to her that the only kind she can have is tomato juice
    4. Tell her that she can't have any kind of juice because she is on a low sodium diet

57. Assuming all of her fresh food involved is cooked without salt, which of the following meal plans would be prohibited on Mrs. Simon's 1000 mg. (1 g.) sodium diet?
    1. Baked chicken, boiled potatoes, broccoli, coffee
    2. Mixed fruit salad bowl with cottage cheese, crackers, relish dish (celery, carrot, olives, sweet pickles), tea
    3. Soft cooked egg, salt free toast, jelly, skim milk
    4. Fillet of sole, baked potato, lettuce and tomato salad, fresh fruit cup, milk

Jim, a 10-month-old boy, is admitted to the hospital for treatment of an iron deficiency anemia. He is a fat baby, who appears very pale. His hemoglobin is 5 g. and he has an enlarged heart. His mother states, "I don't understand what's wrong with him—he doesn't eat any solid foods, but I always see that he gets plenty of milk." Questions 58 to 60 refer to this situation.

58. Jim should have been started on solid foods at least by 4 or 5 months of age because
    1. His fetal reserve of iron was depleted
    2. It would have been wise to start early to teach him how to chew
    3. His bone marrow activity had slacked off
    4. It would have helped to wean him from the bottle

59. Your background knowledge of the basic nutrients that act as partners in building red blood cells will form the basis for a teaching plan. These nutrient partners are iron,
    1. Calcium, and vitamins
    2. Carbohydrates, and thiamin
    3. Proteins, and ascorbic acid
    4. Vitamin D, and riboflavin

60. Which of the following foods would you emphasize to Jim's mother as a source of iron to be included in his diet daily?
    1. Orange juice
    2. Lamb
    3. Egg yolk
    4. Milk

CHAPTER 5

The behavioral sciences

Individuals are constantly interacting with both the internal and the external environment and at any given moment in time stand as a conglomerate of their own and their forebears' experience. Since nursing is concerned with the basic needs of people, the nurse, in order to understand and assist the individual, must be constantly aware of the many factors that influence a person's response. To better understand the factors involved, the nurse must study and review those concepts of anthropology, sociology, and psychology that are applicable to nursing. *Anthropology* studies the origins, physical development, social beliefs, and customs of human beings. *Sociology* studies the organizations, functions, and actions of human societies. *Psychology* studies human behavior and development of the personality.

CULTURE AND THE INDIVIDUAL

BASIC CONCEPTS

A. All people are influenced by the culture into which they are born
B. Cultural factors include race, nationality, and religion
C. Groups that share a common race, nationality, religion, or language are known as ethnic groups
D. Society as a whole frequently develops a fixed set of expected responses for certain ethnic groups
E. When each member of an ethnic group is expected to respond in a specific manner, the expected responses are called stereotypes

THE SIGNIFICANCE OF ANTHROPOLOGY TO NURSING

A. Nursing uses principles of anthropology to understand the influence of culture on the individual
B. Nursing is concerned with
   1. Cross-cultural variation and boundaries within own culture
   2. Different cultural practices serving same functions and indicating variations between groups
   3. Cultural variability in all stages of the life cycle: child rearing, marriage patterns, health maintenance, etc.
   4. Existence of different cultural ways of dealing with illness and death

CULTURAL INFLUENCES
Race

A. Race is defined as a certain combination of physical traits that are transmitted by lineage or heredity
B. Physical traits of a race include skin color; texture and/or color of hair; eye shapes and folds; shape of nose, lips, and cheekbones; contour of the head; and body build
C. Races are frequently labelled by the color of the skin
   1. Yellow—Mongolian
   2. Black—Negro
   3. White—Caucasian
   4. Red—Indian
D. Segregation and discrimination based on race have been reported since history was first recorded
E. History demonstrates many incidents of cruelty associated with racial discrimination
   1. American Indians moved to reservations

2. Blacks enslaved and treated as chattel
3. Hitler's attempts to organize Germany by annihilation and internment of all non-Aryans
4. The United States internment of Japanese-Americans in camps during World War II
5. Repeated incidents of violence associated with attempts to integrate neighborhoods, schools, jobs, and churches
6. Derogatory names such as "Whitey," "Slant-eyes," "Nigger," and "Redskin" are used as epithets to express the negative feelings existing between races

F. Reform movements directed toward integration of racial minority groups
1. Political and economic pressures applied
2. Repeated demonstrations to make public aware of problem
3. Voter registration drives
4. Legislation against racial discrimination enacted into law
5. Violations of integration laws brought to litigation in the courts
6. Publicity
7. Educational programs

G. Of all the factors involved in ethnic group membership, race, which is given a great deal of emphasis, appears to be a biologic phenomenon that seems to contribute few specifics to the cultural background

Nationality

A. Nationality is defined as original or acquired membership in a particular nation
B. Nationalities are usually labelled from the name of the country or an abbreviation of such a name; for example
1. Denmark—Danes or Danish
2. Sweden—Swedes or Swedish
3. Italy—Italian
4. Canada—Canadians
C. The culture of nationalities is passed down through generations in the forms of
1. Beliefs and superstitions
2. Foods and national dishes
3. Festivals and feast days
4. Language and the meanings of certain words
D. Nationality and the culture it imparts frequently become even more important when a group of people immigrate to a new country where the members tend to join together to form a subculture of the new national culture
E. The subculture provides its members with a sense of security by furnishing a collective identity and maintaining the familiar
F. Most people maintain their membership in this subculture even though the size of the group involved may be extremely small
G. These subcultures frequently maintain their native language to foster the differences and resist assimilation into the new nationality
H. Nationalism is extremely important in time of national emergencies such as wars and invasions
I. Incidents of segregation and discrimination based on nationality have been reported throughout history
1. Derogatory names such as "Wop" for the Italian, "Mick" for the Irishman, "Spic" for the Puerto Rican, and "Jap" for the Japanese are used as epithets to express the negative feelings existing between nationalities
2. Ethnic jokes are frequently used to express this hostility in a socially acceptable manner
3. Legislation against discrimination on the basis of national origin has been developed and enacted into law
4. Violations of the law have been brought to litigation in the courts

Religion

A. Religion is defined as the quest for values of the ideal life usually embodied in a particular set of beliefs practiced individually or within an organized system
B. Religious beliefs in some form have existed in every group during every period of history
C. Organized religions have been instrumental in developing an ethical and moral system that has frequently been based on a society's needs
D. Organized religions established churches that have served as religious, cultural, educational, and social institutions
E. The major organized religions of the world are divided into 2 main groups: the monotheistic, which recognizes one god, and the polytheistic, which recognizes more than one god

F. The monotheistic religions are Roman Catholicism, Islam, Protestantism, Eastern Orthodoxy, and Judaism
G. The polytheistic religions are Hinduism, Confucianism, Buddhism, Shintoism, and Taoism
H. Most of the world's religions have developed many rituals as part of their worship and these rituals form the basis of the religious culture that is passed down from generation to generation
I. Recent changes in religions include
   1. A move toward unification of many denominations with the emphasis being placed on similar beliefs rather than unique differences
   2. An attempt to take a more active role in social problems
   3. A relaxation of many of the rituals and a simplification of approach to the basic tenets
J. Incidents of segregation and discrimination based on religion have been reported throughout history

CULTURE AND HEALTH

A. General influences
   1. Cultural background influences the way in which people view both health and disease
   2. The cultural influences seem to be derived from the areas of nationality and religion rather than race
B. Specific influences
   1. National culture may influence an individual's
      a. Response to illness
      b. Response to pain and even the tolerance of pain
      c. Need for superstitions and rituals
      d. Acceptance of dietary change both in type or in consistency of food
      e. Need for support and comfort from the family
      f. Ability to communicate in understandable terms
      g. Response to loss of independence
      h. Feelings about loss of privacy and exposure of parts of the body
      i. Feelings about loss of body parts
      j. Need for specific rites and rituals associated with dying
   2. Religious culture may influence an individual's
      a. Views on conception, birth, and child care
      b. Views about the meaning of pain and suffering
      c. Feelings about the meaning of death
      d. Desire for guidance from the clergy
      e. Acceptance of certain treatments such as immunizations and blood transfusions
      f. Concept of illness as a punishment
      g. Dietary restrictions including the types of food and their preparation
      h. Need for specific rites and rituals associated with dying

SOCIETY AND THE INDIVIDUAL

BASIC CONCEPTS

A. Every human society has institutions for the socialization of its members
   1. Process by which individuals are compelled or induced to conform to the customs of the group
      a. Group establishes rules and codes of conduct governing its members and these become the norms, values, and mores of the group
      b. Role of members includes specified rights, duties, attitudes, and actions
   2. Controls established through a system of rewards and punishment
      a. Reward leads to acceptance as a member of the group
      b. Punishment for antisocial behavior leads to rejection and separation from the group
B. Development of society requires sanction of group members
   1. Growth takes place in social space
      a. Social boundaries separate one group from another
      b. Barriers to participation are established through mores and customs
   2. Leader's influence is always limited to conditions placed on it by the total group
   3. Behavioral roles are established by members of the group
C. A society is a reflection of all the functional relationships that occur between its individual members
   1. Products of group life are a major determinant in an individual's intellect, creativity, memory, thinking, and feeling
      a. Human beings have no memory,

thought, or feeling that does not include society
  b. Intellect and creativity can be enhanced or hampered by society
2. Members of a society have functional and rewarding social contact
  a. Members are accepted and approved and then participate in establishing rules, norms, and values
  b. The nonmembers have, at best, limited social contacts with the members; this causes a segmentation of relationships and provides few rewarding experiences for the nonmembers
D. A society or a group can change because of conflict among members
  1. This conflict is greatest when there is an absence of certain members, an introduction of new members, or a change in leadership
  2. The resulting reorganization goes through 3 stages
    a. Tension stage caused by the conflict
    b. Integration stage during which members learn about "the other's" problem
    c. Resolution of tension stage during which a reconstruction of the group's norms and values takes place
  3. The resolution of conflict and the restoring of equilibrium
    a. This takes place when people interact with one another and the group is dynamic
    b. Conflicts are not resolved when groups are rigid with fixed membership and ideas
E. The family is the primary group
  1. Helps society to establish and maintain its code of behavior
  2. Provides individual members with
    a. Strong emotional ties
      (1) Much sensory contact is present
      (2) Members care about the emotional and physical well-being of each other
      (3) Members are responsive to one another's feelings, acts, and opinions
      (4) Members learn empathy by vicariously reliving the experiences of others

      (5) Members view selves through the eyes of others
    b. A feeling of security by meeting dependent needs
    c. A system of communication
      (1) Overt—words
      (2) Covert—body language
    d. Role identification and intimacy that help to internalize the acceptable behavioral patterns of the group
    e. A spirit of cooperation and competition through sibling interaction
  3. Changes that have influenced the family's ability to indoctrinate children with the norms of society
    a. The Industrial Revolution changed an agrarian society into an industrial one
      (1) Families became nuclear rather than extended
      (2) Families depended more on secondary groups for survival
      (3) New social groups were established to replace the extended family
      (4) Labor unions replaced patriarchal management
        (a) Laws enacted to protect the rights of children and other dependent people of society
        (b) Laws enacted to establish minimum wage and hour benefits
      (5) There was increased mobility of individuals
    b. The altered male and female role patterns
      (1) The changing status of women
        (a) More women go outside the home to work
        (b) Women have an increased role in decision making
      (2) The changing status of men
        (a) More men must assume homemaking responsibilities
        (b) Men have to share decision making with women, thus decreasing dominance
      (3) Increased partnership in home and financial management has resulted in some conflicts

(4) Role confusion has contributed to an increase in separations and divorces

c. Factors resulting in a reduction in the size of families
   (1) Increase in financial cost involved in raising and educating children
   (2) Emphasis on limited population growth
   (3) Wide dissemination of birth control information
   (4) Legalization of abortions

F. Peer groups help youth to establish norms of behavior and assist in the rites of passage from the family group to society
   1. Youth learns about society through contact with the peer group
   2. Youth develops further self-concept in contact with other youths
   3. Society's norms are more readily accepted through peer group interaction and pressure
   4. Peer group interaction can produce change in its individual members
   5. Members have a strong loyalty to the peer group because of the reciprocal relationships and other rewards the group offers
   6. Peer group norms may conflict with family or society's norms
   7. If mores of family and society are not internalized, delinquency and socially unacceptable behavior may develop

G. Group membership may enhance overall function while hindering specific individual performance
   1. Cognitive behavior and verbal associations may improve quantitatively, but qualitative improvement may not follow
   2. Competition may increase muscular activity leading to a more rapid speech pattern and a feeling of vigor, but accuracy may be lessened
   3. An increase in speed of performance may occur, but quality and accuracy may be lowered
   4. Group pressures can create a leveling effect
      a. The poorer worker's performance tends to improve in a group
      b. The superior worker's performance tends to become less superior and more like the rest of the group

H. The type of leadership in a group depends on the needs of the group members as well as the personality of the leader
   1. Authoritarian leader—is rigid and uses leadership role as an instrument of power; the leader makes all the decisions, which are then handed down to the membership; little communication and interrelating between leader and group
   2. Democratic leader—is fair and logical, uses the leadership role to stimulate others to achieve a collective goal; the leader encourages interrelating among members by relating to all members; weaknesses as well as strengths are accepted; the contributions of all members are fostered and utilized
   3. Emotional leader—reflects the feeling tones, norms, and values of the group
   4. Laissez-faire leader—is passive and unproductive; usually assumes the role of a participant-observer and exerts little control or guidance over group behavior
   5. Bureaucratic leader—is rigid and assumes a role that is determined by formal criteria or rules that are inherent in the organization and frequently unrelated to the present group; the leader is not emotionally involved and avoids interrelating with the group members
   6. Charismatic leader—can assume any of the above behaviors since the group places supernatural power in this person or the office and frequently follows directions without question

I. The community is a social organization that is considered the individual's secondary group
   1. Relationships among members are usually more impersonal
   2. Individuals participate in a more delimited manner or in a specific capacity
   3. The group frequently functions as a means to an end
      a. The group enables diversified groups to communicate
      b. The group helps other groups to identify community problems and possible solutions
   4. The secondary group is usually rather large and meets on an intermittent basis; contacts are usually maintained through correspondence

5. Leaders of the community facilitate group interaction
    a. They have a knowledge of the community and its needs
    b. They have the skill to stimulate others to act
6. Secondary groups help establish laws that are necessary to limit antisocial behavior
    a. Laws provide diversified groups with a common base of acceptable behavior
    b. Some laws may favor and protect the vested interests of specific groups within the society

THE SIGNIFICANCE OF SOCIOLOGY TO NURSING

A. Nursing uses principles of sociology in understanding the relationships among persons, families, and communities
B. Nursing is concerned with
    1. Societal factors that determine the way the group's needs are met
    2. Pressure imposed by a given society to ensure conformity to its rules and mores
    3. Society's methods of establishing a hierarchy of values and roles
    4. Societal changes and how they affect values, family, and roles
    5. Society's influence on health practices and illness

SOCIETY AND HEALTH CARE

A. The role of society
    1. Traditionally societies have placed great emphasis on caring for their members when they are ill
    2. Recently society's role in health maintenance and the prevention of disease has been given an increased priority
    3. Society's provision for health maintenance includes
        a. Protection of food, water, and drug supplies
        b. Establishment of public health agencies for the supervision, prevention, and control of disease and illness
        c. Development of public education programs
        d. Awarding scholarship grants for health education and research
        e. Development of unemployment insurance programs
        f. Establishment of Workmen's Compensation insurance

g. Establishment of Social Security and Medicare programs
        h. Establishment of social welfare services and Medicaid programs
        i. Supervision of medical and hospital insurance programs
B. The health agency as a social institution has
    1. A bureaucratic structure
    2. Policies, rules, and regulations governing behavior of its members
    3. An impersonal viewpoint
    4. A status hierarchy
    5. An increasingly specialized subculture
C. The hospital as a subculture of society
    1. The employees develop both written and unwritten hospital policies that
        a. Set standards of acceptable behavior for both patients and staff
        b. Regulate the patient's contact with the primary group by limiting visitors
        c. Force both patients and staff to relate to the secondary group
        d. Punish unacceptable behavior by any members of the group including the patient
    2. The folklores and folkways of the hospital serve to
        a. Maintain the mystique of medicine by fostering the use of a unique language and system of symbols
        b. Attach stigmas to various social illnesses such as venereal disease, mental illness, drug addiction, and alcoholism, which are associated with certain patterns of living and acting that are not acceptable to the group
        c. Perpetuate the roles and values of the health team members and maintain the status quo
    3. The hospital has several functions
        a. The primary functions of the hospital are to help the patient regain health and resume a role in society by providing services directed toward
            (1) The treatment of illness
            (2) Rehabilitation
            (3) The maintenance of health
        b. The secondary functions of the hospital are to help society by providing services directed toward
            (1) The education of health professionals

(2) The education of the general public

(3) Research

D. The delivery of health services—a new responsibility of the community
1. Members of society become active participants in prevention of illness
2. Community health centers care for the ill in the home rather than the hospital
3. Extended care facilities are established with more community and homelike atmosphere
4. Nonmedical community leaders take an active role in establishing health policy for society
5. Lay members of the community become involved with health agencies' policies and decisions
6. Health maintenance and treatment are no longer considered a privilege but the right of all members of society

BEHAVIOR AND THE INDIVIDUAL

BASIC CONCEPTS

A. Human beings must be able to perceive and interpret stimuli in order to interact with the environment
1. Perception and cognitive functioning are influenced by
a. The nature of the stimuli
b. Culture, beliefs, attitudes, and age
c. Past experiences
d. Present physical and emotional needs
2. An individual's personality development is influenced by the ability to perceive and interpret stimuli
a. Through these processes the external world is internalized
b. The external world may in turn be distorted by the individual's perceptions

B. Humans have to communicate in order to interact with the environment
1. Communication is a behavior that is learned through the process of acculturation
2. People have to communicate with others to make needs known
a. The infant uses the cry to bring attention to needs
b. Hearing is essential to the development of good speech for one learns to form words by hearing the words of others
c. The written word usually replaces the spoken word when face to face encounters are impractical or supplements the spoken word when further clarification is necessary
3. Productive communication depends on the consensual validation of all involved
a. To understand the intent of the message, each person must be aware of the meaning of the spoken word as well as the inflections in the speaker's voice
b. Validation can best be accomplished when participants are empathetic
c. The language and channel of communication must be adapted to the person and the purpose for which it is intended
d. Feedback is necessary to evaluate the effectiveness of the words and guide the communication
e. Satisfaction is enhanced for all involved when lines of communication are kept open
4. Barriers to effective communication include
a. Variations in culture, language, and education
b. Problems in hearing, speech, or comprehension
c. A refusal to listen to another point of view
d. The use of selective inattention, which may cause an interruption or distortion of the message
5. Nonverbal behavior communicates the inner feelings of the individual performing the behavior
a. Facial expression, posture, and body movement may express the anxiety, pain, tension, fear, happiness, joy, or satisfaction the individual is experiencing
b. Nonverbal communication may transmit a different message than the individual's verbal communication
c. Confusion arises when there is a difference in the verbal and nonverbal message received

C. Psychologic experiences provide the energy that is transformed into behavior

1. Anxiety frequently provides the push that moves people to action because it
   a. Develops when two goals or needs are in conflict
   b. Is a state of apprehension or tension aroused by impulses from within
   c. Prepares one for action or completely overwhelms and inhibits action
2. Anxiety develops in stages that are referred to as levels
   a. The first level increases alertness and prepares the body for action
   b. The second level increases apprehension and creates an awareness of discomfort
   c. The third level is the stage of free-floating anxiety that creates feelings of impending doom
   d. The fourth level is the stage of panic that creates uncontrolled, unrealistic behavior
3. The sympathetic nervous system prepares the body's physiologic defense for fight or flight by stimulating the adrenal medulla to secrete epinephrine and norepinephrine
   a. The heart beat is accelerated to pump more blood to the muscles
   b. The peripheral blood vessels constrict to provide more blood to the vital organs
   c. The bronchioles dilate and breathing becomes rapid and deep to supply more oxygen to the cells
   d. The pupils dilate to provide increased vision
   e. The liver releases glucose for quick energy
   f. The prothrombin time is lowered to protect the body from loss of blood in the event of injury
4. Seyle's general adaptation syndrome (GAS) is the body's physiologic adaptation to stress (anxiety)
   a. The adrenal cortex secretes cortisone during the emergency stage
   b. When stress continues the increased secretion of cortisone causes the body to go through a resistive stage
   c. If the process continues the last stage is exhaustion and death
5. Defense mechanisms serve to protect the personality by controlling anxiety and reducing emotional pressures; the commonly used normal defense mechanisms that help an individual to deal with reality are
   a. Identification—the individual internalizes the characteristics of an idealized person
   b. Substitution—the individual replaces one goal for another
   c. Compensation—the individual makes up for a perceived lack in one area by emphasizing capabilities in another
   d. Sublimation—a socially acceptable behavior is substituted for an unacceptable instinct; this mechanism is used when the expression of these instincts would prove a threat to the self
   e. Compromise—the reciprocal give-and-take necessary in many relationships to salvage some part of the situation or the goal
   f. Rationalization—the individual makes acceptable excuses for one's behavior and feelings

   NOTE: The other defense mechanisms used to deal with reality appear in Psychiatric nursing, pp. 425-426

THE SIGNIFICANCE OF PSYCHOLOGY TO NURSING

A. Nursing uses principles of psychology in understanding the development of human behavior
B. Nursing is concerned with
   1. Recognizing that all behavior is motivated and has meaning to the performer
   2. The phases of personality development during the life cycle
   3. The role of environment in personality development
   4. The use of behavior to handle emotional stress
   5. The interrelationship between the psyche and the soma

THE DEVELOPMENT OF THE PERSONALITY
Factors involved in personality development

A. Behavior is a learned response that develops as a result of past experiences
B. To protect the individual's emotional

well-being these experiences are organized in the psyche on 3 different levels
1. The conscious level is composed of
past experiences easily recalled to
mind that create little, if any, emotional discomfort
2. The subconscious level of awareness
has been deliberately pushed out of
consciousness but can be recalled with
some effort
3. The unconscious level of awareness
contains the largest body of material
and greatly influences behavior
a. This material cannot be deliberately brought back into awareness
since it is usually unacceptable to
the individual
b. If recalled, this material is usually
disguised or distorted as in dreams;
however, it is still capable of producing a good deal of anxiety
C. According to Freud the personality consists of 3 parts—the id, the ego, and the
superego
1. The id is that part of the personality
that contains the instincts, impulses,
and urges; it is totally self-centered
and unconscious
2. The ego is the conscious self, the "I"
that deals with reality; the part of the
personality that is shown to the environment
3. The superego is that part of the personality that controls, inhibits, and
regulates those impulses and instincts
whose uncontrolled expression would
endanger the emotional well-being of
the individual and the stability of the
society

**Critical periods in the formation
of the personality**

A. The personality of an individual develops
in overlapping stages that shade and
merge together
1. Certain goals must be accomplished
during each stage in the development
from infancy to maturity
2. If these goals are not accomplished
at specific periods, the basic structure
of the personality will be weakened
3. Factors in each stage persist as a
permanent part of the personality
4. Each stage has particular frustrations
and major traumas that must be overcome

5. Successful resolution of the conflicts
associated with each stage is essential
to normal development
6. Unresolved conflicts remain in the unconscious and result in maladaptive
behavior
B. The tasks related to personality development during the period of infancy
1. Freud: oral stage—the infant obtains
gratification by taking everything in;
begins to develop self-concept from
the responses of others
2. Erikson: trust vs. mistrust—trust develops from the inner feeling of self-
worth that is transmitted through maternal care; the child learns to depend
on the satisfaction that is derived
from this care and when the need is
met, trust develops
3. Sullivan: need for security—the infant learns to rely on others to gratify
needs and satisfy wishes; develops a
sense of basic trust, security, and self-
worth when this occurs
C. The tasks related to personality development during the early childhood period
1. Freud: anal stage—the struggle of giving of self and breaking the symbiotic
ties to mother; as the ties are broken,
the child learns independence
2. Erikson: autonomy vs. shame and
doubt—the struggle of holding on to
or letting go; an internal struggle for
self-identity; love vs. hate
3. Sullivan: learning to communicate
needs through the use of words and
the acceptance of delayed gratification
and interference with wish fulfillment
D. The tasks related to personality development during the preschool period
1. Freud: oedipal stage—love for and desire to possess parent of the opposite
sex creates fear and guilt feelings;
desires are repressed and role identification with parent of the same sex
occurs
2. Erikson: initiative vs. guilt—stage of
intensive activity, play, and consum-
ing fantasies where the child inter-
jects parents' social consciousness
3. Sullivan: development of body image
and self-perception—organizes and
uses experiences in terms of approval
and disapproval received; begins using selective inattention and disasso-
ciating those experiences that cause

physical or emotional discomfort and pain

E. The tasks related to personality development during the school age period
   1. Freud: latency stage—the period of low sexual activity and identification with peer groups
   2. Erikson: industry vs. inferiority—the child wants to learn how to make things with others and strives to achieve success
   3. Sullivan: the period of learning to form satisfying relationships with peers by using competition, compromise, and cooperation; in this period the pre-adolescent learns to relate to peers of the same sex

F. The tasks related to personality development during period of adolescence
   1. Freud: genital stage—time when sexual activity increases and sexual identity is strengthened or attacked
   2. Erikson: identity vs. identity diffusion —the developmental task involves integrating childhood identifications with the basic drives, native endowments, and opportunities offered in social roles
   3. Sullivan: learning to be independent and to establish satisfactory relationships with members of the opposite sex

G. The tasks related to personality development during the period of young adulthood
   1. Erikson: intimacy vs. isolation—the developmental task involves moving from the relative security of self-identity to the relative insecurity involved in establishing intimacy with another
   2. Sullivan: becoming economically, intellectually, and emotionally self-sufficient

H. The tasks related to personality development during the period of later adulthood
   1. Erikson: generativity vs. self-absorption—the mature person is interested in establishing and guiding the next generation
   2. Sullivan: learning to be interdependent and assuming responsibility for others

I. The tasks related to personality development during the period of senescence
   1. Erikson: the older person adapts to

triumphs and disappointments with a certain ego integrity
   2. Sullivan: the older person has an acceptance of responsibility for what life is and was and of its place in the flow of history

The influence of basic needs on the development of the personality

A. Humanity has certain basic needs that must be satisfied
   1. The need to communicate
      a. Through communication, humans maintain contact with reality
         (1) The individual needs to validate findings with others to correctly interpret reality
         (2) Validation is enhanced when communication conveys an understanding of feelings
      b. Through communication, the individual develops a concept of self in relation to others
   2. The need for security
      a. The need to feel secure as an assurance of survival is fundamental
      b. Fear emerges when survival is threatened
      c. Initially the infant's security is related to the satisfaction of physical needs
      d. Security is enhanced when the same individual meets the infant's physical needs in a consistent manner
      e. The infant must also perceive love to feel secure
      f. Security is derived from the individual's perception of self in relation to others
      g. How the individual handles these perceptions influences personality development
   3. The need to move from dependence to independence
      a. The infant is dependent on the parents, but through learning acquires faculties for independence
      b. There is no real security or deep assurance of survival in being dependent on others, since uncertainties develop if one's security is totally derived from this source
      c. The infant must feel love and security before reaching out to strug-

gle with the problems in the environment

d. When the need for love and security is met the child is sustained in the failures and hurts associated with learning and independence

e. Denial of the opportunity to learn or frustration in the drive for independence will produce emotional problems

4. The need to develop a self-concept
   a. Self-concept begins to develop early in infancy
   b. The determination of the self-concept develops primarily through interaction with significant persons in the environment
   c. An integral part of the self-concept is the body image
   d. The first and most deeply learned perception of body image develops from the attitudes of significant others, since children view themselves as others view them
   e. The concept of self is the root of security and future developmental needs
   f. Communication enhances the development of self
   g. A person's self-concept is the basis for emotional stability or instability; a secure person has strength and capacity for independence and becomes less anxious when circumstances require the help of others

5. The need to find relief from organic discomfort
   a. Through experience, one learns the most satisfying ways of relieving discomfort
   b. Adjustment to illness depends on how the individual adjusts to life

B. The needs of a specific individual at a given time will vary according to internal and external environmental factors

C. To attain psychologic equilibrium and achieve need satisfaction, the individual attempts to maintain a feeling of safety and comfort in adapting to life's situations; this is often achieved by maintaining a feeling of worth and a feeling of being needed by others

Motivation, learning, and behavior

A. All behavior is motivated
   1. A motive always implies some purpose
   2. Social motives are often changed through learning
   3. Symbolic rewards are the major factors in learning
   4. Social approval is an important form of symbolic reward

B. Behavior and emotions
   1. Emotions act as motives for behavior since they often involve a reaction to some external situation
   2. Behavior is always accompanied and often controlled by the emotions
   3. Emotions may facilitate or hinder the learning process
   4. Emotions exert a strong influence on the thinking process

C. Automatic behavior
   1. Is the predetermined or repetitive type behavior that has been used successfully in prior situations
   2. Requires little effort or thought
   3. Is adapted to definite situations and is difficult to alter if the situation changes
   4. Plays a minor role in the functioning of a mature and independent adult

D. Life is a continually changing process and when these changes occur in areas of significance they often produce rather distinct emotional responses; these changes include
   1. Resistance to change—the individual hesitates to accept or adapt to the change and may attempt to deny its occurrence or reject its outcome
   2. Regression—the individual returns to an earlier type of behavior that, at the time, provided some satisfaction and gratification and now provides an escape from the unacceptable or anxiety-producing situation
   3. Acceptance and progression—the individual adapts to the change and expends energy on outside objects rather than self-centered aims

THE THERAPEUTIC NURSING RELATIONSHIP

A. Fundamental requirements of a therapeutic relationship
   1. The ability to communicate therapeutically requires a basic understanding and use of interviewing techniques such as
      a. Open-ended rather than probing questions

b. Reflection of words and feelings, and paraphrasing
c. Acceptance of the patient's behavior
d. Nonjudgmental objective attitude
e. Focusing on the emotional needs of the patient
f. Having a therapeutic goal for the interview

2. The recognition that an individual has a potential for growth
   a. Individuals need to learn about their own behavior in relation to others
   b. Exchanging experiences with others provides the reassurance that reactions are valid and feelings shared
   c. Participating with groups increases knowledge of interpersonal relationships and helps individuals to identify their strengths and resources
   d. The identification of the individual's strengths and resources helps to convey the expectation of growth

3. The recognition that an individual needs to be accepted
   a. Acceptance is an active process designed to convey respect for another
   b. Acceptance of others implies and requires acceptance of self
   c. To be nonjudgmental, one has to become aware of one's own attitudes and feelings and their effect on perception
   d. Acceptance requires that individuals be permitted and even encouraged to express their feelings and attitudes even though they may be divergent from the general viewpoint
      (1) Individuals should be encouraged to express both positive and negative feelings
      (2) This encouragement must occur on both the verbal and nonverbal level
   e. Acceptance means showing interest in another person; interest requires
      (1) Face to face contact and really listening to what the other person has to say
      (2) Developing an awareness of the other person's likes and dislikes
      (3) Attempting to understand another's point of view
      (4) Using nonverbal as well as verbal expressions of acceptance
   f. Acceptance requires the development of interpersonal techniques that encourage others to express problems; the listener's
      (1) Reflection of feelings, attitudes, and words helps the speaker to identify feelings
      (2) Open-end questions permit the speaker to focus on problems
      (3) Paraphrasing assists the speaker in clarifying statements
      (4) Use of silence provides both the listener and the speaker with the necessary time for thinking over what's being discussed
   g. Acceptance requires the recognition of factors that block communication, including
      (1) Any overt or covert response that conveys a judgmental or superior attitude
      (2) Direct questions that convey an invasive or probing attitude
      (3) Ridicule that conveys a hostile attitude
      (4) Talking about one's own problems and not listening, which conveys a self-serving attitude and loss of interest in the speaker

4. The recognition that both the nurse's and the patient's emotional needs influence the therapeutic process
   a. A knowledge of the nurse's own emotional needs provides the opportunity to exert some control over those needs that may interfere with the relationship
   b. This recognition and knowledge allows the nurse to share feelings with the patient
   c. This recognition and knowledge helps the nurse to function more effectively as the change agent for the patient

B. The recognition of behavioral changes that result from physical illness

1. Anxiety, fear, and depression occur whenever there is a health problem
   a. Body image and feelings of being in control of one's body have their basis in the early developmental period
   b. Anxiety develops whenever a real or imagined threat to the body image occurs
2. Signs of the anxiety, fear, and depression associated with illness are variable and include
   a. Indifference to symptoms—usually related to failure to accept the occurrence of a health problem
   b. Denial of reality—usually related to attempts to maintain stability and integrity of the personality
   c. Reaction formation—usually related to attempts to block the reality from consciousness and acting as if nothing was wrong
   d. Failure to keep appointments and follow physician's or nurse's directions—usually related to fear of finding additional problems or admitting there is something wrong
   e. Overconcern with bodily functions and symptoms—usually related to fear of death
   f. Asking many questions and offering many complaints—usually related to attempts at keeping a staff member by the bedside because of fears associated with illness
3. Emotional needs of the ill person include
   a. The security of continuous relationships with friends and members of their families
   b. Some way of achieving the feeling of self-worth and self-esteem
   c. Assistance in accepting the dependent role of the patient
   d. Assistance in resolving conflicts while maintaining security
   e. Assistance in refocusing inner resources
   f. Contact with the reality of the external world
4. To help the individual maintain the self-concept during illness, the nurse must understand the normal stages of illness
   a. Denial—the individual cannot believe it is happening
   b. Anger—something has happened that one cannot control
   c. Depression—one grieves for loss or expected loss
   d. Acceptance of the illness and learning how to adapt—this stage can only be reached when the individual has resolved the conflicts that develop during the earlier stages
5. Common reactions occur to the change in body image associated with many health problems
   a. Attitudes toward one's body and self-concept greatly influence response
   b. Fear is a universal response; individual may focus on fear of
      (1) Pain
      (2) Incapacitation
      (3) Disfigurement
      (4) Altered self-concept
      (5) Rejection by loved ones
      (6) Death
   c. Questioning is a universal response; individual may focus on
      (1) This can't be happening to me
      (2) Is this really happening to me?
      (3) What did I do to deserve this?
      (4) Why am I being punished?
   d. Grief and mourning are universal responses; individual may focus on
      (1) What was in the past
      (2) What could have been for the future
      (3) Loss of missed opportunities
      (4) A magnified view of the loss
      (5) Avoiding interpersonal contacts

REVIEW QUESTIONS FOR THE BEHAVIORAL SCIENCES

1. Play for the preschool-age child is necessary for the emotional development of
   1. Projection
   2. Competition
   3. Introjection
   4. Independence
2. For an emotional balance the individual always needs
   1. Family, work, and play
   2. Biologic satisfaction and social acceptance
   3. Individual recognition and group acceptance
   4. Security and social recognition
3. The stage of development where a pal is loved more than self is
   1. Early school age
   2. Latency

3. Pre-adolescence
4. Adolescence
4. The emotional leader of a group is one who
   1. Reflects the feeling tone of the group
   2. Has an authoritarian role within the group
   3. Designates the roles within the group
   4. Selects those who are to be members of the group
5. In which stage of growth and development should surgery be delayed, if possible, because of the effects on personality development?
   1. Oral
   2. Anal
   3. Oedipal
   4. Latency
6. In the process of development the individual strives to maintain, protect, and enhance the integrity of the ego. This is normally accomplished through the use of
   1. Ritualistic behavior
   2. Withdrawal patterns
   3. Defense mechanisms
   4. Affective reactions
7. An example of displacement is
   1. Ignoring unpleasant aspects of reality
   2. Imaginative activity to escape reality
   3. Pent-up emotions are directed to other than the primary source
   4. Process of resistance to demand on the individual
8. Sublimation is a defense mechanism that helps the individual to
   1. Act out in reverse something already done or thought
   2. Channel unacceptable sexual desires into socially approved behavior
   3. Return to an earlier less mature stage of development
   4. Exclude from the conscious things that are psychologically disturbing
9. The defense mechanism in which emotional conflicts are expressed through motor, sensory, or somatic disability is identified as
   1. Dissociation
   2. Psychosomatic
   3. Compensation
   4. Conversion
10. The basic emotional task the infant has to learn is to
    1. Feel like others
    2. Count on others
    3. Love others
    4. Identify with others
11. Another term for the superego is
    1. Self
    2. Ideal self
    3. Narcissism
    4. Conscience
12. Personality is unique for every individual for it is the result of the person's
    1. Genetic background, placement in family, and autoimmunity
    2. Biologic constitution, psychologic development, and cultural setting
    3. Childhood experiences, intellectual capacity, and socioeconomic status
    4. Intellectual capacity, race, and socioeconomic status

13. Which relationship is of extreme importance in the formation of the personality?
    1. Parent-child
    2. Sibling
    3. Peer
    4. Heterosexual
14. Physiologically, anxiety is manifested by
    1. Dilated pupils, dilated bronchioles, increased pulse rate, hyperglycemia, and peripheral vasoconstriction
    2. Constricted pupils, constricted bronchioles, increased pulse rate, hypoglycemia, and peripheral vasodilation
    3. Dilated pupils, constricted bronchioles, decreased pulse rate, hypoglycemia, and peripheral vasoconstriction
    4. Constricted pupils, dilated bronchioles, increased pulse rate, hypoglycemia, and peripheral vasodilation
15. Mental experiences operate on different levels of awareness. Which level best portrays one's attitudes, feelings, and desires?
    1. Fore-conscious
    2. Preconscious
    3. Conscious
    4. Unconscious
16. Which part of the nervous system is primarily affected during a fight or flight reaction?
    1. Central
    2. Peripheral
    3. Parasympathetic
    4. Sympathetic
17. Groups are important in the emotional development of the individual because groups
    1. Go through the same developmental phases
    2. Always protect their members
    3. Are easily identified by their members
    4. Identify acceptable behavior for their members
18. The superego is that part of the self that says
    1. I want what I want
    2. I can wait for what I want
    3. I should not want that
    4. I like what I want
19. The family is important in emotional development because the family
    1. Gives rewards and punishment
    2. Helps one to learn identity and roles
    3. Provides support for the young
    4. Reflects the mores of a larger society
20. Communication ties an individual to
    1. Physical surroundings
    2. Environmental surroundings
    3. Social surroundings
    4. Materialistic surroundings
21. Problems with dependency versus independency develop during which stage of growth and development?
    1. Infancy
    2. Toddler
    3. Preschool
    4. School age
22. The college boy who is small in build and unable to participate in sports becomes the life of the party and a mod dresser. This is an example of the mechanism of
    1. Reaction formation
    2. Compensation

3. Sublimation
4. Introjection
23. Unsatisfied needs create anxiety that motivates an individual to action. This action is brought about *mainly* to
    1. Relieve physical discomfort
    2. Reduce tension
    3. Remove the problem
    4. Deny the situation
24. The primary emergence of the personality is demonstrated around the age of
    1. 6 months
    2. 9 months
    3. 2 years
    4. 6 years
25. A person has a mature personality if the
    1. Ego acts as a balance between the id and the superego pressures
    2. Ego responds to the demands of the super-ego
    3. Ego responds to the demands of society
    4. Superego has replaced and increased all of the controls of the parents
26. The most appropriate way to decrease anxiety is by
    1. Prolonged exposure to fearful situations
    2. Introducing an element of pleasure into fearful situations
    3. Avoiding unpleasant objects and events
    4. Acquiring skills with which to face emergencies
27. In applying mental health principles to the care of any person with children, the nurse should be aware that
    1. Many parents experience feelings of resentment in relation to their children
    2. Every parent has inborn feelings of love and acceptance for children
    3. It is pathologic to feel anger and resentment toward a child
    4. It is easier to adjust to the first child than to later ones
28. Many persons who are "well-adjusted" in ordinary daily living become dependent and demanding when physically ill and hospitalized. This is probably an example of the mechanism of
    1. Denial
    2. Compensation
    3. Reaction formation
    4. Regression
29. A 5-year-old boy is constantly found slapping his little sister. This behavior is probably caused by
    1. Sibling rivalry
    2. Unresolved oedipal conflicts
    3. Negativistic id impulses
    4. Overcompensation efforts of superego
30. The problem of separation anxiety initially occurs during the
    1. Oral stage
    2. Anal stage
    3. Phallic stage
    4. Latency stage
31. The basic emotional task for the toddler is
    1. Trust

2. Independence
3. Identification
4. Industry
32. Which level of anxiety best enhances an individual's power of perception?
    1. Mild
    2. Moderate
    3. Severe
    4. Panic
33. The person with socially aggressive behavior needs an environment that
    1. Allows freedom of expression
    2. Is mainly group oriented
    3. Provides controls by setting limits
    4. Can be manipulated
34. Strict toilet training before the child is ready will cause problems in personality development because at this stage the child is learning to
    1. Satisfy parents' needs
    2. Identify own needs
    3. Live up to society's expectations
    4. Satisfy own needs
35. The superego is the
    1. Conscience
    2. Reality testor
    3. Censor of behavior
    4. Stimulus for the id
36. A person who deliberately pretends an illness is usually
    1. Psychotic
    2. Neurotic
    3. Malingering
    4. Using conversion defenses
37. Since people need some gratifying communication to learn, to grow, and to function in a group, all events that significantly curtail communication will eventually produce
    1. Some degree of mental deficiency
    2. Severe disturbances
    3. Further attempts to increase communication
    4. Withdrawal
38. Resolution of the oedipal complex takes place when the child overcomes the castration complex and
    1. Rejects the parent of the same sex
    2. Identifies with the parent of the opposite sex
    3. Identifies with the parent of the same sex
    4. Introjects behaviors of both parents
39. An emotional experience in childhood becomes traumatic when
    1. The ego is overwhelmed by anxiety it can't handle
    2. The superego has not been internalized
    3. The child is unable to verbalize own feelings
    4. The parents are harsh and restrictive
40. The ability to tolerate frustration is an example of one of the functions of the
    1. Id
    2. Superego
    3. Ego
    4. Unconscious

CHAPTER 6

Pharmacology and drug therapy

Modern drug therapy is a culmination of historic experience and extensive research that has made available many drugs and combinations of drugs. The frequency with which drugs are employed and the availability of information about drugs in the news media have involved the public in pharmacology.

The physician, pharmacist, and nurse each bring a particular area of expertise and interest to the planning, administration, and evaluation of the patient's drug regime. Working together, team members can outline plans to protect the patient's resources, support the action of the drug being given, and make optimal use of restored function affected by the drug.

The nurse's participation in planning requires knowledge of the patient's physiologic problem, the predictable pharmacodynamic effect of the drug, and the contribution drug therapy will make to the total plan for the patient.

DEFINITIONS
Common terms

A. Chemotherapy—use of drugs to destroy invading organisms or abnormal tissue in the host
B. Drug—chemical agent that interacts with living systems and is employed to prevent, diagnose, or treat disease
C. Drug legislation—laws that provide the standards for drug manufacture and distribution and protect the public against fraudulent claims about drug action; e.g., Federal Controlled Substances Act, regulations of the Federal Bureau of Narcotics and Dangerous Drugs, and regulations by specific states
D. Drug standards—criteria for drug composition established by chemical or bioassay and published in official publications; e.g., United States Pharmacopeia, National Formulary, Pharmacopoeia Internationalis
E. Pharmacodynamics—the biochemical and physiologic effects of drugs and their mechanisms of action on living tissue
F. Pharmacology—the analysis of properties of chemicals that have a biologic action
G. Pharmacotherapeutics—the planned use and evaluation of the effect of drugs employed to prevent and treat disease
H. Toxicology—the analysis of poisons and poisonings caused by drugs

Terms that describe drug effect

A. Adverse effect—an action differing from the planned effect
B. Side effect—an often predictable outcome that is unrelated to the primary action of the drug
C. Toxic effect—a pathologic extension of the primary action of the drug
D. Cumulation—elevation of circulating levels of a drug consequent to slowing of metabolic pathways or excretory mechanisms
E. Drug dependence—driving need for continued use of a behavior or mood altering drug that leads to abuse
   1. Psychic dependence—craving requiring periodic or continued use of a drug for pleasure or relief of discomfort
   2. Physical dependence—appearance of characteristic symptoms when drug use is suspended or terminated (withdrawal or abstinence symptoms)

205

F. Hypersusceptibility—a response to a drug action that is higher than that occuring when the same dosage is given to 90% of the population

G. Idiosyncrasy—genetically conditioned enzymatic or receptor responsiveness that interferes with metabolic degradation of a drug

H. Paradoxic response—an action of a drug producing a response that contrasts sharply with the usual therapeutic effect obtained with the same dosage of the drug

I. Receptor—cellular site where union between a drug and a cellular constituent produces a reversible action

J. Tolerance—lowering of effect obtained from an established dosage of a drug that necessitates raising the dosage to maintain the effect

K. Tachyphylaxis—rapidly developing tolerance to a drug

L. Drug allergy—response occurring when drugs are from protein sources or combine with body protein and induce an allergen-antibody reaction that releases vasoactive intermediates that cause fluid transudation into tissues
   1. Anaphylaxis—life-threatening episode of bronchial constriction and edema that obstructs the airway and causes generalized vasodilation that depletes circulating blood volume; occurs when a drug allergen is administered to an individual having antibodies produced by prior use of the drug
   2. Urticaria—generalized pruritic skin eruptions or giant hives; occurs when a drug is administered to an individual having antibodies produced by prior use of the drug
   3. Angioedema—fluid accumulation in periorbital, oral, and respiratory tissues with lengthening of the expiratory phase and wheezing as bronchial constriction gradually progresses; occurs when a drug is administered to an individual having antibodies produced by prior use of the drug
   4. Serum sickness—gradually emerging intermittent episodes of dyspnea, hypotension, generalized edema, joint pain, rash, swollen lymph glands; occurs 7 or more days after initial administration of a drug causing gradual low level (titer) production of antibodies that interact with circulating

drug to produce symptoms as long as the drug remains in the body
   5. Arthus reaction—a localized area of tissue necrosis caused by disruption of blood supply; occurs when spasticity, occlusion, and degeneration of blood vessels is precipitated by injection of a drug into a site having large quantities of bivalent antibodies
   6. Delayed-reaction allergies—rash and fever occurring during drug therapy

DRUG ACTIONS
Sites

A. Local—drug acts at the site of application

B. Systemic—drug is distributed to selected internal receptor sites after being absorbed from tissues following administration; these routes include oral, sublingual, buccal, rectal, parenteral (intradermal, subcutaneous, intramuscular, intravenous, intraspinal, intracardiac)

Mechanisms

Drugs modify physiologic activity by replacing, interrupting, or potentiating physiologic processes

A. Replacement—administration of insulin required for cellular utilization of glucose

B. Interruption—antimetabolic drugs trick the cell into utilizing an inactive component in building protein

C. Potentiation—sulfonylurea group of oral hypoglycemic agents stimulate pancreatic beta cells to produce insulin

Factors influencing dosage-response relationships

A. Age, weight, sex, size, physiologic status, genetic and environmental factors affect responses and dosage required for therapeutic effect

B. The ratio between the median toxic dose and the median effective dose (TD50/ED50) of a drug provides the therapeutic index (T.I.), which is used as a guide to the safe dosage range; a low T.I. provides a narrow margin of safety and the patient's status is monitored closely for evidence of drug-related adverse effects; e.g., antineoplastic drugs

C. Concentration of active drug at receptors and duration of drug action is affected by
   1. Characteristics of the drug and the

rate of absorption, distribution, bio-transformation, and excretion

2. Drug affinity for particular tissues, immaturity of enzymes required for metabolism of the drug, or depressed function of tissues naturally metabolizing or excreting the drug

D. Membrane barriers, placental or blood-brain barrier, may block or selectively pass drug from circulating fluids to protected areas

E. Plasma protein binding of drugs maintains tissue levels by liberating drug when stores are lowered and by slowing renal clearance until the drug is freed from binding sites

Drug interactions

A. Drugs and foods may interact to adversely affect the therapeutic plan; e.g., ingestion of foods or vitamin preparations containing vitamin K may inhibit the hypothrombinemic effect of oral anticoagulants

B. Drug antagonism—opposing effects of 2 drugs at receptor sites in body tissues
1. Chemical antagonism—combining or binding of 2 drugs causing inactivation of the chemicals
2. Pharmacologic antagonism—competition of 2 drugs for a receptor that may allow the weaker drug to block access by the more potent drug
3. Physiologic antagonism—opposing action on physiologic systems that allows cancellation of action by either drug

C. Drug action summation—combined or concurrent action of drugs that increases therapeutic effects or incidence of adverse effects
1. Synergism—interaction of drugs at common receptor sites that alters metabolism or excretion and enhances the effect of drugs
2. Addition—action of 2 drugs at different receptors that produces an effect twice that possible when either drug is used alone
3. Potentiation—an intensified action occurring when 2 drugs are administered concurrently that is greater than when either drug is used alone

GENERAL INFORMATION

A. Drug nomenclature
1. Official name (generic, nonproprietary)—designated title under which a drug is listed in official publications
2. Chemical name—descriptive name identifying chemical composition and placement of atoms
3. Trade name (brand, proprietary)—manufacturer's registered and legally owned name for a drug

B. Sources of drugs
1. Active constituents of plants—alkaloids, glycosides, gums, resins, tannins, waxes, volatile or fixed oils
2. Animal sources of biologic products—enzymes, sera, vaccines, antitoxins, toxoids, hormones
3. Mineral sources—iron, iodine, Epsom salt

C. Drug dosage forms
1. Prepared by manufacturers in units for convenience of administration
2. Forms used include capsules, extended-release capsules, tablets (enteric-coated, extended-release), troche, pills, suppositories, powders, ampules, vials, delayed-release (repository) suspensions, prefilled cartridges, liniment, lotion, cream, ointments, pastes
3. Chemical preparations—solutions (waters, true solutions, syrups), aqueous suspensions (mixtures, emulsions, magmas, gels), spirits, elixirs, tinctures, fluidextracts, extracts

NURSING RESPONSIBILITIES

A. Knowledge required
1. Predictable effect of drugs on physiologic and emotional problems
2. Commonalities and variations between the actions of drugs employed for comparable therapeutic effect
3. Adverse effects and interactions of drugs commonly occurring during drug therapy
4. Biopsychosocial factors influencing drug therapy plans

B. Actions required
1. Establish a plan for observation of patient's reaction to medication
2. Establish a plan for drug administration based on the patient's needs
3. Involve the patient in implementing the drug therapy plan
4. Interpret the goals of the drug therapy plan to the patient
5. Employ nursing measures to support drug action
6. Share observations of drug effect with

health team members evaluating the plan

7. Reassess the individual's readiness to maintain the drug therapy plan

8. When necessary prepare for continued drug therapy at home
   a. Plan a specific schedule for drug use within the individual's pattern of living
   b. Explain common adverse effects and factors that may change drug requirements
   c. Describe the problems requiring physician contact

CARDIOPULMONARY DRUGS
Drugs that affect cardiac function

A. Terms describing drug action on the heart
1. Chronotropic—affecting the time or rate of contraction
2. Dromotropic—affecting conductivity of nerve fibers (pacemaker tissue in the heart)
3. Inotropic—affecting the force of muscular contraction

B. Digitalis glycosides
1. Positive inotropic action is achieved by increasing permeability of muscle membranes to the calcium and sodium ions required for contraction of muscle fibrils
   a. Forceful contraction during systole improves peripheral tissue perfusion
   b. Chamber emptying allows additional venous blood to enter cardiac chambers during diastole
2. Negative chronotropic effect is achieved by an action mediated by the vagus nerve that slows firing of the sinoatrial (SA) node and impulse transmission through the atrioventricular (AV) node (negative dromotropic action)
3. Preparations have the same qualitative action on the heart but differ in potency, rate of absorption, amount of drug absorbed, onset of action, speed of elimination
   a. Acetyldigitoxin (Acylanid)
   b. Deslanoside (Cedilanid-D)
   c. Digitalis
   d. Digitoxin (Crystodigin, Digitaline Nativelle, Myodigin, Purodigin)
   e. Digoxin (Davoxin, Lanoxin)
   f. Gitalin (Gitaligin)
   g. Lanatoside C (Cedilanid)
   h. Ouabain

4. Digitalization
   a. Provides an initial loading dose for acute effect on the enlarged heart
   b. After desired effect is achieved, the dosage is lowered to maintenance level replacing drug metabolized and excreted each day

5. Adverse effects
   a. Most frequent—nausea, vomiting, headache, drowsiness, insomnia, vertigo, confusion are all attributable to drug action at central nervous system sites; oral forms also cause nausea and vomiting by irritation of gastric mucosa
   b. Bradycardia attributable to drug induced slowing of SA node firing
   c. Arrythmias are first evidence of toxicity in one third of patients, premature nodal or ventricular impulses, varying degrees of heart block caused by drug action that slows transmission of impulse through the AV node
   d. Xanthopsia (yellow vision) caused by drug effect on visual cones
   e. Gynecomastia (mammary enlargement) in males resulting from estrogen-like steroid portion of digitalis glycosides

6. Considerations during therapy
   a. Premature contractions elevate the audible apical rate and mask the pacemaker conduction rate; apical pulse is taken before administration and drug is withheld when pulse rate drops to 60 in adults or to 90 in children
   b. Immaturity of hepatic and renal systems in premature and newborn infants or depressed hepatic or renal function in adults may result in cumulation
   c. Since potassium ions are required for interaction of digitalis glycosides with sodium-potassium dependent membranes, the lowering of serum levels of potassium ion may foster digitalis toxicity
   d. Since calcium ions act synergistically with digitalis on myocardial membranes, an elevation of serum calcium ion levels may increase

sensitivity of cardiac muscle to digitalis action

7. Drug interactions
   a. Phenobarbital, phenytoin, and phenylbutazone, by induction of hepatic microsomal enzymes, accelerate metabolism of digitalis glycosides, and serum levels are lower when the drugs are used concomitantly
   b. Diuretics that cause hypokalemia may contribute to the incidence of serious arrhythmias when administered concurrently with digitalis glycosides; supplemental potassium may be used for replacement of losses, or potassium-sparing diuretics may be prescribed to prevent potassium ion losses

Drugs that affect cardiac arrhythmias

A. Suppression of parasympathetic nervous system control at SA and AV nodes can be achieved by administering drugs such as atropine sulfate
   1. Atropine sulfate has a positive dromotropic effect by abolishing impulses that slow conduction at the SA or AV nodes when carotid sinus stimulation or drugs (digitalis) induce bradycardia or heart block
   2. Adverse effects caused by concurrent suppression of nerve activity in other tissues—depression of gastrointestinal motility, decreased glandular secretions, decreased bladder emptying
B. Stimulation of sympathetic nerve (beta adrenergic) receptors can be achieved by administering drugs such as isoproterenol hydrochloride (Isuprel Hydrochloride, Proternol)
   1. Has a positive chronotropic and inotropic effect by stimulating AV node transmission
   2. Concurrent stimulation of arterial beta receptors improves peripheral tissue perfusion
   3. Adverse effects—widespread vasodilation, hypotension, SA node stimulation causing tachycardia and palpitation, flushing, headache, nausea, tremor, dizziness, anxiety, restlessness
C. Depression of sympathetic nerve (beta adrenergic) receptors can be achieved by administering drugs such as propranolol hydrochloride (Inderal)

1. Has a negative inotropic effect by depressing cardiac response to sympathetic nervous system stimuli via blocking action at beta receptors
   a. Some vasodilation of coronary arteries occurs
   b. Reduces inotropic and chronotropic effect of exercise and patient may be light-headed, weak, and fatigued with exercise
2. Adverse effects—bradycardia, cardiac arrest; transient episodes of nausea, vomiting, diarrhea, constipation, lethargy, insomnia, dizziness, fatigue; serious problems include fever with myalgia, sore throat, erythematous rash, paresthesia of hands, visual disturbances, and hallucinations
3. Currently used also for therapy of angina pectoris and hypertension
D. Suppression of myocardial irritability by decreasing the permeability of muscle fibers to sodium ion influx can be achieved by administering drugs such as quinidine, lidocaine hydrochloride, procainamide hydrochloride, and phenytoin
   1. Quinidine preparations control atrial arrhythmias by prolonging the effective refractory period and slowing depolarization
      a. Drugs include quinidine gluconate (Quinaglute), quinidine hydrochloride, quinidine polygalacturonate (Cardioquin), quinidine sulfate (Quinidex, Quinora)
      b. Adverse effects—heart block caused by drug depression of AV node and ventricular conduction tissue; accelerated AV conduction or ventricular tachycardia occurring with initial dosage is caused by vagolytic action (may be lessened by digitalis administration); vasodilation with syncope and hypotension caused by depressant effect on all muscle tissue may occur with high dosage or I.V. use; gastric irritation with nausea, vomiting, and diarrhea may occur with oral use; allergic response; cinchonism, which may occur with long-term therapy, is initially seen as diarrhea, hot flushed skin followed by headache, vertigo, tinnitus, syncope, nausea, vomiting, skin rash, or visual disturbances (photophobia, diplopia)

c. Drug interactions
 (1) Quinidine preparations have neuromuscular blocking properties and may produce prolonged apnea when used with neuromuscular blocking drugs or drugs that depress conduction at the myoneural junction (polymyxin B, neomycin, kanamycin)
 (2) Quinidine has a mild depressant effect on the hepatic enzyme system that synthesizes coagulation factors, therefore concomitant use with oral anticoagulants may cause excess hypoprothrombinemia with bleeding
 (3) Quinidine has anticholinergic properties and excess cholinergic blocking (excess dryness of mouth, constipation) may result with concomitant use of belladonna alkaloids or other drugs with anticholinergic properties (phenothiazines, antihistamines, tricyclic antidepressants, procainamide hydrochloride)
2. Lidocaine hydrochloride (Xylocaine Hydrochloride) is administered I.V. by bolus or drip to control ventricular irritability
 a. Adverse effects—drowsiness, nervousness, dizziness, blurred vision, nausea, tremor, hypotension, generalized paresthesias
 b. Dosage exceeding 3 to 4 mg. per minute may depress inhibitor influences on motor pathways and cause convulsions or may depress medullary centers and cause respiratory arrest; I.V. bolus over 100 mg. may depress myocardial contractility
3. Procainamide hydrochloride (Pronestyl) is administered orally to control ventricular irritability
 a. Suppressive levels in blood depend on maintenance of an exact schedule for administration
 b. Adverse effects—decreased motility of the gastrointestinal tract (paralytic ileus), generalized vasodila-

tion caused by vagolytic action, anorexia, vomiting, nausea, bitter taste, asthenia, mental depression, flushing, allergic responses (urticaria, angioedema, fever)
 c. Drug interactions—procainamide hydrochloride has anticholinergic properties and excess cholinergic blocking may result with concomitant use of belladonna alkaloids or other drugs with anticholinergic properties
4. Phenytoin (Dilantin, Toin), formerly diphenylhydantoin, controls atrial or ventricular arrhythmias by reducing automaticity without decreasing conduction
 a. High alkalinity requires infusion of drug in large veins at maximum rate of 50 mg. per minute
 b. Oral drug causes gastric irritation that is lessened by ingestion of copious fluids with drug
 c. Adverse effects—lack of coordination and balance, dizziness, nausea, vomiting, pruritus, rash, nystagmus, constant lethargy, gingival hyperplasia occurs with prolonged use as the drug disrupts fibroblastic activity
 d. Drug interactions—prolonged use of phenytoin may inhibit activity of the intestinal conjugase enzyme that converts polyglutamates to monoglutamates and the reduced absorption of folic acid may cause mild megaloblastic anemia; dicumarol, chloramphenicol, disulfiram, and INH (in individuals who are slow inactivators of isoniazid) inhibit the hepatic microsomal enzymes, slow metabolism of phenytoin, and thereby increase serum levels of phenytoin

Drugs that affect circulating blood volume

A. Drugs that stimulate sympathetic nerve (beta adrenergic) receptors
 1. Site of action
  a. Cardiac beta receptors produce a positive inotropic and chronotropic effect
  b. Bronchial beta receptors dilate the the bronchi
  c. Arterial beta receptors dilate arte-

rioles and arteries in skeletal and cardiac muscle
2. Drugs—used primarily for cardiac and bronchial action
   a. Epinephrine hydrochloride (Adrenalin Chloride) also acts at alpha receptors to constrict capacitance vessels (venules and veins) and resistance vessels (arterioles and arteries) of vital organ beds
   b. Ephedrine sulfate has an effect comparable to epinephrine
   c. Isoproterenol hydrochloride (Isuprel Hydrochloride, Proternol) also dilates arterioles and arteries of the kidneys and intestine
3. Adverse effects—anginal pain when cardiac contractile force improves in patients with subclinical coronary vessel occlusion, inhibition of intestinal motility (gaseous distention, constipation) caused by beta receptor stimulation, elevation of blood glucose levels (transient hyperglycemia), depletion of glycogen stores, central nervous system stimulation (headache, insomnia, hyperexcitability)

B. Drugs that stimulate arterial alpha adrenergic receptors
1. Site of action
   a. Alpha receptors cause constriction that elevates the blood pressure
   b. Increase arterial constriction, which increases the work load of the left ventricle and may reflexly slow cardiac rate causing reduced cardiac output and effective blood flow
2. Drugs
   a. Hydroxyamphetamine hydrobromide (Paredrine)
   b. Methoxamine hydrochloride (Vasoxyl)
   c. Phenylephrine hydrochloride (Neo-Synephrine Hydrochloride)
3. Adverse effects—constriction of resistance vessels without action on capacitance vessels may increase venous pooling and reduce venous return to the heart

C. Drugs that directly stimulate arterial smooth muscles
1. Site of action—constricts resistance vessels to produce pressor effect
2. Drug—angiotensin amide (Hypertensin) has venous pooling and brady-

cardia potential comparable to drugs acting on arterial alpha receptors
3. Adverse effects—dizziness, headache, mild urticaria

D. Drugs that stimulate arterial and venous alpha adrenergic receptors
1. Site of action
   a. Alpha receptors cause constriction that elevates the blood pressure
   b. Venous alpha receptors cause constriction that improves blood flow toward the heart
2. Drugs—used for combined effect on capacitance and resistance vessels
   a. Levarterenol bitartrate (Levophed Bitartrate) also has a positive inotropic and chronotropic effect on the heart
   b. Mephentermine sulfate (Wyamine Sulfate) also stimulates cardiac beta receptors
   c. Metaraminol bitartrate (Aramine) also stimulates cardiac beta receptors
3. Adverse effects
   a. Considerations during therapy—infiltration may cause local vasoconstriction leading to tissue necrosis; I.V. administration is titrated with the blood pressure level to prevent a rise to hypertensive levels
   b. Adrenergic stimulation inhibits intestinal motility and gaseous distention or constipation may occur with prolonged administration

E. Drugs that constrict arterioles and venules
1. Vasopressin (Pitressin) has a direct musculotropic effect that constricts small vessels when infused by a route delivering the drug to bleeding sites
2. Carbazochrome salicylate (Adrenosem, Adrestat, Statimo) is an oxidative product of epinephrine and has a comparable vasoconstrictive action that controls persistent oozing from arterioles and capillaries
3. General adverse effects that may occur with therapeutic doses of the vasopressors—headache, restlessness, anxiety, weakness, pallor, dizziness, tremor, precordial pain, palpitation, respiratory distress; overdose may cause convulsions, cerebral hemorrhage, arrhythmias

F. Plasma volume expanders
1. Osmotic agents to mobilize excess tissue fluid and expand blood volume
    a. Dextran 40 (Rheomacrodex) is used when blood protein levels are within normal limits; it improves capillary blood flow, which decreases stasis of blood and red blood cell aggregation in microcapillaries
    b. Dextran (Expandex) may also be used and is a more effective expander of blood volume; however, it tends to have an adverse effect on blood flow to microcapillaries as it increases blood viscosity
2. Albumin replacement to maintain serum levels and normal oncotic pressure
    a. Types of preparations
        (1) Normal human serum albumin
        (2) Normal human serum albumin (salt-poor)
        (3) Plasma protein fraction (human)
    b. Actions
        (1) Decreases tissue fluid accumulation
        (2) Decreases the hematocrit level
        (3) Elevates the blood pressure to normal levels when administered slowly while restricting oral fluid intake
    c. Adverse effects—allergic reaction (skin rash) may occur during or immediately after administration

Drugs that decrease vasoconstriction

A. Drugs that deplete norepinephrine at arterial sympathetic nerve terminals
1. Site of action
    a. Alpha adrenergic receptors decrease response to sympathetic nervous system stimuli and interrupt vasoconstriction
    b. Cardiac adrenergic receptors slow heart rate
2. Drugs
    a. Rauwolfia alkaloids—work by inhibiting the stimulation of vascular smooth muscles; cross the blood-brain barrier and act on medullary vasomotor centers and on central nervous tissue to cause sedative effect
        (1) Alseroxylon (Rautensin, Rauwiloid)
        (2) Deserpidine (Harmonyl)
        (3) *Rauwolfia serpentina* (Raudixin, Rautina, Wolfina)
        (4) Rescinnamine (Moderil)
        (5) Reserpine (Rau-Sed, Reserpoid, Sandril, Serpasil)
        (6) Syrosingopine (Singoserp)
        (7) Adverse effects—continual drowsiness, bizarre dreams, nasal congestion, gastric ulcers (parenteral drug increases secretion of gastric acid), bradycardia, lethargy, diarrhea (drug increases gastrointestinal tone and motility), episodes of depression that necessitate discontinuance of the drug
        (8) Drug interactions
            (a) Potentiates the depressant effect of barbiturates
            (b) Increases hypotension if given with other drugs causing vasodilation
            (c) Adds to the direct tissue depression of digitalis or quinidine and may result in cardiac asystole
        (9) Considerations during therapy—drugs lower the convulsive threshold, which necessitates lower dosage in epileptic individuals
    b. Guanethidine sulfate (Ismelin)
        (1) Hypotensive effect is most pronounced when sitting or standing
        (2) Adverse effects—orthostatic hypotension and hypotension during exercise, prominence of parasympathetic nerve-controlled visceral activity (increased intestinal motility with uncontrollable diarrhea occurring after eating), bradycardia, inhibits ejaculation
        (3) Drug interactions
            (a) Use with amphetamines, other sympathetic drugs (ephedrine, methylphenidate), chlorpromazines, or mood elevating drugs (amitriptyline hydrochloride—Elavil; imipramine hydrochloride—Tofranil)

decreases the effective-
ness of guanethidine in
reducing blood pressure

(b) Used with thiazide diuretics, enhances hypoten-
sive effect and permits reduction of dosage

c. Methyldopa (Aldomet) depletes
norepinephrine at peripheral and
central sites
(1) Sustains and may increase
renal blood flow
(2) Adverse effects—orthostatic
hypotension, dizziness, weakness, drowsiness, bradycardia,
dryness of mouth, nasal congestion, diarrhea, hypersensitivity reaction (hemolytic
anemia, hepatitis, fever, malaise)

B. Drugs that decelerate norepinephrine
biosynthesis at arterial sympathetic nerve
terminals
1. Site of action—monoamine oxidase inhibitors act at cerebral and peripheral
sites
2. Drug—pargyline hydrochloride (Eu-
tonyl)
a. Latent period of several days before antihypertensive action is evident
b. Adverse effects—psychic depression, mood changes, euphoria, insomnia, headache, nightmares
(caused by central nervous system
stimulation), orthostatic hypotension, edema (caused by sodium
and water retention), gastrointestinal disturbances
c. Drug-food interactions—hypertensive crisis with vascular rupture,
occipital headache, palpitation,
stiffness of neck muscles, emesis,
sweating, photophobia, and cardiac
arrhythmias may occur when neuro-
hormone levels are elevated by
ingestion of foods with high tyramine content (pickled herring, alcoholic beverages, chicken livers,
aged or natural cheese, chocolate)
d. Drug interactions—potentiates the
pressor effect of other adrenergic
drugs (epinephrine, norepinephrine, methyldopa, levodopa, dopamine, amphetamines) and potentiates the effects of sedatives

C. Drugs that have a direct relaxant effect
on arterial smooth muscle
1. Hydralazine hydrochloride (Apreso-
line Hydrochloride, Dralzine, Lopress)
a. Intravenous administration lowers
blood pressure in 15 minutes and
effect is sustained for 3 to 4 hours
b. Sustains or may increase renal
blood flow
c. Reflex stimulation of the heart improves cardiac output
d. Adverse effects—palpitations, localized collections of tissue fluid
(periorbital, ankle, genital tissues),
severe headache, dizziness, anxiety,
depression, tachycardia, gastrointestinal disturbances, flushing, dyspnea on exertion, rash
2. Sodium nitroprusside (Nipride)
a. Short action period necessitates
continuous I.V. infusion
b. Adverse effects—sweating, muscular twitching, nausea, anxiety, apprehension (associated with rapid
reduction in blood pressure), transient restlessness, agitation, retch-
ing, rash; if biotransformation of
nitroprusside to thiocyanate
reaches toxic levels, psychosis and
delirium may occur
3. Diazoxide (Hyperstat)
a. Widespread action on arterioles
leads to blood pressure reduction
to normal levels in 1 to 5 minutes
after single rapid intravenous injection
b. I.V. should be given within a 15-
to 20-second time period to avoid
tenacious protein binding, which
neutralizes the drug
c. Adverse effects—significant temporary hyperglycemia, marked sodium and water retention, gastrointestinal disturbances (nausea, vomiting, anorexia), headache, flushing, supraventricular tachycardia

D. Drugs that act as ganglionic blocking
agents
1. Site of action—interrupts acetylcho-
line-mediated transmission of stimuli
at the sympathetic nerve ganglion by
competitive inhibition
2. Drugs—employed only selectively because they affect acetylcholine action
in the parasympathetic nervous system

a. Chlorisondamine chloride (Ecolid)
b. Mecamylamine hydrochloride (Inversine Hydrochloride) crosses the blood-brain barrier
c. Pentolinium tartrate (Ansolysen)
d. Trimethaphan camsylate (Arfonad) also has a direct vasodilating effect that increases the hypotensive response
3. Adverse effects—blocking of parasympathetic ganglia causes dryness of nose, mouth, and throat, blurred vision, gastrointestinal disturbances (adynamic ileus, anorexia, nausea, vomiting), urine retention, and severe orthostatic hypotension

E. Drugs that reduce sympathetic nerve impulses from the brainstem
1. Site of action—reduce alpha-adrenergic stimulation from cardioaccelerator and vasoconstrictor centers in the medulla
2. Drug—clonidine hydrochloride (Catapres)
3. Decreases cardiac output and reduces peripheral resistance
4. Adverse effects—mild and infrequent orthostatic hypotension, dry mouth, sedation, drowsiness
5. Considerations during therapy—gradual reduction of dosage is required at termination of therapy to avoid rapid rise in blood pressure and associated symptoms (nervousness, agitation, headache)

F. Drugs that lower sensitivity of baroreceptors in the carotid and aortic sinuses
1. Action—improves baroreceptor response to high arterial pressure; the impulses traveling to cardioinhibitory centers in the medulla provide the stimulus for slowing cardiac conduction that decreases cardiac output and lessens hypertensive levels
2. Drugs
a. Alkavervir (Veriloid)
b. Cryptenamine (Unitensen)
3. Adverse effects—persistent nausea and vomiting, bradycardia, epigastric distress, hiccups, salivation, hyperhidrosis, blurred vision, paresthesia, excessive hypotension

G. Drugs that control peripheral vasospasm by alpha adrenergic blocking
1. Action—drugs occupy alpha receptors to prevent activation by norepineph-

rine, which allows epinephrine action at beta receptors and consequent vasodilation
2. Drugs
a. Phenoxybenzamine hydrochloride (Dibenzyline)
b. Phentolamine mesylate (Regitine)
3. Adverse effects—orthostatic hypotension, reflex tachycardia, hypermotility of intestinal tract (diarrhea), nausea, vomiting, nasal congestion

H. Drugs that have a direct relaxant action on smooth muscles of peripheral arteries and lessen constriction or spasticity
1. Azapetine phosphate (Ilidar) also causes some cardiac stimulation
2. Cyclandelate (Cyclospasmol)
3. Isoxsuprine hydrochloride (Vasodilan) also has beta adrenergic stimulation action that increases heart rate and dilates arteries to peripheral muscles
4. Nicotinyl alcohol (Roniacol) acts primarily on dermal vessels in the blush area
5. Nylidrin hydrochloride (Arlidin) improves blood flow to skeletal muscle where anoxia-related muscle cramps exist; action at beta adrenergic receptors in the heart causes palpitations
6. Tolazoline hydrochloride (Priscoline Hydrochloride) has some cardiac stimulation action

I. Drugs relaxing smooth muscle of vessels and having some effect on musculature of major abdominal viscera
1. Drugs
a. Dioxyline phosphate (Paveril Phosphate)
b. Ethaverine hydrochloride (Ethaquin, Laverin, Neopavrin)
c. Papaverine hydrochloride
2. Adverse effects—hypotension, respiratory depression, hepatotoxicity, drowsiness, vertigo, headache, rash

J. Drugs that control angina pectoris—nitrates
1. Action
a. Decreases resistance of smooth muscle of large capacitance vessels (veins, venules) and large resistance vessels, which decreases cardiac work and myocardial oxygen requirements
b. Decreases the incidence of anginal attacks and improves work tolerance

c. Decreases central venous pressure, left ventricle end-diastolic pressure, and pulmonary wedge pressure, and lowers blood pressure causing a reflex increase in heart rate

d. Increases blood flow through coronary arteries and collateral channels with increased blood flow to ischemic areas of the heart

2. Drugs
  a. Nitrates for sublingual use
    (1) Erythrityl tetranitrate (Cardilate)
    (2) Isosorbide dinitrate (Isordil, Sorbitrate)
    (3) Nitroglycerin
        (a) Effect in 1 to 2 minutes; repeat dosage in 5 minutes if pain persists
        (b) When taken 3 minutes before activity known to cause anginal pain, pain-free exercise tolerance increases
        (c) Tablets deteriorate rapidly in heat, light, moisture (potency loss by sublimation)
        (d) Sublingual use causes slight stinging, burning, tingling under the tongue, and absence of these signs can indicate deterioration of the drug
  b. Nitrates for oral use
    (1) Inositol hexanitrate (Tolanate)
    (2) Mannitol hexanitrate (Nitranitol)
    (3) Pentaerythritol tetranitrate (Peritrate)
    (4) Trolnitrate phosphate (Metamine)

3. Adverse effects—concurrent vasodilation in cerebral, splanchnic, and cutaneous vessels may cause headache, facial blushing, hypotension, dizziness, fainting with repeated use; reflex tachycardia; tolerance develops especially with long-acting forms and may cause tolerance to sublingual forms

4. Drug interactions—sudden hypotension may occur when alcohol is ingested close to the time of nitrate use

Drugs that affect pulmonary ventilation

A. Bronchodilators
  1. Theophyllines
    a. Drugs
      (1) Aminophylline
      (2) Dyphylline (Dilor, Neothylline)
      (3) Oxtriphylline (Choledyl)
      (4) Theophylline (Aqualin, Elixophyllin)
    b. Actions
      (1) Act directly on bronchial smooth muscle to decrease spasm and relax smooth muscle of the vasculature
      (2) Direct stimulatory effect on myocardium increases cardiac output, which improves blood flow to kidneys
      (3) Direct action on renal tubules provides diuretic effect by increasing excretion of sodium and chloride ions
    c. Adverse effects—oral forms cause gastric irritation
    d. Considerations during therapy—cumulation of drug can occur unless dosage is regulated; parenteral drug must be administered slowly over a 4- to 5-minute period to avoid peripheral vasodilation (hypotension, facial flushing), cerebral vascular constriction (headache, dizziness), cardiac palpitation, and precordial pain
  2. Epinephrine hydrochloride—the drug of choice in respiratory emergency and anaphylactic reactions
    a. Actions
      (1) Acts at beta adrenergic receptors in bronchus to relax smooth muscle and increase respiratory volume
      (2) Inhalants have a local action causing vasoconstriction that reduces congestion or edema
    b. Adverse effects—cardiac palpitation, overuse of inhalants may cause "congestive rebound"
  3. Isoproterenol hydrochloride (Isuprel Hydrochloride, Proternol)
    a. Action—similar to theophyllines
    b. Adverse effects—action at cardiovascular beta receptors causes tachycardia, peripheral blood vessel dilation (hypotension)

4. Metaproterenol (Alupent, Metaprel)
5. Terbutaline (Bricanyl) has little effect on cardiac tissue
6. Oral drugs that relax bronchi and decrease glandular and tissue fluid in bronchi
   a. Drugs
      (1) Methoxyphenamine hydrochloride (Orthoxine)
      (2) Phenylpropanolamine hydrochloride (Propadrine)
      (3) Pseudoephedrine hydrochloride (Sudafed)
   b. Adverse effects—transient elevation in pulse and systolic blood pressure, dry oral tissues
7. Cromolyn sodium (Aarane, Intal) acts primarily by preventing release of mediators of type I allergic reactions (histamine, slow-reacting substance of anaphylaxis) from sensitized mast cells; prophylactic use by inhaling capsule contents lessens bronchoconstriction
8. Adverse effects common to bronchodilator group—anxiety, nervousness, tremors, nausea, vomiting, headache, dizziness

B. Narcotic antagonists employed to improve respiratory depression or respiratory arrest induced by overdose of addictive analgesics
1. Drugs
   a. Levallorphan tartrate (Lorfan)
   b. Nalorphine hydrochloride (Nalline)
   c. Naloxone hydrochloride (Narcan)
2. Actions
   a. Competes with narcotics for receptors at respiratory center
   b. Lowers threshold for carbon dioxide stimulation of respiration (increases respiratory rate and tidal volume, which decreases blood CO_2 level)
3. Considerations during therapy—inactivation of narcotic action may induce withdrawal symptoms; respiratory depression may recur when action of drug terminates and narcotic activity returns; naloxone hydrochloride action limited to reversal of narcotic, propoxyphene, or pentazocine lactate related depression, but nalorphine hydrochloride or levallorphan tartrate induce respiratory depression in the absence of narcotics

C. Drugs that control cough (antitussives)
1. Narcotic type cough suppressants (limited sedative effect)
   a. Drugs
      (1) Dextromethorphan hydrobromide (Dormethan, Romilar)
      (2) Hydrocodone bitartrate (Dodone, Dicodid)
      (3) Levopropoxyphene napsylate (Novrad)
      (4) Noscapine (Nectadon)
   b. Acts on medullary control center to suppress cough
   c. Adverse effects—hypersensitivity, nausea, drowsiness
2. Antihistaminic cough suppressants
   a. Drugs
      (1) Chlorphedianol hydrochloride (Ulo)
      (2) Diphenhydramine hydrochloride (Benadryl)
   b. Act at tissue level to prevent histamine-induced edema causing irritation of cough-sensitive nerve endings in tracheobronchial structures
   c. Adverse effects—mild sedation
3. Local anesthetic cough suppressants
   a. Drugs
      (1) Benzonatate (Tessalon)
      (2) Carbetapentane citrate (Toclase)
   b. Acts to inhibit cough reflex at afferent endings of vagus nerve and at medullary transmission sites
   c. Adverse effects—occasionally nausea, drowsiness, holding drug in mouth causes slight numbness

D. Expectorants—increase production of thinner, less viscid secretions that protect bronchial tissues
1. Hydriodic acid—administered diluted sipped through straw to avoid damage to teeth
2. Elixir of terpin hydrate—42.5% alcohol content of compounds provides expectorant action

E. Mucolytics
1. Drugs
   a. Calcium iodide
   b. Glyceryl guaiacolate (Robitussin)
   c. Iodinated glycerol (Organidin)
   d. Potassium iodide (Enkide)
2. Act to raise the osmolality of bronchial glandular secretions causing fluids to move to dilute the secretions
3. Adverse effects—nausea, skin erup

tions; long-term use of iodides may cause iodism (inflammation of respiratory tract tissues, skin eruptions, accumulation of fluid in nasal passages, lungs, eyelids)

Drugs that affect red blood cell building

A. Drugs that provide components for protein framework of cells by supplying cofactors for DNA biosynthesis of nucleotides
1. Vitamin B_{12} replacement
   a. Cyanocobalamin
   b. Hydroxocobalamin
   c. Vitamin B_{12} with intrinsic factor concentrate
   d. Liver injection
2. Tetrahydrofolic acid
   a. Folate sodium (Folvite Sodium)
   b. Folic acid (Folvite)
   c. Leucovorin calcium
B. Drugs that provide a component of hemoglobin for erythroblasts
1. Oral iron sources
   a. Drugs
      (1) Ferrocholinate (Chel-Iron, Ferrolip)
      (2) Ferrous fumarate (Ircon, Toleron)
      (3) Ferrous gluconate
      (4) Ferrous lactate (Ferro Drops)
      (5) Ferrous sulfate
   b. Adverse effects—nausea, vomiting, fatalities in children ingesting enteric coated tablets thinking they are candy
   c. Drug interactions—ferrous sulfate binds tetracycline and decreases absorption; magnesium trisilicate decreases absorption of iron preparations
2. Parenteral iron sources
   a. Drugs
      (1) Iron-Dextran injection (Imferon)
      (2) Iron sorbitex (Jectofer)
   b. Adverse effects—tissue staining (use "Z" tract for injection), fever, lymphadenopathy, nausea, vomiting, arthralgia, urticaria, severe peripheral vascular failure, anaphylaxis, secondary hematochromatosis

Drugs that affect blood coagulation

A. Drugs that lower blood lipid levels
1. Aluminum nicotinate (Nicalex)

   a. Action—decreases biosynthesis of cholesterol by interfering with availability of CoA and increasing catabolism and oxidation of cholesterol in the liver
   b. Adverse effects—gastrointestinal disturbances, flushing of facial tissues, pruritus
2. Cholestyramine resin (Cuemid, Questran)
   a. Action—accelerates removal of bile acids in the intestinal lumen and the lowered levels of bile increase hepatic oxidation of cholesterol causing a decrease in circulating cholesterol
   b. Adverse effects—constipation (especially in elderly patients taking high daily doses), nausea, heartburn, diarrhea
   c. Drug interactions—action in intestinal lumen may bind iron or acids or may absorb neutral drugs (digoxin, levothyroxine sodium, liothyronine sodium, warfarin, phenylbutazone, thiazide diuretics); long-term use interferes with absorption of fat-soluble vitamins
3. Clofibrate (Atromid S)
   a. Action—inhibits the rate of biosynthesis of cholesterol by acting on beta lipoproteins
   b. Adverse effect—nausea
   c. Drug interactions—potentiates the hypoprothrombinemic action of anticoagulants by displacing coumarins from albumin-binding sites and reducing liver stores of vitamin K required for coagulation factor synthesis
4. Dextrothyroxine sodium (Choloxin) increases the rate of oxidation or hydroxylation of cholesterol in the liver
5. Sitosterols (Cytellin) interferes with absorption of exogenous cholesterol and reabsorption of endogenous cholesterol
B. Drugs that prevent intravascular clot formation
1. Heparin sodium (Depo-Heparin Sodium, Hepathrom, Lipo-Hepin, Liquaemin Sodium, Meparin, Panheprin) interacts with enzymes of the coagulation process to inhibit prothrombin conversion to thrombin and the conversion of thrombin required for fibrin formation

a. Heparin sodium activity is measured by venous clotting time determination
b. Control of heparin sodium-induced bleeding by use of protamine sulfate, which has a strong positive charge and unites with the negative charge of heparin to form an inert complex
2. Prothrombin inactivators (oral anticoagulants)
   a. Action—interfere with utilization of vitamin K in the liver to interrupt synthesis of prothrombin
   b. Drugs
      (1) Acenocoumarol (Sintrom)
      (2) Anisindione (Miradon)
      (3) Dicumarol
      (4) Diphenadione (Dipaxin)
      (5) Phenindione (Danilone, Hedulin)
      (6) Phenprocoumon (Liquamar)
      (7) Warfarin sodium (Coumadin, Panwarfin)
      (8) Warfarin potassium (Arthrombin-K)
   c. Therapeutic action monitored by tests of prothrombin activity
   d. Adverse effects—external or internal bleeding
   e. Control of excess bleeding—whole blood, plasma; vitamin K_1; menadiol sodium diphosphate (Kappadione, Synkayvite), menadione, menadione sodium bisulfite (Hykinone), phytonadione (AquaMephyton, Konakion, Mephyton), vitamin K_5 (Synkamin)
   f. Drug-food interaction—antagonism occurs with excessive ingestion of foods rich in vitamin K (fish, fish oils, tomatoes, cheese, kale, cauliflower, cabbage, spinach, egg yolk, liver)
   g. Drug interactions
      (1) Action potentiated by impairing platelet function (salicylates, chlorpromazine); by impairing anticoagulant degradation (tolbutamide, chloramphenicol); by interfering with albumin binding (sulfisoxazole, phenylbutazone, indomethacin, clofibrate); by decreasing absorption of vitamin K from the intestine (cholestyramine resin)
      (2) Action inhibition by stimulating enzymes that degrade the drug (barbiturates, chloral hydrate, glutethimide); by decreasing other clotting factors (oral contraceptives)
3. Platelet aggregation inhibitors decrease liberation of thrombin by platelets at tissue sites
   a. Aspirin
   b. Dipyridamole (Persantine)
C. Drugs that replace deficient coagulation factors
   1. Antihemophilic factor (Hemofil)
      a. Obtained from human sources
      b. Provides concentrated factor VIII
   2. Antihemophilic plasma
   3. Factor IX complex (Konȳne) contains factors II, VII, IX, X (concentrated)
D. Clotting factor replacement
   1. Epsilon-aminocaproic acid (Amicar) inhibits the enzyme that destroys formed fibrin and increases fibrinogen activity in clot formation
   2. Fibrinogen (Parenogen) maintains plasma fibrinogen levels required for clotting materials
   3. Thrombin supplies physiologic levels of natural material at superficial bleeding sites to control bleeding

OPHTHALMIC PREPARATIONS

A. Anti-infective agents
   1. Most of the anti-infective drugs used systemically are available in forms for topical use in the eye (lids, conjunctiva, cornea) to treat bacterial, fungal, protozoal, helminthic infections
   2. Concurrent systemic therapy may be planned for severe infections
   3. Use of drugs infrequently prescribed for systemic therapy lessens development of resistant organisms or sensitization of individuals to commonly used drugs
B. Glucocorticoids
   1. Employed for therapy of acute non-pyrogenic ocular inflammation
   2. Decrease inflammation and reduce the scarring that contributes to visual loss
   3. Local suppression of inflammatory responses may mask symptoms of ocular disease

4. Repeated use may slightly raise intraocular pressure by reduction of aqueous humor outflow

C. Miotics
1. Facilitate aqueous humor outflow in control of elevated intraocular pressure
2. Action
   a. Constricts the pupil, pulls the iris away from the filtration angle, and improves outflow of aqueous humor
   b. Direct stimulation of parasympathetic effector cells
      (1) Pilocarpine hydrochloride (or nitrate)
      (2) Carbachol
      (3) Methacholine chloride (Mecholyl)
   c. Indirect action by inhibition of cholinesterase
      (1) Physostigmine
      (2) Neostigmine bromide (Prostigmin)
      (3) Demecarium (Humorsol)
      (4) Isoflurophate (Floropryl)
      (5) Echothiophate (Phospholine)
3. Adverse effects—twitching of eyelids, brow ache, headache, ocular pain, ciliary and conjunctival congestion, accommodative myopia, contact dermatitis, and effects secondary to drug absorption (hypersalivation, sweating, nausea, vomiting, abdominal pain, diarrhea, bradycardia, hypotension, bronchoconstriction)
4. Consideration during therapy—drainage into nose or throat and consequent systemic effect may be lessened by applying pressure at the inner canthus after instillation

D. Carbonic anhydrase inhibitors
1. Action—decrease inflow of aqueous humor in control of intraocular pressure (administered orally or parenterally)
2. Drugs
   a. Acetazolamide (Diamox)
   b. Dichlorphenamide (Daranide, Oratrol)
   c. Ethoxzolamide (Cardrase, Ethamide)
   d. Methazolamide (Neptazane)
3. Adverse effects—diuresis, paresthesia, anorexia, nausea, vomiting, depression, confusion, destruction of the angle

E. Osmotic agents
1. Action employed to reduce volume of intraocular fluids
2. Administered systemically to decrease blood osmolality, which mobilizes fluid from the eye
3. Drugs
   a. Glycerin (Glyrol, Osmoglyn)
   b. Mannitol (Osmitrol)
   c. Urea (Urevert, Ureaphil)
4. Adverse effects—headache, nausea, vomiting

F. Anticholinergic drugs
1. Drugs paralyze accommodation (cycloplegia) and dilate the pupil (mydriasis) by relaxing the ciliary muscle and the sphincter muscle of the iris; used for examination of eye interior
2. Drugs
   a. Atropine and scopolamine provide long action required for children under 6 years of age when the eye has very active accommodation
   b. Homatropine hydrobromide
   c. Cyclopentolate (Cyclogyl)
   d. Eucatropine
   e. Tropicamide (Mydriacyl)
3. Adverse effects—systemic reactions (primarily in children and elderly) are dryness of mouth and skin, flushing, fever, rash, thirst, tachycardia, irritability, hyperactivity, ataxia, confusion, somnolence, hallucination, delirium

G. Adrenergic drugs providing mydriasis without cycloplegia
1. Dilate pupil (mydriasis) by causing contraction of dilator muscle of the iris with minimal effect on ciliary muscle, which lessens effect on accommodation
2. Drugs
   a. Phenylephrine (Efricel, Neo-Synephrine)
   b. Epinephrine
   c. Hydroxyamphetamine (Paredrine)
3. Adverse effects—brow ache, headache, blurred vision, pain, lacrimation, allergic reactions; systemic effects include tachycardia, premature ventricular contractions, hypertension, hyperhidrosis, tremors, blanching

CENTRAL NERVOUS SYSTEM DRUGS
Drugs that affect emotional responses

A. Action—affect behavioral responses by modifying neurohormonal levels in the

thalamus, hypothalamus, reticular formation, and limbic system
B. Types of drugs
1. Antidepressant drugs—increase the level of norepinephrine at subcortical neuroeffector sites
    a. Monoamine oxidase (MAO) inhibitors—elevate norepinephrine levels in brain tissues by interference with the enzyme MAO; act as psychic energizers
        (1) Drugs
            (a) Isocarboxazid (Marplan)
            (b) Phenelzine sulfate (Nardil)
            (c) Tranylcypromine sulfate (Parnate)
        (2) Drug interactions—MAOI potentiate the effects of alcohol, barbiturates, anesthetic agents (cocaine), antihistamines, narcotics, corticoids, anticholinergics, sympathomimetic drugs
        (3) Drug-food interactions—hypertensive crisis with vascular rupture, occipital headache, palpitation, stiffness of neck muscles, emesis, sweating, photophobia, and cardiac arrhythmias may occur when neurohormonal levels are elevated by ingestion of foods with high tyramine content (pickled herring, beer, wine, chicken livers, aged or natural cheese, chocolate)
        (4) Adverse effects—central nervous system stimulation (headache, restlessness, insomnia), peripheral edema, orthostatic hypotension, dry mouth, constipation, urine retention, transient impotence, anorexia, nausea
    b. Norepinephrine blockers provide elevated levels of the neurohormone by preventing reuptake and storage at the axon (tricyclic compounds)
        (1) Drugs
            (a) Amitriptyline hydrochloride (Elavil)
            (b) Desipramine hydrochloride (Norpramin, Pertofrane)
            (c) Doxepin hydrochloride (Adapin, Sinequan)
            (d) Imipramine hydrochloride (Presamine, Tofranil)
            (e) Nortriptyline hydrochloride (Aventyl)
            (f) Protriptyline hydrochloride (Vivactil)
        (2) Drug interactions—potentiate effects of anticholinergic drugs and central nervous system depressants; e.g., alcohol and sedatives
        (3) Adverse effects—orthostatic hypotension, skin rash, drowsiness, dry mouth, blurred vision, constipation, urine retention, tachycardia, central nervous system stimulation in elderly patients (excitement, restlessness, incoordination, fine tremor)
    c. Norepinephrine release stimulators (cerebral stimulants)—improve productivity by decreasing psychomotor activity or response to environmental stimuli
        (1) Drugs
            (a) Methylphenidate hydrochloride (Ritalin)
            (b) Pipradrol hydrochloride (Meratran)
        (2) Adverse effects—hyperexcitability, irritability, restlessness
    d. Norepinephrine uptake accelerator—alters sodium transport in nerve and muscle cells and affects a shift in intraneural metabolism of norepinephrine
        (1) Drug—lithium carbonate (Eskalith, Lithane, Lithonate)
        (2) Drug-food interaction—restriction of sodium intake increases drug substitution for sodium ions, which causes signs of hyponatremia (nausea, vomiting, diarrhea, muscle fasciculations, stupor, convulsions)
        (3) Adverse effects—excess voiding and extreme thirst caused by drug suppression of antidiuretic hormone (ADH) function, which causes dehydration

2. Antipsychotic drugs (major tranquilizers)—control behavior when the patient's uncontrolled actions are destructive to self, others, or the environment
   a. Types of drugs
   (1) Phenothiazine derivatives
   (a) Drugs
   (1) Acetophenazine maleate (Tindal)
   (2) Chlorpromazine hydrochloride (Thorazine)
   (3) Fluphenazine hydrochloride (Prolixin)
   (4) Perphenazine (Trilafon)
   (5) Prochlorperazine (Compazine)
   (6) Promazine hydrochloride (Sparine)
   (7) Thioridazine hydrochloride (Mellaril)
   (8) Trifluoperazine (Stelazine)
   (9) Triflupromazine hydrochloride (Vesprin)
   (b) Adverse effects—incoordination of voluntary muscle action (dyskinesia) in children (speech, swallowing, tongue or facial muscle control problems, and clonic muscle contractions); pseudoparkinsonism syndrome in elderly patients on long-term therapy (shuffling gait, masklike facies, drooling of excessive saliva, rigid muscles with continual tremor subsiding on intentional movement, pill-rolling movements of fingers)
   (2) Butyrophenones
   (a) Drugs
   (1) Droperidol (Inapsine)
   (2) Haloperidol (Haldol)
   (b) Adverse effects—similar to phenothiazines
   (3) Dihydroindolone
   (a) Drug—molidone hydrochloride (Moban)
   (b) Adverse effects—similar to phenothiazines
   (4) Thioxanthenes
   (a) Drugs
   (1) Chlorprothixene (Taractan)
   (2) Thiothixene
   (b) Adverse effects—similar to phenothiazines
   b. General adverse effects of major tranquilizers—manifestations of extrapyramidal tract irritation, drowsiness (highest incidence in initial days of therapy), orthostatic hypotension, constipation, urinary retention, anorexia, hypersensitivity reactions (tissue fluid accumulation, photoallergic reaction, impotence, cessation of menses or ovulation)

3. Antianxiety drugs (minor tranquilizers)—used when individuals are incapable of coping with environmental stresses and accomplishing daily activities
   a. Types of drugs
   (1) Propanediol compounds
   (a) Drugs
   (1) Meprobamate (Equanil, Meprospan, Meprotabs)
   (2) Phenaglycodol (Ultran)
   (3) Tybamate (Solacen)
   (b) Drugs have some effect on skeletal muscle relaxation by action on interneurons
   (c) Adverse effects—hypotension (caused by depressive effect on vasomotor centers), headache, insomnia, hypersensitivity reactions
   (2) Benzodiazepine group
   (a) Drugs
   (1) Chlordiazepoxide hydrochloride (Librium)
   (2) Clorazepate dipotassium (Tranxene)
   (3) Diazepam (Valium)
   (4) Oxazepam (Serax)
   (b) Produce significant relaxant effect on skeletal muscles by depression of

polysynaptic reflex arcs of
the spinal cord (useful
in convulsions of alcohol
withdrawal or status epi-
lepticus)
    (c) Adverse effects—hypo-
    tension incidence high
    with parenteral adminis-
    tration
(3) Nonphenothiazine compounds
(resemble antihistamines)
    (a) Drugs
        (1) Hydroxyzine hydro-
        chloride (Atarax)
        (2) Hydroxyzine pa-
        moate (Vistaril)
    (b) Adverse effects—similar
    to antihistamines and
    atropine
b. General drug interactions—potentiation of depressant effects of alcohol or sedatives
c. General adverse effects of minor
tranquilizers—drowsiness, hypotension, muscle relaxation, decreased
ability to concentrate occur frequently in initial days of therapy;
hypersensitivity reactions

Drugs that affect cerebrocortical activity

A. Anticonvulsant drugs modify bioelec-
tric activity at subcortical and cortical sites and raise the threshold response
to stimuli precipitating seizure activity
1. Grand mal seizure control
    a. Carbamazepine (Tegretol)—also
    used for psychomotor seizure con-
    trol
    b. Phenytoin (Dihycon, Di-Lan, Di-
    lantin, EKKO)—also used for psy-
    chomotor seizure control
    c. Ethotoin (Peganone)—also used
    for psychomotor seizure control
    d. Magnesium sulfate 50%
    e. Mephenytoin (Mesantoin)
    f. Mephobarbital (Mebaral)
    g. Metharbital (Gemonil)
    h. Primidone (Mysoline)—also used
    for psychomotor seizure control
2. Petit mal seizure control
    a. Ethosuximide (Zarontin)
    b. Methsuximide (Celontin)
    c. Paramethadione (Paradione)
    d. Trimethadione (Tridione)
3. Adverse effects—dizziness, drowsiness,
nausea, vomiting, skin rash; other ad-

verse effects related to the drugs
    a. The succinimides (ethosuximide,
    methsuximide, phensuximide)—
    apathy, nervousness, headache,
    blurred vision, albuminuria
    b. The barbiturates (methobarbital,
    metharbital, primidone)—head-
    ache, irritability
    c. Magnesium sulfate 50%—cardiac
    or respiratory center depression
    (calcium salts used to compete
    with drug initiated depression of
    vital centers)
    d. The oxazolidinediones (parametha-
    dione, trimethadione)—depression
    of leukocytes (swollen glands, per-
    sistent cutaneous eruptions), blur-
    ring of vision in bright light, photo-
    sensitivity
    e. The hydantoins (phenytoin, etho-
    toin, mephenytoin)—high alkalin-
    ity (pH = 12) causes tissue irri-
    tation by all routes (slow intrave-
    nous administration required to
    avoid irritation, acute respiratory
    and cardiovascular depression; oral
    drug with copious fluids), inco-
    ordination, ataxia, fine muscle
    tremor, gingivitis and hyperplasia
    of gums (caused by decreased fi-
    broblastic activity), or hirsuitism
    in adolescents on long-term ther-
    apy
4. Drug interactions
    a. Phenytoin potentiates the action of
    oral anticoagulants
    b. Phenytoin inhibits absorption of
    dietary folic acid (may precipitate
    mild megaloblastic anemia)
B. Anti-parkinsonism drugs
1. Levodopa (Dopar, L-dopa) supplies
dopamine required for norepinephrine
synthesis and maintenance of the
neurohormonal balance at subcortical,
cortical, and reticular sites that control motor function
    a. Initial therapy involves increasing
    dosage until adverse effects emerge
    or maximum dosage (8 g. per 24
    hours) is attained
    b. Adverse effects—nausea, anorexia,
    vomiting, weakness, psychic dis-
    turbances (hallucinations, emo-
    tional changes), orthostatic hypo-
    tension, hypersexuality, hypergly-
    cemia, cardiac arrhythmias

c. Drug-food interactions
(1) Production of dopamine may be suppressed during therapy by foods with high tyramine content (pickled herring, Chianti wine, natural or aged cheese, chocolate, chicken livers)
(2) Pyridoxine (vitamin B$_6$) rapidly causes decarboxylation of levodopa in peripheral tissues and vitamin preparations or foods with high pyridoxine content are avoided (dried beans, dry milk, whole grain products, salmon, tuna, pork, and beef liver or kidneys)
d. Considerations during therapy—levodopa metabolites produce false positive reactions to ketone tests done with sodium nitroprusside reagent (Acetest, Ketostix, Labstix)
2. Amantadine hydrochloride (Symmetrel)—believed to release dopamine and other catecholamines from neural storage sites, which decreases severity of symptoms and improves functional capacity (often used with levodopa or anticholinergic drugs)
a. Adverse effects—edema of ankles caused by increased vascular permeability, dizziness, irritability, tremor, slurred speech, ataxia, mental depression, lethargy, cutaneous reaction (livedo reticularis)
b. Drug interactions—potentiates action of anticholinergic drugs and levodopa unless dosage of drugs is decreased
3. Anticholinergic drugs act at central sites to inhibit cerebral motor impulses and to block efferent impulses causing rigidity of the musculature
a. Drugs
(1) Benztropine mesylate (Cogentin)
(2) Cycrimine hydrochloride (Pagitane)
(3) Ethopropazine hydrochloride (Parsidol)
(4) Procyclidine hydrochloride (Kemadrin)
(5) Trihexyphenidyl hydrochloride (Artane, Pipanol, Tremin)
b. Adverse effects—drowsiness, dry mouth, blurred vision, dizziness, nausea, central nervous system stimulation, tachycardia, headache; ethopropazine hydrochloride may also cause euphoria, hostility, paranoia, hypotension, paresthesia

Drugs that affect skeletal muscle contraction

A. Cholinesterase inhibitors—prevent enzymatic conversion of acetylcholine to acetate and choline, which allows accumulation of the neurotransmitter at the myoneural junction and higher level stimulation of muscle contraction; e.g., therapy of myasthenia gravis
1. Drugs
a. Neostigmine bromide (Prostigmine Bromide)—also used for stimulation of smooth muscle contraction in abdominal viscera (uterus, bladder)
b. Ambenonium chloride (Mytelase)
c. Pyridostigmine bromide (Mestinon)
2. Administration on an around-the-clock basis is required to maintain myoneural transmission in the patient with myasthenia gravis (extended-release forms may be used)
3. Therapy improves strength of contraction in all muscles, but a primary concern is maintenance of contractile strength of respiratory muscles to improve vital capacity
4. Adverse effects—sustained depolarization of the muscle membrane caused by the drug prevents repolarization and the patient becomes extremely weak and breathing is shallow; other problems include excess tearing, copious secretions in nose and mouth, profuse perspiration, incontinence of feces or urine
5. Drug interactions—atropine sulfate antagonizes the action of cholinesterase inhibitors and can be used for treatment of overdose
B. Skeletal muscle relaxants—act at varying levels on the multisynaptic neural pathways in the spinal cord and subcortical areas to interrupt transmission of

reflex stimuli causing hypertonicity of muscles
1. Drugs
   a. Carisoprodol (Rela, Soma)
   b. Chlormezanone (Trancopal)
   c. Chlorphenesin carbamate (Maolate)
   d. Chlorzoxazone (Paraflex)
   e. Mephenesin (Mephson, Romeph, Tolax, Tolserol)
   f. Metaxalone (Skelaxin)
   g. Methocarbamol (Robaxin)
2. Adverse effects—analgesia, lassitude, weakness of noninvolved muscle groups, drowsiness, incoordination, hepatotoxicity, dermatitis
3. Drug interactions—potentiate action of other sedatives or central nervous system depressants
4. Considerations during therapy—metabolites of chlorzoxazone color urine orange or purple-red and use of ferric chloride reagent for bile content testing shows a false positive reaction; metaxalone produces a reducing agent causing a false positive reaction for glycosuria when Benedict's reagent or Clinitest is used
C. Motor end-plate transmission inhibitors
1. Actions
   a. Interfere with acetylcholine transmission by competitively binding to the receptor sites
   b. Paralysis of muscles follows a predictable progression
     (1) Eyelids become heavy, swallowing and talking become difficult; muscle weakness in extremities, neck, trunk, spine, intercostals, diaphragm (artificial ventilation required)
     (2) Return of function follows a reverse order of the initiation pattern
2. Types of drugs
   a. Drugs causing depolarization with initial contraction and inhibiting repolarization
     (1) Decamethonium bromide (Syncurine)
     (2) Succinylcholine chloride (Anectine, Quelicin, Sucostrin)
   b. Drugs preventing depolarization by acting at the end-plate, leaving muscles in relaxed state—curariform, nondepolarizing or neuromuscular blocking drugs
     (1) Dimethyl-tubocurarine iodide (Metubine)
     (2) Dimethyl-tubocurarine chloride (Mecostrin)
     (3) Gallamine triethiodide (Flaxedil)
     (4) Pancuronium bromide (Pavulon)
     (5) Tubocurarine chloride
3. Drug interactions
   a. Hexafluorenium bromide (Mylaxen) prolongs action of succinylcholine chloride (may be administered concurrently to replace drug hydrolyzed by cholinesterase)
   b. Edrophonium chloride (Tensilon) antagonizes the effect of curariform drugs by acting as an acetylcholine substitute to displace drug from the end-plate

Drugs that produce anesthesia

A. Classic stages of anesthesia occurring with inhalant anesthetic drugs
1. Stage I—euphoria, gradual loss of consciousness
2. Stage II—hyperexcitement (thrashing of extremities), hyperactivity of reflexes (eyelids, swallowing), dilation of pupils
3. Stage III—depression of corneal reflex and pupillary response to light, voluntary control absent, muscle tone decreased
4. Stage IV—medullary paralysis, death
B. Balanced anesthesia includes use of several drugs and provides control of analgesia, consciousness, and muscle relaxation
C. Agents commonly used for inhalation anesthesia
1. Cyclopropane (Trimethylene)
2. Enflurane (Ethrane)
3. Ether (diethyl ether)
4. Ethyl chloride
5. Ethylene
6. Fluroxene (Fluoromar)
7. Halothane (Fluothane)
8. Methoxyflurane (Penthrane)
9. Nitrous oxide (Nitrogen Monoxide)
10. Trichloroethylene (Trilene)
11. Vinyl ether (Vinethene)
D. Barbiturates used as anesthetic agents (administered intravenously)

1. Action—high lipoid affinity provides prompt effect on cerebral tissue and rapid induction with ultra-short action
2. Drugs
    a. Methohexital sodium (Brevital Sodium)
    b. Thiamylal sodium (Surital Sodium)
    c. Thiopental sodium (Pentothal Sodium)
E. Nonbarbiturate used as anesthetic agents (administered intravenously or intramuscularly)
    1. Action—induces a cataleptic state (patient appears to be awake but dissociated from the environment), aborts pain response, amnesia for the procedure
    2. Drugs—ketamine hydrochloride (Ketalar, Ketaject)
F. Local anesthetics accomplish their effect primarily by decreasing the permeability of the nerve membrane to the influx of sodium ions required for depolarization of the neuron
    1. Sites of induction of local anesthetic agents include
        a. Surface (topical)
        b. Infiltration (local)—solution injected in limited area where nerve fibers have no sheath and weak solution blocks nerve endings
        c. Field block—solution injected close to nerves around area to be anesthetized
        d. Nerve block—solution injected at perineural site distant from desired anesthesia site; stronger solutions required to allow filtration through the nerve sheath
        e. Peridural (epidural, extradural, caudal)—solution is injected at a site blocking the paravertebral and peridural sections of spinal nerves controlling sensory stimuli at manipulation site
        f. Spinal (intrathecal, subarachnoid)—solution is injected into the spinal subarachnoid space to anesthetize nerve roots emerging from the spinal cord; hypobaric solutions (drug diluted with distilled water) gravitate caudad and hyperbaric solutions (drug diluted with dextrose) gravitate cephalad
    2. General adverse effects—allergic reactions, convulsions, cardiopulmonary arrest; hypotension during peridural or spinal anesthesia (drug action increases vascular capacitance by blocking tonic constrictor impulses to the veins, which allows pooling of blood in veins, reduced venous return to the heart, decreased cardiac output)
    3. Drugs
        a. Local anesthetics used topically
            (1) Benoxinate hydrochloride (Dorsacaine)
            (2) Benzocaine
            (3) Butacaine sulfate (Butyn Sulfate)
            (4) Butyl aminobenzoate picrate (Butesin Picrate)
            (5) Cocaine
            (6) Cyclomethycaine (Surfacaine)
            (7) Dibucaine (Nupercaine) also used for spinal anesthesia
            (8) Dimethisoquin hydrochloride (Quotane Hydrochloride)
            (9) Diperodon hydrochloride (Diothane Hydrochloride)
            (10) Dyclonine hydrochloride (Dyclone)
            (11) Hexylcaine hydrochloride (Cyclaine Hydrochloride) also used for nerve block
            (12) Lidocaine hydrochloride (Xylocaine) also used for nerve block
            (13) Phenacaine hydrochloride (Holocaine Hydrochloride)
            (14) Piperocaine hydrochloride (Metycaine Hydrochloride) also used for nerve block
            (15) Pramoxine hydrochloride (Tronothane Hydrochloride)
            (16) Proparacaine hydrochloride (Ophthetic, Ophthaine)
            (17) Tetracaine hydrochloride (BudOpto Anacel, Pontocaine Hydrochloride) also used for nerve block
        b. Local anesthetics used primarily for nerve block
            (1) Bupivacaine hydrochloride (Marcaine Hydrochloride)
            (2) Chloroprocaine hydrochloride (Nesacaine, Nesacaine-CE)
            (3) Mepivacaine hydrochloride (Carbocaine Hydrochloride)
            (4) Prilocaine hydrochloride (Citanest Hydrochloride)

(5) Procaine hydrochloride (Novocain)

(6) Propoxycaine hydrochloride (Blockain Hydrochloride)

Drugs that produce sedation and sleep

A. Drug action—suppresses interneuronal activity between the thalamus and the cerebral cortex to reduce motor activity and produce sleep

B. Types of drugs
1. Trichloroacetic acid—produces natural sleep
   a. Drugs
      (1) Chloral betaine (Beta-Chlor)
      (2) Chloral hydrate (Felsules, Lorinal, Noctec, Somnos)
      (3) Petrichloral (Periclor)
   b. Adverse effects—gastric irritation causing diarrhea
   c. Drug interactions—potentiates the effects of alcohol taken concurrently causing sudden loss of consciousness
   d. Considerations during therapy—drug metabolites cause false positive reaction for glycosuria when Benedict's reagent is used for testing
2. Paraldehyde primarily is used to control hyperactivity of alcoholics or to control convulsions; drug has a pungent odor and taste and elimination of drug from lungs maintains environmental odor
3. Phenothiazine derivatives (act like antihistamines) used for sleep induction in anxious patients
   a. Drugs
      (1) Methotrimeprazine hydrochloride (Levoprome)
      (2) Promazine hydrochloride (Sparine)
      (3) Propiomazine hydrochloride (Largon)
   b. Adverse effects—hypotension, dizziness, dry mouth, cardiac palpitation, pseudoparkinsonism symptoms, cholestatic jaundice, agranulocytosis
4. Barbiturate sedatives—most frequently used hypnotics
   a. Barbiturates with high lipoid tissue affinity producing rapid response
      (1) Hexobarbital (Sombucaps, Sombulex)

(2) Pentobarbital sodium (Nembutal)

(3) Secobarbital (Seconal)
   b. Barbiturates with moderate lipoid tissue affinity producing moderately slow response
      (1) Amobarbital (Amytal)
      (2) Aprobarbital (Alurate)
      (3) Butabarbital sodium (Bubartal Sodium, Butisol Sodium)
      (4) Probarbital calcium (Ipral)
      (5) Talbutal (Lotusate)
   c. Barbiturates with low lipoid tissue affinity producing slow response
      (1) Barbital (Neuronidia)
      (2) Phenobarbital (Luminal)
   d. Adverse effects—morning drowsiness, hypersensitivity reactions (photosensitivity, dermatologic reactions), respiratory depression, and hypotension (most frequent with parenteral use)
   e. Fatalities from overdosage are affected by differences in lipoid tissue affinity
      (1) High lipotropic group rapidly produces respiratory depression and marked hypotension after ingestion of excess drug
      (2) Moderate lipotropic group produces a protracted period of sedation but allows timelapse for resuscitation or reconsideration
      (3) Low lipotropic group allows excretion concurrent with slow action and is least popular for self-induced overdosage
   f. Drug interactions—barbiturates lower blood levels of orally administered griseofulvin and decrease the therapeutic effect; barbiturates increase activity of hepatic microsomal enzymes and accelerated metabolism of oral anticoagulants lowers their hypoprothrombinemic effect
5. Other sedatives and hypnotics
   a. Ethchlorvynol (Placidyl)—adverse effects include morning drowsiness, blurring vision, transient hypotension
   b. Ethinamate (Valmid)—adverse effects include morning drowsiness
   c. Flurazepam hydrochloride (Dal-

mane)—adverse effects include dizziness, tachycardia, gastrointestinal disturbances
  d. Methaqualone (Quaalude, Sopor) —adverse effects include morning drowsiness, gastrointestinal disturbances
  e. Methyprylon (Noludar)—adverse effects include morning drowsiness, gastrointestinal disturbances
  f. Sodium bromide used primarily for daytime sedation—adverse effects include gastric irritation, generalized rash, tremulousness of hands, lips, and tongue, impaired mental processes, auditory and visual hallucinations, or coma with long-term use allowing excess levels of drug
  g. Glutethimide (Doriden)
    (1) Adverse effects—morning drowsiness, transient hypotension, and infrequently produces pharyngeal and laryngeal reflex depression
    (2) Drug interactions—acts synergistically with oral anticoagulants to decrease their effectiveness
C. Excess ingestion
  1. Any of the sedative-hypnotics may cause unconsciousness, coma, death
  2. Addiction to these drugs alone or in combination has increased
  3. Removal of gastric content of drug by aspiration, resuscitative measures (assisted ventilation, cardiac massage), hemodialysis of diffusible drug, vasopressor administration to counteract vascular collapse, and correction of acidosis
  4. Follow-up supervision to avoid repetition of the problem
D. These drugs are habit-forming and withdrawal after long-term use may precipitate severe symptoms—anxiety, tremor, insomnia, confusion, perceptual distortions, agitation, delirium, gastrointestinal disturbances, orthostatic hypotension, convulsions leading to cardiovascular collapse and death

Drugs that control pain

A. Antipyretic analgesics
  1. Action unclear but involves many mechanisms
  2. Antipyretic activity—lowers hypothalamic "thermostat" and dissipates heat by vasodilation and diaphoresis
  3. Salicylates—commonly used and also have anti-inflammatory properties
    a. Drugs
      (1) Acetylsalicylic acid (A.S.A., Aspirin, Asteric, Ecotrin)
      (2) Carbaspirin calcium (Calurin)
      (3) Choline salicylate (Arthropan)
      (4) Salicylamide (Amid-Sal, Liquiprin, Rasperin, Salamide, Salicim, Salrin)
      (5) Sodium salicylate
    b. Adverse effects—gastric irritation, salicylism with long-term use (visual disturbances, tinnitus, dizziness, mental confusion, diaphoresis, nausea, vomiting, intense thirst)
    c. Drug interactions
      (1) Salicylates have an intrinsic hypoglycemic effect and require a decrease in the dosage of oral hypoglycemics for diabetics (they displace sulfonylurea hypoglycemics from protein binding sites, which causes a greater hypoglycemic effect)
      (2) Salicylates decrease absorption of indomethacin from the intestinal tract and lower its effective circulating level
      (3) Salicylates antagonize the effect of sulfinpyrazone and probenecid in reducing serum uric acid levels by inhibiting tubular secretion of uric acid
      (4) Salicylates have a hypoprothrombinemic action and potentiate effect of oral anticoagulants primarily by inhibiting platelet aggregation
  4. Nonsalicylates employed for patients with salicylate allergy, gastric ulcers, and those receiving anticoagulant therapy
    a. Drugs
      (1) Acetaminophen (Apamide, Febrolin, Fendon, Lyteca, Nebs, Tempra, Tylenol) also has muscle relaxant properties
      (2) Acetophenetidin (used as component of preparations to allow lower dosage because

higher dosage causes agranulocytosis, anemia, hepatotoxicity, methemaglobinemia)
   (3) Dipyrone (Dimethone, Narone, Nartate, Novaldin, Pydirone, Pyral, Pyrilgin)
   (4) Mefenamic acid (Ponstel) also has anti-inflammatory properties
   b. Adverse effects—vertigo, skin rash, depression of leukocyte and erthyrocyte production
B. Anti-inflammatory analgesics
   1. Salicylates may be used at high dosage levels for joint pain and for action that increases excretion of uric acid by competitive blocking of uric acid reabsorption in renal tubules (decreases deposits in joints causing pain and deformity)
   2. Indomethacin (Indocin) is used for articular pain
      a. Inhibits cellular exudates and suppresses vascular permeability to relieve joint pain
      b. Adverse effects—gastric irritation (administered with an antacid), throbbing morning headache, disturbed equilibrium, psychiatric disturbances, blood dyscrasias
   3. Colchicine (Colchin) is used for therapy of gout—onset of diarrhea terminates therapy, but articular pain usually abates prior to diarrhea onset
   4. Ibuprofen (Motrin)
   5. Oxyphenbutazone (Tandearil); phenylbutazone (Butazolidin)
      a. Adverse effects—drug action at renal tubule sites increases absorption of sodium and water (dietary sodium intake is restricted to prevent edema), gastric irritation, hypersensitivity reactions (skin rash, fever, edema), thrombocytopenia
      b. Drug interactions—drugs displace coumarin-type drugs from albumin binding sites and potentiate bleeding
C. Analgesics for minor pain control
   1. Ethoheptazine citrate (Zactane)
   2. Pentazocine hydrochloride (Talwin)
      a. Withdrawal symptoms occur when chronic users abstain
      b. Adverse effects—respiratory depression, increased cardiac rate, hypotension

3. Propoxyphene hydrochloride (Darvon)—chronic use causes constipation, drowsiness, skin rash, and psychic dependence
D. Unclassified analgesics
   1. Carbamazepine (Tegretol)
      a. Controls trigeminal neuralgia by action that decreases synaptic transmission in the nerve nucleus
      b. Has sedative, anticholinergic, and muscle relaxant properties
   2. Cobra venom extract (Cobroxin, Nyloxin)
      a. Administered parenterally for intractable pain when narcotics have only a limited effect
      b. Peak effect may take 16 weeks
      c. Protein origin may cause allergic responses
E. Addictive analgesics
   1. Action
      a. Raise the pain threshold and interfere with pain perception centers
      b. Have antitussive and sedative actions
   2. Drugs
      a. Codeine sulfate
      b. Hydromorphone hydrochloride (Dilaudid)
      c. Levorphanol tartrate (Levo-Dromoran)
      d. Meperidine hydrochloride (Demerol)
      e. Morphine sulfate
      f. Oxycodone (used in Percodan)
      g. Oxymorphone hydrochloride (Numorphan)
      h. Pantopium (Pantopon)
   3. Adverse effects—antispasmotic action on smooth muscle may decrease motility of gastrointestinal tract; euphoria, nausea, drowsiness, miosis, urine retention, hypotension with position changes, tolerance, respiratory depression
   4. Overdose of addictive analgesics—action of drugs at medullary centers causes depression of respiration (decreased depth and rate of respiratory cycles)
      a. Morphine sulfate at therapeutic dosage depresses respiration and the drug should be withheld if respirations are below 12
      b. Assisted ventilation and narcotic

antagonists required; levallorphan tartrate (Lorfan), nalorphine hydrochloride (Nalline), or naloxone hydrochloride (Narcan) compete with narcotic for receptors in respiratory center to lower threshold for carbon dioxide stimulus to respiration

5. Withdrawal of addictive drugs
   a. Early signs include uncontrollable lacrimation, rhinorrhea, diaphoresis, yawning
   b. Progression seen as violent gastrointestinal disturbances, muscle spasms, joint pain, gradual increase of metabolic activity (may be halted by use of narcotic)
6. Methadone maintenance
   a. Addiction transferred from "illegal hard drugs" to "legal hard drugs"
   b. Proved effective with long-term, hard-core addicts
   c. Program has been controversial since its inception because it is not therapeutic, but merely switches addiction

Drugs for appetite suppression (anorexiants)

A. Action
   1. Primary drugs are amphetamines or drugs with comparable action, which act at hypothalamic appetite centers to suppress desire for food
   2. Amine oxidase inhibition in cerebrocortical and reticular-activating structures provides elevated mood and increased mental acuity
B. Drugs
   1. Amphetamine sulfate (Benzedrine)
   2. Benzphetamine hydrochloride (Didrex)
   3. Chlorphentermine hydrochloride (Presate)
   4. Chlortermine hydrochloride (Voranil)
   5. Dextroamphetamine sulfate (Dexedrine)
   6. Diethylpropion hydrochloride (Tenuate, Tepanil)
   7. Fenfluramine hydrochloride (Pondimin)
   8. Mazindol (Sanorex)
   9. Methamphetamine hydrochloride (Desoxyn, Syndrox)
   10. Phendimetrazine tartrate (Plegine)
   11. Phenmetrazine hydrochloride (Preludin)
   12. Phentermine hydrochloride (Wilpo)
C. Adverse effects—constipation, blurred vision, nausea, vomiting, oral dryness, metallic taste, tenacious saliva, tachycardia, insomnia, irritability, urticaria, rebound depression
D. Drug interactions—hypertensive crisis if used by patients taking MAO inhibitors; cancels guanethidine action by displacing it from its binding site in adrenergic neuron

DRUGS THAT AFFECT THE GASTROINTESTINAL SYSTEM
Emesis control

A. Antiemetics
   1. Drugs decreasing labyrinthine excitability and the conduction of vestibular-cerebellar stimuli (motion sickness control)
      a. Cyclizine hydrochloride (Marezine Hydrochloride)
      b. Dimenhydrinate (Dramamine)
      c. Diphenidol hydrochloride (Vontrol)
      d. Hydroxyzine hydrochloride (Atarax, Vistaril)
      e. Meclizine hydrochloride (Bonine)
   2. Drugs diminishing sensitivity of the chemoreceptor trigger zone to irritants; e.g., drugs, radiation therapy
      a. Pipamazine (Mornidine)
      b. Promethazine hydrochloride (Fellozine, Ganphen, Phenergan)
      c. Pyrathiazine hydrochloride (Pyrrolazote)
      d. Thiethylperazine maleate (Torecan)
      e. Trimethobenzamide hydrochloride (Tigan)
   3. General adverse effects—drowsiness, concurrent effect on vasomotor centers causing hypotension (dizziness), dryness of oral mucosa, blurring of vision, slight incoordination, tinnitus, fatigue, headache
   4. Drug interactions—potentiate effect of central nervous system depressants
B. Emetics
   1. Drugs causing ejection of gastric contents by irritation of the stomach, which results in stimulation of medullar vomiting center

a. Black mustard
b. Cupric sulfate
2. Drugs causing emesis by direct stimulation of chemoreceptor trigger zone of the medulla; e.g., apomorphine hydrochloride
3. Drugs causing emesis by action as gastric irritants and as stimulants of the chemoreceptor trigger zone; e.g., ipecac
4. Alcohol sensitization—disulfiram therapy
   a. Disulfiram (Antabuse) used as planned abstinence program for consenting alcoholics
   b. Drug inhibits formation of liver enzymes required for alcohol degradation and acetaldehyde blood levels increase to provide the stimulus for violent vomiting, severe hypotension, extreme discomfort
   c. Adverse effects—drowsiness, easy fatigability, metallic taste in mouth, impotence, headache, skin eruptions, peripheral neuritis
   d. Drug interactions—ingestion of alcohol from any source (e.g., tinctures) precipitates vomiting sequence

Gastric antacids

Neutralize gastric hydrochloric acid
A. Coating antacids
   1. Action
      a. Provide a protective film on the stomach lining
      b. Lower gastric acid level, which allows more rapid movement of stomach contents into the duodenum
      c. Drugs containing aluminum, magnesium, and calcium have minimal absorptive tendency
   2. Drugs
      a. Aluminum carbonate gel, basic (Basaljel)
      b. Aluminum hydroxide gel (Amphojel)
      c. Aluminum hydroxide with magnesium trisilicate (Gelusil)
      d. Aluminum and magnesium hydroxides (Maalox)
      e. Aluminum phosphate gel (Phosphaljel)
      f. Calcium carbonate (Titralac)
      g. Dihydroxyaluminum aminoacetate (Robalate)

h. Magaldrate (Riopan)
i. Magnesium (carbonate, oxide, or trisilicate)
3. Adverse effects—constipation caused by combination of aluminum chloride component with phosphate ions to form insoluble complex in intestine; diarrhea caused by magnesium component of antacids
B. Noncoating antacids
   1. Sodium bicarbonate is absorbed from the intestine and high ingestion may cause alkalosis
   2. Rapid action in the stomach causes "rebound acidity" and loud eructation

Gastric motility suppressants

A. Anticholinergic drugs block acetylcholine action at gastrointestinal neuroeffector sites, which decreases production of glandular (salivary, gastric, pancreatic) secretions and digestive tract motility controlled by the parasympathetic nervous system
   1. Belladonna alkaloids and derivatives
      a. Atropine sulfate
      b. Belladonna leaf, tincture
      c. Homatropine methylbromide (Mesopin, Novatrin)
      d. Methscopolamine bromide (Lescopine, Pamine, Proscomide)
      e. Methyl atropine nitrate (Metropine)
      f. Scopolamine hydrobromide
   2. Synthetic substitutes for belladonna alkaloids
      a. Isopropamide (Darbid)
      b. Mepenzolate methyl bromide (Cantil)
      c. Methantheline bromide (Banthine)
      d. Oxyphenonium bromide (Antrenyl)
      e. Poldine methylsulfate (Nacton)
      f. Propantheline bromide (Pro-Banthine)
   3. General adverse effects—abdominal distention, constipation, urinary retention
B. Anticholinergic drugs with a direct effect on smooth muscle action caused by their local anesthetic property
   1. Drugs
      a. Dicyclomine hydrochloride (Bentyl)
      b. Methixene hydrochloride (Trest)
      c. Oxyphencyclimine hydrochloride (Daricon, Vio-Thene)

d. Thiphenamil hydrochloride (Trocinate)
2. Adverse effect—tachycardia
C. Drugs with minimal anticholinergic effect that provide smooth muscle relaxation by antispasmodic action
   1. Adiphenine hydrochloride (Trasentine)
   2. Alverine citrate (Profenil, Spacolin)
   3. Flavoxate hydrochloride (Urispas)
   4. Piperidolate hydrochloride (Dactil)
D. Acetylcholine substitution providing stimuli when major abdominal visceral hypomotility slows function
   1. Bethanechol chloride (Urecholine)—primary use is for relaxation of sphincter and increasing contraction of the urinary bladder
   2. Adverse effects—dilation of bronchi and blood vessels, bradycardia, hypermotility of the gastrointestinal tract, bladder spasm, hypersecretion of glands occurring primarily with subcutaneous injection

Antidiarrheals

A. Absorbents soak up intestinal liquid
   1. Nonabsorbable drug taken after each loose bowel movement until control is established
   2. Drugs
      a. Activated attapulgite (Claysorb, Pharmasorb)
      b. Bismuth subcarbonate
      c. Kaolin and pectin (Kaopectate)
B. Enteric bacteria replacement
   1. Used when prolonged use of antibiotics has suppressed natural bacterial flora and overgrowth of pathogenic bacteria has occurred
   2. *Lactobacillus acidophilus* and *L. bulgaricus*
      a. Enhance production of lactic acid from carbohydrates in intestinal lumen and acidity suppresses pathogenic bacterial overgrowth
      b. *L. acidophilus* is a natural commensal of the intestine
C. Motility suppressants
   1. Increase tone of intestinal musculature, ileocecal valve, and anal sphincter to slow expulsion of intestinal content, and larger amounts of water are absorbed from the intestine
   2. Drugs
      a. Diphenoxylate hydrochloride (Lomotil)

b. Tincture of opium (1% opium content)
c. Camphorated opium tincture (0.04% opium content)
3. Drug interactions—potentiation of action of central nervous system depressants

Cathartics

A. Intestinal lubricant—mineral oil
   1. Nonabsorbable oil that decreases dehydration of feces and lubricates the intestinal tract
   2. Adverse effects—anal leaking of oil with continued use
   3. Drug interactions—interferes with absorption of fat-soluble vitamins from foods and drug sources
B. Fecal softeners
   1. Act in the colon to lower surface tension of feces, which allows water and fats to penetrate feces and ease evacuation of softer stool
      a. Dioctyl calcium sulfosuccinate (Surfak)
      b. Dioctyl sodium sulfosuccinate (Colace, Doxinate)
      c. Poloxamer 188 (Pluronic F68)
   2. Increasing bulk by addition of gel to feces—increased bulk in intestinal lumen stimulates propulsive movements by pressure on mucosal lining
      a. Drugs
         (1) Methylcellulose (Cellothyl, Cologel, Hydrolose, Melozets, Methulose, Premocel, Syncelose)
         (2) Sodium carboxymethylcellulose (Bu-lax, C.M.C.)
         (3) Psyllium hydrophilic mucilloid (Metamucil, Mucilose)
      b. Considerations during therapy—full glass of fluid is required to assure that gel reaches the stomach before swelling
C. Colon irritants—stimulate peristalsis by reflex response to irritation caused by drug contacting the mucosa of the intestinal lumen
   1. Defecation stimulus in 6 to 24 hours
      a. Aloin (Alophen)
      b. Cascara sagrada (Peristaltin, Peristim)
      c. Danthron (Danivac, Dorbane)
      d. Senna (Senokot)
      e. Sennosides A and B (Glysennid)
   2. Defecation stimulus in 6 to 8 hours

　　a. Bisacodyl (Dulcolax)
　　b. Oxyphenisatin acetate (Isocrin, Lavema, Prulet)
　　c. Phenolphthalein (Phenolax)
3. Defecation stimulus in 3 hours
　　a. Castor oil (Neoloid)
　　b. Rapid action by concurrent stimulation of motor activity in small intestine
　　c. Offensive taste may be disguised by chilled fruit juice, coffee, root beer
4. General adverse effects—increased peristalsis may cause cramping until completion of evacuation; nursing infants may have diarrhea if mother takes the drug

D. Saline cathartics
1. Act by increasing the osmolality of content in the intestinal lumen; high water content moves rapidly to provide evacuation in 1 to 3 hours
2. Drugs
　　a. Magnesium citrate
　　b. Magnesium sulfate
　　c. Sodium biphosphate
　　d. Sodium phosphate
3. Considerations during therapy—drugs produce copious watery stool, propulsive flatus, sudden urge to defecate; complete evacuation of intestine may be followed by 2 to 3 days without bowel movement
4. Other drug—magnesium hydroxide (Milk of Magnesia) is frequently used for its smooth laxative effect

DRUGS THAT AFFECT THE BODY'S FLUID AND ELECTROLYTE BALANCE
Drugs that control fluid balance

A. Antidiuretic hormone (ADH) replacement
1. Vasopressin is an extract of the posterior pituitary gland hormone, pitressin
　　a. Drug effect on water conservation evidenced as concentration of urine (higher specific gravity)
　　b. Adverse effects—concurrent action on smooth muscle of vasculature causing hypertension, gastrointestinal and urinary tract smooth muscle contraction
2. Lypressin (Diapid) is a synthetic ADH substitute used as a nasal spray
　　a. Used when urinary frequency or thirst increases

　　b. Adverse effects—excessive use causes vasoconstriction
B. Aldosterone replacement
1. Action
　　a. Drugs stimulate reabsorption of sodium ions from the renal tubules and decrease glandular elimination of sodium ions (salivary, sweat, gastrointestinal glands)
　　b. Drug action restores sodium and potassium ion balance and extracellular and intracellular fluid levels, which has a positive effect on hemodynamic function, nutrient utilization, nitrogen excretion
2. Drugs
　　a. Desoxycorticosterone acetate (Doca Acetate, Percorten Acetate)
　　b. Fludrocortisone (Florinef)
3. Adverse effects—edema (excessive retention of sodium and water), hypertension, cardiac hypertrophy, hypokalemia
4. Considerations during therapy—sodium intake encouraged at a high level to lower drug requirement
C. Diuretics
1. Aldosterone activity antagonists
　　a. Action—interfere with aldosterone-induced reabsorption of sodium ions at distal nephron sites to increase sodium chloride excretion and decrease potassium ion loss (potassium-sparing)
　　b. Drugs
　　　(1) Spironolactone (Aldactone)
　　　(2) Triamterene (Dyrenium) causes gastric irritation
　　c. Adverse effects—mild headache, hyponatremia, tissue dehydration, mild acidosis resulting from decreased excretion of ammonium; long-term use causes low serum sodium ion concentrations that stimulate aldosterone secretion
　　d. Drug interactions—additive effect when used with diuretics causing sodium ion excretion
2. Carbonic anhydrase inhibitors (sulfonamide diuretics)
　　a. Action
　　　(1) Prevent carbonic anhydrase hydration of carbon dioxide and dehydration of carbonic acid that maintains acid-base ratio of circulating fluids by

exchange of hydrogen and sodium ions to allow formation of bicarbonate in tubules

(2) Elevated tubule sodium content holds water and promotes diuresis

b. Drugs
  (1) Acetazolamide (Diamox)
  (2) Dichlorphenamide (Daranide, Oratrol)
  (3) Ethoxzolamide (Cardrase, Ethamide)
  (4) Methazolamide (Neptazane)
c. Adverse effects—hypokalemia resulting from elevated sodium ion content of tubule urine at distal nephron, which raises exchange rate of potassium ions; fever; skin rash; depression of bone marrow, crystalluria and renal calculi may occur with long-term use; gastrointestinal disturbances; paresthesia in face and extremities

3. Sodium transport inhibitors
  a. Action
    (1) Mercurial diuretics block sulfhydryl-containing enzymes that control tubule transport systems for sodium ions in the nephron by release of mercurial ions in tubule cells
    (2) Act chiefly at proximal and distal tubule sites for active transport and the action also affects passive transport of chloride and water
  b. Drug—mercaptomerin sodium (Diucardin, Thiomerin)
  c. Adverse effects—hypokalemic alkalosis caused by potassium and hydrogen ion exchange for sodium ions at collecting tubules, which increases output of K^+ and H^+ with prolonged therapy; destruction of tubule cells with excess use, hypersensitivity reactions (pruritus, skin rash, gastrointestinal disturbances, stomatitis, vertigo, headache)

4. Thiazides and drugs with similar action
  a. Action
    (1) Wide use includes therapy of hypertension to decrease circulating blood volume, counteract sodium-retaining effects of antihypertensives, and im-

prove blood flow from capillaries

(2) Interfere with sodium ion transport at ascending limb of Henle's loop and inhibit carbonic anhydrase activity at distal tubule sites

b. Drugs
  (1) Bendroflumethiazide (Benuron, Naturetin)
  (2) Benzthiazide (Aquatag, Exna)
  (3) Chlorothiazide (Diuril)
  (4) Chlorthalidone (Hygroton)
  (5) Hydrochlorothiazide (Esidrix, Hydro-Diuril, Oretic)
  (6) Methyclothiazide (Enduron)
  (7) Quinethazone (Hydromox)
  (8) Trichlormethiazide (Methahydrin, Naqua)
c. Adverse effects—hypokalemia caused by rapid exchange of potassium ions for sodium ions at collecting tubules; initial diuresis may cause weakness, fatigue, dizziness; drug-induced hyperglycemia may convert prediabetic to diabetic state; gastrointestinal irritation, dizziness, vertigo, paresthesia, headache, skin rash, urticaria; long-term therapy may induce symptoms of gout secondary to increased uric acid reabsorption and asymptomatic hyperuricemia

5. Dual action sites providing potent diuresis
  a. Action
    (1) Interfere with active transport of sodium ions in ascending limb of Henle's loop
    (2) Action at proximal tubule sites inhibits sodium chloride and water reabsorption
  b. Drugs
    (1) Ethacrynic acid (Edecrin)
    (2) Furosemide (Lasix)
    (3) Metolazone (Zaroxolyn)
  c. Adverse effects—hypokalemia and alkalosis (drugs exchange sodium ions at collecting tubules causing K^+ and H^+ loss), hyperuricemia with long-term oral use, elevated blood urea nitrogen, ototoxicity (rare)

6. Increase renal blood flow
  a. Action
    (1) Theophyllines (xanthines)

have a direct stimulatory effect on the myocardium that increases cardiac output and increased blood flow accelerates glomerular filtration rate

(2) Direct action on renal afferent arterioles increases the excretion rate of sodium and chloride ions

b. Drugs
(1) Theophylline-calcium salicylate (Phyllicin)
(2) Theobromine calcium salicylate (Theocalcin)

c. Adverse effects—dizziness, syncope, palpitation, hypotension

d. Drug interactions—salicylate component and oral anticoagulants act at similar sites in hepatic coagulation process that affects prothrombin level control

7. Osmotics
a. Action
(1) Act by increasing osmolality of plasma that causes osmotic movement of fluid from tissues to intravascular bed
(2) Transient expansion of plasma volume reversed by renal excretion of excess fluid

b. Drugs
(1) Dextrose 50%—increases fluid output by action in tubules; short duration of action because drug is actively reabsorbed in proximal tubule
(2) Glycerine 50% (Glyrol, Ophthalgan, Osmoglyn)—may cause vomiting and headache, which may be relieved by lying down after ingestion
(3) Mannitol (Osmitrol)—increases osmotic pressure of glomerular filtrate and tubule content and a large amount of dilute urine is excreted; may cause changes in hydration of cerebral centers that may cause nausea, vomiting, transient headache, thirst
(4) Sterile urea (Ureaphil, Urevert)—acts by elevation of the osmotic pressure of glomerular filtrate; may cause hyponatremia, hypokalemia

(lethargy and muscle weakness), tissue dehydration

Electrolyte deficits caused by diuretics

A. Potassium ion deficit
1. Shift of sodium ions to intracellular content occurs when potassium ions are lowered; the shift of cation leads to hyperpolarization of membrane fibers causing lethargy, muscle paralysis
2. Potassium ion replacement
a. Foods with high potassium content; e.g., meats, bananas, raisins, citrus fruits, melons
b. Drugs
(1) Potassium gluconate (Kaon)
(2) Randall's solution (Potassium Triplex)
(3) Potassium chloride (K-Lyte, Kay Ciel)

B. Sodium ion deficit
1. Persistent diaphoresis (fever, hot environment) during diuretic therapy may deplete sodium excessively
2. Patient's self-induced restriction of sodium intake below prescribed levels may cause hyponatremia
3. Excess sodium ion depletion has a cancellation effect on diuretics dependent on inhibition of sodium transport in the nephron; absence of sodium ions allows reabsorption of water to proceed and edema may persist; therapy includes hypertonic sodium chloride with water restriction to reinstitute effective diuresis
4. Problems evident as weakness, nausea, dryness of mouth, drowsiness, asthenia, leg cramps related to decreased isotonicity and electrodynamic activity

Drugs that control elevated metabolic product levels

A. Removal of excess potassium ions from serum
1. Hypertonic glucose and insulin rapidly move potassium into cells and lower serum levels; this may occur when inadvertent rapid infusion of KCl causes transient hyperkalemia
2. Sodium polystyrene sulfonate (Kayexalate)
a. Cation exchange resin acting in intact intestinal lumen by liberation

of sodium ions in exchange for potassium ions to form a new resin (moves 50 mEq. K$^+$/hour)

b. Oral administration with sorbital, a sugar, to improve palatability and act as osmotic cathartic

c. Adverse effects—hypokalemia, anorexia, nausea, prolonged use depletes calcium, magnesium ions

B. Drugs removing urea by blocking urate reabsorption in renal tubules (uricosuric agents)

1. High level of urate elimination (700 mg./24 hours) lowers serum urea levels and moves urea from tophaceous deposits

2. Drugs
   a. Probenecid (Benemid)
   b. Sulfinpyrazone (Anturane)

3. Adverse effects—hypersensitivity reactions, headache, gastrointestinal disturbances

4. Drug interactions—the action of salicylates that compete for the same renal tubule transport sites for elimination antagonizes the uricosuric effect

5. Considerations during therapy—high fluid intake required to avoid precipitation of crystals in nephrons; metabolites of the drugs cause a false positive glucose reaction with Benedict's test and Clinitest

C. Drugs removing urea by providing alternate excretory pathways

1. Allopurinol (Zyloprim)
   a. Acts as a substrate for xanthine oxidase and converts purines to more soluble oxypurinol
   b. Decreases hyperuricemia and tophaceous deposits in joints

2. Adverse effects—hypersensitivity reactions, pruritic skin rash, fever, gastrointestinal disturbances, malaise

3. Considerations during therapy—high fluid intake required to provide solvent for xanthine, hypoxathine, uric acid in nephrons

D. Drugs removing ammonia from circulating fluids

1. Action—increase hepatic conversion of ammonia to urea

2. Drugs
   a. Arginine glutamate (Modumate)
   b. Arginine hydrochloride (R-Gene)

3. Adverse effects—transient nausea,

blushing, salivation, increased respiratory depth

E. Drugs removing bile salts from tissues

1. Cholestyramine resin (Cuemid, Questran)—acts as an anion exchange resin in the intestinal lumen to remove bile acids (raises elimination of bile acids to 10 times normal level)

2. Adverse effects—nausea, heartburn, diarrhea

3. Drug-food interaction—interferes with absorption of fat-soluble vitamins in food or drugs; resin may bind acids or absorb neutral drugs (digoxin, levothyroxine sodium, liothyronine sodium, warfarin, phenylbutazone, thiazide diuretics) and decrease absorption from intestine (resin administered 1 hour after other drugs)

4. Considerations during therapy—unpleasant odor disguised by fruit juices, pulpy or pureed fruits, thin soups

F. Drugs removing localized collections of fluid from tissues

1. Alpha amylase (Buclamase, Fortizyme)—carbohydrase used for control of inflammatory, edematous problems around traumatized joints

2. Adenosine phosphate (Cardiomone, My-B-Den)—decreases edema, erythema, dermatitis, pruritus at site of venous ulcers by vasodilating action

G. Enzymes removing intravascular clots (proteolytic enzymes)

1. Used systemically to degrade the fibrin network and trapped cells forming the clots to make a pathway for blood flow; topically in cavities to remove necrotic tissue and exudate

2. Drugs
   a. Tromelains (Ananase)
   b. Chymotrypsin (Chymar, Cytolav, Enzeon)
   c. Fibrinolysin (Actase, Thrombolysin)
   d. Papain (Papase)
   e. Streptokinase
   f. Trypsin crystallized (Parenzyme, Tryptar)
   g. Urokinase

3. Adverse effects—hypersensitivity reactions, pain at injection site, dizziness, headache, nausea, hypotension; intravenous administration of fibrinolysin causes high incidence of adverse effects and febrile reactions

Drugs that control calcium ion balance
A. Intestinal absorption inhibitor
   1. Sodium phytate (Rencal)
   2. Acts as cation exchange agent in intestinal lumen
   3. Used in hyperparathyroidism
B. Intestinal absorption enhancer (vitamin D replacement)
   1. Calciferol (Drisdol)
   2. Used in vitamin D replacement therapy
C. Calcium ion replacement
   1. Calcium gluconate
   2. Calcium lactate
   3. Dibasic calcium phosphate
D. Osteoclastic activity control (parathyroid hormone substitution)—parathyroid hormone for replacement

DRUGS THAT AFFECT THE BODY'S HORMONAL BALANCE
Drugs that affect glucose assimilation

A. Insulin replacement for natural hormone
   1. Types of insulin (Table 6-1)
   2. Administration consideration
      a. All forms of insulin are administered subcutaneously
      b. Only regular insulin can be used for intravenous administration
      c. Some insulin preparations can be combined in the same syringe with the physician's approval
      d. When mixing insulins, the regular insulin should be drawn into the syringe first
      e. Sites of administration should be rotated

   3. Adverse effects—insulin excess (internal sources of glucagon may delay the onset of insulin shock symptoms by liberation of glucose from hepatic storage sites), irritability, mental confusion, disorientation, convulsions, unconsciousness, tremor, tachycardia, weakness, pallor, cold and moist skin surface, headache, hunger
   4. Drug interactions—hypoglycemic effects of insulin antagonized by growth hormone, corticotropin, glucocorticoids, thyroid hormone, glucagon, epinephrine
B. Oral hypoglycemic drugs
   1. Drugs that stimulate pancreatic beta cells to produce insulin in adults with residual functioning cells (sulfonylurea group)
      a. Acetohexamide (Dymelor)
      b. Chlorpropamide (Diabinese)
      c. Tolazamide (Tolinase)
      d. Tolbutamide (Orinase)
   2. Drugs that facilitate utilization of endogenous insulin at cell level—phenformin hydrochloride (DBI, Meltrol)
   3. General adverse effects—hypersensitivity reactions (sulfonylurea group causes skin eruptions), jaundice, pruritus, headache, weakness, paresthesia
   4. Drug interactions—tolbutamide decreases tolerance to alcohol; thiazides, corticoids interfere with hypoglycemic action; sulfaphenazole, phenylbutazone, MAO inhibitors enhance hypoglycemic activity of oral hypoglycemics

Table 6-1. Types of insulin

Insulin	Onset	Peak	Duration
Rapid acting			
Insulin injection (regular insulin)	½ to 1 hr.	2 to 6 hrs.	5 to 8 hrs.
Prompt insulin zinc suspension (Semilente)	½ to 1 hr.	3 to 9 hrs.	12 to 16 hrs.
Intermediate acting			
Globin zinc insulin injection	1 to 4 hrs.	6 to 16 hrs.	16 to 24 hrs.
Insulin zinc suspension (Lente)	1 to 4 hrs.	7 to 12 hrs.	24 to 30 hrs.
Isophane insulin suspension (NPH)	1 to 2 hrs.	7 to 12 hrs.	24 to 30 hrs.
Long acting			
Extended insulin zinc suspension (Ultralente)	4 to 8 hrs.	10 to 30 hrs.	34 to 46 hrs.
Protamine zinc insulin suspension (PZI)	1 to 8 hrs.	12 to 24 hrs.	30 to 36 hrs.

Drugs that control the thyroid hormone

A. Drugs inhibiting oxidation of iodides to prevent their combination with tyrosine in formation of thyroxine
   1. Drugs
      a. Methylthiouracil (Methiocil, Muracil)
      b. Propylthiouracil
      c. Methimazole (Tapazole)
   2. Adverse effects—hypothyroidism in fetus, allergic reactions (skin rash, urticaria), agranulocytosis
B. Thyroid hormone activity enhancers
   1. Thyrotropin (Thytropar) provides hormone when pituitary production is deficient
   2. Protirelin (Thypinone) is a thyrotropin-releasing hormone (synthetic prohormone)
C. Hormone substitutes
   1. Action—cause suppression of feedback production by pituitary
   2. Drugs
      a. Levothyroxine sodium (Letter, Levoid, Synthroid, Titroid)
      b. Liothyronine sodium (Cytomel)
      c. Thyroglobulin (Endothyrin, Proloid)
      d. Thyroid (Thyrar)
   3. Adverse effects—physical hyperactivity, accelerated metabolism
D. Precursor for thyroid hormone formation
   1. Strong iodine solution (Lugol's solution)
   2. Adverse effects—hypersensitivity reactions (swelling and hypersecretion of glands, laryngeal edema)

Drugs that affect gonadal function and fertility

A. Androgens are used to replace deficient hormones in males postpuberty and preclimacteric to improve development of secondary sex characteristics or as single-incident therapy controlling lactogenic activity in the nonnursing mother
   1. Drugs
      a. Fluoxymesterone (Halotestin, Ora-Testryl, Ultandren)
      b. Methyltestosterone (Metandren, Neo-Hombreol-M, Oreton-M)
      c. Testosterone (Androlan, Andronaq, Hormale Aqueous, Malogen, Neo-Hombreol-F, Oreton, Sterotate)
      d. Testosterone cypionate (Depo-Testosterone, Durandro, Malogen CYP, T-Ionate-P.A.)
      e. Testosterone enanthate (Delatestryl, Malogen LA, Repo-Test, Testate, Testostroval-P.A.)
      f. Testosterone propionate (Hormale Oil, Neo-Hombreol, Oreton Propionate, Testonate)
   2. Adverse effects—adolescent males may have premature epiphyseal closure (decreased skeletal development, height stops increasing)
B. Estrogens primarily used to replace deficient hormones to control hormonal balance in menopausal or postmenopausal women or to maintain menses and fertility in females during reproductive years
   1. Drugs
      a. Chlorotrianisene (Tace)
      b. Conjugated estrogens (Conestron, Conjutab, Equgen, Menotabs, Premarin, Theogen)
      c. Dienestrol (DV, Synestrol)
      d. Diethylstilbestrol (DES)
      e. Esterified estrogens (Amnestrogen, Estrifol, Evex, Femogen, Glyestrin, Menest, SK-Estrogens, Trocosone, Zeste)
      f. Estradiol (Aquadiol, Progynon)
      g. Estrone (Estrusol, Menformon [A], Theelin, Wynestron)
      h. Ethinyl estradiol (Estinyl, Feminone, Lynoral, Palonyl)
      i. Hexestrol
      j. Methallenestril (Vallestril)
      k. Promethestrol dipropionate (Meprane Dipropionate)
   2. Adverse effects—anorexia, nausea, vomiting, tissue fluid accumulation
C. Progestogen replacement provides the stimulus for desquamation of the uterine lining required for completion of the menstrual cycle or for maintenance of the uterine lining during pregnancy
   1. Drugs
      a. Dydrogesterone (Duphaston, Gynorest)
      b. Ethisterone
      c. Hydroxyprogesterone caproate (Delalutin)
      d. Medroxyprogesterone acetate (Depo-Provera, Provera)
      e. Norethindrone (Norlutin)
      f. Norethindrone acetate (Norlutate)

g. Progesterone (Gesterol, Lipo-Lutin, Proluton)

2. Adverse effects—initial use causes profuse vaginal flow (shedding of accumulations of endometrial tissue), spotting, irregular bleeding, nausea, lethargy, jaundice

D. Conception inhibition

1. Fixed combination program provides the estrogen component of the combination tablet to suppress secretion of FSH and the progestogen inhibits midcycle release of LH from the pituitary when tablets are taken from the fifth to the twenty-fifth day and a placebo tablet is taken the remaining 7 days

a. Ethinyl estradiol–ethynodiol diacetate (Demulen)

b. Ethinyl estradiol–norethindrone acetate (Norlestrin)

c. Ethinyl estradiol–norgestrel (Ovral)

d. Mestranol–ethynodiol diacetate (Ovulen)

e. Mestranol–norethindrone (Norinyl, Ortho-Novum)

f. Mestranol-norethynodrel (Enovid)

2. Sequential program provides estrogen for 14 to 16 days (fifth to eighteenth or twentieth day) and a combination of estrogen and progestogen is used for 6 days in a plan that provides estrogen for control of ovulation and progestogen to induce endometrial shedding

a. Ethinyl estradiol–dimethisterone (Oracon)

b. Mestranol-norethindrone (Norquen, Ortho-Novum SQ)

3. Adverse effects—thrombophlebitis; during the first 4 months—headache, nausea, vomiting, breast fullness, depression, fatigue, brownish facial pigmentation, fluid retention, intermenstrual spotting

E. Abortion induction

1. Estrogen in high dosage after ovulation disrupts the estrogen-progesterone balance that usually maintains the dense endometrial nutrient bed for fertilized ova

2. Saline instillation produces a mascerated fetus

3. Dinoprost tromethamine (Prostin F_2 Alpha)

a. Action—used during second trimester to trigger vasoconstriction and uterine contractions that interfere with endocrine function of placenta

b. Adverse effects—nausea, vomiting, diarrhea, pain at extrauterine sites, allergic reactions (not administered to patients with history of asthma)

F. Conception enhancers

1. Menotropins (Pergonal) stimulates growth and maturation of ovarian follicles in women with deficient ovum production by creating an effect on ovarian follicles comparable to that of natural FSH and LH

2. Chorionic gonadotropin (A.P.L., Almetropin, Antuitrin-S, Chorex, Chorigon, Follutein, Glucotropin-Forte, Khorion, Libigen, Luton, Pregnyl, Riogon, Stemultrolin)

a. Administered concurrently to support LH effect on ovulation when follicle maturation has occurred

b. Adverse effects—20% of patients have multiple births

3. Clomiphene citrate (Clomid)

a. Used during the fifth to the tenth day of the menstrual cycle to stimulate release of FSH and LH in anovulatory women

b. Adverse effects—multiple births, visual changes, dizziness, lightheadedness

G. Induction and control of uterine contractions

1. Oxytocin (Pitocin, Syntocinon, Uteracon)

a. Used to induce labor by stimulation of characteristic rhythmic contraction and relaxation of uterine muscles

b. Administered I.M. after delivery of the anterior shoulder or I.V. after delivery of the baby to provide uterine contractions that complete expulsion of uterine contents and decrease bleeding from endometrial sites

2. Sparteine sulfate (Spartocin, Tocosamine)

a. Used to stimulate uterine muscle contraction when inertia occurs during labor

b. Adverse effects—lengthens refractory period of cardiac muscle and may cause bradycardia

H. Drugs promoting involution of the uterus in the puerperium
1. Ergonovine maleate (Ergotrate Maleate)
2. Methylergonovine maleate (Methergine)
3. Maintain the uterus in slightly contracted state that controls bleeding from intrauterine sites and maintains tone, rate, and amplitude of rhythmic contractions required for involution of the uterus

Anabolic steroids (androgens)

A. Action related to inducing retention of nitrogen, potassium, and phosphorus required for tissue building; drug action is dependent on availability of carbohydrates and proteins
B. Drugs
1. Ethylestrenol (Maxibolin)
2. Methandriol (Androdiol, Diolandrone, Dostene, Methostan, Nabadial, Neostene, Stenediol)
3. Methandrostenolone (Dianabol)
4. Nandrolone decanoate (Deca-Durabolin)
5. Oxandrolone (Anavar)
6. Oxymetholone (Adroyd, Anadrol)
7. Stanozolol (Winstrol)
C. Adverse effects—bone maturation may proceed faster than linear bone growth in children; women may have irreversible deepening of the voice or hirsutism, clitoral enlargement that may be reversible, acne, stimulation of libido, menstrual irregularities, sodium and water retention; prepuberty males have growth of pubic hair, phallic enlargement, and increased frequency of erections

Pituitary hormone

A. Used when the adrenal gland is functioning normally for hormonal stimulation of glucocorticoid production in control of inflammation, immune response
B. Used when pituitary function is deficient to replace natural hormone
C. Corticotropin (Actest, Acthar, Cortigel, Cortrophin, Cortrophin Zinc) stimulates adrenal release of aldosterone, cortisol, androgen at an accelerated rate
1. Negative feedback lowers endogenous production of pituitary hormone when circulating glucocorticoid level is elevated
2. Adverse effects—increased liberation of mineralocorticoid (aldosterone) may cause electrolyte disturbances as a result of sodium ion retention and potassium ion losses, excess androgen release results in signs of masculinization in women (hirsutism, acne, amenorrhea), acute allergic reactions

Glucocorticoids

A. May be used in physiologic dosage to correct deficiency of the hormone
B. Most frequently used to produce high plasma levels of hormone for suppression of inflammation and immune responses by interfering with the physiologic factors that promote and maintain sequestration of fluid and irritants in tissues; e.g., allergy and collagen disorders
1. Stabilizes lysosome membranes, which decreases spilling of tissue enzymes that propagate inflammation
2. Suppresses antibody production after an initial brief increase in antibody release and the process may mask signs of infection
3. Protein catabolism and gluconeogenesis increase available nutrients for tissue needs
C. The plasma level of glucocorticoids is raised after administration, which decreases ACTH and glucocorticoid production
1. Inactivity of adrenals necessitates maintenance of uninterrupted administration schedule
2. Gradual decrease in dosage is planned as therapy terminates to allow return of adrenal cortical function
D. Some effect on target tissues within 24 to 48 hours with feeling of well-being, improvement in appetite, and weight gain
E. Drugs possessing variable amounts of mineralocorticoid activity
1. Cortisone acetate (Cortone Acetate)
2. Hydrocortisone (Cortef, Hydrocortone)
3. Prednisolone (Delta-Cortef, Hydeltrasol, Meticortelone, Sterane)
4. Prednisone (Delta-Dome, Deltasone, Deltra, Meticorten, Paracort, Servisone)
F. Drugs with negligible mineralocorticoid activity

Betamethasone (Celestone)
Dexamethasone (Decadron, Deronil, Dexameth, Hexadrol, Gammacorten)
3. Fluprednisolone (Alphadrol)
4. Meprednisone (Betapar)
5. Methylprednisolone (Medrol)
6. Paramethasone acetate (Haldrone, Stemex)
7. Triamcinolone (Aristocort, Kenacort)
G. Adverse effects
1. Catabolic effect on muscle protein and bone matrix weakens musculoskeletal structures (osteoporosis, muscle wasting, weakness)
2. Glucose mobilization burdens pancreatic production of insulin causing lability in diabetics and precipitation of symptoms in prediabetics
3. Glyconeogenesis increases deposition of lipids in mandibular tissues (moon-face), cervicothoracic and abdominal tissue
4. Atrophy of lymphoid tissue lowers normal defense mechanisms controlling pathogens and infections occur without usual warning signs
5. Gastric hyperacidity increases ulcer incidence
6. Central nervous system stimulation may progress to euphoria, psychosis, insomnia
7. Sudden withdrawal after long-term use causes weakness, abdominal pain, circulatory collapse, nausea, vomiting

ANTINEOPLASTIC DRUGS
General information
A. Drugs act primarily by action on malignant cells during reproduction of proteins
B. One drug or a combination of drugs may be used to increase specificity of action and decrease drug tolerance
C. Administration routes delivering drug to involved organs
1. Isolation or regional perfusion that requires extracorporeal perfusion
2. Intra-arterial infusion at organ site that allows uptake of drug before it enters the venous route
3. Intracavity instillation
D. Antineoplastic drugs have a low therapeutic index (T.I.) and evidence of cytotoxic effects occur in normal tissues
E. General adverse effects—anorexia, nausea, vomiting, lassitude, hyperuricemia

(caused by rapid breakdown of tumor tissue), epithelial tissue lesions (stomatitis, abdominal cramps, diarrhea), bone marrow depression (bleeding, infections), alopecia

Types of drugs
A. Sex hormones—change hormonal balance and slow growth rate of certain tumors; e.g., estrogen to males with prostatic cancer
1. Estrogens—used in treatment of postmenopausal patients with metastatic breast cancer or males with cancer of the prostate
a. Drugs
(1) Conjugated estrogens (Premarin)
(2) Diethylstilbestrol
(3) Esterified estrogens (Amnestrogen, Menest, SK-Estrogens)
(4) Ethinyl estradiol (Estinyl, Feminone, Lynoral, Novestrol)
b. Adverse effects—females have edema, nausea, anorexia, changes in libido, breast tenderness, abdominal cramps, dizziness, irritability, pigmentation of nipples and areola, uterine bleeding, stress incontinence; males have gynecomastia, impotence
2. Androgens—used in treatment of postmenopausal patients with disseminated tumor cells from breast cancer
a. Drugs
(1) Calusterone (Methosarb)
(2) Dromostanolone propionate (Drolban)
(3) Fluoxymesterone (Halotestin, Ora-Testryl, Ultandren)
(4) Testolactone (Teslac)
(5) Testosterone (Neo-Hombreol-F, Oreton)
b. Adverse effects—virilism (enlargement of clitoris, hirsutism), edema, erythrocythemia; virilism seldom occurs with testolactone because it is hormonally inert
3. Progestogens—used for metastatic and recurrent endometrial carcinoma
a. Drugs
(1) Hydroxyprogesterone (Delalutin)
(2) Medroxyprogesterone (Depo-Provera, Provera)

(3) Megestrol acetate (Megace)
    b. Adverse effects—emergence of characteristics of opposite sex
B. Antimetabolites—interfere with production of purine precursors (guanine, adenine) required for DNA or RNA synthesis; pyrimidine precursors (cytosine, thymine) required for DNA synthesis or the precursors (cytosine, uracil) required for RNA synthesis; or the folic acid conversion required for DNA or RNA protein construction
  1. Purine antagonist (adenine analog)
    a. Azathioprine (Imuran) action as sulfhydryl enzyme inhibitor makes it useful as immunosuppressive drug
    b. Mercaptopurine (Purinethol)
  2. Purine antagonist (guanine analog)—Thioguanine
  3. Pyrimidine antagonist (thymine analog)
    a. Fluorouracil (also uracil analog)
    b. Floxuridine (also uracil analog)
    c. Hydroxyurea (Hydrea)
  4. Pyrimidine antagonist (cytosine analog)—Cytarabine (Cytosar)
  5. Folic acid antagonist—methotrexate
C. Alkylating agents—cause chromatin disruptive effects similar to X rays by transferring their side chains to molecules in the cell and reacting selectively with phosphate groups of DNA
  1. Drugs
    a. Busulfan (Myleran)
    b. Carmustine
    c. Chlorambucil (Leukeran)
    d. Cyclophosphamide (Cytoxan, Endoxan)
    e. Mechlorethamine hydrochloride (Caryolysine, Mustargen)
    f. Melphalan (Alkeran)
    g. Pipobroman (Vercyte)
    h. Thio-tepa (Thio-TEPA)
    i. Triethylenemelamine
    j. Uracil mustard
  2. Adverse effects—stimulation of vomiting centers causes persistent vomiting; powerful central nervous system stimulant causes ataxia, intermittent convulsions; toxic metabolites in bladder cause hemorrhagic cystitis requiring an increased fluid intake
D. Plant alkaloids—disorganize the mitotic spindle to decrease cell reproduction
  1. Drugs

    a. Vinblastine sulfate (Velban) crosses blood-brain barrier
    b. Vincristine sulfate (Oncovin)
  2. Adverse effects—constipation, diarrhea, peripheral neuropathy (central neuropathy highest with vinblastine sulfate), ataxia, muscle weakness, paresthesia (tingling, numbness, tremor of extremities); problems common to other antineoplastics such as gastrointestinal tract symptoms, cutaneous lesions, and suppression of bone marrow are infrequent with these drugs
E. Antibiotics—act by binding to DNA to slow RNA production and interfere with cell building (these drugs are highly toxic and are not useful as anti-infectives)
  1. Dactinomycin (Cosmegen)
  2. Daunomycin
  3. Mithramycin (Mithracin)
  4. Mitomycin (Mutamycin)
  5. Forms with high incidence of adverse effect on heart and lung tissue
    a. Daunorubicin
    b. Adriamycin
    c. Bleomycin sulfate (Blenoxane)
F. Radioactive agents
  1. Gold (^{198}Au) used for pleural effusions and ascites secondary to cancer
  2. Sodium iodide (^{131}I) avidly taken up by thyroid cells
  3. Sodium phosphate (^{32}P) reduces the erythrocyte count; e.g., in polycythemia vera
G. Other drugs
  1. L-asparaginase enzymatically hydrolyzes 1-asparagine and deprives leukemic cells of the amino acid required for cell building
  2. Mitotane (Lysodren) acts on malignant cell in the adrenal cortex to suppress functional and nonfunctional tissue to decrease excess glucocorticoids
  3. Procarbazine hydrochloride (Matulane) interferes with amino acid synthesis in cells; may cause central and peripheral neuropathy (behavioral changes, changes in sleep patterns, peripheral nerve dysfunction)

DRUGS THAT CHELATE HEAVY METALS

A. Action—drugs form a chemical union with metals by mutual sharing of valence forces to form inactive water-soluble complexes with little ionizing potential

B. Drugs
1. Disodium edetate (Endrate)
   a. Chelation of calcium removes the ions from serum, deposits, nodules
   b. One gram of drug chelates 120 mg. calcium ions
   c. Adverse effects—hypocalcemia-induced cardiopulmonary arrest or convulsions, hypotension, nausea, diarrhea, skin rash in facial area
2. Calcium disodium edetate (Calcium Disodium Versenate)
   a. Chief use is for chelation of lead, but also acts on cadmium, chromium, copper, iron, manganese, nickel, zinc
   b. Urine lead content monitored; peak excretion in 24 to 48 hours
   c. Adverse effects—acute tubule necrosis, malaise, fatigue, numbness of extremities, gastrointestinal disturbances, fever, pain in muscles and joints
3. Deferoxamine mesylate (Desferal)
   a. Chelates iron
   b. Renal excretion of chelate (ferrioxamine) causes reddish coloring of urine
   c. Adverse effects—pain at injection site, skin rash, blurred vision, abdominal pain, leg cramps, tachycardia, fever; long-term use causes allergic reactions
4. Penicillamine (Cuprimine)
   a. Chelates copper, iron, mercury, lead
   b. Chief use is for copper chelation in Wilson's disease (hereditary defect in copper metabolism causing copper accumulation in liver, brain)
   c. Adverse effects—hypersensitivity reactions, leukopenia, thrombocytopenia, hyperpyrexia (caused by depletion of copper in thalamic temperature control center)
5. Dimercaprol (BAL)
   a. Chleates arsenic, mercury, gold, copper, lead
   b. Adverse effects—local pain at site of injection; may cause persistent fever in children receiving therapy; rise in blood pressure accompanied by tachycardia following injection

DRUGS THAT CONTROL ALLERGIC AND INFLAMMATORY RESPONSES

A. Antihistamines
1. Actions
   a. Interfere with histaminic action by competing for extravascular receptors at arteriole sites
   b. Block histamine-induced irritation of nerve endings causing itching or burning, dilation of arterioles, and constriction of venules causing transudation of fluid into tissues
   c. Prevent progression but has no effect on existing problems
   d. Also have antiemetic, anticholinergic, and central nervous system depressant effect
2. Drugs
   a. Ethanolamine derivatives are the most potent and highly sedating drugs
      (1) Carbinoxamine maleate (Clistin)
      (2) Diphenhydramine hydrochloride (Benadryl)
      (3) Doxylamine succinate (Decapryn)
   b. Ethylenediamine derivatives have intermediate sedative effects (sometimes cause excitement and mild to moderate dizziness is common)
      (1) Chlorothen citrate (Tagathen)
      (2) Methapyrilene hydrochloride (Histadyl)
      (3) Pyrilamine maleate
      (4) Tripelennamine citrate (Pyribenzamine Citrate)
   c. Phenothiazine derivatives are highly sedating
      (1) Cyproheptadine hydrochloride (Periactin Hydrochloride)
      (2) Methdilazine hydrochloride (Tacaryl)
      (3) Trimeprazine tartrate (Temaril)
   d. Propylamine derivatives have a low sedative effect
      (1) Brompheniramine maleate (Dimetane)
      (2) Chlorpheniramine maleate (Chlor-Trimeton, Histaspan, Teldrin)
      (3) Dexbrompheniramine maleate (Disomer)
      (4) Dexchlorpheniramine maleate (Polarmine)

(5) Dimethindene maleate (Forhistal Maleate, Triten)

(6) Pheniramine maleate (Trimeton)

(7) Pyrrobutamine phosphate (Co-Pyronil)

(8) Triprolidine hydrochloride (Actidil)

3. General adverse effects—inability to concentrate, ataxia, excitation, irritability, palpitation, insomnia, tremors, nervousness (anticholinergic predominance symptoms frequently occurring in children or elderly), headache, hypotension, dryness of mouth, nausea, vomiting, anorexia, diarrhea, or constipation

4. Drug interactions—potentiation of central nervous system depressant effects of alcohol, sedatives, hypnotics

B. Glucocorticoids are used as anti-inflammatory agents (see pp. 239-240)

C. Other drugs that have an anti-inflammatory effect (see pp. 243-248)

DRUGS THAT CONTROL INFECTION
Definition of terms

A. Antibiotic—a metabolic product of an organism used to destroy another organism

B. Bactericidal effect—capable of destroying bacteria at low concentrations; e.g., disrupt building of cell membrane or wall and allow leak of cytoplasm

C. Bacteriostatic effect—slows reproduction of bacteria; natural physiologic mechanisms are required for phagocytic abolition of the bacteria

D. Superinfection—emergence of microorganism growth; e.g., yeast and fungi, when natural protective flora is destroyed by anti-infective drug

E. Bacterial resistance—a natural characteristic of an organism or one acquired by mutation preventing destruction by a drug to which it was previously susceptible

Types of drugs

A. Penicillin preparations
1. Disrupt bacterial cell wall synthesis when new cells are forming by interfering with the synthesis and cross-linkage of mucopeptides in the final stage of cell wall synthesis
2. Broad spectrum of pathogen suscepti-

bility except to *Staphylococcus aureus* —liberating penicillinase
   a. Amoxicillin (Amoxil, Larocin)
   b. Ampicillin (Omnipen, Penbritin, Polycillin, Principen)
   c. Carbenicillin disodium (Geopen, Pyopen)
   d. Hetacillin (Versapen-K)
   e. Penicillin G benzathine (Bicillin, Permapen)
   f. Penicillin G potassium (Dramicillin, Pedacillin, Pentids, Pfizerpen)
   g. Penicillin G procaine (Crysticillin A.S., Diurnal-Penicillin, Duracillin A.S., Pentids-P, Wycillin)
   h. Penicillin V (Pen-Vee, V-Cillin)
   i. Potassium phenethicillin (Darcil, Maxipen, Syncillin)

3. Semisynthetic forms resistant to penicillinase liberated by *Staphylococcus aureus*
   a. Cloxacillin sodium monohydrate (Tegopen)
   b. Dicloxacillin sodium monohydrate (Dynapen, Pathocil, Veracillin)
   c. Methicillin sodium (Staphcillin)
   d. Nafcillin sodium (Unipen)
   e. Oxacillin sodium (Bactocill, Prostaphlin)

4. Adverse effects—allergic reactions (highest incidence with parenteral administration)
   a. Penicillinase (Neutrapen) used to inactivate circulating penicillin by its enzymatic action that converts the drug to penicilloic acid
   b. Superinfection; e.g., *Candida, Pseudomonas*, in vagina, respiratory and intestinal tracts

5. Drug interactions—salicylates and sulfonamides compete with penicillin for nephron tubule transport sites for secretion from the blood, blocking may cause high blood levels of penicillin; probenecid (Benemid) is a sulfonamide used therapeutically with penicillin to slow tubule secretion and allow lower dosage of penicillin

B. Cephalosporins
1. Disrupt synthesis of bacterial cell wall by inactivating transpeptidase required for cross-linkage of peptidoglycan chains
2. Minor structural difference from penicillin allows therapy for penicillin-sensitized patients

3. Broad spectrum limited by sensitivity to action of cephalosporinase of some gram-negative rods (*Enterobacter, Pseudomonas*)
   a. Cefazolin sodium (Ancef, Kefzol)
   b. Cephacetrile (Celospor)
   c. Cephalexin monohydrate (Keflex)
   d. Cephaloglycin (Kafocin)
   e. Cephaloridine (Loridine)
   f. Cephalothin sodium (Keflin)
   g. Cephradine (Velosef, Anspor)
4. Adverse effects—allergic reactions (minor rashes, urticaria, fever, eosinophilia), superinfection, dizziness, fatigue, headache, severe diarrhea, nephrotoxicity with large dosage
5. Considerations during therapy—metabolites cause a false positive reaction for glycosuria in tests with Benedict's, Clinitest, Fehling's solution

C. Erythromycins and similar drugs
1. Compete for receptor sites on the ribosome unit to inhibit mRNA synthesis of protein required for reproduction
2. Excretion route is in the bile through the intestine (90%), which allows use with compromised renal function
3. Drugs
   a. Clindamycin hydrochloride (Cleocin Hydrochloride)
   b. Erythromycin (E-Mycin, Erythrocin, Ilotycin)
   c. Erythromycin ethylsuccinate (Erythrocin Ethylsuccinate, Pediamycin)
   d. Lincomycin hydrochloride monohydrate (Lincocin)
   e. Oleandomycin phosphate (Matromycin)
   f. Troleandomycin (Cyclamycin, TAO)
4. Adverse effects—gastrointestinal disturbances (nausea, vomiting, pyrosis, diarrhea, abdominal pain, stomatitis, black tongue)
5. Drug interactions—decrease tolerance to alcohol ingestion

D. Tetracyclines
1. Block tRNA attachment to ribosomes to inhibit protein synthesis
2. Drugs
   a. Chlortetracycline hydrochloride (Aureomycin)
   b. Demeclocycline (Declomycin)
   c. Doxycycline hyclate (Vibramycin Hyclate)

d. Methacycline hydrochloride (Rondomycin)
e. Oxytetracycline (Terramycin)
f. Tetracycline (Achromycin, Panmycin, Sumycin, Tetracyn)
3. Adverse effects—gastroenteritis (fever, liquid stools) caused by superinfection; hepatotoxicity (lethargy, anorexia, behavioral changes, jaundice, fatty necrosis); phototoxicity (exaggerated sunburn, pigmentation); enamel hypoplasia, dental caries, bone defects in children under 8 years of age and in fetus after fourth month gestation; nephrotoxicity; hyperuricemia; pseudotumor cerebri (in infants)
4. Drug interactions
   a. Drugs delay blood coagulation and potentiate effect of oral anticoagulants
   b. Oral drug forms insoluble mixture with iron and the calcium, magnesium, and aluminum salts of foods and drugs; e.g., milk and antacids and absorption of drug is erratic when taken concurrently
   c. Sodium bicarbonate orally decreases dissolution of capsules that require acid media in stomach
5. Considerations during therapy—parenteral drugs contain ascorbic acid causing false positive test with Benedict's and Clinitest and a false negative test with Clinistix and Tes-Tape

E. Other antibiotics
1. Streptomycin group
   a. Disrupt protein synthesis by providing substitute for essential nucleotide required by mRNA
   b. Drugs
      (1) Gentamicin sulfate (Garamycin)
      (2) Kanamycin sulfate (Kantrex)
      (3) Neomycin sulfate (Mycifradin Sulfate, Neobiotic)
      (4) Paromomycin (Humatin)
      (5) Spectinomycin dihydrochloride (Trobicin)
      (6) Streptomycin sulfate (Strycin)
      (7) Vancomycin hydrochloride (Vancocin Hydrochloride)
   c. Adverse effects—rapid emergence of resistant bacteria
2. Polymyxin group
   a. Detergent effect on bacterial cell

membrane increases permeability, which disrupts intracellular osmotic gradient
  b. Drugs
    (1) Colistimethate sodium (Coly-Mycin M)
    (2) Colistin sulfate (Coly-Mycin S)
    (3) Polymyxin B sulfate (Aerosporin)
3. Oral forms of both drug groups are used to suppress bacterial growth in the intestine (decrease ammonia production or "sterilize bowel")
4. General adverse effects—high incidence of neurotoxicity (circumoral or lingual paresthesias, injury to auditory branch of the eighth cranial nerve or to vestibular branch of the eighth cranial nerve), nephrotoxicity
5. Drug interactions
  a. Potentiation of neuromuscular blocking agents, general anesthetics, or parenterally administered magnesium
  b. Suppression of intestinal bacteria that synthesize vitamin K by oral forms decreases available vitamin K and potentiates action of oral anticoagulants
F. Reserve antibiotics used only in severe drug resistant infections
  1. Chloramphenicol (Amphicol, Chloromax, Chloromycetin, Mychel)
    a. Substitutes for essential amino acid phenylalanine, which prevents mRNA activity
    b. Adverse effects—single dose may cause aplastic anemia with pancytopenia especially in children and premenopausal women; leukopenia, thrombocytopenia, anemia, gray syndrome (feeding disturbances, abdominal distention, pallid cyanosis, vasomotor collapse, ashen gray color, death) in premature and newborn infants resulting from deficient mechanisms for renal and hepatic glucuronide conjugation, allergic reactions, superinfection, nausea, vomiting, diarrhea, abdominal pain, neuritis, coolness and weakness of extremities, headache, confusion, mental depression, enterocolitis, stomatitis
    c. Drug interactions—inhibits bio-

transformation of tolbutamide, diphenylhydantoin, dicumarol
  2. Novobiocin sodium (Albamycin sodium)—may cause bone marrow depression, intrahepatic biliary obstruction, allergic reactions
  3. Ristocetin (Spontin)—may cause high incidence of blood dyscrasias
  4. Bacitracin (Baciguent)—used topically (or intracavity) may cause nephrotoxicity with systemic use
G. Antiviral—amantadine hydrochloride (Symmetrel)
  1. Primary use is prophylaxis when exposure to viral infection; e.g., A_2 influenza virus has occurred
  2. Drug acts by preventing entrance of virus into host cells
  3. Adverse effects—insomnia, dizziness, irritability, tremor, slurred speech, ataxia, mental depression
H. Sulfonamides
  1. Actions
    a. Act by substitution of a false metabolite for para-aminobenzoic acid required for bacterial synthesis of folic acid
    b. Plasma protein binding maintains tissue levels by liberating drug when tissue levels are low
    c. Tenacious plasma protein-binding may hold drug until it reaches renal sites producing high levels in tubule urine
    d. Many forms require alkalinization of urine and high fluid intake to maintain urine volume and decrease incidence of nephron crystals
    e. Recycling of drug in nephron delays excretion and maintains blood levels of drug
      (1) Tubule cells excrete drug into tubule urine after removal from plasma protein-binding sites
      (2) Tubule cells also reabsorb drug from tubule urine and it returns to tissue and liver sites to be metabolized
      (3) Alkalinization of urine slows recycling and increases excretion rate
  2. Drugs
    a. Drugs used for intraintestinal therapy

(1) Phthalylsulfathiazole (Cremo-thalidine, Rothalid, Sulfathali-dine)

(2) Succinylsulfathiazole (Rolsul, Sulfasuxidine)

(3) Sulfasalazine (Azulfidine)

b. Drugs with 24 hour duration of action

(1) Sulfadimethoxine (Madribon)

(2) Sulfameter (Sulla)

(3) Sulfamethoxypyridazine (Midicel)

c. Drugs requiring equally spaced administration schedules

(1) Sulfachlorpyridazine (Soni-lyn)

(2) Sulfadiazine

(3) Sulfamethizole (Thiosulfil)

(4) Sulfamethoxazole (Gantanol)

(5) Sulfaphenazole (Sulfabid)

(6) Sulfisomidine (Elkosin)

(7) Sulfisoxazole (Gantrisin, SK-Soxazole, Sodizole, Sosol, Soxomide, Sulfisocon, Unisulf)

3. Adverse effects—anorexia, nausea, vomiting (caused by gastric irritation and action at vomiting centers in medulla), malaise, blood dyscrasias (leukopenia, thrombocytopenia, erythrocytopenia) and hypoprothrombinemia, allergic reactions (generalized skin eruptions, high fever, severe headache, stomatitis, conjunctivitis, rhinitis, destructive skin lesions, death can result), hepatotoxicity, kernicterus in fetus (replaces protein-bound bilirubin)

4. Drug interactions—enhances action of oral anticoagulants and methotrexate

I. Kidney-specific drugs

1. Nalidixic acid (NegGram)—a urinary bactericidal that provides high concentration in nephron for therapy

a. Adverse effects—nausea, vomiting, rash, urticaria, dizziness, pruritus, diplopia, weakness, headache, drowsiness

b. Considerations during therapy—metabolites cause a false positive reaction with Benedict's or Clinitest

2. Nitrofurantoin (Cyantin, Furachel, Furadantin, Furalan, Macrodantin, N-Toin, Trantoin)

a. Acts as a diffusible acid when tubule urine is acid; provides a high concentration of drug in nephrons for antibacterial action

b. Adverse effects—nausea, vomiting, gastritis, skin rashes (frequent in children), hemolytic anemia

c. Drug interactions—concurrent use of gastric antacids decreases oral drug availability

3. Methenamines exert antibacterial activity by liberation of ammonia and formaldehyde by hydrolysis in an acid urine

a. Drugs

(1) Methenamine (Uritone)

(2) Methenamine hippurate (Hiprex)

(3) Methenamine mandelate (Mandelamine)

b. Adverse effects—nausea, vomiting, pruritus, skin rash

c. Considerations during therapy—drug action is dependent on acid urine (pH 5.5 or lower) and concurrent citrus juices, ascorbic acid; arginine hydrochloride, ammonium chloride is required; sulfamethizole and sulfathiazole may form insoluble precipitates with formaldehyde

4. Drugs providing soothing effect (local anesthetic action) on irritated urinary tract tissues

a. Drugs

(1) Ethoxazene hydrochloride (Serenium)

(2) Phenazopyridine hydrochloride (Pyridium)

b. Urine tinted bright orange-red by azo dye origin of drugs

5. Sulfisoxazole (Gantrisin) and sulfamethoxazole (Gantanol) are sulfa drugs used primarily for urinary tract infections

a. Adverse effects—same as other sulfa products

b. Considerations during therapy—do not administer to patients receiving methenamines; encourage patient to drink fluids since these drugs can cause crystals

J. Sulfones that control *Mycobacterium leprae* (Hansen's disease)

1. Action

a. Deprives bacteria of the nucleotide required for folic acid synthesis and growth

b. Slow elimination and wide tissue

distribution of the drug permits daily administration; mucosal lesions improve in 3 to 6 months; nerve tenderness decreases in 6 to 9 months; however, skin lesions require 1 to 3 years for bacilli clearance

2. Drugs
  a. Acedapsone (repository form with few adverse effects)
  b. Acetosulfone sodium (Promacetin)
  c. Clofazimine (Lamprene)—a red compound that colors the skin, conjunctiva, urine, sputum, and sweat red-brown
  d. Dapsone (Avlosulfon)
  e. Sulfoxone sodium (Diasone Sodium)
  f. Thiazolsulfone (Promizole)

3. Adverse effects—hemolytic anemia at start of therapy, gastrointestinal disturbances, allergic reactions with serum sickness–like symptoms and exacerbation of lesions

K. Drugs that control *Mycobacterium tuberculosis*

1. Primary triad of drugs for therapy includes isoniazid, streptomycin sulfate, aminosalicylic acid or ethambutol; bacterial resistance to single drugs develops rapidly and combination decreases resistance and adverse effects

2. Drugs
  a. Isoniazid or INH (Hyzyd, Niconyl, Nydrazid)
    (1) Interferes with synthesis of the lipoprotein cell wall of *Mycobacterium*
    (2) Competes for enzyme required for synthesis of pyridoxine, resulting in a vitamin B_6 deficiency causing neurologic symptoms (hyperreflexia, paresthesia of extremities, vertigo) unless this vitamin is supplied during therapy
    (3) Used for prophylaxis of 1 year's duration for individuals who change from a negative to a positive reaction to the tuberculin test and to individuals living with a newly diagnosed tubercular patient
    (4) Adverse effects—hepatotoxicity in alcoholics, depression of bone marrow, skin rash
    (5) Considerations during therapy—drug causes false positive reactions for glycosuria with Benedict's and sometimes with Clinitest; drug may exacerbate symptoms of rheumatoid arthritis
    (6) Drug interactions—aminosalicylic acid decreases rate of isoniazid inactivation; isoniazid may interfere with metabolism of phenytoin and potentiate its effect to toxic levels

  b. Aminosalicylic acid preparations
    (1) Interfere with bacterial synthesis of folic acid by providing a substitute nucleotide
    (2) Adverse effects—gastric irritation, abdominal pain, nausea, vomiting, diarrhea
    (3) Considerations during therapy—metabolites cause a false positive reaction for glycosuria with Benedict's test
    (4) Drug interactions—potentiation of phenytoin action by interfering with its metabolism

  c. Streptomycin sulfate (pp. 244-245)

  d. Drugs used as substitutes for streptomycin sulfate
    (1) Drugs
      (a) Capreomycin sulfate (Capastat Sulfate)
      (b) Cycloserine (Seromycin)
      (c) Rifampin (Rifadin, Rimactane)
      (d) Viomycin sulfate (Viocin)
    (2) Dosage spacing (2 to 3 times per week) after initial intensive therapy decreases incidence of neurotoxicity to these drugs
    (3) Drug interactions with rifampin—absorption delayed by aminosalicylates (drugs administered on a schedule allowing 8 to 12 hours between them); inhibits activity of oral anticoagulants; phenobarbital interferes with rifampin ac-

tivity when used concomitantly
e. Second-line drugs used in therapy
    (1) Bind bacteria to inhibit cell metabolism and prevent multiplication
    (2) Ethambutol hydrochloride (Myambutol)
    (3) Ethionamide (Trecator S.C.)
    (4) Pyrazinamide (PZA)
3. Therapy effect may be seen as improvement in x-ray films and sputum cultures in 1 month, cavitation regression in 8 months

ANTIFUNGAL AND ANTIPARASITIC DRUGS

A. Antifungals
  1. Therapy may include topical and systemic use of the drugs to control fungi in tissue
  2. Drugs
     a. Griseofulvin, micronized (Fulvicin-U/F, Grifulvin V, Grisactin)
        (1) Acts as an analog of purine and is incorporated into new epithelial cells during synthesis of nucleic acids
        (2) Adverse effects—peripheral neuritis, vertigo, fever, dryness of mouth, arthralgia, mild transient urticaria, nausea, diarrhea, headache (may disappear as therapy continues), drowsiness, fatigue
     b. Nystatin (Mycostatin, Nilstat)
        (1) Binds tenaciously to cell wall sterols and causes a detergent effect that increases permeability of membrane and causes cell to rupture
        (2) Adverse effects—oral use causes transient nausea, vomiting
     c. Amphotericin B (Fungizone)
        (1) Detergent-like effect on cell wall that increases permeability of membrane and causes cell to rupture
        (2) Adverse effects—paresthesia and muscle weakness (caused by drug effect on normal cells containing sterols), chills, marked hyperpyrexia, nephrotoxicity, nausea, vomiting, flushing of skin, generalized pain, allergic reactions, convulsions
        (3) Considerations during therapy—deteriorates rapidly in light, so intravenous bottle and tubing should be covered during the 6-hour administration period
     d. Flucytosine (Ancobon)
        (1) Interferes with DNA synthesis by disrupting pyrimidine production when drug analog is used by fungi
        (2) Adverse effects—depression or dysfunction of normal tissues with rapid rate of proliferation (bone marrow, reticuloendothelial, intestinal, gonadal, epidermal tissues), skin rash, nausea, vomiting, diarrhea
B. Antiparasitics
  1. Flagellate control
     a. Furazolidone (Furoxone, Tricofuron)
        (1) Adverse effects—frequently causes nausea, vomiting
        (2) Drug interactions—inhibits activity of monoamine oxidase and use with adrenergic drugs or tyramine-containing foods may cause hypertensive crisis; concomitant ingestion of alcohol produces nausea, vomiting, headache, and hypotension
        (3) Considerations during therapy—degradation products may tint urine brown
     b. Metronidazole (Flagyl)
        (1) Adverse effects—nausea, headache, anorexia, vomiting, diarrhea, epigastric distress, abdominal cramping and metallic, sharp, unpleasant taste in mouth
        (2) Drug interactions—concomitant ingestion of alcohol produces nausea, vomiting, headache, and hypotension
  2. Extraintestinal amebicides—emetine hydrochloride
     a. Causes degeneration of the nucleus and reticulation of the ameba cytoplasm
     b. Adverse effects—nausea, vomiting,

dizziness, tachycardia, slight increase in systolic blood pressure, skeletal muscle weakness, activity-related dyspnea, regional myositis at injection site
3. Intestinal amebicides
   a. Glycobiarsol (Amoebicon, Broxolin, Milibis)—has arsenical component (low intestinal absorption) and bismuth component that slows peristalsis
   b. Iodine-containing drugs (minimal intestinal absorption)
      (1) High iodine content has lethal effect on trophozoites that decreases production of cysts
      (2) Drugs
         (a) Chiniofon (Anayodin, Quinoxyl)
         (b) Diiodohydroxyquin (Diodoquin, Floraquin, Ioquin, Yodoxin)
      (3) Adverse effects—nausea, vomiting, rash, acne, pruritus ani, abdominal cramping
   c. Intestinal amebicides with minimal adverse effects
      (1) Diloxanide (Entamide)
      (2) Diloxanide furoate (Furamide)
      (3) Glaucarubin (Glarubin)
4. Antimalarial drugs
   a. Definition of terms
      (1) Causal prophylaxis—drugs used to intercede at primary tissue sites to eradicate *Plasmodium* before it begins reproduction cycles
      (2) Radical cure—drugs used to destroy tissue parasites
      (3) Suppressive prophylaxis and suppressive cure—drugs used to interrupt the blood cycle phase
      (4) Clinical cure—drugs provide relief of symptoms in an acute exacerbation of malaria
   b. Primaquine phosphate
      (1) Primary drug for radical cure of *Plasmodium vivax* and also has a gametocytocide action in 3 days
      (2) Control requires 14 days; therapy is continued for 8 weeks
   c. Chloroquine phosphate (Aralen Phosphate, Roquine) and hydroxy-chloroquine sulfate (Plaquenil Sulfate)
      (1) Inhibit oxygen uptake and interfere with nucleic acid synthesis in plasmodia
      (2) Modify gametocytes of *P. vivax* to prevent completion of reproduction cycle
      (3) Used with primaquine phosphate for suppressive prophylaxis of *P. vivax* for individuals traveling to endemic areas
   d. Amodiaquine hydrochloride (Camoquin Hydrochloride)
      (1) Used with chloroquine hydrochloride for clinical cure of *P. vivax* or *P. falciparum*
      (2) Rapid acting schizonticide providing negative peripheral blood samples in 48 to 72 hours; afebrile in 24 to 48 hours; continuation of therapy provides suppressive cure of *P. falciparum*
   e. Trimethoprim (Syraprim)
      (1) Acts as a dihydrofolate reductase inhibitor
      (2) Used for *P. falciparum* strains resistant to other drugs
   f. Chloroguanide hydrochloride (Paludrine) and pyrimethamine (Daraprim) used for suppressive prophylaxis
      (1) Act as folic acid antagonists and prevent nucleic acid synthesis by plasmodia; sterilizing effect that inhibits gametocyte development in mosquito breeder of *P. falciparum* and *P. vivax*
      (2) Slow acting; therapy continued 4 weeks after last exposure
   g. Reserve plasmodicidals (quinine alkaloids) used when strains are resistant to other drugs
      (1) Quinine sulfate, quinine dihydrochloride, quinacrine hydrochloride (Atabrine Hydrochloride) act as schizonticidal and gametocidal agents
      (2) High affinity for nucleoproteins of liver and muscles; provides tissue levels for parasite control

(3) Adverse effects—yellow pigmentation of all tissues, prolonged use causes cinchonism (tinnitus, headache, altered auditory acuity, blurred vision, nausea) irritation of cardiac tissue (tachycardia), headache, gastrointestinal disturbances occur frequently

h. General adverse effects—decreased corneal sensitivity with high dosage, peripheral retinal pigmentation, blind gaps in visual field, skin dryness, pruritus, photosensitivity (exaggerated sunburn), peripheral muscle weakness, paresthesia

5. Antihelmintics—used to combat worm infestation

a. Aspidium oleoresin
(1) Paralyzes muscle of tapeworms and segments are excreted
(2) Adverse effects—nausea, vomiting, bloody diarrhea, uterine stimulation, depression of cardiac muscle, blindness

b. Bephenium hydroxynaphthoate (Alcopara)—blocks neuromuscular transmission, glucose transport, anaerobic glycolysis in hookworms, roundworms, whipworms

c. Dichlorophen (Anthiphen)
(1) Causes tapeworm scolex to detach from intestinal wall and disintegrates worm segments almost completely
(2) Adverse effects—abdominal cramps, colicky pain

d. Hexylresorcinol (Caprokol, Crystoids)
(1) Paralyzes worms (hookworms, roundworms, pinworms, whipworms, threadworms, tapeworms, intestinal flukes) and worms are inactive when excreted
(2) Adverse effects—burning sensation of skin, oral and anal mucous membrane

e. Methylrosaniline chloride—paralyzes pinworms, threadworms, and liver flukes

f. Piperazine citrate (Antepar Citrate, Multifuge, Ta-Verm, Vermidol)
(1) Paralyzes musculature of pin-

worms and roundworms by curare-like action
(2) Within 3 days pinworms are passed active and alive; roundworms paralyzed and alive

g. Pyrantel pamoate (Antiminth)
(1) Blocks neuromuscular transmission in roundworms, hookworms, pinworms
(2) Adverse effects—anorexia, nausea, vomiting, diarrhea, abdominal cramps, headache, dizziness, drowsiness, rash

h. Pyrvinium pamoate (Povan)
(1) Inhibits respiratory enzymes and anaerobic metabolism to inactivate pinworms, threadworms
(2) Adverse effects—nausea, vomiting, abdominal cramps, cyanine dye origin of drug colors stool bright red

i. Stibophen (Fuadin)
(1) Used for eradication of schistosomes, blood flukes
(2) Adverse effects—nausea, vomiting, diarrhea, arthralgia, headache, abdominal pain, drop in cardiac rate of 10 beats per minute at time of injection, hepatic necrosis

j. Thiabendazole (Mintezol)
(1) Interferes with metabolic pathways of hookworms, roundworms, pinworms, whipworms, threadworms, *Trichinella spiralis* larvae
(2) Absorbed from intestine and major portion excreted in urine within 48 hours
(3) Adverse effects—transient headache, weakness, dizziness, nausea, vomiting, anorexia

REVIEW QUESTIONS FOR PHARMACOLOGY AND DRUG THERAPY

1. As a general rule, which of the following tests is most valuable in the selection of an antibiotic?
   1. Susceptibility test
   2. Tissue culture test
   3. Serologic test
   4. Sensitivity test of organism
2. Nancy, age 3, is receiving tetracycline (Achromycin). Her fever is down and secretions have

lessened, but she is eating poorly, withdrawn, lethargic, irritable, and sobs readily. The nurse would promptly discuss the problem with the physician because
1. She needs a higher food intake to fight the infection
2. Anemia is a frequent occurrence after infection and treatment with antibiotics
3. Concurrent bladder infection may be present as an extension of her gram-negative infection
4. Generalized physical symptoms and behavior problems may precede drug-induced liver damage

3. Mrs. Herman has diminished urine output after cardiac surgery. Her serum potassium level is elevated and the physician has prescribed polystyrene sodium sulfonate (Kayexalate) sorbitol orally. The drug combination will
1. Remove potassium ions from serum and provide carbohydrate for nutrition
2. Stimulate transfer of potassium ions and increase coupling with the resin
3. Allow exchange of sodium ions for potassium ions and increase intestinal water content
4. Increase solubility of polystyrene sodium sulfonate and facilitate its absorption

4. Mr. Andrews will be taking sulfisoxazole (Gantrisin) at home. The nurse will instruct the patient to
1. Measure and record urine output
2. Strain urine for crystals and stones
3. Maintain the exact time schedule for drug-taking
4. Stop the drug if his urinary output increases

5. A patient with a urinary tract infection is receiving methenamine mandelate (Mandelamine) and ascorbic acid. The primary reason for administering the two drugs concurrently is that ascorbic acid
1. Improves methenamine mandelate effect on bacteria by acidifying the urine
2. Promotes healing of irritated bladder mucosa
3. Interacts with methenamine mandelate to decrease crystal and stone formation
4. Decreases bladder irritation by acidifying the urine

6. Postural changes immediately after spinal anesthesia may result in hypotension because there is
1. Dilation of capacitance vessels
2. Decreased response of baroreceptors
3. Interruption of cardiac accelerator pathways
4. Decreased strength of cardiac contractions

7. Susan is found by her mother playing with an open bottle of diuretic tablets. The physician tells Susan's mother to give syrup of ipecac to Susan. The effect of the drug will be enhanced by
1. Resting until vomiting occurs
2. Drinking 2 to 3 glasses of water
3. Actively playing until vomiting occurs
4. Stimulating the gag reflex

8. A patient with tuberculosis has been receiving streptomycin sulfate daily for 1 week. He is being discharged and the physician plans to have him come to the clinic for administration of the drug twice a week. The spaced dosage is planned to
1. Increase compliance with the therapy plan
2. Lessen risk of adverse effects of the drug on neural tissue
3. Minimize disruption of the rest hours required for recovery
4. Lessen tissue trauma from injections while resistance is low

9. Vitamin B_6 is given with isoniazid (INH) because it
1. Improves the nutritional status of the patient
2. Enhances tuberculostatic effect of isoniazid
3. Provides the vitamin when isoniazid is interfering with natural vitamin synthesis
4. Accelerates destruction of remaining organisms after inhibition of their reproduction by isoniazid

10. Mrs. Legere and her son Johnny are seen at the clinic. They both have severe upper respiratory infections and the physician plans to prescribe tetracycline (Achromycin). The nurse reminds him that Johnny is 6 years old and that Mrs. Legere is in her eighteenth week of pregnancy. The data are important because the drug may cause
1. Persistent vomiting when given to small children and pregnant women
2. Tooth enamel defects in children under 8 years of age and in the maturing fetus
3. Lower red blood cell production at times in their development when anemia is a common problem
4. Changes in the bone structure of young children and pregnant women

11. Patients receiving propranolol hydrochloride (Inderal) should be told that they may
1. Experience dizziness with strenuous activity
2. Have a flushing sensation for a few minutes after taking the drug
3. Notice acceleration of the heart rate after eating a heavy meal
4. Have pounding of the heart for a few minutes after taking the drug

12. Mr. Peters has been receiving streptomycin sulfate for 2 weeks. He states that he is "walking like a drunken seaman." The nurse would withhold the drug and promptly report the problem to the physician because the signs may be a result of drug effect on the
1. Cerebellar tissue
2. Peripheral motor end plates
3. Vestibular branch of the eighth cranial nerve
4. Internal capsule and pyramidal tracts

13. Mr. Paulson has been on home care with chlorpromazine hydrochloride (Thorazine) for nearly a year and is managing well. The nurse's assessment is directed at seeking evidence of adverse effects of the drug. She would
1. Examine his eyeballs and question him about the color of his stools

2. Take his temperature and ask him if he has frequent colds
3. Take his blood pressure and ask if he has headaches
4. Examine his skin and ask if he has numbness or coldness of his feet

14. Photosensitization is a side effect associated with the use of
    1. Chlorpromazine
    2. Thioridazine
    3. Ritalin
    4. Stelazine

15. Mrs. Smith is admitted with a diagnosis of partial occlusion of the left common carotid artery. She is an epileptic and has been taking phenytoin (Dilantin) for 10 years. In planning her care the nurse would
    1. Place an airway, suction, and restraints at her bedside
    2. Ask her to remove her dental bridge and eyeglasses
    3. Observe her for evidence of increased restlessness and agitation
    4. Obtain a history of seizure incidence

16. Mrs. Smith is scheduled for an arteriogram at 10 A.M. and is to have nothing by mouth before the test. Her phenytoin (Dilantin) is scheduled for administration at 9 A.M. The nurse would
    1. Administer the drug with 30 ml. of water at 9 A.M.
    2. Give the same dosage of the drug rectally
    3. Omit the 9 A.M. dose of the drug
    4. Ask the physician if the drug can be given intramuscularly

17. Mrs. Smith is scheduled to receive phenytoin (Dilantin) 100 mg. orally at 6 P.M. She is having difficulty swallowing capsules since the arteriogram. The nurse would
    1. Open the capsule and sprinkle the powder on pureed fruit
    2. Give her 4 ml. of phenytoin suspension containing 125 mg./5 ml.
    3. Obtain a change in the prescribed administration route to allow I.M. administration
    4. Insert a rectal suppository containing 100 mg. phenytoin

18. The nursing history indicates that Mrs. Smith neglects her personal hygiene. The nurse plans health teaching and emphasizes meticulous oral hygiene because phenytoin (Dilantin)
    1. Causes hypertrophy of the gums
    2. Irritates the gingiva and destroys tooth enamel
    3. Increases alkalinity of the oral secretions
    4. Increases plaque and bacterial growth at the gum lines

19. Mrs. Smith will continue receiving folic acid at home. The reason for continuing the drug is
    1. Folic acid will prevent neuropathy caused by phenytoin
    2. Folic acid improves absorption of iron from foods
    3. Folic acid content of common foods is inadequate to meet her needs
    4. Phenytoin inhibits folic acid absorption from foods

20. Mrs. Smith now is receiving heparin sodium intravenously and oral coumadin concurrently. When the patient expresses concern about why she needs both drugs, the nurse's explanation is based on knowledge that the plan
    1. Immediately provides maximum protection against clot formation
    2. Allows clot dissolution and prevents new clot formation
    3. Maintains levels of circulating anticoagulant during the periods when the oral drug is being absorbed
    4. Provides anticoagulant intravenously until the oral drug reaches its peak effect

21. After Mrs. Smith has received I.V. heparin sodium for 3 days, the drug is discontinued. The nurse continues to observe her closely during the early days of treatment with coumadin because
    1. Coumadin action is greater in patients with epilepsy
    2. Seizures increase the metabolic degradation rate of coumadin
    3. Coumadin affects the metabolism of phenytoin
    4. Phenytoin increases the clotting potential

22. Mrs. Smith is being discharged from the hospital at the end of the week. When discussing problems that relate to adverse effects of coumadin, the nurse will tell her to consult with the physician if the following problem occurs
    1. Increased incidence of transient ischemic attacks
    2. Excess menstrual flow
    3. Swelling of ankles
    4. Decreased ability to concentrate

23. Mrs. Smith's prothrombin levels have been somewhat unstable when done in the clinic laboratory. The nurse would interview the patient to identify factors contributing to the problem. She first would ask her about
    1. Intake of vitamin tablets or capsules
    2. Use of sleeping medications
    3. Use of analgesics
    4. Compliance with the plan for taking coumadin

24. Mrs. Smith calls the clinic nurse after her weekly prothrombin test to find out if her oral anticoagulant dosage is to be changed. She mentions that her sleeping medication, secobarbital sodium (Seconal), is gone, but she plans to get more when she comes for her appointment in 3 days. The nurse tells her to come for a refill today because
    1. Absence of sleep may precipitate seizures
    2. Discontinuance of the drug may affect the prothrombin level
    3. She may have withdrawal symptoms because she has been taking the drug for 3 weeks
    4. Her seizure control is dependent on the combined action of Dilantin and the barbiturate

25. When teaching Mr. James how to use nitroglycerin, the nurse would tell him to place 1 tablet under his tongue when he has pain and

to repeat the dosage in 5 minutes if pain persists. She also would tell him to
1. Place 2 tablets under his tongue when intense pain occurs
2. Place 1 tablet under his tongue 3 minutes before activity and repeat the dosage in 5 minutes if pain occurs
3. Swallow 1 tablet and place 1 tablet under his tongue when pain is intense
4. Place 1 tablet under his tongue when pain occurs and use an additional tablet after the attack to prevent recurrence

26. The nurse would tell Mr. James that he should suspect that his nitroglycerin tablets have lost their potency when
1. Slight tingling is absent when the tablet is placed under his tongue
2. Onset of relief is delayed but duration of relief is unchanged
3. Pain occurs even after taking the tablet prophylactically to prevent its onset
4. Pain is unrelieved but facial flushing is increased

27. Mrs. Gray is receiving neostigmine bromide (Prostigmin) for control of myasthenia gravis. In the middle of the night, the nurse finds her weak, unable to move, barely breathing. Assessment that would identify that the problems are related to overactivity of neostigmine bromide are
1. High-pitched, gurgling bowel sounds
2. Rapid pulse with occasional ectopic beats
3. Distention of the bladder
4. Fine tremor of the fingers and eyelids

28. The problems are related to action of the drug that
1. Increases the production of acetylcholine
2. Decreases the activity of cholinesterase
3. Stimulates production of norepinephrine
4. Enhances the activity of epinephrine

29. Mr. Dowd is taking isocarboxazid (Marplan). The nurse will seek evidence of drug effect on body tissues, which causes
1. Hypotension, edema
2. Increased psychomotor activity and appetite
3. Diarrhea, anorexia
4. Flushing of face and neck, increased salivation

30. During the interview, Mr. Dowd tells the nurse that he is going to a cocktail party later in the day. The nurse would advise him to
1. Drink only wines or diluted drinks
2. Have a snack with milk before going to the party
3. Avoid participation in heavy discussions
4. Avoid drinking wines or eating cheeses

31. The nurse's advice is based on knowledge of precautionary measures that should be observed by patients during isocarboxazid (Marplan) therapy to prevent
1. Vomiting, hyperexcitability
2. Cardiac palpitation, hypertension
3. Gastric hemorrhage, abdominal distention
4. Excess fatigue, return of depression symptoms

32. Mr. James is receiving isophane insulin suspension (NPH) daily and he also is to receive insulin injection (regular insulin) because his urine test was positive. In preparing the insulin for administration, the nurse would
1. Mix the insulins in any required proportion in the same syringe
2. Give the insulins separately unless the ratio of dosage is greater than 1:1
3. Give the insulins in the same syringe when the ratio is 1:1
4. Administer the insulins in separate syringes using different sites for injection

33. Mr. James has a cough. He tells the nurse that he takes Robitussin cough syrup about every 2 hours when he has a cold. The nurse would tell him that
1. He may take the cough syrup if his urine test remains negative
2. He must calculate the sugar in his daily carbohydrate allowance
3. He can substitute an elixir for the syrup
4. He can increase his fluid intake and humidify his bedroom to control the cough

34. When glucagon is administered for reversal of hypoglycemic state, it acts by
1. Liberating glucose from hepatic stores of glycogen
2. Competing for insulin and blocking its action at tissue sites
3. Providing a glucose substitute for rapid replacement of deficits
4. Supplying glycogen to the brain and other vital organs

35. A patient has an anaphylactic reaction within the first half hour after an intravenous infusion containing penicillin is started. Problems occurring during an anaphylactic reaction are the result of
1. Decreased cardiac output and dilation of major blood vessels
2. Bronchial constriction and decreased blood volume
3. Respiratory depression and cardiac standstill
4. Constriction of capillaries and decreased cardiac output

36. Epinephrine hydrochloride (Adrenalin) is administered immediately. The therapeutic effect of the drug is an outcome of action at
1. Beta adrenergic receptors in the bronchus and heart
2. Alpha adrenergic receptors in arteries and veins
3. Beta adrenergic receptors in arteries and veins
4. Alpha adrenergic receptors in bronchus and heart

37. Occurrence of an anaphylactic reaction indicates that a patient has
1. An acquired atopic sensitization
2. Passive immunity to the penicillin allergen
3. Antibodies to penicillin acquired after prior use of the drug
4. Potent bivalent antibodies developed when the intravenous was started

38. A patient is receiving methotrexate by infusion into the hepatic artery. The infusion method provides a high concentration of drug for destruction of hepatic cancer cells and

1. Delivers the drug to cancer cells in adjacent biliary structures
2. Allows dilution of drug by blood in hepatic sinusoids and delivery of dilute drug to metastases
3. Minimizes the quantity of drug released into the systemic circulation
4. Provides concentrated drug for destruction of metastatic sites distal to the liver

39. A form of folic acid, Calcium Leucovorin, is being administered intramuscularly during intra-arterial chemotherapy with methotrexate. The drug is being administered intramuscularly to
   1. Provide levels of folic acid required by blood-forming organs
   2. Provide the metabolite required for destruction of cancer cells
   3. Provide folic acid, which acts synergistically with antineoplastic drugs to destroy cancer cells
   4. Increase production of phagocytic cells required to remove debris liberated by disintegrating cancer cells

40. A patient in shock is receiving levarterenol bitartrate (Levophed) intravenously for regulation of blood pressure. The planned effect of the drug is based on action that
   1. Stimulates adrenergic receptors at arterial sites
   2. Stimulates adrenergic receptors in the heart
   3. Depresses cholinergic receptors in the arteries
   4. Increases adrenal output of epinephrine

41. The reason a second clamp is placed on the intravenous infusion tubing when levoproterenol hydrochloride (Levophed) is being administered is
   1. The drug must be infused slowly because it is irritating to the vein
   2. Administration of the drug above the established rate may cause generalized arterial constriction
   3. Extravasation of the drug into subcutaneous tissues causes sloughing
   4. Headache and cerebral hemorrhage occur when the infusion runs rapidly

42. A patient has an urticarial response after taking ampicillin (Polycillin) orally for 3 days. Diphenhydramine hydrochloride (Benadryl) is administered to
   1. Destroy histamine in tissues and reverse the urticarial response
   2. Inhibit release of vasoactive substances and dilate tissue capillaries
   3. Metabolize histamine and inhibit release of substances causing intense itching
   4. Compete with histamine for receptors and interfere with vasodilation action

43. This patient may also be given penicillinase (Neutrapen) to
   1. Displace penicillin from receptor sites
   2. Counteract the effects of penicillin in tissues
   3. Destroy the penicillin allergen
   4. Maintain therapy with a nonallergic form of penicillin

44. Mr. Rush is receiving digoxin (Lanoxin). While he is receiving the drug, the nurse is primarily concerned with
   1. Taking his apical pulse before drug administration and teaching him how to count his pulse rate
   2. Observing him for return of normal cardiac conduction patterns and for adverse effects of the drug
   3. Observing him for changes in cardiac rhythm and planning activity based on his tolerance
   4. Monitoring vital signs and encouraging gradual increase in activities of daily living

45. Mr. Rush has atrial fibrillation. The physician has prescribed quinidine sulfate (Quinicardine) and digoxin (Lanoxin). The goal of the drug therapy plan is to
   1. Decrease atrial irritability and slow transmission of impulses through the atrioventricular node
   2. Stimulate sinoatrial node control of conduction and shorten the refractory period of atrial tissue
   3. Suppress irritability of atrial and ventricular myocardial tissue
   4. Slow sinoatrial node firing rate and decrease irritability of the atrial myocardial tissue

46. Mr. Rush now is receiving digitoxin (Purodigin) I.M. at 10 A.M. daily. At 9:30 A.M. he states that he has been nauseated since awaking. He has a p.r.n. order for trimethobenzamide (Tigan) and he receives Amphojel every 2 hours. The nurse would
   1. Give the Amphojel now and give the digitoxin at 10 A.M.
   2. Give the trimethobenzamide now, the Amphojel at 10 A.M., and withhold the digitoxin
   3. Hold the digitoxin for 1 hour and give the Amphojel now
   4. Give the Amphojel and trimethobenzamide now and give the digitoxin at 10 A.M.

47. Mr. Rush is receiving hydrochlorothiazide (Diuril) and spironolactone (Aldactone) to relieve edema. The nurse will observe him for evidence of
   1. Excessive loss of sodium ions
   2. Elevation of the urine specific gravity
   3. Negative nitrogen balance
   4. Excessive retention of potassium ions

48. While Mr. Rush has gluteal edema, the nurse will use the deltoid muscle for administration of drugs I.M. mainly because at edematous sites
   1. Deposition of injected drug causes pain
   2. Blood supply is insufficient for drug absorption
   3. Fluid leaks from the site for long periods after injection
   4. Tissue fluid dilutes the drug before it enters the circulation

49. The nurse goes to Mr. Rush's bedside to give his 10 A.M. digitoxin (Purodigin). He has a lidocaine hydrochloride (Xylocaine) intravenous drip running at 3 mg./minute for control of premature ventricular contractions. The cardiac monitor shows 20 PVC's per minute,

and his heart rate is 78. The nurse's first actions would be to

1. Increase the lidocaine hydrochloride flow rate and check for sources of excess neural stimuli
2. Check the availability of the defibrillator and run an EKG rhythm strip
3. Administer the digitoxin and increase the lidocaine hydrochloride flow rate
4. Run an EKG rhythm strip and administer the digitoxin

50. Mr. Rush is being discharged from the hospital. He has a prescription for procainamide hydrochloride (Pronestyl) that he is to take for control of ventricular irritability. He should be told that

1. His heart rate will be slower and he may experience fatigue
2. The drug must be taken at exact time intervals prescribed to maintain the therapeutic effect
3. He should plan a schedule for taking the drug during highest periods of activity
4. The total daily dosage of drug must be maintained, but he may modify the schedule to allow taking the drug with meals

History and trends in nursing and nursing education in the United States and Canada

Nursing as it is known today has had a relatively short history—only slightly over 100 years. Modern nursing is usually said to have begun with the work of Florence Nightingale. However, nursing has its roots in ancient days, and many would claim that nursing really antedates all other kinds of health and medical care. Nursing has a history, the knowledge of which should serve to make the modern nurse proud of nursing's heritage and determined to make contemporary nursing meet modern challenges.

Knowledge of how nursing developed and the progress it has made should help in viewing the current problems of nursing in perspective. History should illuminate the present while it tells of the past. As each generation enters the nursing field, failure to recognize what has gone before will cause that generation to repeat the mistakes of the past. As knowledge advances, as societies change, as economic situations differ, so will nursing if it is to meet society's needs. The history of nursing then reflects how the leaders in nursing have attempted to meet new demands in new ways without losing sight of the original and fundamental goals of nursing. Modern nursing is fortunate in having as its founder a woman of the stature and wisdom of Florence Nightingale. Continued study of her writings brings new insights and appreciations of her work and its influence. The study of nursing is a rewarding experience.

In the material that follows, some reference is made to the ancient and medieval world, but more emphasis is placed on the modern world, particularly the twentieth century. The various movements that have occurred are treated chronologically because in this way changes and trends can be viewed more easily. Sometimes it would appear that changes go in cycles and that the cycles seem to repeat themselves. It should be remembered that nursing cannot be seen in isolation. It reflects the moods and modes of the period and in turn helps to influence the times as well. Nursing acts on society and is acted upon by society. So, nursing changes, and the more it changes, the more it remains the same.

THE ANCIENT WORLD

A. Care of the sick
   1. Hospitality was evident even in primitive societies when strangers were provided food, clothing, and shelter

2. The welfare of individuals was seen as necessary for group survival
   a. Children were cared for even though infanticide was practiced as economic necessity

b. The tribes cared for the aged and ill
B. Concept of disease
1. Primitive peoples believed spirits caused diseases, hence many superstitions developed, some of which still persist
2. Treatment followed the cause; the evil spirits must be driven out
3. Magic rites were performed by medicine men
4. Amulets and other similar objects were believed to have healing power
5. Potions were used from which some current drugs developed
6. Some of the methods used were forerunners of modern therapies (massage, therapeutic baths)
7. Until relatively recent times the mentally ill were considered to be possessed of demons or evil spirits
C. Medicine and nursing in the Ancient World
1. Egypt
a. Medical papers described both the diseases and the surgical treatments used
(1) Ebers Papyrus (medical)
(2) Smith Papyrus (surgical)
b. Pharmacy was well developed using injections, pills, capsules, powders, inhalations, inunctions, and other forms still in use today
c. Dentistry was well developed
d. Women had a good status in comparison to other societies
e. No evidence that nurses as such were recognized
2. India
a. References to nurses were to male nurses
(1) Required to know how to compound drugs
(2) Had to know what is now called hygienic care and assisted with moving
b. Women were generally restricted to the work of the home
3. Greece
a. Greek mythology included Asklepios, a renowned physician who was the son of Apollo
(1) Two sons, one a surgeon, the other an internist
(2) Six daughters, one of whom was Hygeia, the goddess of

health, another Panacea, the goddess who restored health
(3) The caduceus, the modern symbol of medicine, stems from Asklepios
b. Hippocrates (460 b.c.)
(1) Considered the father of medicine
(2) Writings included description of nursing activities that were taught
4. Rome
a. Especially noted for sanitation as evidenced by baths and aqueducts
b. Military hospitals were developed

THE MEDIEVAL PERIOD

A. Influences predominant in medicine
1. The Roman tradition in lay medicine
2. The ecclesiastical as practiced in the monasteries
B. Nursing
1. Greatly influenced by both military and religious
2. These influences are still visible to some extent today
C. Important military nursing orders
1. Knights Hospitalers of St. John of Jerusalem, Rhodes, and Malta, commonly called Knights of St. John
a. Secular at first, later strictly religious, finally military and aristocratic
b. Built hospitals
c. Had branches in many countries
d. Gave excellent nursing care including that of the mentally ill
e. Nursing efficiency waned after expulsion of Christians from Palestine
f. Traditions still influential today in form of ambulance corps and nursing associations
2. Teutonic Knights—similar to Knights of St. John but less extensive and influential
3. Knights of St. Lazarus—especially concerned with care of lepers
D. The secular orders
1. The Third Order or Tertiaries—worked with the poor and the sick in the community
2. The Beguines—hospital work a chief interest but not the only one
3. Santo Spirito—a nursing order of men
4. The Oblates—did excellent work in the hospitals of Florence

5. Order of St. Vincent de Paul—of great influence all over the world as a fine nursing order
E. Revival in medicine
This period was the forerunner of great medical developments as evidenced by the work of such men as
  1. Leonardo da Vinci—classic anatomic studies and sketches
  2. Vesalius—founder of the science of anatomy
  3. Harvey—the discoverer of the circulation of blood
  4. Sydenham—the introducer of the clinical method
  5. John Locke—physician-philosopher

THE DARK PERIOD

A. Deterioration in hospitals and nursing
  1. The decline in monastic orders resulted in closing many hospitals
  2. Secular organizations were not willing or able to take over responsibility for the sick
  3. The status of women was low and, with convents closed, girls had little opportunity for education
  4. Hospitals were staffed by paid attendants
  5. Religious hospitals also suffered from poor nursing standards; servants did the nursing while the nuns concentrated on administrative and housekeeping functions; religious exercises also took precedence over other activities
B. Reform was beginning
  1. Writers were beginning to write about nursing and the care of the sick
  2. The Society of Friends had great influence in the idea of service
  3. Position of women was beginning to improve; influential women, while not concerned with nursing per se, did influence public opinion from which nursing ultimately benefited
  4. The Duchess d'Aiguillon established the Hotel Dieu Hospital in Quebec City, Canada in 1639 and staffed it with nursing sisters from France
  5. Jeanne Mance, a celebrated woman in Canadian history, was instrumental in founding the city of Montreal itself and then established and administered the Hotel Dieu Hospital of Montreal for the remainder of her life

6. By the end of the seventeenth century, the number of Canadian-born nursing sisters outnumbered those of French birth
7. The first Canadian order of nuns (the Grey Nuns), founded in 1738 by Marguerite d'Youville, introduced visiting nursing in Canada, and established hospitals and missions in western Canada
8. The Seven Years' War (1756-1763) created significant changes in the nursing environment since all of the hospitals at this time were governed by the French religious orders who were abandoned by the French after Quebec fell to British rule
9. Many health problems occurred as a result of the mass immigration of British following the Seven Years' War and these problems became the thrust for the development of nursing in English-speaking Canada
10. Nonsecular English-speaking hospitals were established but the conditions for patient care were less than desirable
11. New religious orders (both French and English) were influenced by Mother Elizabeth Seton's Sisters of Charity
12. The number of professional nurses was minimal and by the end of the eighteenth century there still were none at the Government House Hospital in upper Canada
13. Loyalist pioneers in Nova Scotia and New Brunswick depended on self-taught practical nurses for care of the sick
14. Nursing in English-speaking Canada remained primitive and, outside of the religious orders, little was done to attract intelligent laywomen into nursing

THE NIGHTINGALE ERA

A. Forerunners
  1. Decline in hospital nursing in England and elsewhere as monastic orders were dissolved
  2. Secular nurses were from lowest social order, often illiterate, cruel, and addicted to drinking
  3. Sairey Gamp in Dickens' *Martin Chuzzlewit* depicted the nurse of the times

4. Elizabeth Fry, a Quaker, led in prison reform and founded a society of visiting nurses
5. The deaconess movement was revived
6. Pastor Fliedner and his wife began a place for discharged prisoners that ultimately culminated in Kaiserwerth, where young women were trained in the care of the sick
7. The deaconesses they trained were intelligent, moral in character, and devoted to their work but lacked sound training

B. Florence Nightingale (1820-1910)
1. The daughter of wealthy parents, she was gifted, religious, and socially conscious
2. She was well travelled and highly educated in the languages, literature, science, and mathematics, which was unusual for young women of her day
3. She insisted on studying nursing and over the opposition of her parents spent 3 months at Kaiserwerth
4. Her competence as a nurse was evident in her work in London as superintendent of a nursing home for governesses and during a cholera epidemic at Middlesex Hospital
5. She was consulted by others concerned with social reform because of her interest in reform for nurses

C. The Crimean War
1. The poor care of the wounded and sick soldiers stirred up the emotions of people at home
2. Sir Sidney Herdest, Secretary of War and a personal friend of Miss Nightingale, asked her to go to Crimea; her letter requesting permission to go to Crimea crossed his request in the mail
3. Miss Nightingale with 40 nurses went to Scutari where they found that a barracks had been converted into a hospital; the conditions were terrible —there were no supplies, no sewage system, and vermin abounded; patients were in a horrible state of neglect and mortality rates were very high
4. Though she had no military rank she was able to reorganize the medical service of the British Army; her reforms were responsible for reducing the mortality rates in the army to a level lower than had ever been achieved

D. The postwar years
1. Miss Nightingale worked for and finally succeeded in having a Royal commission appointed to investigate the medical services of the army
2. She made a study of the sanitary conditions in India, a land she never visited, and became an expert in that field
3. Grateful relatives and friends of soldiers of the Crimean War raised a fund for Miss Nightingale in appreciation of her efforts
4. This fund was used to establish a nursing school to train nurses as she thought they should be trained
5. The school was established in 1860 at St. Thomas Hospital, London
   a. A qualified woman was appointed as superintendent
   b. It was not under the control of the hospital, but a separate institution
   c. Both theoretical and practical training were included
   d. Strict discipline was enforced, probably an outgrowth of military and religious influence
   e. Only well-qualified applicants were accepted
6. Miss Nightingale was in close contact with the school but was never an actual participant in it
7. A chronic illness kept Miss Nightingale an invalid for nearly 50 years; this did not deter her from wielding a tremendous influence on nursing and related health affairs
8. Interestingly, she consistently opposed the germ theory and the registration of nurses, but in all other matters concerning nursing and health she was in the forefront
9. She wrote extensively and through these writings and her accomplishments her influence remains strong today

NURSING IN THE UNITED STATES
The colonial period

A. Indian tribes had medicine men who cast out evil spirits by various means
B. There is evidence that medicinal plants were used, also some treatments such as massage

C. Early hospitals
1. 1658—a hospital now known as Belle-vue, Manhattan Island
2. 1731—"Old Blockley," now know as Philadelphia General Hospital
3. 1751—Pennsylvania Hospital, Phila-delphia, founded by Benjamin Frank-lin and Dr. Thomas Bond
4. 1771—New York Hospital
5. Those who cared for the sick were not trained though the hospitals did have a paid staff

The nineteenth century

A. Religious orders active in nursing
1. Sisters of Charity, especially in the South
2. Protestant sisterhoods developed as outgrowths of European groups
B. Nursing during the Civil War
1. There were no prepared nurses and no organized groups to care for wounded and ill soldiers
2. Miss Nightingale's advice was sought because of her work in the Crimean War
3. Laymen and laywomen volunteered, including well known individuals such as Louisa May Alcott, Walt Whitman, Clara Barton, and Dorothea Linde Dix
4. Dorthea Linde Dix
a. Appointed Superintendent of Fe-male Nurses of the Army
b. Known for her investigations of the care of the mentally ill
5. In 1881 following her work in the Civil War, Clara Barton persuaded the United States to ratify the Geneva Treaty of the Red Cross and thus be-came known as the founder of the American Red Cross
C. Early nursing schools
1. First schools followed the Nightin-gale plan
a. Bellevue, New York, 1873
b. Connecticut Training School, New Haven, 1873
c. Boston Training School, later Mas-sachusetts General Hospital Train-ing School, 1873
2. Confusion existed from the beginning as to the primary purpose of the schools—whether to educate nurses or to provide better nursing in the hospitals

3. Financing the schools became an early problem; the students soon became the only staff, doing the housekeeping and whatever else was required, and learning what they could as they cared for patients
4. Control was transferred from an inde-pendent committee to the hospital board, thus departing from the Night-ingale plan
D. Growth of schools
1. 1882—first school in a mental hospital
2. 1886—first school for Catholic Sisters
3. 1888—first school for male students
4. 1891—first school for Negro students
5. Rapid growth of schools accompanied the growth of hospitals
a. 1880—15 schools, 323 students
b. 1890—35 schools, 1552 students
c. 1890 to 1900—342 schools, 1200% increase
6. Rapid growth led to lessening of standards and many hospitals be-came interested in profit from their schools
E. Movement toward organization
1. Beginnings of registration
a. 1903—first legislation governing practice of nursing and nursing education
b. 1913—20 states had legislation and though the laws were unequal they did exercise some control
2. Development of nursing organizations
a. 1893—American Society of Super-intendents of Training Schools (later National League for Nursing Education) organized to set and maintain standards
b. 1896—Nurses' Associated Alumnae of the United States and Canada (later the American Nurses' Asso-ciation and the Canadian Nurses' Association) was organized for in-dividual nurses
c. 1899—The International Council of Nurses was founded in Boston; it is composed of nursing associations throughout the world
F. 1899—a course in Hospital Economics at Teachers College, Columbia University was developed as a move toward improv-ing the administration and teaching in nursing schools
G. The beginning of public health nursing
1. Lillian Wald began her work in New

York at the Henry Street Settlement House

2. Nursing of the sick in the home was begun in Boston, Chicago, and other cities as visiting nurse societies were organized

H. Nursing in the Spanish American War
1. Again there was no plan to use trained nurses and those employed were unprepared and unsuitable
2. Finally the American Red Cross was able to convince Washington that a trained staff was essential and sent experienced nurse superintendents and trained staff to hospitals with commendable results
3. The success of the trained nurses in this war resulted in the authorization for an Army Nurse Corps with a nurse director in 1901

The twentieth century
Studies affecting nursing and nursing education

A. *Nursing and Nursing Education in the United States*—1923
1. Study resulted from a conference sponsored by the Rockefeller Foundation for the purpose of discussing the status of public health nursing
2. Committee for the Study of Public Health Nursing Education was formed with C. E. A. Winslow as chairman
3. Josephine Goldmark was chosen as director of the study and the report is popularly called *The Goldmark Report*
4. Original intent was to study only public health nursing but later expanded to include all nursing
5. Report included recommendations relative to
   a. The desirability of establishing university schools of nursing that would be adequately financed, administered by a qualified dean, and include liberal arts in the curriculum
   b. The inadequacy of many schools and disadvantages of the apprenticeship system
   c. The need for 2 types of workers in nursing
   d. Admission requirements in hospital schools and curriculum and teaching needs

e. The kind of training needed by nurses in public health
f. Postgraduate courses

B. *Nursing Schools Today and Tomorrow*—1934
1. Committee on the Grading of Nursing Schools was initiated by the National League of Nursing Education but supported by the American Nurses' Association, National Organization of Public Health Nurses, and American Medical Association; this report is popularly called *The Grading Committee Report*
2. Dr. May Aynes Burgess directed the study
3. Two "gradings" of schools were done in 1929 and in 1932
4. Two thirds of all schools participated
5. Recommendations included
   a. Employment of graduate nurses to replace students
   b. The closing of inadequate schools
   c. Collegiate level education with enriched curriculum
   d. Better prepared students
   e. Better prepared faculty

C. *Nursing for the Future*—1948
1. Sponsored by the National Nursing Council, the successor to the National Nursing Council for War Service
2. Directed by Dr. Esther Lucile Brown and popularly called *The Brown Report*
3. Included nursing service and nursing education in terms of what was best for the public not for the profession
4. Director made visits to schools all around the United States assuring participation of many individuals
5. Used lay and professional advisory committees extensively
6. Recommendations included
   a. Term *professional* to be used only by those graduated from professional schools or by achievement in some system of examination
   b. Both academic and professional training and basic alterations in the curriculum
   c. Requirements relative to administrative structure, facilities, faculty, and financing of nursing education
   d. Mandatory free accreditation of schools of nursing

e. Improved training for practical nurses
7. As a result of this study, Margaret Bridgman was employed by the National League for Nursing as a consultant to university nursing schools; this service was financed by the Russell Sage Foundation and a report was published as *Collegiate Education for Nursing* in 1953

D. *A Program for the Nursing Profession*—1949
1. A Committee on the Function of Nursing was formed under the aegis of the Division of Nursing Education, Teachers College, Columbia University
2. Eli Ginsberg, economist, was chosen as chairman; the report is popularly called *The Ginsberg Report*
3. A deliberative committee rather than a research group
4. Recommendations in many ways paralleled those of *Nursing for the Future*, which was going on concurrently

E. *Liberal Education and Nursing*—1959
1. A study done under the aegis of the Institute of Higher Education, Teachers College, Columbia University as part of a series covering those professions that admit students directly from high school
2. Findings included
   a. More lip service than reality to inclusion of liberal arts
   b. Some confusion as to what constitutes liberal arts

F. *Community College Education for Nursing*—1959
1. The Cooperative Research Project in Junior and Community College Education for Nursing, sponsored by the Division of Nursing Education, Teachers College, Columbia University, studied the possibility of 2-year, associate degree programs, to prepare for the technical practice of nursing
2. Dr. Mildred L. Montag, whose dissertation, *The Education of Nursing Technicians,* laid the foundations for the associate degree program, was named project director
3. Financed by an anonymous donor
4. Cooperated with 7 community colleges and 1 hospital school
5. Findings included
   a. Graduates passed licensing examinations
   b. Evaluated by employers as satisfactory in practice
   c. Colleges could support these programs financially

G. *Abstract for Action*—1970
1. National Commission for the Study of Nursing and Nursing Education established by the American Nurses' Association and National League for Nursing as a result of the recommendation of the Surgeon General's Consultant Group in Nursing
2. Distributed questionnaires to many schools and nurse educators relative to role, function, goals, and future of nursing
3. Compiled data that had been secured through many studies, large and small
4. Recommendations included
   a. Desirability of regional planning
   b. Necessity of research
   c. Single licensure for all in nursing occupation
   d. Academies to recognize excellence in the several specialized areas
   e. Preparation for episodic and distributive nursing
5. Following the report the Commission assumed the responsibility for implementation of its recommendations

Changes in nursing organizations

A. The American Nurses' Association
1. 1911—name changed from Nurses' Associated Alumnae of United States and Canada
2. 1952—restatement of functions following a study of various nursing organizations; all concerns of individual professional nurses retained by American Nurses' Association
3. 1962—the House of Delegates of the American Nurses' Association amended the purposes of the organization
4. 1964—Study Committee appointed to recommend organizational structure in order to carry out functions
5. 1966—new structure adapted
   a. Three commissions formed
      (1) Economic and General Welfare
      (2) Nursing Education
      (3) Nursing Service
6. 1970—a Commision on Research added
7. Individual members may choose to belong to a division of practice

a. Medical-surgical nursing
b. Maternal and child health nursing
c. Psychiatric and mental health nursing
d. Geriatric nursing
e. Community health nursing
8. Academy for Nursing Practice, established 1970—its members, known as Fellows, are certified as qualified
9. Academy of Nursing established in 1973
   a. Purpose is to explore broad issues and problems concerning nursing and health care
   b. Charter members named in January, 1974
10. Congress of Nursing Practice established in 1968
11. Structure of American Nurses' Association
    a. President
    b. Three Vice-Presidents
    c. Secretary
    d. Treasurer
    e. Ten Directors
    f. House of Delegates
    g. Ten standing committees
    h. Four commissions
    i. Five divisions of practice
    j. Ten occupational forums
12. Membership available to all registered professional nurses
13. State associations are divided into districts and are constituent associations of the American Nurses' Association
14. American Nurses' Foundation—founded in 1955 by American Nurses' Association
    a. Supported by public funds as well as contributions by nurses
    b. Sponsors and conducts research, disseminates research, and gives consultation
15. *American Journal of Nursing*, published by American Journal of Nursing Company, official journal
16. American Nurses' Association headquarters in Kansas City, Missouri
17. Conventions held biennially
B. National League for Nursing Education
   1. Name changed from American Society of Superintendents of Training Schools for Nurses in 1912
   2. Membership limited to those involved in nursing education until 1943 when lay members were admitted

3. Served as the education committee of the American Nurses' Association
4. Sponsored curriculum studies and reports
   a. 1917—Standard Curriculum for Nursing Schools
   b. 1927—Curriculum for Schools of Nursing
   c. 1937—Curriculum Guide for Schools of Nursing
5. 1952—became part of the new organization, National League for Nursing
C. National Association for Colored Graduate Nurses
   1. Organized in 1908
   2. In some states black graduates were not eligible for membership in district, state, and national associations
   3. Dissolved in 1951 after American Nurses' Association (1950) absorbed its functions and responsibilities
D. National Organization of Public Health Nursing
   1. Organized in 1912
   2. Promotion of public health nursing—coordination and standardization of public health nursing was major interest
   3. Nurse and lay membership even though it was primarily a nursing organization
   4. The official publication was *Public Health Nursing*
   5. 1952—became part of the new National League for Nursing
E. Association of Collegiate Schools of Nursing
   1. Organized in 1932
   2. Membership open only to those accredited programs offering college degrees
   3. Purpose was to
      a. Develop nursing on professional and collegiate level
      b. Strengthen relationships between schools of nursing and institutions of higher education
      c. Stimulate research and experimentation
   4. Had total of 37 members
   5. Dissolved in 1952, becoming a part of the new National League for Nursing
F. American Association of Industrial Nurses
   1. Organized in 1942

2. Growth of industry, especially in war time, prompted greater attention to welfare of workers and their families
3. American Nurses' Association had industrial nurse section from 1946 to 1952
4. Was 1 of 6 national organizations that participated in reorganization study but withdrew in 1952 maintaining its own organization

G. National League for Nursing
1. Organized in 1952 as a result of structure study combining the functions and activities of
    a. National League of Nursing Education
    b. National Organization of Public Health Nursing
    c. Association of Collegiate Schools of Nursing
2. Membership included
    a. Individual members—anyone interested in nursing (registered nurses, practical nurses, nurses aides, and lay people)
    b. Agency members—hospitals, nursing homes, public health agencies, educational programs, and public schools
3. Functions included
    a. Identifying needs of society and fostering programs designed to meet these needs
    b. Developing and supporting services to improve nursing care and nursing service
    c. Working with American Nurses' Association for advancement of nursing
    d. Working with governmental agencies toward achievement of comprehensive health care
4. Structure made provision for
    a. Officers
        (1) One President and President-Elect
        (2) Two Vice-Presidents
        (3) Treasurer
        (4) Board of Directors
    b. Two divisions
        (1) Division of Individual Members—forms Council on Community Planning for Nursing
        (2) Division of Agency Members with the following councils
            (a) Associate Degree Programs

            (b) Baccalaureate and Higher Degree Programs
            (c) Diploma Programs
            (d) Practical Nursing Programs
            (e) Hospital and Institutional Nursing Services
            (f) Public Health Nursing Services
5. Services provided
    a. Shares responsibility for recruitment with American Nurses' Association
    b. Accreditation of nursing programs
    c. Test construction
        (1) Selection tests
        (2) Achievement tests
        (3) Participates with the American Nurses' Association State Board Committee in construction of licensing examinations
    d. *Nursing Outlook,* published by American Journal of Nursing Company, official journal
    e. Biennial convention
    f. Headquarters at 10 Columbus Circle, New York 10019

H. National Student Nurses' Association
1. Organized in 1953
2. Individual membership preferred
3. Purpose is chiefly that of preparing for membership in the American Nurses' Association upon graduation
4. Annual conventions
5. Headquarters at 10 Columbus Circle, New York 10019

I. National Association for Practical Nurse Education and Service, Inc.
1. Organized in 1940
2. Active in stimulating interest in practical nursing, accrediting programs, and seeking financial support for practical nursing

J. National Federation of Licensed Practical Nurses, Inc.
1. Founded in 1949
2. Membership limited to licensed practical nurses
3. Recognized by American Nurses' Association as official organization for practical nurses

Special interest organizations

A. Association of Operating Room Nurses
1. Founded in 1957
2. Membership includes nurses engaged in operating room work at all levels

3. Interested in new practices and developments in operating room nursing
4. Holds annual congress

B. American Association of Nurse Anesthetists
1. Founded in 1931
2. Membership open to registered nurses who have taken a 12-month course and passed a qualifying examination
3. Purpose is to further art of anesthesiology and develop educational standards
4. Accredits schools of nurse anesthetists

C. American Association of Colleges of Nursing
1. Founded in 1969
2. Purpose is to promote university nursing programs and to take positions on issues relevant to higher education in nursing

D. Other specialty associations form as specializations increase

International organizations

A. International Council of Nurses
1. Founded in 1899 in Boston
2. A federation of National Nursing Organizations of which American Nurses' Association is a member
3. Membership automatic for individual nurses belonging to national organizations
4. Congress meets every 4 years—1973 in Mexico City; 1977 in Tokyo
5. Purposes are to raise worldwide standards of nursing education and promote general welfare of nurses
6. Oldest continually functioning international council
7. Headquarters at Geneva, Switzerland

B. International Red Cross
1. Founded by Henri Dunant, a Swiss, in 1863
2. Geneva Convention of 1864 confirmed Dunant's original principles
3. International Red Cross Committee coordinates national committees
4. The Florence Nightingale medal was authorized to be given to nurses of special distinction in 1912
5. American Red Cross—a component part of the International Red Cross
   a. Any graduate nurse may be a member of the Red Cross Nursing Service
   b. The services include
      (1) Teaching home nursing
      (2) Blood collection
      (3) Disaster nursing
      (4) Providing educational materials

C. World Health Organization
1. Organized in 1946 as an agency of the United Nations
2. Nursing recognized as integral part
3. Influential in showing nursing as an essential part of medical and health teams
4. Expert Committees on Nursing organized in 1950 and still serving
5. Nurses of many nationalities have worked in many projects all over the world
6. Influenced national governments to establish nursing divisions in health departments
7. Reports of Expert Committees, guides for nursing surveys, reports of regional conferences, and seminars help to disseminate knowledge and recommendations about nursing

Advances in education

A. Early developments in collegiate education
1. First nursing program in the world that was an integral part of a university was developed by the University of Minnesota in 1909
2. Two 5-year programs leading to bachelor of science degrees established in 1916
   a. Teachers College, Columbia University in cooperation with the Presbyterian Hospital School of Nursing (discontinued in 1924)
   b. University of Cincinnati
3. By 1931, there were 67 schools of nursing with some connection to a college or university
4. Collegiate programs for graduates of diploma programs were also developed
   a. Teachers College program for public health nurses—1910
   b. Western Reserve University School of Applied Arts and Sciences program for public health nurses—1911
   c. Simmons College (Boston) program for public health nurses—1912
5. The Association of Collegiate Schools of Nursing organized in 1928

6. Curriculum influenced by publication of 3 works on curriculum—1917, 1927, 1937—plus additional works relative to faculty and other essentials required for a good school of nursing
7. Accreditation of schools of nursing began in 1939 by the National League of Nursing Education in cooperation with the North Central Association of Colleges and Secondary Schools; first list of accredited schools was issued in 1941 and contained 70 schools
8. Nursing schools responded in 2 war crises
   a. World War I
      (1) Increased enrollment of students
      (2) Improved educational background of applicants
      (3) Vassar Training Camp during the summer of 1918 prepared 400 college graduates to transfer to nursing schools in the fall
      (4) System of nursing education was shown to have many defects needing correction
      (5) Army School of Nursing developed
   b. World War II
      (1) Increased enrollments both in the prewar and war periods
      (2) Authorization by Congress of the Cadet Nurse Corps (Bolton Act) in 1943 (discontinued in 1948)
      (3) Accelerated program mandated, all essential theory and practice within 2½-year period with 6 months experience in military, federal, civilian hospitals, or public health agencies
      (4) Tuition and fees paid to nursing school by federal government
      (5) Students received monthly stipends
B. Developments in the second half of the century
   1. Development of the associate degree nursing program
      a. The Cooperative Research Program in Junior and Community College Education for Nurses resulted from a proposal in M. Montag's *The*

Education of Nursing Technicians (1952-1957)
   (1) Purpose was to develop and test a new program preparing for those functions commonly associated with the registered nurse
   (2) Seven colleges and 1 hospital program cooperated
   (3) Results of the 5-year project published in *Community College Education for Nursing* and stated
      (a) Graduates capable of passing licensing examinations
      (b) Graduates rated by employers as good or better than other graduates of similar experience
b. The program developed differed greatly from existing programs and had the following characteristics
   (1) Controlled and financed by community college
   (2) Faculty employed by the college
   (3) Curriculum developed by the faculty with at least one third of total credits in general education, with remainder in nursing
   (4) Broad grouping of subject matter in contrast to many small courses
   (5) Students met admission and graduation requirements of the college
   (6) Faculty met college requirements for appointment and enjoyed all faculty privileges and responsibilities
   (7) Students eligible for associate degree
   (8) Graduates eligible to take state licensing examinations
   (9) Students provided own housing
c. These programs had very rapid growth, on the average of 50 per year
d. In 1974 the number of programs was 610, enrolling an estimated 88,469 students, a growth rate of 1.12% over 1973
e. Over one third of the students en-

rolled in nursing programs are in associate degree programs
2. Developments in baccalaureate degree nursing programs
    a. Designation of the baccalaureate degree as the minimal preparation for the practice of professional nursing resulted from a recommendation in *Nursing for the Future*
    b. All specialized programs leading to a baccalaureate degree were discontinued in 1957
    c. Graduates of diploma programs seeking a baccalaureate degree are admitted to the generic program with advanced standing (usually verified by examination)
    d. Curriculum changed to include
        (1) More emphasis on liberal arts
        (2) Reorganization of the nursing major
        (3) More selective clinical laboratory experiences
        (4) More independent study
    e. Better qualified faculties
    f. The control of the programs is now fully by the universities
    g. Federal funding of construction, special projects, grants to programs, and scholarships and loans to students have helped these programs appreciably
    h. Accreditation of programs has tended to improve quality
    i. The number of programs has increased and in 1974 was 314, enrolling an estimated 94,379 students, a growth rate of 1.11% over 1973
3. Growth of higher degree nursing programs
    a. Master's degree nursing programs
        (1) While graduate programs existed before 1959 they have received increased attention since that date
        (2) Programs include those that
            (a) Provide functional preparation for teaching or administration in addition to clinical study
            (b) Provide only a clinical nursing specialty
        (3) Federal funding of students through traineeships has assisted in preparing nurses for careers in teaching, administration, or a clinical specialty
        (4) Programs numbered 92 in 1974 and enrolled 4462 full-time students
    b. Doctoral degree nursing programs
        (1) Increased recognition that doctoral preparation is necessary if nursing is to develop true professional status
        (2) University faculty positions often require doctoral preparation
        (3) Research essential to a profession requires doctoral preparation
        (4) Number of nurses holding earned doctorates has increased greatly since 1950, however, the exact number holding doctorates can only be estimated because many nurses receive doctorates in areas other than nursing
4. Diploma nursing programs
    a. The number has declined since 1955
    b. In 1974 the number of programs was 495, enrolling an estimated 64,494 students, a growth rate of 0.94% over 1973
    c. Changes in curriculum have occurred as a result of the influence of college-based programs, especially the associate degree program
    d. Length has been shortened from 36 months to 27 or 24 months, often following the academic year pattern
    e. Tuition is usually charged
    f. Required living in nurses' dormitories declining with students usually choosing own place of residence
    g. More flexible admission requirements are common
    h. The term *generalist* for these graduates voted by National League for Nursing Council of Diploma Programs because of emphasis on the term professional for the baccalaureate degree graduate
5. Practical nurse programs
    a. Practical nursing defined by American Nurses' Association in 1959 as

(1) The care of the ill, infirm, or injured under the direction of a registered professional nurse, licensed physician, or dentist

(2) Requiring less specialized skill, judgment, and knowledge than that of the professional nurse

b. Functions stated by American Nurses' Association and National Federation of Licensed Practical Nurses, Inc.

(1) Personal and environmental hygiene, comfort and safety, spiritual needs, observing and recording signs and symptoms not requiring professional judgment

(2) Contribution to the understanding of the employing institution and staff relationships

(3) Personal growth

c. Most programs are now 12 months in length

d. Integrated programs of study and clinical experience the pattern by the mid 1960s

e. The number of programs has increased considerably caused, in large measure, by federal and state financial assistance

(1) 1951—W. K. Kellogg Foundation gave funds for 5 years to 5 states to expand practical nursing programs (number of programs increased from 5 to 41)

(2) 1956—the Health Amendments Act provided $5,000,000 for improvement and expansion of practical nursing programs in public vocational schools

(3) 1962—Manpower Development and Training Act provided funds for retraining the unemployed and by 1963, 129 practical nurse projects were in operation

f. 1974—the programs number 1294, enrolling an estimated 58,266 students, a growth rate of 1.01% over 1973

6. American Nurses' Association Position Paper on Nursing Education—1965

a. All nursing programs to be within the organized educational system of the United States

b. Recognized 2 types of practice

(1) Technical—preparation in the associate degree program

(2) Professional—preparation in the baccalaureate degree program

c. Aides to be prepared in vocational schools or adult programs instead of on-the-job training

7. American Nurses' Association's statement on diploma programs in 1973 really nullified its earlier stand on education although some attempts were made to change the wording after criticism

Advances in nursing service

A. Early developments

1. Employing graduate nurses as part of nursing staff and thus relieving students from total responsibility for patient care began in 1930s partly as a a result of

a. Closing of small and poor schools resulting from *Grading Committee Study*

b. Decrease in private duty nurses as a result of the depression

2. Study of nursing service administration sponsored by W. K. Kellogg Foundation in 1951

a. Fourteen universities developed master's degree programs preparing for nursing service administration

b. Few of these programs remain in operation today

3. Introduction of team nursing

a. Result of a combination of recommendations in *Nursing for the Future* and *A Program for the Nursing Profession*

b. Nursing team organized to meet the needs of the patient rather than relying on acuteness of illness or techniques needed

(1) Professional nurse—team leader—plans, directs, participates in implementation and evaluates care

(2) Other nursing personnel—

practical nurses and aides—
contribute to planning
and give such care as
delegated
(3) Daily team conference held to
plan, delegate, and evaluate
care
c. First team implemented at Teachers College, Columbia University,
in cooperation with Morrisania
Hospital and later Woman's Hospital and Frances Delafield Hospital
d. Courses included in program for
registered nurses seeking baccalaureate degree at Teachers College
e. The term is still used but the
concept has been so misunderstood and misused that it has
lost its original purpose; where
properly interpreted, it can be a
useful way of organizing nursing
care
4. Proliferation of workers in nursing
a. Increased use of auxiliary workers
during war years
b. Increased development of practical
nursing programs
c. Redefinition of practical nursing
makes it seem virtually like that of
registered nursing
B. Later developments
1. Introduction of clinical specialists
a. Engaged in giving nursing care
b. Assisting as consultants
2. Changing baccalaureate curricula produced nurses better prepared for professional practice
3. Increased numbers of nurses with baccalaureate degrees
4. Introduction of associate degree graduate pointed out the obvious need for
orientation of new staff and in-service
education
5. Emphasis on economic security and
welfare by American Nurses' Association
a. Increased salaries and benefits
b. Introduced collective bargaining
c. Produced possibility of strikes
6. Primary nursing—one way of organizing nursing service to permit the
nurse to give total care to the patient and to be held accountable for
it

Legislation related to nurses and nursing

A. Licensure to practice nursing
1. Purpose of licensure is to protect the
public
2. American Nurses' Association, from
the time of its inception, saw need
for legislation to set standards for
nursing
3. First states to have nurse licensing
laws were
a. North Carolina—1903
b. New York—1903
c. New Jersey—1903
4. 1952—all states and territories had
nurse practice acts
5. Early laws were permissive, with
New York the first state to pass a mandatory licensing law in 1938 that, because of the war, did not become effective until 1948
6. All but a few states now have mandatory laws
7. The laws are administered by a state
board of nursing either as a department of state government or as an
autonomous agency
8. The definition of the practice of nursing is included in the law
9. The individual state boards of nursing
are organized under the American
Nurses' Association as the Committee
of State Boards of Nursing
a. Composed of 1 professional employee from each state board
b. Concerned with specific problems
related to licensing
10. The State Board Test Pool Examination was begun in 1944 and is now
used by all jurisdictions
a. Each state board agrees to adopt
the Test Pool Examination as its
licensing examination
b. Blueprint Committee, a subcommittee of the Committee on State
Boards of Nursing develops the
plan for the tests
(1) Uses item writers nominated
by state boards to write the
questions
(2) Reviews the final drafts of
examinations
c. Each state board reviews and accepts each examination
d. Examination administered by each
state board of nursing

e. Passing score determined by each state board of nursing
f. The National League for Nursing Test Construction Unit works with the Blueprint Committee in the test construction
g. Facilitates the licensing of nurses as they move from state to state
    (1) Renewal of licenses usually required every 2 or 3 years
    (2) Different licensing laws and examinations are required for practical nursing
    (3) Licenses can be revoked for cause by the state board of nursing
B. Federal legislation
    1. Works Progress Administration (1935) —depression resulted in many nurses being unemployed and this Act made employment possible
    2. Federal Security Agency Appropriations Act—1941
        a. Administered by United States Public Health Service
        b. $1,200,000 appropriated to assist in training nurses for national defense
        c. Appropriation increased to $3,500,000 in 1942
    3. Nurse Training Act (The Bolton Act) (1943) established the Cadet Nurse Corps
    4. Health Amendments Act (1956) provided traineeships for those preparing for teaching, supervision and administration, and public health nursing
    5. Nurse Training Acts
        a. 1964—first comprehensive federal legislation to provide for increase in supply of nurses and to assist in modernizing nursing education
        b. 1968—Title II of the Health Manpower Act provided aid to students and to schools of nursing
        c. 1971—Nurse Training Act expanded and extended federal aid until 1974
        d. 1965 to 1971—over 334 million dollars awarded for
            (1) Scholarships and loans
            (2) Traineeships
            (3) Construction
            (4) Support for nursing schools
            (5) Projects to improve nursing education and recruitment

C. Legislation affecting nurses and nursing
    1. Social Security Act—1935
        a. Nurses became eligible for benefits—1951
        b. Amendments in 1965 provided for hospital and medical care for persons 65 years of age and older (Medicare)
        c. Some funds concerned with maternal-child care, blind and crippled children, and the training and employment of nurses in this care
    2. Hill-Burton Act (1947) provided financial aid for construction of hospitals, nursing homes, and other health facilities

Accreditation of nursing programs

A. State Board of Nursing approval of schools is a form of accreditation but it is mandatory rather than voluntary; no school of nursing can function without state approval under nurse practice acts
B. National League for Nursing has had responsibilty for the accrediting of schools of nursing since 1952
    1. Forerunners in the voluntary accreditation of schools were
        a. National Organization of Public Health Nursing
        b. National League of Nursing Education
        c. National Nursing Accrediting Service
    2. Purpose was to improve standards and to make available to the public the names of schools meeting approved criteria
    3. Criteria are set for each type of program
        a. Baccalaureate and higher degree
        b. Associate degree
        c. Diploma
        d. Practical nurse
    4. Period of accreditation—6 to 8 years, with reevaluation required if school is to continue on accredited list
    5. National League for Nursing recognized as approved agency for accrediting by the National Commission on Accreditation
    6. The Nurse Training Act of 1964 recognized the National League for Nursing as the accrediting agency for those programs desiring federal funds
    7. The American Association of Junior

Colleges has opposed specialized accreditation in the colleges and prefers that nursing programs be included in the regional accreditation of the institution
  a. Associate degree programs were approved for federal funds if accredited by another agency
  b. National League for Nursing recognized as auxiliary accrediting agency for these programs
8. List of accredited schools published annually in *Nursing Outlook*

Nursing publications

A. *The American Journal of Nursing*
  1. Founded in 1900 under aegis of the Associated Alumnae of United States and Canada
  2. Company organized with stock sold only to nurses and alumni associations, thus keeping professional control
  3. Produced and published by J. B. Lippincott Co. for 20 years
  4. 1912—American Nurses' Association became sole owner of all stock and the American Journal of Nursing Company was organized
  5. Published monthly by the Journal Company
  6. Official organ of the American Nurses' Association
B. *Nursing Outlook*
  1. Absorbed assets of the journal, *Public Health Nursing,* in 1953
  2. Published monthly by the Journal Company
  3. Official organ of the National League for Nursing
C. *Nursing Research*
  1. Launched under aegis of Association of Collegiate Schools of Nursing in 1952
  2. National League for Nursing, after its reorganization, assumed responsibility for publication
  3. Published bimonthly by the Journal Company
D. *Nursing Imprint*
  1. Published 4 times yearly by National Student Nurses Association
  2. Official organ of the Association
E. Publications of interest to nurses
  1. *International Nursing Review,* official organ of International Council of Nurses

2. *World Health,* published monthly by World Health Organization
3. *Hospitals,* published monthly by American Hospital Association
4. *Nursing Forum,* published quarterly under independent auspices
5. *Journal of Nursing Service Administration,* published monthly under independent auspices
6. *Nursing '76,* published monthly under independent auspices

Nursing service in the federal government

A. The commissioned services
  1. The Army Nurse Corps
    a. Established in 1901 under Army Reorganization Act as Army Nurse Corps, Female
    b. American Red Cross maintained reserve corps of nurses for army until 1947
    c. 1920—nurses received relative rank with range from second lieutenant to major with fewer benefits than men's ranks
    d. 1947—received permanent rank
    e. 1955—male nurses given commissions in reserve corps; in regular army in 1966
    f. 1965—legislation provided same standards relative to promotion as men
    g. Scholarship program for students in nursing
    h. Ranks now include general
  2. Navy Nurse Corps
    a. Established in 1908 under Navy Appropriations Act
    b. American Red Cross recruited as they did for the army
    c. 1947—received permanent rank
    d. Scholarship program for students in nursing
    e. Ranks now include rear admiral
  3. Air Force Nurse Corps
    a. Established in 1949 as part of Air Force Medical Service
    b. Ranks now include general
    c. Aerospace nursing—a new specialty
  4. United States Public Health Service
    a. Has a commissioned corps with ranks as in the Navy Nurse Corps
    b. Also employs under federal civil service

B. Other nursing services
   1. Veteran's Administration
      a. Transferred to Veteran's Bureau (later named Veteran's Administration) from United States Public Health Service in 1922
      b. Employs a large number of nurses in hospitals located throughout the United States
      c. Nurses now classified as professionals in civil service
   2. Department of Health, Education and Welfare
      a. Indian Service
      b. National Institutes of Health Clinical Center

Current developments

A. Changes in the legal definition of nursing
   1. 1972—New York state law for the registered professional nurse was changed to include
      a. Diagnosing and treating human response to actual or potential health problems through
         (1) Case finding
         (2) Health teaching
         (3) Health counseling
      b. Providing care supportive to or restorative of life and well-being
      c. Executing the medical regimen prescribed by a licensed physician or dentist
   2. Several other states are broadening their laws in similar fashion; e.g., Nevada, California, Colorado, Pennsylvania, New Jersey
B. Mandatory continuing education for relicensure being advocated in several states to ensure current competency; bills have been introduced in some state legislatures to mandate this requirement
C. American Nurses' Association's move to organize for collective action
   1. Emphasis to be on achieving quality care
   2. Assure the public of accountability of nurses
   3. Increase accessibility of health services
   4. Interest in economic welfare not abandoned but emphasis decreased
D. Commission on Education of the American Nurses' Association after a period of relative inactivity becoming more aggressive by

1. Reiterating the stand of the position paper
2. Proposing that American Nurses' Association assume responsibility for accreditation of nursing programs
E. Increasing numbers of professional nurses are going into private practice as individual practitioners or in groups under partnership arrangements
   1. Conduct screening
   2. Give nursing care
   3. Teach preventive health measures
F. Nurses Coalition for Action in Politics (N-CAP) organized in 1974
   1. Purpose is to promote health care of people by encouraging nurses to take a more active and effective part in government
   2. Voluntary, nonprofit organization
   3. Membership available through contributions
G. Nursing education
   1. The career ladder
      a. Advocates of this concept desire a curriculum that begins at either practical nurse or associate degree level and articulates with each succeeding level up to master's degree level
      b. Opponents of this concept contend that this would virtually destroy the integrity of each program and further confuse the use of the products of each program
      c. Several programs have been designed to carry out the idea; the success of these programs remains to be proved
   2. The external degree program
      a. A nontraditional program that does not require enrollment in or attendance at any nursing program
      b. Competency validated by both written and performance examinations
      c. Examinations include those in general education and nursing
      d. Performance examinations given in a hospital setting with actual patients
      e. Program attractiveness can be judged by the number of applicants enrolled
      f. Presently offered only in New York State
   3. Curriculum change in baccalaureate programs

a. Focus of organization changing from the traditional "Big 5" to emphasis on nursing process and nursing functions

b. Changes necessary to implement the role of nurses as described in the new definitions of nursing

c. Enlarging to include the expanded role of the nurse in
(1) Health maintenance
(2) Primary care
(3) Screening
(4) Community health

d. Increasing use of independent study

4. Increasing number of practitioner programs
a. Nurse practitioner—one skilled in assessment and management of psychosocial and developmental problems and able to function independently
b. Specialty nurse practitioner; e.g., family nurse practitioner, pediatric nurse practitioner

5. Increasing number of programs leading to doctorates in nursing

H. Nursing service
1. Primary nursing
a. A plan of organization by which a nurse is responsible for total care of the patient or a group of patients using the nursing process
b. Primary nurse—plans and carries out plan of care
c. Requires greater attention to nurse's comments regarding patient, and integrating nurses' notes with notes of other health professionals

2. Problem Oriented Medical Records (POMR)
a. Increasing use of this method of categorizing patient's problems rather than using diagnostic classification
b. Method is criticized by some physicians and nurses
(1) No panacea for poorly written notes by physicians or nurses
(2) Too well defined and categorized problems
(3) Repetitive

3. Peer review
a. Nurses actively engaged in nursing appraise the quality of individual nursing care according to established standards of practice
b. Essential if nurses are to be held accountable for care given
c. Useful in helping individual nurses improve their own practice
d. Useful in recommending nurses for advancement or merit increases

4. Clinical specialist
a. High degree of knowledge, skill, and competence in a specialized area
b. Use is increasing as more nurses are prepared in master's degree programs

I. Institutional licensure
1. Proposal that health care facilities would have the authority to determine proper utilization of personnel according to specific job descriptions
2. Individual licensing laws for nurses and other health workers except physicians and dentists would be eliminated
3. Proponents argue this would increase flexibility, permit better utilization of personnel, and improve health care
4. Opponents contend that while new ways are needed in institutions this proposal would not improve the situation
a. Knowledge and judgment needed because the tasks rather than the mechanics of the tasks should be the controlling factor
b. Job descriptions already present
c. Educators cannot prepare workers unless they know what is needed
d. Competency is an individual responsibility, not exclusively the responsibility of the employer
5. Several projects now underway to study effects of such a plan

J. Developments related to and influencing nursing
1. Moves toward national health insurance
a. For several years bills have been introduced but none has become law
b. Believed inevitable within a few years
2. Social and economic factors
a. Increased cost of medical care
b. Increase in persons over 65 years of age in population
c. Declining birth rate

d. Family planning
e. Need for consideration of minority groups in education and employment
f. Housing needs
g. Hunger and malnutrition
3. Increase in number and types of health professionals; e.g., respiratory therapists, operating room technicians, emergency technicians
4. Changes in medical practice include
    a. Increased specialization
    b. Increased skill in organ transplants
    c. Improved anesthetic agents increasing safety of surgical intervention
    d. Drug research and screening—more scrutiny of drugs reaching the market
    e. Introduction of physician's assistants
5. Increase in hospital beds with concurrent emphasis on ambulatory care
6. Proliferation of nursing homes and extended care centers
7. Shortage of nurses—a controversial subject
    a. Largest number of registered nurses employed in history—800,000
    b. Maldistribution a factor in supply and demand
    c. Economic situation in the nation influences employment
    d. The existence of an oversupply and overuse of practical nurses is a debatable subject
8. The Patient's Bill of Rights—American Hospital Association—a bill of particulars designed to protect patients by establishing standards governing the hospital's and professional staff's responsibility to patients and their families

NURSING IN CANADA
Nightingale influence

A. Florence Nightingale's influence ultimately led to the development of a training system for nurses that provided the thrust for establishing nursing as a profession
B. Because of the lack of adequate training facilities in Canada, Canadians such as Isabel Hampton, M. Adelaide Nutting, and Isabel Maitland Stewart came to the United States to study nursing and remained to become leaders in the field

C. First training school for nurses organized under the Nightingale system was opened at the General and Marine Hospital in 1874, in Saint Catharines, Ontario; the school, under the direction of Dr. Theophilus Mack, became the Mack Training School for Nurses
D. Hospitals soon discovered that their expenses were decreased by the use of student nurses on staff; this discovery led to the establishment of hospital-based schools of nursing and continued into the late 1960s

The nineteenth century

A. Religious orders active in nursing
    1. Grey Nuns active in western provinces
    2. Hospitallers of St. Joseph active in Acadia
    3. Sisters of Charity active in Prince Edward Island
    4. Sisters of Providence active in Quebec
B. Nursing during the Northwest Rebellion (Riel Rebellion)
    1. Military leaders recognized the importance of professional nursing skills when civilian nurses cared for the wounded and ill soldiers in Saskatchewan
    2. In 1896, Dr. George Sterling Ryerson, a medical officer during the Riel Rebellion, organized the Canadian Red Cross
    3. In 1898 the government attached a group of volunteer nurses (V.O.N.) to the Yukon Military Force
C. Early nursing schools
    1. First school to open and follow the Nightingale plan was the Mack Training School at the General and Marine Hospital in Saint Catharines, Ontario, which began in 1874
    2. Introduction of training schools for nurses was almost automatic in progressive hospitals after 1880
    3. From the beginning, educational needs of students were subordinated to nursing needs of patients and many conflicts developed
    4. Hospital boards maintained control over schools and succeeded in keeping them dependent rather than allowing the independence advocated by Florence Nightingale
    5. As new schools opened they did tend

to follow some of the Nightingale principles

   a. Women were in charge of the programs

   b. Courses were extended over a 2- or 3-year period

   c. Incidental instruction accompanied extended practice (work) periods

D. Growth of schools

  1. 1881—The Toronto General Hospital School opened

  2. 1886—The Hospital for Sick Children in Toronto opened a school; in 1896 it became the first to introduce training in theory with practical demonstrations preceding ward work

  3. 1887—Winnipeg General Hospital became the first hospital in Western Canada to start a training program

  4. 1890—Lady Stanley Institute became the first school to open independent of a hospital

  5. 1894—The Royal Victoria Hospital in Montreal opened a school

  6. By 1900, 20 hospital schools were in operation as compared to 342 in the United States

E. Movement toward organization

  1. Under the British North American Act, education and health became provincial responsibilities

  2. Nursing affairs and organization came under provincial control as an area of general health

  3. Prior to 1909, 3 unsuccessful attempts were made by nursing leaders to initiate Dominion registration for nurses

  4. Development of nursing organizations

   a. 1896—American Superintendents' Society in the United States organized alumnae groups in both Canada and the United States into the Nurses Associated Alumnae of the United States and Canada

   b. 1908—the first national organization for nurses was established when alumni and local and provincial associations joined together as the Canadian National Association of Trained Nurses (CNATN)

F. 1928—first course in teaching and administration offered by Extension Department of the University of Toronto (Ontario), followed by 1-year certificate courses and postgraduate courses in clinical nursing

G. The beginning of public health nursing

  1. The Victorian Order of Nurses for Canada

   a. Organized by Lady Aberdeen in 1897 to meet the needs of the Canadian outpost settlers who were experiencing both a total lack of facilities and appropriately trained nurses

   b. Developed and staffed Cottage Hospitals, which served as district nursing stations in remote, pioneer areas

   c. Operated special training centers for nurses until courses in public health nursing were started in 5 universities with the financial support of the Canadian Red Cross

   d. Offers bursaries to help nurses undertake graduate courses in public health nursing

  2. St. Elizabeth's Visiting Nurse Association

   a. Organized as a Catholic visiting nurse service in 1908

   b. Pioneered in selling immunization and medical examination services for children to separate school boards

  3. Public Health Nursing

   a. Officially established in Toronto in 1912 by Dr. C. J. Hastings and Miss Eunice Dyke to amalgamate maternal and child care with communicable disease control

   b. Supported by Canadian Red Cross Society after World War I

   c. By 1919, Provincial Boards of Health and a Department of Health in Ottawa had been established

   d. Quebec became one of the first provinces to develop rural health units

  4. Nursing Service of the Metropolitan Life Insurance Company

   a. In 1909, especially in Quebec, this organization became associated with public health nursing through the efforts of Lillian D. Wald

   b. Inaugurated an experimental campaign in Quebec to combine health teaching and supervision in an attempt to reduce infant mortality rate

   c. Assisted in establishing a School

of Public Health Nursing at the University of Montreal

H. Nursing in the Boer War
1. 1899—nurses in South Africa were granted the rank, allowances, and pay of a lieutenant in the Army
2. Reserve of Nursing Sisters incorporated with the Canadian Army Medical Corps
3. 1906—Nursing Sisters Georgina Pope and Margaret Macdonald were appointed to Permanent Army Medical Corps, thus Canada became the first country to give military rank to women

The twentieth century
Studies affecting nursing and nursing education

A. *Special Committee on Nurse Education* —1916
1. Report presented to the Canadian National Association of Trained Nurses
2. Recommendations included
   a. Nurse training schools or colleges should be established within the educational system of each province
   b. Nurse training schools should be separated in organization from hospitals that were still to be used for practical training
B. *Report on Nursing Service*—1926
1. Report by the Canadian Nurses' Association to the Federal Department of Health
2. Contained information on
   a. Issues and trends in nursing
   b. Problems related to recruitment of nurses and attrition from programs
   c. Issues related to conserving nurse power
C. *Survey of Nursing Education in Canada (the Weir Report)*—1932
1. A study of nursing education in Canada jointly sponsored by the Canadian Nurses' Association and The Canadian Medical Association under the chairmanship of Dr. Stewart Cameron
2. Purpose was to investigate growing criticism about nursing and its training system across the 5 main sections of Canada
3. Surveyed the economic, educational, and sociologic problems of nurses and nursing

4. Report contained recommendations on
   a. Delivery of health care; e.g., the need for a comprehensive system of supervision and control of nursing personnel
   b. Nursing as a profession; e.g., Provincial Registration Acts required amendments in areas related to nursing education
   c. Private duty nursing; e.g., only registered graduates should be allowed to use the title *nurse*
   d. Institutional nursing; e.g., training schools should be established within educational institutions
   e. Student nurses; e.g., a period of internship as part of regular nurses' training may be desirable
   f. Teachers of nursing; e.g., the number of full-time qualified teachers should be increased
   g. Examination system; e.g., only graduates of approved training schools should be permitted to write the examination
D. *Proposed Curriculum for Schools of Nursing*—Canadian Nurses' Association
1. The 1939 curriculum proposal and a 1940 supplement, *Improvement of Nursing Education in the Clinical Field,* arose from recommendations in the Weir Report; purpose was to serve as a guide to administrative, supervisory, and teaching responsibilities relative to students on wards
2. The 1946 guide approved a demonstration program in nurse education at the Metropolitan School of Nursing in Windsor, Ontario
E. *Evaluation of the Metropolitan School of Nursing (the Lord Report)*—1952
1. A study to examine all aspects of this demonstration program (less than 3 years in length) jointly sponsored by the Canadian Nurses' Association and the Canadian Red Cross under the direction of Nettie Fidler
2. Purpose was to see if skilled clinical nurses could be prepared in less than 3 years if school controlled student's clinical time
3. Concluded that
   a. The average graduate of this program compared with the average graduate of the control school in both bedside skills and achieve-

ment on the Registered Nurse Examination

b. Schools with complete control of students can prepare nurses in 2 years as well as those prepared in 3 years

F. *Report on the Experiment in Nursing Education at the Atkinson School of Nursing of the Toronto Western Hospital*—1955

1. Before the project at the Metropolitan School was completed, a project under the direction of W. Stewart Wallace was begun at the Toronto Hospital
2. Program was to follow the same curriculum as Metropolitan School but an "intern" third year under the control of Nursing Service was added
3. Study showed problems developed because of the 2 plus 1 nonintegrated pattern of the program and the division of authority between the school and hospital

G. *Study of Nursing Education in New Brunswick*—1956

1. Sponsored by the New Brunswick Department of Health and Social Service and reported by Kathleen Russell
2. Recommendations included
   a. Hospital schools should reorganize to become independent by 1957
   b. Students should be assured more direct patient care during clinical experience
   c. Interprovincial reciprocal registration should be established
   d. The establishment of a School of Nursing at the University of New Brunswick
   e. The inclusion of a 3-month psychiatric affiliation in all nursing programs
   f. The Provincial Association should hold 3-month institutes for the preparation of clinical instructors until postgraduate courses can be established
   g. Policies for the organization and preparation of nursing assistant groups should be written

H. *Report of the Pilot Project for the Evaluation of Schools of Nursing in Canada (Spotlight on Nursing Education)*—1960

1. Sponsored by the nursing profession through the Canadian Nurses' Association under the direction of Helen K. Mussallem
2. Purpose was to examine status of schools of nursing to determine their readiness for a program of voluntary national accreditation
3. Study showed that 21 of the 25 schools surveyed would not have passed accreditation
4. Recommendations included
   a. A reexamination of nursing education in Canada be undertaken
   b. An improvement program to upgrade programs be started
   c. The evaluation of the quality of nursing service in clinical agencies be established
   d. An accreditation program for schools be established by the Canadian Nurses' Association

I. *Royal Commission on Health Services Briefs*—1961

1. Indicated unanimity for change in nursing education
2. Projected evolvement of 2 levels of nurses—those required for leadership roles and those technically skilled for bedside nursing

J. *Report of Royal Commission on Health Services*

1. Suggested expansion of university schools of nursing especially at masters and doctoral level
2. Recommended that baccalaureate programs in nursing develop integrated curriculum
3. Recommended establishment of a comprehensive, compulsory, universal, health service program for all Canadians
   a. Requested examination of an extension of the role of the nurse
   b. Projected number of additional nurses required by 1971
4. Specifically recommended that
   a. Schools of nursing have budgets separate from nursing service
   b. Diploma nurses be registered and graduated from 2-year nursing programs
   c. Salaries comparable with education and responsibility in other fields be paid nurses
5. Recommendations that were implemented as a result included new patterns of nursing curricula, home care

programs, health councils, and group practices

K. *Report of the Nursing Education Survey Committee for the Province of Alberta (Scarlett Report)*—1961-1963
   1. Sponsored by the Department of Health in Alberta
   2. Recommendations included that
      a. A Provincial Council of Nursing be established for licensing of all nursing personnel; licensure be mandatory for those who nurse for hire in Alberta
      b. Nursing education remain under the aegis of the University of Alberta and the program be shortened to 4 years
      c. The 2-year program as demonstrated by the Nightingale School in Toronto not be instituted in Alberta because of the costs of such a program

L. *Report on the Canadian Nurses' Association School Improvement Program* (Glenna S. Rowsell)—1961-1964
   1. Report emerged from recommendation of *The Report of the Pilot Project for the Evaluation of Schools of Nursing in Canada* in 1960; examined 168 diploma schools (98% of all such schools in Canada)
   2. Reaffirmed impracticality of an accreditation program of schools of nursing at this time; based on task force recommendations
   3. Task force also made following recommendations relative to the School Improvement Program
      a. The Canadian Nurses' Association create a Department of Nursing Education to act in consultant capacity to new programs and in nursing research
      b. The Canadian Nurses' Association clarify beliefs about nursing education and nurses' roles in society
   4. Indicated need for continued study in areas of philosophy and school objectives, organization and administration, curriculum, facilities, and residence living

M. *A Study of the Development of a Diploma Program in Nursing at the Ryerson Institute of Technology, Toronto*—1963
   1. Submissions were made to the Royal Commission on Health Services by nursing leaders that a nursing program be conducted at a level after high school under the jurisdiction of an educational institution; program approved in 1963 by College of Nurses of Ontario and conducted at Ryerson Institute of Technology
   2. The 5-year experimental program had its own governing body and budget, a well-qualified teaching staff, 1 full-time teacher per 10 students, and control of student time and experience over a maximum 30 hour week
   3. In 1973, the success of the program was made evident as provision was made for its continuance following an evaluation by Moyra Allen

N. *Plan for the Development of Nursing Education Programs Within the General Educational System of Canada*—1964
   1. Sponsored by the Canadian Nurses' Association under the direction of Helen K. Mussallem and popularly called *A Path to Quality*
   2. Overall purpose of the study was the preparation of a plan for basic nursing education programs within general educational systems
   3. Basic elements advocated by the project and rebuffed by the Canadian Hospital Association were that
      a. Nursing programs be developed within educational systems
      b. Two categories of nursing personnel be prepared
         (1) The professional nurse to be prepared in a 4-year university program
         (2) The technical nurse to be prepared in a 2-year program under educational auspices
      c. Two categories to be prepared in a ratio of 1 professional to 3 technical nurses

O. *Royal Commission on Health Services Nursing Education in Canada* (Dr. Helen K. Mussallem)—1964
   1. Purpose was to examine and analyze all types of formal educational programs for personnel providing nursing care with emphasis primarily on those preparing nurses for registration in the provinces
   2. Recommended that
      a. Deplorable lack of qualified teach

ers be remedied as soon as possible

b. Diploma schools of nursing be part of the provinces' systems after high school

c. Educational programs be revised to prepare 2 levels of nurses—the university and diploma nurses, with the former providing leadership in nursing practice and the latter assisting the professional nurse

d. More graduate programs be designed to prepare nurses in research, consultation, and nursing specialties

P. *A Plan for the Education of Nurses in the Province of New Brunswick (Portrait of Nursing)*—1965

1. Sponsored by the New Brunswick Association of Registered Nurses and directed by Katherine MacLaggan

2. Purposes of the undertaking were

  a. To project a plan for educating 2 categories of nurses

  b. To present a plan for nurse education

    (1) To those in the general educational system of the province

    (2) To those responsible for nursing education and its development

3. The Canadian Hospital Association wanted hospitals to continue operation of nursing schools even though 84 junior college programs had been initiated in the United States by this time

4. Recommendations included that

  a. Federal, provincial, and local governments finance nurse education at Institutes of Health Sciences

  b. Four health service groups be formed with clearly written levels of function (nurses Grades I and II, secretaries, wardkeepers)

5. That Provincial Councils on Education for Health Services be formed and be responsible to the Ministry of Education

6. Local management boards be responsible for

  a. Setting and receiving tuition

  b. Approving personnel appointments

  c. Approving all programs of education prior to submission to the Provincial Council for consideration

  d. Contracting for clinical experience

Q. *Committee on the Healing Arts*

1. Established by Province of Ontario, July, 1966

2. Study investigated role and function of nursing personnel, nature of nursing activities, supply and demand, curriculum, teaching staff requirements

3. Recommendations included

  a. That the provincial association merge with the Ontario Association of Registered Nursing Assistants

  b. That studies be done to improve nurse resource utilization

  c. That activities representing the practice of nursing be defined

  d. That Labor Relations Act be amended according to the British Columbia model

  e. That Canadian Nurses' Association continue to develop uniform standards of registration

R. *Report on the Project for the Evaluation of the Quality of Nursing Service* (sponsored by Canadian Nurses' Association)—1966

1. First attempt to evaluate the quality of nursing service, administration, and nursing care being provided within the concept of total patient care

2. Findings were summarized according to

  a. Nursing care

  b. Philosophy and objectives

  c. Nursing service administration

  d. Nursing personnel

  e. Medical-nursing relationships

  f. Nursing students and nursing service

3. Recommendations were that

  a. Nursing service departments evaluate care given

  b. Roles, functions, and relationships of physicians, nurses, and administrators within patient care area be defined

  c. Standards for nursing service and hospital accreditation programs be set

  d. Nursing personnel be used more economically

  e. Individual nursing care plans be implemented

f. More challenging clinical experiences be structured for students using problem solving approaches

S. *Ad Hoc Committee on Nursing Education, Department of Public Health, Province of Saskatchewan*—1966
1. Formed after the recommendation of the Royal Commission on Health Services that Nursing Education Planning Committees be established provincially
2. Submitted basic guidelines for a system of educating nurses in Saskatchewan based on the belief that authority and responsibility for nurse education belonged to an agency whose primary concern was education
3. Recommendations included
   a. That Department of Education be responsible for education of nurses including the diploma level
   b. That Provincial Nurses' Association determine minimum admission standards and standards for registration
   c. That 2 central schools be established by Department of Education and hospital schools be phased into these
   d. That present 5-year university program be altered to 4-year integrated baccalaureate program and enrollment be increased by 50%
   e. That university certificate courses be eventually phased out

T. *Community Colleges and Nursing Education in Ontario* (R. G. Quittendon)—1968
1. Study initiated to provide data for optimum development of nurse training in relation to community needs
2. Findings were that
   a. Nonuniversity, postsecondary school enrollments increased 400% between 1955 and 1966 in Canada
   b. Ontario University enrollments increased 250% between 1955 and 1965
   c. Diploma nursing enrollment in Ontario increased 35% between 1955 and 1965 while nursing assistant enrollment increased 100%
   d. Health science divisions needed to be developed in community colleges for training health team members

U. *Ontario Council of Health Report*—1969
1. Ontario Council of Health received legislative approval in 1968 becoming Senior Advisory body to Minister of Health
2. Guidelines for study were inherent in The Royal Commission on Health Services and included health care delivery, health manpower, education of health disciplines, and regional organization of health services

V. *Report of the Ontario Health Council on Health Care Delivery Systems*—1970
1. Prepared by a subcommittee on community health and presented to the Ontario Council of Health
2. Recommendations included
   a. Urgent need to make primary care more accessible from existing health workers
   b. Development of ambulatory care facilities
   c. Involvement of health science centers and professional faculties in primary health care delivery
   d. Examination of the role of the community health nurse in health services
   e. Establishment of health resource centers

W. *Task Force Reports on Cost of Health Services in Canada-Public Health Services*—1970
1. Suggested that public health practice was not as effective or economically sound as it might be
2. Recommendations included that
   a. Health services be regionalized
   b. Levels of community care be available to the public
   c. Home care programs be expanded
   d. University programs in public health be strengthened
   e. Community health centers be constructed
   f. Governments subsidize group practice by physicians
   g. Studies be done in use of physician-associates

X. *Task Force Reports on Cost of Health Service in Canada*—1970
1. Established by Conference of Ministers of Health of Canada in 1968 to inquire into ways of restraining escalating health services expenditures

2. Areas of inquiry related to hospital services
3. Recommendations included that
   a. Nursing units not be staffed for maximum nursing care loads adding personnel as required
   b. A uniform classification of care functions be established for Canada
   c. Specialized service units be encouraged
   d. Ambulatory care facilities be developed, along with community health centers
   e. Home care programs be expanded
   f. Standards for nursing care be formulated and measured
   g. Accreditation be mandatory for all hospitals of a national, nongovernmental nature
   h. Community mental health clinics be developed
   i. Further studies related to use of physician-associates be done
Y. *National Conference on Assistance to the Physician*—1971
   1. Sponsored by Department of National Health and Welfare, Canadian Medical Association, Canadian Nurses' Association, Consumers Association of Canada, and L'Association des Medecins de Langue Française du Canada
   2. Recommendations included expansion of Outpost Nursing Programs; a system of national portability for those educated in expanded roles; development of community health care services (health centers for ambulatory care)

Changes in nursing organizations

A. Canadian Nurses' Association
   1. In 1951, *Structure Study of the Canadian Nurses' Association* was undertaken by Dr. Pauline Jewett and the structure was changed in 1954
   2. Changes included
      a. Number of National Standing Committees reduced from 11 to 5
         (1) Nursing Service Committee
         (2) Nursing Education Committee
         (3) Public Relations Committee
         (4) Legislation and By-Laws Committee
         (5) Finance Committee
      b. Authority and responsibility for directing and operating the Canadian Nurses' Association delegated by its members to the board of directors composed of
         (1) A representative from each of the 10 provincial associations
         (2) Chairmen of the standing committees
         (3) Two members from nursing sisterhood
         (4) The President-elect
         (5) Two Vice-Presidents
         (6) The President
      c. The functions of the board of directors were to
         (1) Establish and revise policies
         (2) Appoint the executive director
         (3) Approve unusual expenditures
         (4) Implement the organization's program as determined at the annual meeting open to all members
   3. Objectives of the Canadian Nurses' Association as stated in the Constitution are to
      a. Promote the best interests of the members of the nursing profession and the general public
      b. Formulate policies in the fields of nursing service, nursing education, and employment relations, for the purpose of advising provincial associations with regard to the maintenance and improvement of the ethical and professional standards of nursing education and nursing service, and the economic standards of nursing employment
      c. Provide effective media for the exchange of information within the National Association and with other organizations
   4. Activities of the Canadian Nurses' Association include
      a. Acting as voice of the Canadian nursing profession at both national and international levels
      b. Being active internationally through the International Council of Nurses
   5. Canadian Nurses' Association celebrated its 50th anniversary in 1958, the year in which the first French-Canadian, Alice M. Girard, was elected President
   6. After a study of the administration

and organizational structure of the Canadian Nurses' Association in 1962, the following changes occurred
   a. The standing committees were reduced from 5 to 3 in 1966; Nursing Service, Nursing Education, and Social and Economic Welfare
   b. The Executive Committee became the Board of Directors
   c. The subcommittee of the Executive Committee became the Executive Committee
   d. The advisory and research functions were expanded
7. Activities included
   a. 1927—*Weir Report*
   b. 1936 and 1944—*Proposed Curricula for Schools of Nursing in Canada*
   c. 1947—published a Canadian Nursing History: *Three Centuries of Canadian Nursing*
   d. 1948 to 1952—supported project at Metropolitan Demonstration School of Nursing in Windsor, Ontario
   e. 1957—first Canadian Conference on Nursing held
   f. 1958—promoted development of Canadian Nurses' Association Retirement Fund
   g. 1960—*Spotlight on Nursing Education* published
   h. 1961—evaluation of quality of nursing service developed
   i. 1961—Canadian Nurses' Association and Kellogg Foundation established bilingual Nursing Unit Administration Extension Program
   j. 1962—established Canadian Nurses' Foundation
   k. 1965—carried out first national inventory of registered nurses
   l. 1967—undertook development of Canadian Nurses' Association Testing Service (CNATS) to be used by provincial associations for registration and for licensing purposes instead of the National League for Nursing Examinations
B. Student Nurses' Association—first organized system of student government in Canadian schools of nursing was established in 1917 at the Toronto General Hospital
C. Canadian University Nursing Student Association

D. Canadian Association of University Schools of Nursing (C.A.U.S.N.)
   1. Originally formed as Canadian Conference of University Schools of Nursing
   2. An association of 22 university schools from 9 provinces and a member of the Association of Universities and Colleges of Canada
   3. Concerned with health of the nation and university preparation of nurses
   4. In 1971, name was changed from Canadian Conference of University Schools of Nursing to allow for French translation—"Association Canadienne des Écoles Univérsitaires de Nursing"

Special interest organizations

A. The Canadian Association of Neurological and Neurosurgical Nurses (C.A.N.N.N.)
B. Canadian Council of Cardiovascular Nurses (C.C.C.N.)
C. Ontario Nurse Midwives Association
   1. Organized in 1974 and recognized as an affiliated group of Registered Nurses' Association of Ontario in 1975
   2. Membership open to nurses currently registered in any province of Canada who have successfully completed a prescribed midwifery course in a recognized educational program
   3. Purposes are to
      a. Promote care of mother and child during the maternity cycle
      b. Promote the education, licensure, and practice of the nurse midwife in Canada
      c. Function as liaison with other professional groups and the public
      d. Promote common interests of members of the Association
D. Canadian Red Cross—a national voluntary health and welfare organization that has been significantly involved with nursing
   1. After World War I—provided financial support for nurses and universities for higher education in nursing; supported public health nurses directly and through the Victorian Order of Nurses
   2. 1919—initiated training of public health nurses for work in rural and more isolated areas of Canada by

establishing programs in Nursing Station and Outpost Hospital Nursing
3. 1920—offered funds for developing public health nursing in universities (British Columbia, McGill, Dalhousie, Toronto, and Western Ontario)
4. After World War II—financially supported the Demonstration School of Nursing at Windsor, Ontario, the pioneer of independent diploma schools of nursing in Canada

International organizations

A. International Council of Nurses
1. A federation of National Nursing Associations of which Canada became the fourth member in 1909
2. Congress meets every 4 years and has met twice in Canada (1929 and 1969 in Montreal)
3. Canadian involvement with the International Congress
   a. 1924—Jean Gunn elected Second Vice-President serving until 1933, then as First Vice-President until 1939
   b. 1933—Florence Emory appointed Chairman of Membership Committee until 1953
   c. 1965—Alice Girard elected as President; first Canadian to hold this position
B. Order of St. John (St. John Ambulance Brigade)
1. Appeared as a formal organization in Canada in 1890
2. Linked to Canadian Nurses' Association through the presence of a member or officer on the Nursing Advisory Committee of the Order
3. Publishing activities include
   a. 1930—*St. John Home Nursing Manual*—a Canadian rather than a British edition
   b. 1951—*What the Home Nursing Auxiliary Should Know About Civil Defense and Child Care in the Home*
   c. 1954—*St. John Home Nursing Manual* revised to *Home Nursing Manual*
   d. *Patient Care in the Home*
C. World Health Organization—Canada's relationship closely parallels the United States' association with this organization

Advances in education

A. Early developments in university education
1. Several trends strengthened need for more advanced education for nurses
   a. Rapid, widening scope of medical practice
   b. General public concern regarding health and social welfare
   c. Increasingly critical evaluation of professional education
2. University of British Columbia offered the first baccalaureate degree course in nursing in the British Empire in 1919; patterned on the 2+2+1 pattern already established at the University of Minnesota
3. 1920—6 universities began certificate or diploma courses of 1-year duration in public health nursing and teaching and administration with grants from the Canadian Red Cross
   a. First course in public health nursing at Dalhousie University in Halifax
   b. First course in teaching and administration established at McGill University, Montreal
4. 1924—Grey Nuns organized first French language course in nursing education and ward administration for graduate nurses at University of Montreal
5. 1925—first French language public health nursing course in Canada established at University of Montreal
6. 1933—University of Toronto received Rockefeller Grant utilized in establishment of 4-year, integrated basic baccalaureate degree program that prepared graduates for varied types of nursing service (first program of this nature in Canada)
7. 1941—first joint conference of the Canadian Nurses' Association Executive Committee and directors of Canadian University Schools of Nursing
8. Problems in establishing university programming for nurses continued even in the 1940s because of
   a. Ambivalent approach of many nurses
   b. Lack of qualified staff
   c. Unwillingness of hospitals to accept loss of student time and service

d. Increased costs involved in higher education programs
9. No parallel development in graduate nursing education was occurring with the result that Canadian nurses went to the United States for postgraduate studies, a move that further delayed postgraduate programming in Canada

B. Developments in the second half of the century
1. Esther Lucile Brown's study, *Nursing for the Future* (published in the United States in 1948) had implications for nursing education in Canada
2. Only 2 significant national studies in nursing education had been done by the Canadian Nurses' Association
3. Hospitals owned and operated 90% of schools of nursing
4. Major development in the late 1950s was the establishment of a prepaid hospital insurance program that included the cost of operating nursing schools in hospitals despite the opposition of the nursing profession
5. Various types of nursing programs leading to the diploma rather than the baccalaureate degree exist in Canada today
   a. The traditional course in a hospital school of nursing in Alberta, British Columbia, Manitoba, New Brunswick (to be phased out in 1976), Nova Scotia, and Newfoundland
   b. The community college system in Quebec (Colleges d'Enseignement Général et Professional; the CEGEP Programs), Ontario, Alberta, Saskatchewan (Institutes of Applied Arts and Sciences), Newfoundland (started in 1975), British Columbia, and Manitoba
   c. The system of Regional and Independent Schools of Nursing in Prince Edward Island and New Brunswick
   d. The Programs for Psychiatric Nurses in British Columbia and Manitoba
6. Nightingale School of Nursing— Toronto
   a. Began in 1960
   b. A regional school that controlled the educational program and util-

ized resources within a given geographic area
   c. Supported by the Board of Governors of New Mount Sinai Hospital, Toronto
   d. Operating costs borne by the government of Ontario, with monies derived from the health insurance program
   e. Nightingale School was an alternative to the centralized school system in Alberta and the community college system in Quebec and British Columbia
7. Quo Vadis Nursing Program
   a. Founded in Toronto in 1964 somewhat as a result of a recommendation made by Dr. Mussallem in *Nursing Education in Canada* (1962)
   b. A nursing education for women between 30 and 50 years of age with privileges of living at home, and working a regular workday for 5 days per week
   c. First students graduated in 1966
   d. Program transferred into the community college system in 1973
8. Development of diploma programs in Ontario after 1965
   a. Minister of Health challenged pattern of diploma programs in Ontario by announcing that
      (1) Annual number of graduates would be doubled
      (2) Length of program would be reduced to 2 years within regional schools
      (3) A third internship year in a hospital nursing service would be required from 1965 to 1975
      (4) Schools would have own budgets with monies supplied by the Department of Health
   b. In 1969, the Provincial Association supported the abolition of the internship year as well as urging the financing of nurse education in the same way as other postsecondary programs
   c. In 1971, the internship program was phased out leaving nursing with a 2-year program pattern
   d. By 1973, all nursing education programs at the diploma level had

been transferred to the system of Colleges of Applied Arts and Technology

9. Accelerated nursing program at Grey Nun's Hospital School of Nursing—1966
   a. An experimental 2-year nursing program in the general educational system
   b. System for which students paid tuition
   c. Students were not used for hospital service
   d. Structured liberal education component was included
   e. Students wrote registration examinations at end of 2 years

10. 1966—Saskatchewan became first province in Canada to transfer authority for hospital schools of nursing from Department of Public Health to Department of Education

11. The Colleges d'Enseignement Général et Professional (CEGEP) Schools
    a. *Report of the Royal Commission of Inquiry on Education* (Parent Report) in Quebec suggested that nursing education move into the general educational system, a transfer approved by the Association of Nurses for the Province of Quebec (A.N.P.Q.)
    b. Provincial legislature adopted the *Criteria for College Education* from the Parent Report in 1964; among these were
       (1) All college teachers to have appropriate academic preparation
       (2) System of accreditation be established
       (3) Definite student-teacher ratio to be used
    c. 1966—Concept of nursing education in Colleges d'Enseignement Général et Professional (CEGEP) introduced with 3 colleges starting nursing options in 1967
    d. In 1972, last of schools of nursing based within hospitals closed their doors ending three fourths of a century of history
    e. 1972—after 5 years in the CEGEP system
       (1) Strengths are
           (a) Establishment of in-spector/consultant system to ensure unity and coordination of programs
           (b) An accreditation program for colleges
           (c) An interdisciplinary approach within a shortened program
           (d) A selective, meaningful clinical experience
       (2) Weaknesses are
           (a) Academic preparation of teaching staff (1972—52.2% of nursing teachers held less than baccalaureate degree in nursing)
           (b) No system of scholarships or study leave for teachers
           (c) Student-teacher clinical ratio

12. Diploma nursing programs in community college settings (including CEGEP programs)
    a. 1970—119 community colleges across Canada had 100,701 students enrolled in nursing programs —32,426 in university *stream* courses, 68,275 in vocational courses
    b. Distribution of male and female students in both vocational and university parallel courses is becoming equal
    c. A 2-year, unique educational program distinct from both secondary and higher levels of education is offered by 35 Quebec CEGEP schools
    d. Issues still unresolved include
       (1) Lack of employment for graduates of technical programs
       (2) Lack of space in university systems for students wishing higher education
       (3) Need for upgrading of teaching methods and curricula
       (4) Lack of clinical experiences of a desirable quality
       (5) Lack of prepared teachers in nursing

13. Development of baccalaureate degree programs
    a. 1961—in a brief presented to the *Royal Commission on Health Services in Canada,* The Canadian As-

sociation of University Schools of Nursing stated that a baccalaureate degree provided generalized preparation while masters and doctoral programs would prepare nursing consultants, experts in the clinical fields, and researchers

b. 1961—beginning of Extension Course in Nursing Unit Administration in Toronto, sponsored by the Canadian Nurses' Association with the financial support of the Kellogg Foundation, to assist head nurses in upgrading their skills in administration

c. 1963—similar course taught in French at the University of Montreal

d. 1962—University of Montreal became first university in Canada to establish a faculty of nursing with Alice M. Girard as Dean

e. First basic integrated degree program taught in French in the world instituted at Institut Marguerite d'Youville, Montreal, in 1962

f. 1966—awards made possible through the Canadian Nurses' Foundation for those pursuing baccalaureate degree programs

g. 1967—Institut Marguerite d'Youville amalgamated with the University of Montreal becoming the first university in the world to offer both undergraduate and graduate degrees in nursing taught in French

h. Trend was for the 3-year diploma graduates to enroll in supplementary university courses in nursing education, nursing service (special clinical courses), and public health

i. Some universities have phased out 1-year certificate courses in lieu of courses offering specialization in either clinical or functional areas of nursing or those offering a broad degree without a nursing specialty

j. Following *Royal Commission on Health Services in Canada,* nursing education began a new era with the major development being the general increase in the numbers of basic integrated baccalaureate programs
   (1) 1963—16 programs—8 integrated and 8 nonintegrated

   (2) 1967—26 programs—19 integrated and 7 nonintegrated

14. Baccalaureate program changes
    a. In 1973, the ratio of degree nurses to diploma nurses was 1:12
    b. 1973—University of British Columbia
       (1) Preparing students in degree programs for work in community, hospital, and acute and long-term care centers
       (2) Program permits students to become registered nurses on completion of first 2 years of baccalaureate program
    c. 1974—Canadian Association of University Schools of Nursing developed and tested criteria for the evaluation of University nursing programs
       (1) Focus in curriculum is nursing process, nursing functions, role definition, and expansion to include nurses' role in expanded functions such as health maintenance, primary assessment, and community health
       (2) Increasing utilization of self-study approaches

15. Higher degree programs
    a. Nurses wanting to pursue graduate study in nursing beyond baccalaureate degree until 1959 were required to do so in the United States (majority enrolled at Teachers' College, Columbia University)
    b. Masters programs in Canada could not evolve until sufficient numbers of baccalaureate programs and graduates had been produced
    c. 1959—University of Western Ontario established the first Canadian masters degree program in nursing followed by McGill University
    d. 1962—Canadian Nurses' Foundation was incorporated to provide monies for study at masters and doctoral levels, and for research in nursing service
    e. 1974—McGill University School of Nursing revised the masters program to offer 2 options: nurse clinician and nurse researcher programs
    f. Masters programs offered in 1974 include University of Western On-

tario, McGill University, University of Montreal, University of Toronto, and McMaster University at Hamilton

g. No doctorate programs are yet available in Canada but plans are being drawn up to provide for these in the near future

16. University programs offered through schools of nursing as of 1973 according to *The Canadian Nurse Journal* (January, 1973)
   a. Baccalaureate degree courses
      (1) Integrated, 4-year courses for studies following high school offered by 22 universities
      (2) Baccalaureate degree courses for registered nurses offered by 14 universities
   b. Masters degree programs
      (1) Two-year offered by 7 universities
      (2) One-year offered by 1 university
   c. Certificate courses offered by 5 universities
   d. Family practice nurse program offered by 1 university
   e. Outpost nursing program offered by 1 university
   f. Doctorate programs not offered in any Canadian university
   g. Health science centers are integrated with nursing programs at 2 universities

17. Nonuniversity programs for preparation of nursing personnel as per Canadian Hospital Directory 1974
   a. Hospital schools offering a diploma in nursing—26
   b. Diploma nursing programs in provincial educational systems—76
   c. Diploma nursing programs in regional and independent schools —5
   d. Psychiatric nurse preparation programs in British Columbia, Alberta, Saskatchewan, and Manitoba—7
   e. Nursing assistant programs—71 in all provinces except Quebec where this level of health worker is prepared in Polyvalent schools administered by regional school boards, and licensed by the Professional Corporation of Nursing Assistants of Quebec (P.C.N.A.Q.)

   f. Postdiploma programs for registered nursing assistants available in
      (1) Operating room technician at Humber College, Toronto, Ontario
      (2) Operating room nursing and techniques at the Wascana Institute of Applied Arts and Sciences, Regina, Saskatchewan
   g. Program for registered nursing assistants certificate of achievement in the practice and supervision of care in long-term facilities at Centennial College, Scarborough, Ontario

18. Licensed practical nurse programs
   a. Uncommon in Canada
   b. Nursing orderlies in some provinces are certified on completion of programs; e.g., Alberta Association of Registered Nursing Orderlies, Manitoba Association of Certified Nursing Orderlies
   c. Graduates eligible for licensure as practical nurses (LPN) are those from nursing orderly program and the Nursing Assistant Program at Camosun College, Victoria, British Columbia

19. *Canadian Nurses' Association Position Paper on Nursing Education* (1960s)—supported the following
   a. All nursing education programs should be under the jurisdiction of institutes whose primary aim is education
   b. Two types of nurses be prepared— university and nonuniversity
   c. Graduates of diploma programs to possess high degree of technical skill and to be prepared to assist in assessment of nursing needs and problems
   d. A merging of the roles of the diploma program registered nurse and registered nursing assistant be considered

20. Canadian Testing Service Examinations
   a. Established in 1970 by the Canadian Nurses' Association Testing Service (CNATS); now used in all jurisdictions
   b. Membership of Canadian Nurses'

Association are involved in all phases of test construction

c. Operation of testing service is directed by Test Service Board

d. Examination planning committee coordinates planning of the master blueprint committee with test service board objectives

e. Master blueprint committee constructs overall plan for examinations

f. Blueprint subcommittees have representatives from Canada's main regions—Atlantic, Ontario, Quebec, West, and French language representatives

g. Item writers prepare items on the basis of shared knowledge, current thinking, and practice patterns in various nursing regions

h. Jurisdictional appraisal committee (provincial) review test items to ensure that content meets their legal requirements for registration

i. By 1976, all jurisdictions will accept 350 as a passing score

j. The Canadian Testing Service has facilitated interprovincial registration for nurses (registration is annual)

Advances in nursing service

A. During the early 1930s the majority of nurses were employed in private practice and most of the hospital nursing service was provided by student nurses as part of the training program

B. Employment of graduate nurses for staff nursing in hospitals increased in the late 1930s after the publication of the *Weir Report* in 1932 and as a result of the economic depression

C. The crisis after World War II
   1. World War II left nursing in an even greater state of chaos than World War I because the demands for nursing service were rapidly increased (as a result of newer treatment methods and social changes), while students entering nursing programs declined
   2. Nurses with leadership preparation were lacking as a direct result of the economic depression following the war and the absence of educational programs above the basic level

D. A study of head nurse activities in the

general hospital was carried out by the Department of National Health and Welfare in 1953
   1. Head nurses were not in control of the work situation and felt inadequately equipped to handle the job by training, authority, and experience
   2. Precipitated the development and implementation of certificate courses related to nursing service administration at some universities

E. In 1961, the Canadian Nurses' Association in cooperation with the Canadian Hospital Association sponsored an extension course in Nursing Unit Administration in Toronto; financial support for the project was provided by the W. K. Kellogg Foundation

F. Development of programs for nursing assistants
   1. First formal acknowledgment of the need for auxiliary workers was made on behalf of hospitals when expanding pressures forced an examination of the jobs being done by various hospital workers
   2. This beginning fragmentation laid the foundation for the present partitioning of hospital nursing services and the numbers and categories of workers providing these services
   3. A large group of young women needed to be absorbed from women's military forces into civilian life, and government funds were used to organize schools for the preparation of nursing assistants from the group of ex-service women
   4. Approval and support of the nursing profession was given to the proposal to initiate courses of 9- to 12-month duration in educational settings
   5. Title for new worker suggested by the Canadian Nurses' Association was "nursing assistant" and with it came the thrust of the nursing assistant program across Canada
   6. In 1960, 43 nursing assistant programs were operating with certification or registration of the graduate on completion of the program and writing of examination administered through the Provincial Department of Health, the Provincial Registered Nurses' Associations, and the Boards of Registration of Nursing Assistants

7. The categories of workers in nursing proliferated in the 1960s and included
   a. Registered nurses (university and diploma programs)
   b. Nursing assistants
   c. Psychiatric nurses
   d. Orderlies and attendants
   e. Operating room technicians
8. Problems with proliferation included
   a. A great deal of direct nursing care being given by nursing assistants
   b. A blurring of roles between the registered nurse and the registered nursing assistant
   c. Increasing need for nurses to spend time in teaching and supervisory functions
   d. Increasing desire of nursing assistants for advancement
9. In 1968 at the general meeting of the Canadian Nurses' Association, the recommendation to gradually phase out programs from which practitioners on graduation were not eligible for licensure as registered nurses was approved

G. Definition of nursing, nursing roles, and levels of function
   1. At least 7 provincial associations have position papers related to the definition of nursing, nursing roles, and levels of function
   2. In 1967, the Canadian Nurses' Association published a paper on the roles, functions, and educational preparation for the practice of nursing and proposed a ratio of 1 professional to 3 technical nurses

H. In its *Statement of Delivery of Nursing Care* the Nurses' Association recommended that
   1. Standards of determining the levels of nursing care be formulated from within the nursing profession
   2. A clear distinction be made between nursing and nonnursing activities
   3. Objectives of the health agency as well as the means for achieving stated goals be defined by the nursing service

I. Team nursing
   1. See background material under American section, pp. 268-269
   2. In 1968, Registered Nurses' Association of Ontario offered practical experience in team nursing in a demonstration center supported by Ontario Hospital Services Commission, Ontario Department of Health, and Ontario Public Health Association
      a. Project involved 8 hospitals, an official public health agency, and a voluntary nursing agency
      b. Implementation of team nursing in a controlled situation occurred after participants learned to prepare nursing care plans, conduct team conferences, delegate activities to other nursing personnel
      c. Team nursing development project served to teach nurses how to coordinate care of patients in hospitals, but more important how to coordinate care by involving hospitals, voluntary agencies, and public health teams to promote continuity of patient care

J. Employment of nurses
   1. In the early 1970s, 70% of employed nurses
      a. Were employed in hospital settings
      b. Lacked any additional preparation beyond basic diploma program training (only 5% showed evidence of added preparation)
      c. Were unable with their preparation to initiate any substantial change in a rigid, outmoded system of care
   2. Nursing leaders suggested
      a. A systematic study of the relationship between general duty nurse turnover rates and their opportunity to utilize their knowledge and make independent judgments
      b. Research into nursing care to establish criteria for measuring quality of care being given
      c. An extension of the role of the nurse as a real possibility in the profession's development

K. Accreditation of health care facilities
   1. In 1970, Canadian Council on Hospital Accreditation expanded its program to include accreditation of the 3000 extended care facilities across Canada
   2. In 1974, the Canadian Nurses' Association withdrew its official support for mandatory accreditation of all health agencies and joined with the Canadian Hospital Association in supporting voluntary accreditation

Legislation related to nurses and nursing

A. Economic security and nurse welfare
1. Labor relations and collective bargaining
   a. 1944—Canadian Nurses' Association recognized collective bargaining as a useful process in bettering socioeconomic status of nurses
   b. 1946—British Columbia became first province to introduce collective bargaining
   c. 1970s—nurses in British Columbia, Alberta, Manitoba, Ontario, Quebec, New Brunswick, and Nova Scotia had become organized and certified under provincial labor legislation
   d. "Strike right"—some Canadian nurses have right to strike according to provincial legislation in Quebec, Ontario (except for hospitals), Nova Scotia, British Columbia
   e. Provincial Nurses' Association in Quebec does not bargain for nurses, as a collective bargaining unit; Quebec nurses are members of professional syndicates—English Chapter formed the United Nurses of Montreal in 1966 and La Fédération des Syndicats Professionels d'Infirmières du Quebec, which includes nurses, physiotherapists, etc.
2. Federal Government Employees Compensation Act
   a. Provides coverage for federal government employees injured in the course of their employment
   b. In most instances, collective agreements for nurses contain clauses incorporating workmen's compensation benefits
3. Pension plans
   a. 1958—Canadian Nurses' Association implemented a retirement plan
   b. Canada Pension Plan, established in 1965 by an act of Parliament, makes financial provision for retirement and protects against loss of income in event of severe disability (Quebec nurses eligible under the Quebec Pension Plan)
   c. Approximately 92% of Canada's labor force contributes to either Canada or Quebec Pension Plan

4. Unemployment insurance benefits
   a. Nurses in Ontario became eligible as contributors to the Unemployment Insurance Plan in 1972
   b. Since that time coverage for nurses has been expanded to include pregnancy leave
5. Liability insurance plan for nurses
   a. Development of a national liability insurance plan deferred since only 3 provincial nurses' associations lack a plan of this type
   b. Manitoba Association of Registered Nurses was the latest provincial association to obtain group professional liability insurance in 1974

B. National Health Insurance
1. 1966—following a recommendation from the *Royal Commission on Health Services* (1961), the Medical Care Act received royal assent
2. 1971—all provinces are participants in National Health Insurance except Northwest and Yukon territories, which implemented programs by 1972
3. 1973—Hospital Insurance and Diagnostic Services and Medical Care Directorates amalgamated to administer the 2 national health insurance schemes—Hospital Insurance and Medicare
4. National Health Insurance increased the demand for medical and nursing services in agencies other than hospitals and institutions; e.g., health clinics

C. The Health Disciplines Act—Ontario
1. Received royal assent in 1974 but was not proclaimed law until July, 1975
2. Incorporated recommendations from Committee on the Healing Arts and *Royal Commission Inquiry into Civil Rights*
3. Allowed for lay representation in the professional governing council
4. Created health disciplines board to conduct hearings related to complaints and applications for licensing
5. Gave Council of the College of Nurses of Ontario authority to
   a. Initially register new members and renew registration of standing members
   b. Require nursing personnel to be currently registered with College of Nurses

c. Discipline any person granted initial registration
d. Protect titles—Registered Nurse, Nurse, and Registered Nursing Assistant
e. Establish, maintain, and develop standards of knowledge, skill, and professional ethics

D. Nurse practice acts
1. Nursing is recognized by provincial statutes (Nurses' Acts)
2. Purpose of registration
   a. Registration allows for protection of the general public by distinguishing the trained nurse from the untrained nurse
   b. Protects title of "registered nurse" for persons who have successfully passed registration examinations
3. Enactment
   a. Was first enacted in Nova Scotia (1910), followed by Manitoba (1913), New Brunswick and Alberta (1916), Ontario (1922)
   b. Is administered by provincial associations except in Ontario where College of Nurses registers nurses and in Quebec where Order of Nurses of Province of Quebec licenses nurses for nursing practice
4. Control
   a. In Ontario, with the Nurses' Act of 1961 amended, the College of Nurses of Ontario was established as the governing body of nursing with provision also for governing of nursing assistants (now titled Registered Nursing Assistant)
   b. As of February 1974 only 1 nurses' association had right of appeal to a legal definition of nursing written into law—the Order of Nurses of Quebec
   c. Other 9 provinces have permissive licensure/registration based on inspection and approval of nursing programs
   d. The Order of Nurses of Quebec
      (1) Professional Code of the Province of Quebec proclaimed in February 1974 the changing of the title of Association of the Nurses of the Province of Quebec (A.N.P.Q.) to the Order of Nurses of Quebec (O.N.Q.)

whose chief purpose is protection of the public
      (2) Passage of the Professional Code created professional groups of which 11 have exclusive rights to practice while 10 regulate only title of the health worker
      (3) Quebec Nurses' Act now defines profession of nursing as identification of persons' health needs, assisting with diagnosis, employing nursing interventions, and communication of health problems to clients
   e. Northwest Territories Registered Nurses' Association (N.W.T.R.N.A.)
      (1) January, 1975 the Ordinance Respecting the Nursing Profession in the Northwest Territories was approved by Territorial Council
      (2) Gave Northwest Territories Registered Nurses' Association the authority to
         (a) Join with the Canadian Nurses' Association
         (b) Grant and/or revoke certificates of registration to nurses practicing in the Northwest Territories
         (c) Discipline members of the nursing profession
         (d) Lay claim to being the first professional group north of the sixtieth parallel to acquire registration control over its members
5. Purposes of Nurses' Acts
   a. In most provinces Acts do not define legal boundaries in terms of nursing functions although there is concerted effort by provincial associations to define nursing practice
   b. Provide for interprovincial registration if credentials are equivalent
   c. In some provinces, provide for the licensing of nursing assistants

Accreditation of nursing programs

A. Approval of programs
1. Nursing programs are provincially

controlled within the general health category

2. Provincial associations establish minimum standards and approve nursing programs upon satisfactory inspection
3. Some provinces utilize other approval channels
   a. In Manitoba, an accrediting committee of nurses and nonnurses establishes minimum standards that are approved by the Board of the Provincial Association
   b. In Ontario, the Council of the College of Nurses establishes regulations for programs and inspects nursing centers
4. Approved nursing programs listed in the *Canadian Hospital Directory* and Canadian Nurses' Association publications
5. Association of Community Colleges in Canada is implementing a process by which National Standards for Health Science Programs will be promoted
6. Nursing programs cannot function without approval as specified under individual provincial Nurses' Acts

B. Accreditation
1. 1967—Executive Director of Canadian Nurses' Association consulted with the National League for Nursing on the accreditation process
2. 1972—publication of *Canadian Nurses' Association Position on Accreditation*
3. 1973—self-evaluation tools formulated on which criteria for accreditation will be based
4. 1974—optimum standards for nursing education developed by Canadian Nurses' Association
5. 1975—no system of accreditation provincially or nationally has been established although the majority of provinces favor national accreditation with leadership being provided by Canadian Nurses' Association

Nursing publications

A. *The Canadian Nurse* (1955) (*L'infirmière Canadienne*)
1. Began under sponsorship of the Alumnae Association of Toronto General Hospital; later purchased by the Canadian Nurses' Association
2. The French language journal, *L'infirmière Canadienne*, began in 1959

3. Full-time editors for the English and French journals were appointed in 1965; the Executive Director of the Canadian Nurses' Association is responsible for management and production
4. Published monthly and cost has been included in membership fee since 1966

B. *Three Centuries of Canadian Nursing* (1947)
1. A text sponsored by the Canadian Nurses' Association
2. Written by John Murray Gibbon and Mary S. Mathewson

C. *Countdown: Canadian Nursing Statistics* (1968)
1. Published by Canadian Nurses' Association
2. Based on data collected by the research unit of the Association

D. *The Leaf and the Lamp* (1968)
1. A sequel to the Canadian Nurses' Association publication, *The First Fifty Years* (1958)
2. Published as the organization approached its diamond anniversary
3. A text that presents a contemporary and historic sketch of the organization over its first 60 years

E. *Nursing Papers* (1969)
1. A publication of the School for Graduate Nurses, McGill University
2. Functions as an invitation to nurses to discuss, make critical comments, and express views; mailed to subscribers, university schools of nursing, diploma schools, and agencies interested in nurse education

F. Other publications—see publications under American section, p. 271

Nursing service in the federal government

A. Department of National Health and Welfare
1. Founded in 1919 as the Department of Pensions and National Health
2. Current title adapted in 1944
3. In 1945, nursing positions were established within the Department
   a. Dorothy Percy, Chief Nursing Consultant (1953-1967)
   b. Verna Hoffman (1967 to present) serves as Nursing Advisor to Deputy Minister of Health

4. Since 1960, the Department has co-sponsored 6 nursing conferences with the provinces at which major concerns to nurses were discussed
5. Medical Services Branch of the Department of National Health and Welfare includes these activity areas
   a. Indian Health Services
   b. Northern Health Services
   c. Civil Aviation Medicine
   d. Public Service Health
   e. Immigration Medical Services
   f. Quarantine and Regulatory Services
   g. Prosthetic Services
   h. Emergency Health Services
6. Nurses are employed in Indian and Northern Health Services, Public Service Health, Quarantine and Emergency Health Activities
   a. Indian Health Service
      (1) Program focus shifted from merely treatment to include prevention and teaching
      (2) Programs include immunization, chronic disease control, alcohol abuse correction program, personal health and sanitation, maternal and child care, nutrition
   b. Northern Health Services
      (1) Joint program supported by both federal and territorial governments
      (2) Uses the community health aide as well as the Northern Health Service nurse to carry out program
B. Military services
   1. Royal Canadian Army Medical Corps (R.C.A.M.C.)
      a. Small number served as Canadian Army Medical Corps Reserve Nursing Sisters prior to World War I
      b. Numbers were enlarged during the war and decreased at the conclusion
      c. Expanded during World War II and in 1945, 3600 nurses served with the Royal Canadian Army in military hospitals in Canada and overseas
      d. Nursing sisters from the Royal Canadian Army Medical Corps also served with the Royal Canadian

Air Force and by 1945 the total reached 373
   2. Royal Canadian Naval Nursing Service
      a. Established in 1941
      b. Nursing sisters became sub-Lieutenants after 6 months of service
   3. Canadian Armed Forces Medical Service
      a. Established in 1959
      b. Integrated medical service of army, navy, and air force
      c. Lieutenant Commander Mary Nesbitt was named first Matron-in-Chief
      d. Male nurses were commissioned in 1968
C. Department of Veterans' Affairs—established in 1944 to provide dental, medical, and prosthetic services for veterans
D. Principal Nursing Officer
   1. Serves in an advisory capacity to Deputy Minister of Health on local, national, or international nursing matters
   2. Provides for nursing representation at the Federal Provincial Meeting on Health Standards
   3. Distributes position papers prepared by federal nursing consultants

Current developments

A. Need for a clear legal definition of nursing
   1. Canadian Health Manpower statistics in 1974 showed 14 professional classifications engaged in health care with a fragmentation of care and a clouding of roles
   2. New definition of nursing must
      a. Establish a well-defined role
      b. Provide for accountability
B. Mandatory versus voluntary continuing education for nurses
   1. Debate continues as to whether continuing education should be a mandatory or voluntary requirement for nurse registration and licensure
   2. The pressure for continuing education as a prerequisite for renewal of the license to practice nursing is becoming more urgent
C. The Canadian Nurses' Association—continuing leadership for the present and the future
   1. With a 1975 membership of 104,000

nurses, the Canadian Nurses' Association continues to

a. Promote highest possible standards of nursing care
b. Strive for structure that will assure nurse accountability
c. Encourage preparation of guidelines for standards of nurse preparation, continuing competence in practice, and legal protection especially in areas of expanded nurse roles
d. Explore ways of raising the level of nurse awareness to life-styles that foster optimum health
e. Explore development of standards for ongoing education as a requirement for registration/licensure
f. Stimulate and develop interest in ongoing research in nursing

2. The established priorities for 1974 to 1976 are
a. Evaluation of nursing care
b. Evaluation of educational programs for nurses
c. Evaluation of nurse competence
d. Advancement of nursing research
e. Advancement of the health and rights of the individual

3. Code of Ethics, uniquely Canadian, will be developed by the Association utilizing as a base
a. The International Council of Nurses' Code of Ethics (1973)
b. The Canadian Nurses' Association Statement Related to Ethics of Nursing Research (1972)
c. Provincial legislation and policies

4. Economic welfare for members of the nursing profession remains a major concern of the Association

D. Research in nursing—Canadian Council of Nurse Researchers
1. 1974—Third National Conference on Research in Nursing, projecting that numbers of nurse researchers would increase at all levels, appointed a task force to explore development of a Canadian Council of Nurse Researchers
2. 1974—research unit set up by McGill University in nursing and health care to develop, study, and evaluate the nurse's expanded function especially in primary care
3. 1975—Fourth National Conference on Nursing Research focused on developing indicators for nursing research

E. Nursing education
1. Career ladder concept
a. Supports curriculum that allows articulation with succeeding levels so that one may proceed from nursing assistant level to diploma level etc.; a program is available in Saskatchewan where practical nurses can become diploma graduates
b. Report of a Royal Commission headed by Dr. Leonard Miller strongly supports the career ladder in Newfoundland
c. Humber College of Applied Arts and Technology in Toronto has developed an experimental curriculum that
(1) Offers core courses for nurses and allied health workers
(2) Allows students to elect to continue toward a nursing diploma or a registered nursing assistant certificate after the common initial semester
d. Success of the career ladder approach still remains unproved

2. Changes in curriculum
a. Revision of baccalaureate degree programs to include increased content on community health
b. Graduation of larger numbers of 2-year diploma (community college) and baccalaureate students
c. Specialization at masters level has resulted in the introduction of clinical specialists into health care agencies
d. 1972—Canadian Nurses' Association issued *Statement of the Expanded Role of the Nurse* urging modification of educational programs to allow nurses to enter a variety of health care settings

3. Nurse practitioner programs
a. 1971—The National Conference on Assistance to the Physician recommended that Canada not develop programs to produce "physician's assistants" but rather to augment nursing programs to develop nurse practitioners
b. *Report of the Committee on Nurse Practitioners* (Boudreau Report) (1972)—special Committee estab-

lished by Minister of National Health and Welfare to study role of the nurse practitioner; offered description of nurse practitioners' role and recommended

(1) The delegation of specific, defined tasks by physicians to appropriately prepared nurses

(2) That nurse practitioner preparation be eventually incorporated within baccalaureate programs

(3) That development of nurse practitioner programs become a priority

(4) That basic preparations of nurses at diploma and university levels reflect broadened concept of nursing

(5) That nurse practitioners receive courses in educational institutions affiliated with university health science centers; by 1972, 1 pilot project in nurse practitioner programs was operating; several universities were conducting ad hoc classes for family practice nurses; 6 universities were providing outpost nursing courses; Quebec nurses were exploring the *community nurse* concept

c. 1973—Canadian Nurses' Association issued *Statement on Specialization in Nursing* supporting degrees or levels of specialization in nursing after a basic diploma or baccalaureate program

F. Nursing service

1. Expanded role

a. Four patterns of expanding role of nurse in primary care are emerging

(1) Physician's associate

(2) Community health nurse

(3) Northern Health Service nurse

(4) Primary health care worker

b. Definitions of nurse practitioner are drafted in 7 provinces while 4 provinces (Alberta, Saskatchewan, Ontario, Manitoba) are amending their Nurse Practice Acts to provide for the nurse's expanded role

2. Problem oriented medical records

a. Approach to health records that re-quires a patient-centered focus to define presenting problems

b. 1974—Science Council of Canada submitted a report, *Science for Health Services,* recommending that health care be organized into an integrated system using computer-based health information systems and standardized health records

c. Canadian Nurses' Association recognized value of application of science technology to the health care system (problem-oriented medical records) but deferred endorsement of a single approach as the solution to problems in the health care system

3. Peer review

a. Quality of nursing care given to clients is evaluated in terms of formulated standards of nursing practice

b. A useful evaluation tool for assisting individual nurses to improve their care and for assessing nurses for advancement

c. Essential for nurse accountability for care provided

4. Clinical specialists

a. Definition—nurses prepared at the masters level who possess advanced knowledge, skill, and clinical competence in specialized areas

b. Use—it is predicted that use will increase as more nurses are prepared

G. Developments related to and influencing nursing

1. *Community Health Center Project* (The Hasting Report) (1972)

a. Initiated by Minister of National Health and Welfare to describe community health centers and to determine problems in health center development

b. Recommendations included that

(1) Provinces develop community health centers

(2) Patient-centered, problem-solving approaches be used by all health personnel

(3) A comprehensive system for evaluation of community health centers be instituted

(4) Public health functions continue as a vital part of the health services system
2. *A New Perspective on the Health of Canadians* (1974)— published by the Minister of National Health and Welfare
   a. A document that presents policies to be developed in the health care system within the next 10 to 15 years
   b. Report presented a study of the major causes of death and illness and from these identified the major health problems of the Canadian population
   c. Major focus is on the *health field concept* composed of 4 principal parts—human biology, environment, life-style, and health care organization
   d. Recommendations included that
      (1) The value system of health care organizations be revised
      (2) Programs be initiated to create safer environments and life-styles that foster good health
      (3) Programs geared to the reduction of self-imposed health risks be implemented through government involvement in public education programs
      (4) Programs directed at "neglected" areas of Canadian population be initiated; i.e., programs for the aged, mentally ill, economically deprived, chronically ill, troubled parents and children, etc.
   e. Key proposition for nursing related to
      (1) Reduction of environmental hazards and self-imposed health risks in the population
      (2) Family counselling
      (3) Care of the mentally and chronically ill
      (4) Care of the aged population
      (5) Provision of home care
3. Proliferation of personnel in health care field
   a. Increasing number of health workers and/or professionals who have roles in provision of health services; e.g., operating room technicians, respiratory technicians, nutritionists, dental assistants, etc.
   b. Need for role reevaluation, role modifications, role definitions, and curricular evaluation and change
4. Changes in medical practice patterns such as
   a. Emergence of group practice
   b. Use of the family practice physicians in family practice settings
   c. Increasing specialization
   d. Increasing use of organ transplants
   e. Involvement in research in drug and alcohol use
   f. Increasing safety of surgical interventions including anesthesia
   g. Regionalization of services
   h. Planning for and reevaluation of abortion practices
   i. Addition of the nurse practitioner; e.g., family nurse practitioner, pediatric nurse practitioner
   j. Increasing use of electronic prostheses and computerized assistance with diagnosis
   k. Expanded immunization programs for viral and bacterial diseases
   l. Addition of clinical nurse specialists
5. Other social and economic factors that will influence the delivery of health care include
   a. Spiralling costs of health care
   b. Increasing number of aged
   c. Malnutrition
   d. Cost of housing
   e. Unemployment
H. Nursing manpower
   1. Controversy still exists as to whether or not there is a shortage of nurses
   2. Need for a study on nurse employment and nurse utilization has been recognized and the Health Manpower Directorate has requested the Center for Economic Studies at the University of Montreal to develop such a project

REVIEW QUESTIONS FOR HISTORY AND TRENDS IN NURSING AND NURSING EDUCATION IN THE UNITED STATES AND CANADA

1. Hippocrates is known as
   1. A god in Greek mythology
   2. The father of modern medicine
   3. A Greek military leader
   4. The founder of psychology
2. Florence Nightingale is best known for
   1. The nursing of wounded and ill soldiers in the Crimean War
   2. The reform of prisons in England

3. Being Superintendent of the Training School, St. Thomas Hospital
4. Being the leader of a religious order devoted to nursing

3. Nursing schools in the United States developed under the Nightingale plan soon changed because
   1. The plan was inappropriate for the United States
   2. Financial problems soon affected the schools and hospitals assumed control
   3. Nursing leaders felt hospital control would improve programs
   4. There were insufficient numbers of students in the schools under this plan

4. The first trained nurse in America was
   1. Clara Barton
   2. Dorothea Dix
   3. Linda Richards
   4. Jeanne Mance

5. The first school of nursing in the United States was
   1. Bellevue Hospital Training School
   2. Illinois Training School
   3. Johns Hopkins Training School
   4. St. Luke's Hospital Training School for Nurses

6. The American Red Cross was founded by
   1. Clara Barton
   2. Lillian Wald
   3. Jane Delano
   4. Isabel Hampton Robb

7. The first nurse to hold a university professorship was
   1. Annie Goodrich
   2. Isabel Stewart
   3. Lillian Wald
   4. Adelaide Nutting

8. The first school of nursing to be organized as an integral part of a university was
   1. Vanderbilt University School of Nursing
   2. Western Reserve School of Nursing
   3. Yale University School of Nursing
   4. The University of Minnesota School of Nursing

9. Nursing programs are accredited by
   1. The American Nurses' Association
   2. The National League for Nursing
   3. The American Hospital Association
   4. Regional accrediting agencies

10. The American Nurses' Association's stated priority is
    1. Improved education for nursing practitioners
    2. Collective action for quality of nursing care
    3. Cooperation with other health professionals
    4. Legislative action for nursing and nursing education

11. The American Nurses' Foundation
    1. Raises funds for nursing education
    2. Promotes research and studies in nursing
    3. Is a lay organization interested in nursing
    4. Is a part of the Florence Nightingale Foundation

12. Membership in the National Student Nurses' Association
    1. Is open to all nursing students, individually
    2. Is required by each nursing school

3. Provides membership in the Student Health Association
4. Is available only to collegiate program students

13. Membership in the International Council of Nurses
    1. Is automatic if a member of American Nurses' Association
    2. Is limited only to national professional organizations
    3. Is available to anyone who applies for it
    4. Includes lay as well as nurse members

14. The World Health Organization (W.H.O.)
    1. Organized Expert Committees on Nursing (1950)
    2. Recognizes only physicians as health workers
    3. Makes no provision for nursing or nurses
    4. Uses services of lay people only

15. Nurses in the military nurse corps have
    1. Permanent rank including general and admiral
    2. Relative ranking up to the rank of captain and major
    3. No commissions, but are warrant officers
    4. No commissions, but are civil service

16. The National League for Nursing is
    1. For hospitals and health agencies only
    2. A nursing interest organization
    3. For registered nurses only
    4. Limited to lay members only

17. Membership in the American Nurses' Association
    1. Is required for employment in areas of specialization
    2. Is available to any currently registered professional nurse
    3. Includes both professional and practical nurses
    4. Includes full-time students enrolled in nursing programs

18. The National Federation of Licensed Practical Nurses, Inc. is
    1. A branch of the American Nurses' Association
    2. Recognized by American Nurses' Association as an official organization
    3. Now a part of the National League for Nursing
    4. Concerned only with education of practical nurses

19. The list of National League for Nursing accredited schools is published annually in
    1. *Nursing Outlook*
    2. *American Journal of Nursing*
    3. *Nursing Research*
    4. *Journal of Practical Nursing*

20. Extended role of the nurse includes being
    1. A physician's assistant
    2. Capable of primary care
    3. A nurse anesthetist
    4. A nurse midwife

21. Baccalaureate degree nursing programs prepare for
    1. Professional practice of nursing
    2. Practice as clinical specialists
    3. Technical practice of nursing
    4. Any kind of nursing practice

22. The associate degree nursing program enrolls
    1. One fourth of all students in nursing programs
    2. One half of all students in nursing programs
    3. One third of all students in nursing programs
    4. Three fourths of all students in nursing programs
23. The associate degree nursing program
    1. Was developed through the Cooperative Research Project
    2. Is a variation of the hospital diploma program
    3. Is an upgrading of the practical nurse program
    4. Includes only theory given in a college
24. The number of diploma nursing programs has
    1. Paralleled the growth in hospitals
    2. Increased annually since 1900
    3. Remains relatively constant
    4. Been declining since 1955
25. The functions of the practical nurse are
    1. Similar to those of the professional nurse
    2. Specifically controlled by law
    3. More limited than those of the professional nurse
    4. Within the jurisdiction of the employing agency
26. Nurses employed in the Veterans Administration are
    1. Commissioned officers
    2. Classified as professionals
    3. Classified as paraprofessionals
    4. Members of the military corps
27. The National Committee for the Study of Nursing and Nursing Education Report recommended
    1. Single licensing of all in nursing occupation
    2. Separate licensing for technical and professional nursing
    3. Institutional licensure, which includes nursing
    4. Elimination of licensing of individual nurses
28. Peer review is essential if nurses are
    1. To circumvent evaluation by supervisors
    2. To be accountable for quality of nursing care
    3. Not well qualified for their positions
    4. Not to fall under medical control
29. Primary nursing is a way of organizing nursing service so that a nurse
    1. Is responsible for total care of patient
    2. Serves as a team leader
    3. Plans but does not carry out care
    4. Oversees the nursing care done by others
30. The external degree nursing program makes it possible for individuals to
    1. Become eligible for licensure without preparation
    2. Validate knowledge and competency in nursing by examination
    3. Practice nursing without licensure by examination
    4. Secure a degree without preparation for nursing
31. The first official statement recognizing technical nursing and professional nursing practice was the
    1. American Nurses' Association Position Paper on Education
    2. Report of Esther Lucile Brown, *Nursing For the Future*
    3. Curriculum Guide for schools of nursing
    4. National League for Nursing statement on open curriculum
32. The Position Paper on Education of the American Nurses' Association
    1. Advocated accreditation of nursing programs
    2. Recognized 2 types of nursing practice
    3. Set standards for faculty members
    4. Recommended student admission qualifications
33. The *American Journal of Nursing* is the official organ of the
    1. International Congress of Nurses
    2. National League for Nursing
    3. Committee on State Boards of Nursing
    4. American Nurses' Association
34. The Hill-Burton Act provided for
    1. Scholarships and loans for students
    2. The construction of hospitals and health agencies
    3. The construction of nursing school facilities
    4. Hospital and medical care for persons 65 years of age or older
35. The licensing of nurses to practice nursing is
    1. The responsibility of the National League for Nursing
    2. Under jurisdiction of the American Nurses' Association
    3. Controlled by federal legislation
    4. A function of the state
36. Institutional licensure makes it possible for an institution
    1. To employ even those who are licensed under specific acts
    2. To set up plans and procedures for peer review
    3. To determine which individuals are competent for the kinds of positions needed
    4. To use unqualified individuals to perform tasks required by hospitals
37. The Nurse Training Acts of 1964, 1968, and 1971 provided
    1. Financial aid to schools of nursing
    2. Consultation service to schools of nursing
    3. Requirements for accreditation of schools of nursing
    4. Licensing requirements for graduate nurses
38. The redefining of nursing in Nurse Practice Acts is essential if nurses are to
    1. Function in the expanded role
    2. Be controlled under institutional licensure
    3. Be involved in peer review
    4. Obtain the status of a profession
39. The first comprehensive legislation for nursing education was
    1. The Nurse Training Act, 1943
    2. The Bolton Act, 1943
    3. The Works Progress Administration, 1935
    4. The Nurse Training Act, 1964
40. Licensing the practice of nursing has as its purpose
    1. Protection of the public
    2. Protection of the nurse

3. Assuring high levels of practice
4. Control of education of nurses

41. The interstate movement of nursing is facilitated by
   1. The requirement of mandatory licensing
   2. The nurse practice acts in each state
   3. The use of the State Board Test Pool Examinations
   4. A federal law governing nursing practice

42. Advocates of mandatory continuing education state that it is necessary to
   1. Ensure current competency of nurses
   2. Increase nurses' prestige
   3. Make nursing a profession
   4. Acquire an advanced degree

43. Arguments opposing mandatory continuing education include
   1. Mandatory education should be completed in nursing programs
   2. Learning cannot be made mandatory

3. Nurses haven't time for classes when employed
4. Nursing doesn't change so no additional learning is needed

44. The first state to enact legislation for the registration of nurses was
   1. New York
   2. North Carolina
   3. Mississippi
   4. New Jersey

45. A study of nursing in the United States in 1923 emphasized the need for university schools of nursing; this report is known as
   1. *Nursing and Nursing Education in the United States*
   2. *Committee on the Grading of Nursing Schools*
   3. *The Brown Report*
   4. *The Rich Report*

PART TWO

NURSING AREAS

Fundamentals of nursing

Family-centered nursing

Psychiatric nursing

Medical-surgical nursing

Rehabilitation nursing

CHAPTER 8

Fundamentals of nursing

Fundamentals of nursing are those aspects of nursing common to all clinical nursing areas. The arena in which an individual's health needs are met is constantly changing and expanding. Therefore, the concepts, principles, and skills presented are broad enough to be utilized in any setting in which the nurse may function.

Mastery of the basic concepts and principles involves primarily the use of intellectual processes. Additionally, skills should only be employed when they are thoroughly grounded in knowledge and that knowlegde is applied to provide safe, effective nursing care for patients.

The concepts included are not unique to nursing. Adapted from the social, biologic, and physical sciences, they form the foundation upon which nursing is structured. Their value is centered mainly within the capacity of nurses to apply these concepts and their inherent theory to the provision of total, personalized patient care.

Organization of the procedures that are included is based on their relatedness to basic nursing concepts, their prevalence for use in a variety of health problems, and their commonalities based on scientific knowledge and safe, effective practice. Some of these the nurse carries out directly, while others are carried out interdependently with the physician. Independent function requires both knowledge and judgment while interdependent function adds the requirement of medical direction. The nurse has specific responsibility involving judgment and decision in initiating, maintaining, or terminating many kinds of procedures.

HEALTH
Introduction
A. Health is a generally accepted right; well-being is the norm toward which most governments and all health personnel direct their efforts
B. One of the primary functions of the nursing and medical professions is to help individuals, families, and groups reach the highest level of wellness of which they are capable

Definition
A. The World Health Organization states, "Health is a state of complete physical, mental and social well-being and not just the absence of disease or infirmity"
B. This definition implies there is

1. Interaction between self and environment
2. Preservation of structure and function
3. Maintenance of adaptive potential
C. Significance of definition
   1. Accepted right of all rather than privilege
   2. Reciprocal relationships between individual health and community health
   3. Increasing public expectation of government support for health services and the extent of care provided
   4. Need for nursing and medical practice to move toward maintenance and promotion of health and rehabilitation of the ill rather than merely focusing on provision of episodic care

Basic concepts

A. Health is a continually changing phenomenon
  1. Moves on a continuum between optimal wellness (where potential is maximized and used with purpose) and death
  2. Change may be gradual or abrupt
  3. Level of health attainable depends on adaptive energy, genetic, and environmental factors
    a. Fluctuates throughout life cycle
    b. Varies among individuals
  4. Individual may or may not be aware of change
  5. A person's position on the continuum is determined by
    a. Ability to adapt
    b. Level of adaptation
    c. Culture's view of health
    d. Ability to carry out social, family, and job responsibilities
B. A variety of stresses affect physical, emotional, and social health
  1. May be internal or external
  2. Can be beneficial or detrimental to life
    a. Tension is essential to life
    b. Stress of life and living cause wear and tear
      (1) Produces a nonspecific response that Hans Selye identifies as the general adaptation syndrome (GAS)
      (2) Three stages—alarm, resistance, and exhaustion
  3. They elicit some response from or change in the individual
  4. Sources of stress vary widely for different individuals or within the same individual at different times
  5. Tolerance for stress is individual
  6. Stress may be
    a. Physical—e.g., thermal, accoustic
    b. Chemical—e.g., gas, hormone, nutrient
    c. Microbiologic—e.g., virus, bacteria
    d. Physiologic—e.g., neoplasms, hypofunctions, hyperfunctions
    e. Developmental—e.g., genetic, aging
    f. Psychologic—e.g., values, self-image
C. The ability to maintain a high level of wellness is affected by an individual's ideas, attitudes, and knowledge relative to maintenance and promotion of health; health is thus influenced by many factors, such as
  1. Social
    a. Local or extended community
    b. Socioeconomic status
    c. Geophysical environment
    d. Agencies and resources available
    e. Sociocultural deterrents
  2. Individual
    a. Socioeconomic, cultural background
    b. Educational level
    c. Effects of mass media
    d. Personal resources and values
D. Humanity's internal and external environments are a challenge requiring continual adaptations on a conscious or unconscious level
  1. A person's ability to adapt is affected by
    a. Nature of the stress—its intensity, duration, and character
    b. Nature of the individual—genetic endowment, developmental level, and energy potential
    c. Number of stresses that are present simultaneously
  2. The success of adaptation will determine the nature and degree of assistance required to maintain homeostasis or equilibrium
E. A human being reacts as a unified whole to a stress effecting any aspect of social, emotional, or physical health
  1. An individual is an open system since there is reciprocal interaction between the person and the environment
  2. An individual is made of many interrelated subsystems; e.g., urinary, circulatory
  3. There is reciprocal response between the biologic and psychosocial being
F. Patient needs determine necessary care
  1. Basic needs may be
    a. Physiologic; e.g., oxygen, nutrition, elimination, comfort
    b. Psychologic
    c. Social; e.g., communication, environment
    d. Spiritual
  2. Needs must be satisfied if a person is to carry on activities of life
  3. Health problems that manifest themselves as a result of frustration of these needs may
    a. Be easily compensated

b. Cause other problems

c. Require modification in life style

d. Be a direct threat to life

e. Cause high degrees of anxiety and fear

4. Health problems manifest themselves differently in each individual

5. Psychologic and physiologic responses to health problems vary among individuals

Delivery of health services

A. Purpose—to promote and maintain health, prevent, detect, and treat disease, and rehabilitate the individual

B. Classification of agencies

1. According to control

a. Official or public—government

b. Nonofficial or voluntary—community, religious

c. Proprietary—private (profit-making)

2. According to geographic sphere—city, county, state, or medical region

3. According to services available

a. General—variety of medical services

b. Specialized—specific type of patient or service; e.g., psychiatric, maternity, cancer

C. Changing patterns of service

1. Increasing participation of community

a. Consumer membership on agency boards

b. Agency meetings open to community

c. Demands for accountability

2. Shifting focus to community rather than institution

a. Community health departments

b. Community health centers

c. Community residential facilities; e.g., halfway houses for drug related and mental health problems, walk-in clinics

d. Mobile health stations

e. Teaching of community health aids

f. Home care

3. Crisis intervention groups

a. Suicide prevention

b. Drug addiction control

c. Walk-in mental clinics

d. Professional direction at the scene of an emergency through communication networks

4. Large hospital centers and comprehensive care facilities supplying a wide area

5. Evolving use of hospital emergency rooms for nonemergency ambulatory care

6. Increasing federal involvement; e.g., Medicare, Medicaid, health planning, regional medical planning, funds, grants

D. Health services personnel

1. Roles and functions are blurred

a. Rapid emergence of new types of personnel; e.g., physician's assistant, inhalation therapist, clinical specialist, nurse clinician, paramedics

b. Affects quality care and requires

(1) Clarification of role and function

(2) Development of standards for licensure

(3) Better utilization of personnel

(4) Enforcement of present health practice acts

c. Fragmentation of patient care

2. Team approach often used—provides optimal, unified care to the patient who is the focus of the team

a. Professional health team includes registered professional nurse and physician as colleagues

b. Other members—social worker, nutritionist, therapists, chaplains, etc., utilized as necessary

c. The registered nurse leads the nursing team

d. Nurse functions as

(1) Collaborator with other team members

(2) Liaison between teams

(3) Interpreter to patient and others

(4) Advocate for patient

3. Innovation in the delivery of nursing care

a. Team nursing—see above

b. Primary nursing care (primex, nurse practitioner)

(1) Presents potential for maximum autonomy, authority, and accountability

(2) Suitable for community and hospital settings

(a) Assessment and care in community to prevent illness and maintain health status

(b) Assessment and planning for individual care with responsibility for entire hospital stay on 24-hour basis

(c) Practice independently or in groups

E. Environmental factors in health agencies
1. Quality of health care provided by members of health team influences extent to which health needs are met
2. Conditions responsible for interference with adequate health care of patients in hospitals
   a. Lack of knowledge
   b. Administrative limitations
   c. Lack of commitment

Nursing responsibilities related to health care

A. Generally, the nurse must
1. Recognize the right of persons to receive necessary help
2. Recognize the community's responsibility in providing help
3. Be aware of available agencies in the community and the services they provide
4. Identify potential and present health problems
5. Assess the patient continuously to determine wellness level
6. Encourage participation of the patient in care

B. Specific to individuals, the nurse must
1. Recognize the individual intrinsic worth of each person
   a. Listen, consider wishes when possible, explain when necessary
   b. Avoid stereotyping, snap judgments, unjustified comparisons
   c. Be nonjudgmental and nonpunitive in response and behavior
2. Be aware that each individual must be treated as a whole person
3. Recognize that all behavior has meaning and usually results from coping with stress or anxiety
   a. Be aware of importance of value systems
   b. Be aware of significance of cultural differences
   c. Be sensitive to personal meaning of experiences to patients
   d. Recognize that giving information may not alter patient's behavior

e. Search for patterns of adaptation on which to base action
f. Recognize that adequate behavior patterns may become inadequate under stress
   (1) Health problems may produce a change in family or community constellations
   (2) Health problems may lead to change in self-perception and role identity
g. Be aware that behavioral changes are possible only when the individual has a replacement behavior to maintain equilibrium
4. Help the patient to accept the health problem and its consequences
5. Identify the individual's needs and determine their priority for care

C. Relative to stress, anxiety, and adaptation, the nurse must
1. Recognize the high stress–anxiety potential of most health settings created in part by
   a. The health problem itself
   b. Treatments and procedures
   c. Exclusive behavior of personnel
   d. Foreign environment
   e. Change in life style, body image, and self-concept
2. Take action to minimize or limit anxiety when possible
   a. Listen to patient
   b. Explain what, how, when, where, and why at patient's level
   c. Set limits
   d. Provide opportunities for patient to ventilate
   e. Accept that anxiety cannot always be relieved
   f. Recognize that use of medical jargon can isolate the patient
   g. Recognize own anxiety and cope with it
3. Recognize the defense mechanisms the individual is using
4. Accept the variation in individual responses (physiologic and psychologic) to stress
5. Assess the patient's level of adaptation
   a. Level I—defensive
   b. Level II—compensatory
   c. Level III—overt signs and symptoms of disease

d. Level IV—adaptation has become secondary stress
e. Level V—death
6. Assist patient realistically through varying levels of adaptation as patient attempts to compensate for loss of vital capacity
a. Support adaptation or defense
b. Limit patient's adaptation if inappropriate
c. Alter the signs and symptoms
d. Interrupt the adaptation when it is causing additional stress
e. Supplement the patient's adaptive efforts when necessary
7. Be aware of own emotional responses to patient health problems and patient needs
8. Be aware that nurse-patient interaction is a nursing tool to be directed toward patient well-being

COMMUNICATION

A. Introduction
1. The need to communicate is universal
2. People communicate to satisfy needs
3. Recognition of what is communicated is basic for the establishment of a therapeutic nurse-patient relationship
4. Clear, accurate communication among members of the health team, including the patient is vital to support the patient's welfare
B. Concepts (the major concepts related to communication are presented in the chapter on Behavioral sciences)
C. Nursing responsibilities in promotion of productive communication—the nurse must
1. Be aware that effective communication requires skill in both sending and receiving messages
a. Verbal—words, tone of voice, etc.
b. Written
c. Nonverbal—facial expression, eye contact, posture, tension, etc.
2. Be aware that communication is influenced by many factors other than what is said or how it is said
3. Keep channels of communication open by
a. Focusing on patient
b. Listening with interest
c. Encouraging patient's verbalization by use of interpersonal techniques
d. Being available

e. Being honest
f. Attending to detail
g. Accepting
h. Encouraging participation in care
4. Understand that productive communication is an effective means of promoting a therapeutic change in behavior
5. Be aware that effectiveness of communication cannot be assumed and must be validated by feedback from the patient
6. Understand that stereotyped responses are ineffective in communicating with patients
7. Recognize that the true meaning of communication is not always obvious
8. Be aware that the capacity of the patient (learning, language barriers, etc.) may require adaptations in communication
9. Establish and use channels of communication with relevant members of the health team

THE PROBLEM-SOLVING PROCESS

A. Introduction
1. The basis of personalized patient care is planned rather than intuitive intervention
2. The most efficient way to accomplish this in a future of exploding knowledge and rapid social change is by the use of the problem-solving process
a. A theoretical framework used by the nurse
b. Assists in solving or alleviating both simple and complex nursing problems
B. Need
1. A changing, expanding, more responsible role demands knowledgeably planned, purposeful, and accountable action by nurses
2. Better prepared health professionals and more efficient use of health facilities can meet increasing demands for health care
3. A decision-making process that systematically selects and uses relevant information is a requisite for individualized patient care
4. The composite of cognitive, affective, and activity components that is nursing can best be integrated by the problem-solving process

5. Nursing intervention is directed toward assisting the individual to meet personal needs or solve particular problems
6. A sound basis for continuous learning is necessary

C. Characteristics
1. Dynamic process requiring judgment
2. Scientific, systematic use of validated facts
3. Requires pattern of critical thinking
4. Precludes unwarranted assumptions
5. Provides reasonable alternative solutions

D. Nursing responsibilities
1. Assessment includes
   a. Collection of personal, social, medical, and general data
      (1) Sources—primary (patient, family, and chart) and secondary (colleagues, Kardex, literature)
      (2) Methods
         (a) Interviewing formally (nursing health history) or informally during various nurse-patient interactions
         (b) Observation
         (c) Review of records
   b. Classification of data—screening, organizing, and grouping significant and related information
   c. Definition of problem—making a nursing diagnosis that is the scientific identification of patient needs
      (1) Use of judgment
         (a) Inductive reasoning— specific data to generalizations
         (b) Deductive reasoning— generalizations to specific data
      (2) Identification of stresses in environments (external and internal)
      (3) Awareness of patient and patient's reactions to stress
2. Intervention includes
   a. Making a hypothesis or formulating a nursing care plan—a blueprint for action
      (1) Individualized prescription for care
      (2) Synonymous with nursing orders

   b. Implementation of plan or chosen solution
      (1) Actual administration of planned care
      (2) Adjusted as necessary to immediate needs
   c. Awareness that nursing functions are both independent and interdependent
3. Evaluation and revision includes nursing prognosis as to effectiveness of and response to care

E. Advantages
1. Makes allowance for individual responses to problems
2. Determines priority of care, permitting organization of individual needs in order of importance
3. Permits independent, creative, and flexible nursing intervention
4. Facilitates team cooperation by promoting
   a. Communication between team members
   b. Contribution of team members
   c. Coordination of care
   d. Continuity of approach
5. Provides for patient input

F. Extension to medical records
1. Problem oriented medical record (POMR) consists of standardized data base, problem list, assessment and plan for each problem, and progress notes
   a. Updated by appropriate team members on single progress note
   b. Each problem described according to specific format, which includes *s*ubjective data, *o*bjective findings, *a*ssessment, and a *p*lan for diagnosis, therapy, or teaching (SOAP)
2. Problem oriented records have become the basis for peer review
3. Justifies nursing function
4. Focuses on patient rather than task
5. Improves patient care

ASSESSMENT
Introduction

A. Assessment is necessary to effectively meet patient health needs
B. Personalized nursing intervention is dependent on the ability to make exact, comprehensive appraisal of the individual's health-illness state, as well as on

recognizing the interrelationship of physical and psychosocial needs

Significance

A. Without adequate assessment any plan for nursing action is inadequate, perhaps even detrimental
B. Accurate assessment makes a positive contribution to the quality of nursing care

Basic skills

A. Observation
B. Communication
C. Specific procedures

Scientific observation

A. Definition—the knowledgeable, objective, and systematic gathering of information
B. Depends on
   1. Understanding normal body functions and human behavior, both general and specific for the individual
   2. Knowledge of abnormal changes that may occur evidenced by
      a. Objective signs supplied by laboratory data
      b. Objective symptoms observable to nurse
      c. Subjective symptoms reported by patient; e.g., pain, vertigo, nausea
   3. Recognition of emerging patterns
      a. Clustering of signs and symptoms indicative of specific diseases
      b. Interrelated data; e.g., elevated temperature accompanied by tachycardia
C. Methods
   1. Use of senses to visualize, palpate, manipulate, hear, smell
   2. Use of instruments to percuss, depress, inspect, measure, auscultate, and monitor

Plan for biologic and physical areas

A. Vital signs
   1. Temperature, pulse, respiration
   2. Arterial blood pressure
B. Color
   1. Specific for the individual patient—complexion, etc.
   2. Deviations both general and local
      a. Pallor, cyanosis (extended or circumscribed), blanching (fingernails, etc.)

   b. Ashen or gray
   c. Flushed or ruddy
   d. Jaundiced
   e. Mottled
C. Skin
   1. Turgor, texture
   2. Lesions, rashes
   3. Abrasions, contusions, wounds
      a. Size, shape, depth, location
      b. Presence of drainage—serous, sanguineous, serosanguineous, purulent
   4. Discolorations—ecchymosis, hematomas
   5. Temperature—moistness or dryness
D. Sensory function—sight, hearing, touch, taste, smell, position sense
E. Motor function
   1. Locomotion—standing, sitting, walking
   2. Body mechanics—reaching, turning, lifting, grasping, and balancing
   3. Body posture—relationship of body parts
   4. Speech
   5. Use of prosthetics
F. Rest, sleep, and activity
   1. Restlessness—tossing, undue movement, hyperactivity
   2. Inadequate capacity or lack of vigor
   3. Sleeplessness (insomnia)
   4. Patterns of sleep—both usual and present patterns
G. Levels of consciousness and orientation
   1. Response to stimuli—visual, auditory, tactile or painful; note if patient is alert, somnolent, stuporous, semicomatose, or comatose
   2. Mental status—awareness to time, place, persons, circumstances; note if patient is oriented or disoriented
H. Nutrition
   1. Appetite—desire for or revulsion to food (anorexia, pica, nausea, polyphagia)
   2. Ability to ingest, masticate, and swallow food (dental caries, dysphagia, stricture, atresia)
   3. Capacity to digest food (gastric distress, regurgitation, eructation, vomiting)
   4. Food preferences
   5. Food allergies, sensitivities
I. Elimination
   1. Skin
      a. Excessive perspiration (diaphoresis)

b. Excessive dryness (cracking, scaling)
c. Edema—weeping, pitting
d. Unusual odor; e.g., uremic
2. Respiratory tract
   a. Rate of respirations
   b. Unusual characteristics (stertorous, moist)
   c. Presence of rales, rhonchi, wheezing
   d. Position and excursion of chest
   e. Unusual odor; e.g., fruity breath
3. Urinary and intestinal systems
   a. Characteristics of urine and fecal material—color, odor, consistency
   b. Quantity in relation to intake
   c. Frequency
   d. Facility of elimination—pain, burning, distress
   e. Presence of abnormal constituents, either gross or occult—glycosuria, hematuria, albuminuria, melena, parasites

Plan for psychosocial areas

A. Socioeconomic background
B. Religion
C. Major aspects of value system
D. Attitudes toward health
E. Level of education—formal and self-education
F. Occupation
G. Behavior patterns
   1. Moods—emotional tone
   2. Response to stress
   3. Appropriateness—relative to individual and the situation
H. Family and the individual's place in the constellation
I. Resources within the individual
J. Nonverbal communication—facial expression, movements, position

Nursing responsibilities

A. Accurate and comprehensive observation
   1. How to observe
   2. What to observe
B. Interpretation of findings
   1. Significance
   2. Screening and selection of relevant information
C. Planning a course of action—immediate and long-term
D. Establishing priorities relative to intervention

E. Reporting and recording relevant data concisely, completely, and legibly
F. Measurement of vital signs
   1. General concepts
      a. While vital signs are generally constant, they are sensitive to stresses and respond readily to them
      b. Vital signs indicate vital capacity and function
      c. Variations in norms are related to individual physical constitution as well as health problems
      d. Change in one vital sign is usually accompanied by change in the others
      e. Deviations in vital signs are frequently compensatory as patient adapts to stress and are indicative of physiologic and psychologic imbalance
   2. Nursing responsibilities common to all vital signs
      a. Accuracy of measurement
         (1) Instruments in good working order
         (2) Reading or counting precisely
      b. Elements related to time
         (1) Vital signs taken on admission to help establish base
         (2) Taken during same period of day
         (3) Awareness of biofeedback and relation to vital signs
         (4) Thermometer left in place sufficient length of time according to method used
         (5) Pulse and respirations counted for 1 full minute
         (6) Blood pressure taken regularly as required; e.g., q.½h., q.i.d., o.d., and as status changes
      c. Elements of safety
         (1) Explain to patient
         (2) Know individual's base or usual readings as well as general accepted standard or norm
         (3) Assess significance of changes
G. Temperature
   1. Basic concepts
      a. Balance between heat production and heat loss
      b. Temperature varies in different organs of the body
      c. Close contact with mucosa or skin

and exclusion of circulating air increase accuracy with which thermometer reflects body temperature
(1) Oral temperature—97°F. to
99°F. (approximately 36°C.
to 37.2°C.)
(2) Rectal temperature—slightly
higher
(3) Axillary temperature—slightly
lower
d. Temperature reading can be affected by hot or cold intake or
applications
e. When temperature-regulating
mechanisms of vasoconstriction,
vasodilation, activity of sweat
glands, etc., are inadequate in relation to heat production
(1) Fever or pyrexia develops
(2) Hypothermia or subnormal
temperature occurs
f. The more immature a person's
nervous system, the more pronounced the response to environmental conditions or infections
2. Nursing responsibilities
a. Use appropriate clinical thermometer (oral, rectal) or electronic
probe
b. Take measures to ensure patient
safety
(1) Thermometer clean and intact
(2) Disposable cover on electronic
probe or thermometer
(3) Stay with patient
c. Determine correct route using
parameters such as age, state of
consciousness, nature of health
problem
d. Take measures to lower elevated
temperature
(1) Independent
(a) Manipulate environment
—covers, clothing, room
temperature
(b) Regulate activity to provide rest
(c) Encourage fluids to replace loss
(2) Dependent
(a) Antipyretic, antibiotic,
anti-inflammatory drugs
(b) Alcohol or tepid sponge
(c) Hypothermia blanket

H. Pulse
1. Basic concepts
a. Pulse reflects health in relation to
circulatory system
b. Pulse is a direct reflection of heartbeat
(1) Can be palpated wherever
artery can be compressed
(2) Can be visualized on a monitor
(3) Can be auscultated at apex of
heart (apical beat)
(4) A difference between apical
beat and palpated pulse is the
pulse deficit
c. Pulse rhythm, strength, and rate
can be altered by medications—
cardiotonics
d. Pulse rate is higher during infancy
and senescence
e. When function is impaired, auscultation of apical beat is preferable
2. Nursing responsibilities
a. Evaluate quality of beat—weak,
thready, strong, feeble
b. Identify characteristics in rhythm
—arrhythmias, intermittent, dicrot-
ic
c. Elicit character of vessel
d. Evaluate in relation to other vital
signs
e. Recognize significance of deviation
(1) From average norm of 60 to
100 beats per minute usually
accepted for adults
(a) Below 60—bradycardia
(b) Above 100—tachycardia
(2) From normal baseline established for individual
I. Respiration
1. Basic concepts
a. Respiratory system is vital to life
(1) Humans can live only a few
minutes without oxygen
(2) Rate and rhythm of respirations are involuntary and can
be consciously controlled only
to a degree
(3) Tract has many protective
mechanisms; e.g., cilia, epiglottis
b. Respirations under neural and
chemical regulation
c. Respirations respond to
(1) Factors such as emotions,
activities

(2) Quality of oxygenation in the body
    (a) Anoxia—lack of oxygen
    (b) Hypoxia—inadequate oxygen in tissues for metabolic needs
    (c) Hypoxemia—reduction of arterial oxygen
    (d) Hypocapnia—deficiency of carbon dioxide
(3) Medications such as narcotics

2. Nursing responsibilities
  a. Evaluate quality of ventilation—shallow, deep
  b. Identify difficulties such as dyspnea, orthopnea
  c. Identify significant sounds—rales, stertor, wheezing
  d. Identify irregularities in rhythm—periods of apnea, hyperpnea, Cheyne-Stokes respiration
  e. Recognize whether character of respirations has been affected by pain or emotions
  f. Count respirations without awareness on part of patient
  g. Evaluate rate in relation to pulse, color, etc.

J. Arterial blood pressure
1. Basic concepts
  a. Blood pressure is the pressure exerted by blood against arterial walls
  b. Measurement is possible by use of sphygmomanometer and stethoscope or electronic monitors of arterial pressure
    (1) Highest point of pressure (systole)—corresponds to working phase of cardiac cycle and is first sound heard
    (2) Lowest point of pressure constantly present in vessels (diastole)—corresponds to relaxation phase of cardiac cycle and is last sound heard
    (3) Recorded as systolic over diastolic; e.g., 120/80
    (4) Difference between systolic and diastolic readings in pulse pressure—normally 30 to 50 mm. Hg
  c. Blood pressure is maintained by
    (1) Peripheral resistance affected by vasoconstriction and vasodilation

(2) The cardiac output affected by blood volume and pumping action of heart
(3) Viscosity of blood
(4) Elasticity of vessel walls
  d. Blood pressure is affected by
    (1) Factors such as emotions, age, activity, postural changes, size, and weight
    (2) Chemicals such as hormones, medications
  e. Blood pressure usually measured over brachial artery
    (1) Average pressures of adults are 90 to 140 systolic and 50 to 100 diastolic
    (2) Deviations below this are termed hypotension
    (3) Deviations above this are termed hypertension

2. Nursing responsibilities
  a. If possible, use same arm for consistency after comparing readings in each arm
  b. Use correct size cuff, applied correctly (if cuff is too large it lowers the reading; if too small it elevates the reading)
  c. Locate pulse digitally before inflating cuff
  d. Read manometer at eye level

K. Preparation for diagnostic procedures
1. Basic concepts
  a. The body must maintain relative constancy in its internal environment
  b. All body structures play some role in maintaining homeostasis
  c. Specific conditions are required to get specific results
  d. Reliability of test results is directly proportional to the accuracy with which a procedure is carried out

2. Nursing responsibilities
  a. Obtain and care for specimens of body fluids—gastric analysis, blood chemistries, etc.
  b. Obtain and care for samples of secretions for analysis—urine, stool, sputum, fractional urine specimens, etc.
  c. Measure pressure within body chambers; e.g., arterial and venous pressure
  d. Prepare patient for specific diagnostic procedures; e.g.,

(1) X-ray series—gallbladder, gastrointestinal, barium enema, arteriogram, encephalogram, etc.
(2) Scans—thyroid, brain, liver
(3) Scopic exams—bronchoscopy, proctoscopy
(4) Measurement of pressures— cardiac catheterizations, lumbar puncture
(5) Biopsies
e. Assist in monitoring procedures
(1) Monitors physiologic function by measurement of secretions, excretions, abnormal constituents
(a) Urinalysis—glycosuria, acetone, specific gravity, hematuria by test tape
(b) Stool—blood in stool by test tape
(2) Monitors cardiac function
(a) Recognizes normal configuration of cardiac conduction represented by a P wave, QRS complex, and T wave
(b) Recognizes deviations from regular rate, rhythm, and force of contraction
f. Carries out each activity correctly
g. Recognizes significance of deviations and takes appropriate action
3. Common basic elements
a. Dietary modifications
(1) Withholding food or fluid
(2) Giving special types of food or fluid
b. Administration of medication by nurse or physician
(1) Locally—anesthesia
(2) Parenterally—intravenous dyes, narcotics
(3) Orally—systemic dyes, sedatives
c. Administration of agents that permit visualization of organs—barium, radioactive isotopes
d. Elements relative to time
(1) When preparation begins
(2) When samples and specimens are collected
(3) When specimens can or must be sent to laboratory
(4) When patient may resume

usual activities of daily living —eating, ambulation, elimination
e. Techniques in collecting and handling
(1) Sterile or clean
(2) Correct storage or disposal
(3) Adequate samples for testing
(4) Proper labelling
f. Physiologic factors
(1) Adequate cleansing of intestinal tract—enemas, cathartics
(2) Emptying the bladder (voiding, "clean-catch," catheterizing)
g. Psychologic factors
(1) Explain how and why a procedure is done—at patient's level of understanding and need
(2) Allow time for questions
(3) Support patient during procedure verbally and nonverbally (touch, presence)
h. Positioning
(1) Place patient in correct position, using support as necessary for comfort
(2) Drape patient for privacy

ENVIRONMENT
Introduction

A. A therapeutic environment is concerned with the social, physical, and emotional well-being of the individual
B. To maintain and promote health, it is essential for the nurse to modify both the tangible and intangible aspects of the environment

Concepts

A. Psychosocial
1. Quality care is often affected by the hidden value systems of the health agency as evidenced by governing policies, methods of operation, and power controls
a. Rigid policies and routines often conflict with needs and interests of both patients and personnel
b. Values of the system often emphasize "getting things done" and "patient control" rather than patient needs
2. Interpersonal relationships and com-

munications among team members affect the quality of patient care
   a. Increase in personnel groups leads to overlapping roles
   b. Unclear delineation of responsibilities results in conflict among groups
   c. Nurses are often asked to assume responsibility without having the authority needed to control factors that affect their functioning
3. Diversional and recreational activities are a positive adjunct to a therapeutic atmosphere
4. An environment permeated by courteous and accepting attitudes encourages meaningful communication
5. Recognition of the uniqueness of each individual contributes to a therapeutic atmosphere
6. Hospitalization affects the independence, self-image, and privacy of an individual

B. Physical
1. Comfort, cleanliness, order, control of temperature, ventilation, and light are positive aspects of a patient's environment
2. Control of noxious stimuli such as noise, odors, and unpleasant sights contributes to a therapeutic atmosphere
3. Individuals have the right to expect freedom from superimposed mechanical, physical, bacteriologic, chemical, and immunologic injury

Nursing responsibilities in providing a therapeutic environment

A. Psychosocial
1. Analyze the real goals of a social setting as opposed to verbalized goals
2. Use available influence in the patient's interest rather than enforce conformity to the stereotyped "good patient" role
3. Have "the serenity to accept the things that cannot be changed, courage to change the things that can, and wisdom to know the difference"
   a. Be an agent for change when necessary by identifying needs for change, developing alternatives, involving those who must implement the change, and securing authorization for it

   b. Support the implementation of change
4. Work effectively with health team colleagues
   a. Maintain cooperative relationships
   b. Bring conflicts out into the open for resolution by discussion
   c. Respect another's point of view
5. Maintain an accepting, open environment
   a. Permissive rather than authoritarian
   b. Identify and face problems honestly
   c. Value the expression of feelings
   d. Be nonjudgmental
6. Where possible, encourage patient participation in decision making
7. Recognize the patient as a person
   a. Use names rather than labels such as room numbers or diagnoses
   b. Maintain patient's dignity
   c. Be courteous toward patient, family, and visitors
   d. Protect privacy by use of curtains, avoidance of probing
   e. Permit personal possessions where practical; e.g., own nightclothes, pictures, toys, etc.
   f. Explain at patient's level of understanding and tolerance
   g. Encourage expression of feelings
   h. Approach the patient as a person with difficulties not as a "difficult" person
8. Support a social environment that focuses on patient needs
   a. Use problem-solving techniques in assessment, intervention, and recording
   b. Be flexible in carrying out routines and policies
   c. Be discrete in use of power

B. Physical
1. Regulate and control the physical environment in accordance with patient needs (noise, temperature, etc.)
2. Safeguard patients against physical and mechanical hazards in the environment by application of scientific principles, mechanical and practical knowledge
   a. Maintain equipment in good working order and operate it correctly
   b. Use supportive and protective devices correctly; e.g., side rails, restraints, etc.

c. Take measures to prevent accidents; e.g., clean hallways, dry floors, use of assistance when needed, provision of a signal system for patient
d. Enforce fire prevention rules
3. Recognize that individuals can be sensitized to a variety of substances (food, pollen, chemicals, proteins, etc.)
   a. Elicit history and alert others to the presence of allergies
   b. Eliminate allergens from environment if possible or use barrier; e.g., plastic covers
   c. Recognize symptoms of allergy; e.g., rashes, urticaria, pruritis, dyspnea, etc.
4. Prevent cross-infection
   a. Recognize that microorganisms can be transferred directly by fomites and insects and indirectly by airborne particles
   b. Use medical aseptic techniques
     (1) Handwashing before and after patient care, after handling excreta, etc.
     (2) Bacteriostatic chemicals— antiseptics and disinfectants
       (a) To inhibit or destroy pathogens
       (b) In concurrent and terminal disinfections of contaminated articles
     (3) Barriers such as gowns, gloves, and masks to protect personnel when caring for persons with infections
     (4) Correct disposal of contaminated materials; e.g., linens, tissues, dressings, secretions, and excretions
   c. Use surgical aseptic techniques
     (1) Sterilize by autoclaving, boiling, etc. to destroy all microorganisms
     (2) Barriers such as gowns, gloves, and masks to protect the patient against microbiologic hazards in the environment
     (3) Sterile equipment and technique when caring for wounds, irrigating sterile cavities, giving injections, inserting instruments or devices into body cavities or areas that are normally sterile

5. Eliminate self as a hazard in the environment
   a. Use correct body mechanics to prevent injuries when lifting, turning, or moving patient
   b. Secure physical assistance when necessary to lift or move helpless individuals to prevent dropping or falls
   c. Avoid direct patient contact when the nurse has a local or systemic infection
   d. Assure self of patient identity prior to providing nursing services

COMFORT AND HYGIENE
Introduction
A. The amount of stress and anxiety an individual experiences is proportional to the degree of comfort and control possessed
B. An individual's adaptation to stress is enhanced when physical, emotional, and social ease are present

Definition
A. Comfort is a sense of emotional and physical well-being with freedom from distress
B. Comfort is a
   1. Subjective state evidenced by the absence of pain, anxiety, want, or disease
   2. Relative state of balance
   3. Presence of realistic self-identity and self-image
   4. Productive interaction with others

Concepts related to comfort
A. Discomfort may have a variety of physical and psychosocial causes
   1. Symptoms of adaptation to stress— pain, fever, dyspnea, nausea, vomiting, distention, tension, anxiety
   2. Enforced inactivity necessitated as therapy for health problems
   3. Impairment of body mechanics, caused by either injury or disease
   4. Improperly fitted or misused protective or supportive devices or appliances
   5. Muscle tension or fatigue caused by weakness and debilitation
   6. Local areas of pressure and decubiti resulting from prolonged retention of position

7. Inadequate provision for hygienic needs—cleanliness, nutrition, elimination, etc.
8. Rough, insensitive, or incompetent physical manipulation by health personnel
9. Apprehension related to treatments or procedures necessitated by the health problem

B. Any change or anticipated change in usual or normal physiologic function may be perceived as a threat to life
C. Comfort has a high priority in situations creating the greatest threat to physiologic and psychosocial equilibrium
   1. When signs and symptoms cause undue physical distress—pain, restlessness, insomnia, etc.
      a. May indicate injury or impending injury to the body
      b. May interfere with rest that is essential for cellular function
   2. When discomfort cannot be communicated; e.g., aphasia, language barriers, etc.
   3. When patient is dying
D. Pain and discomfort are subjective and influenced by psychosocial and cultural factors
E. The ability to adapt and maintain comfort is dependent on the support an individual receives from significant people in the environment

Concepts related to hygiene

A. The ability to carry out personal practices related to hygiene influences comfort
   1. Persons differ in hygienic values and practice
   2. Patient's condition may indicate modification of hygienic measures
      a. Health problems may intensify some needs; e.g., foot care in diabetes, oral care in fever, modification of bath, etc.
      b. High level of anxiety may cause regression and dependency
B. The skin and oral cavity reflect an individual's general state of health
C. Unbroken skin and mucosa serve as the first line of defense against injurious agents
   1. Adequate circulation is required to maintain tissue resistance
   2. Resistance to injury differs among individuals

3. Texture of skin alters during various developmental stages
4. Response to injurious agents is inflammation

Nursing responsibilities

A. Accurate assessment and communication of the degree and extent of distress and discomfort, both physical and psychologic
B. Awareness of the significance of discomfort or distress related to the health problem and the individual
C. Recognition that anticipation of pain or discomfort can prolong or intensify the distress
   1. Prompt and judicious use of specific measures to prevent, reduce, or alleviate discomfort
      a. Manipulation of environment to decrease noxious stimuli
      b. Positioning, adjusting pillows, back rub, etc.
      c. Keeping individual's important belongings readily accessible
      d. Treatments; e.g., hot and cold applications
      e. Medications—analgesics, sedatives, tranquilizers
   2. Sensitivity to the individual patient's response to touch, both psychologically and physically
D. Planning and instituting nursing measures related to hygiene and comfort (bathing, oral and back care, care of appendages, etc.) with consideration for individual needs and preferences
E. Early and regular institution of nursing measures to prevent or minimize potential complications
   1. Turning and repositioning as necessary
   2. Maintaining body alignment
   3. Use of supportive devices
   4. Massage and lubrication of skin
F. Recognition that attitudes, individual and social, toward death may vary from acceptance and honesty to evasion, denial, and indifference
   1. Be aware that personal feelings and attitudes (the patient's, the family's, and the nurse's) are an important factor in the situation when an individual is dying
   2. Be readily available to the patient
   3. Listen if the patient wishes to talk but honor the desire to remain silent

G. Be aware that the patient's behavior is an adaptation to dying and may be expressed as denial, anger, bargaining, depression, acceptance

RESPIRATION—THE NEED FOR OXYGEN
Basic concepts

A. Respiration allows for the exchange of oxygen (O_2) and carbon dioxide (CO_2) in the body through the phases of external respiration, which allows for gaseous exchange between atmospheric air and lungs across a semipermeable membrane, and internal respiration, which allows for gaseous exchange between the blood and the cells

B. Oxygen constitutes 20% of atmospheric air

C. Oxygen is essential for life and any interference with cell oxygenation locally or systemically poses a threat to the life of a part of the body or to the entire organism

D. The body has no reserve of oxygen and is not capable of storing it

E. Normally, oxygen is diffused into circulating blood by the respiratory system and is supplied to body cells by the circulation of blood

F. Oxygen is carried in blood in both a physical solution and chemical combination with hemoglobin of red blood cells

G. A prolonged cellular loss of oxygen results in loss of cellular function that is irreversible and that can be life threatening since lack of oxygen affects cells of the brain, heart, and kidneys in that order

H. Oxygen is carried to tissues primarily to oxidize foodstuffs absorbed through the digestive tract

I. Blood does not give up all the transported oxygen to the tissues, nor carbon dioxide to the lungs; carbon dioxide stimulates the respiratory center by increasing the hydrogen concentration of cells in that center

J. To maintain an adequate oxygen supply at the cellular level, certain physiologic necessities are essential
1. An adequate oxygen source
2. A patent airway to allow for oxygen intake and distribution
3. An adequate surface area for absorption of oxygen in the lungs
4. An adequate transport system to deliver oxygen to cells
5. Body cells capable of utilizing the oxygen delivered to them

K. An intact respiratory system, cardiovascular system, and central nervous system are essential for respiratory functioning

L. Respiratory interferences cause difficult breathing (dyspnea), which is defined as an awareness of the need to exert greater respiratory effort to meet oxygen demands of the body

Interferences with sufficient oxygenation of the body cells

A. Complete or partial obstruction of the airway at any point along the respiratory system; e.g., neoplasms, infections, congenital defects

B. Reduction of lung space and efficiency of internal respiration, which complicates free exchange of oxygen and carbon dioxide between alveoli and blood; e.g., pneumonia, lung tumors, tuberculosis, heart failure with pulmonary edema, bronchiectasis, pleurisy, pneumothorax

C. Disruption in the process of union of oxygen and hemoglobin; e.g., blood loss, anemia, decreased red blood cell production

D. Decreased formation of oxyhemoglobin caused by chemicals, which form a stable union with hemoglobin so that the latter is unable to combine with and transport oxygen; e.g., carbon monoxide, cyanide

E. Decreased effectiveness of heart pump action or integrity of arteries, capillaries, and veins; e.g., varicose veins, heart failure, coronary heart disease

F. Decreased efficiency of vital centers controlling respiration and cardiovascular function; e.g., brain injury, meningitis

G. Inadequate utilization of oxygen by individual body cells because of cellular injury and/or destruction; e.g., infections, trauma, change in pH of tissue fluids

Oxygen lack (hypoxia)

May be manifested by
A. Increased pulse rate
B. Rapid, shallow breathing
C. Decrease in ability to concentrate
D. Unstable emotions, apprehension
E. Fainting
F. Muscular incoordination
G. Cyanosis
H. Unconsciousness
I. Extremely difficult breathing
J. Change in position; e.g., restlessness, orthopnea

Overoxygenation

A. When oxygen concentration in blood and tissues is raised carbon dioxide concentration is lowered
B. Overoxygenation is manifested by
1. A fall in blood pressure
2. Decreased vital capacity
3. Fatigue
4. Errors in judgment
5. Paresthesia in hands and feet
6. Anorexia, nausea, and vomiting
7. Hyperemia

Oxygen therapy

A. When an oxygen lack occurs, a commercially prepared oxygen gas may be administered by inhalation
B. Purpose—improves breathing and supplies additional oxygen to body tissues

Basic concepts

A. Oxygen, a therapeutic gas, is colorless, odorless, tasteless, and heavier than air
B. As a gas, it is slightly soluble in water, is drying to mucous membranes and tissues, and supports combustion; therefore oxygen requires humidification in its administration and the mandatory institution and enforcement of safety measures
C. As a form of therapy for respiratory support, oxygen under pressure
1. Decreases apprehension and acute anxiety manifested by patients with brain anoxia
2. Forces the diffusion of oxygen into the blood more readily in proportion to the pressure used
3. Supplies added oxygen to alveolar air to relieve anoxia and/or lack of oxygen in tissues
D. Oxygen may be administered in different concentrations using
1. An oxygen tent for a concentration of up to 55% oxygen
2. Oropharyngeal catheters for a concentration of 35% to 50% oxygen
3. Oxygen masks for a concentration approaching 100% oxygen
E. Selection of the method for administration of oxygen is determined by the physician (except in emergency, life-saving situations when a physician may not be present) on the basis of
1. The patient's need for oxygen concentration
2. The cause of oxygen lack

3. The patient's ability to cooperate with the treatment approach
F. Oxygen equipment can be supplied for home use through the home service division of oxygen supply companies once referral is made by the physician

Nursing responsibilities

A. Since oxygen has the chemical characteristic of supporting combustion, the nurse eliminates open flames and sparks from the environment in which oxygen is being administered; e.g., no smoking signs; use of only grounded electric machines; removal of electric devices such as heating pads, electric call bells; restriction of wool, silk, rayon, or nylon goods; elimination of oils, lotions, and alcohol from care
B. Since oxygen enters lungs under pressure higher than that in the atmosphere, causing rapid evaporation of surface fluids on mucous membranes, the nurse uses methods of humidifying the oxygen; e.g., bottle of water connected to oxygen source or passing oxygen over ice so water is picked up from the ice surface
C. Since oxygen is considered a therapeutic gas and is a medical treatment, the nurse administers oxygen with a physician's order except in
1. Emergency situations when giving oxygen is a life-saving measure
2. Situations when carbon dioxide narcosis is present and, since the low level oxygen in the blood may be the only stimulus for respiration, oxygen is not administered
D. Since oxygen is heavier than air, it will escape through open areas, thus necessitating that the nurse effectively tuck in oxygen canopies when using oxygen tents
E. Since impairment of respiratory, cardiovascular, and central nervous system functions can present threats to cellular oxygenation, the nurse must make patient assessments before oxygen therapy is commenced and during its administration in relation to
1. Color—local and general
2. Skin temperature
3. Mechanics of breathing and character of respirations
4. Character of cough
5. Character and rate of pulse

F. Since general diagnostic tests such as x-rays, sputum examination, determination of vital capacity, bronchoscopy, bronchograms, blood gas evaluations are often ordered in an effort to determine oxygen deficiency, the nurse assumes responsibilities for patient preparation, explanation, and supportive care before, during, and after tests are performed

G. Nursing measures are based on the following objectives
1. To maintain a patent airway
2. To promote optimum rest and minimize patient anxiety to reduce oxygen requirements of the body
3. To assist with diagnostic examinations and provide related nursing care
4. To protect the patient from infection
5. To maintain or promote hydration
6. To administer sufficiently high concentrations of oxygen to overcome or relieve manifestations of oxygen want
7. To provide a safe environment for oxygen administration
8. To observe, assess, record, and report the patient's reaction to oxygen therapy and effectiveness of the treatment approach

Supportive measures to meet oxygen needs

A. Oxygen mask
1. Purpose—to administer therapeutic concentrations of oxygen approaching 100%, which allows for the removal of expired carbon dioxide and for the mixing of air with oxygen
2. Types—oronasal mask covers nose and mouth during administration, accommodating both nose and mouth breathers; nasal mask covers only the nose, permitting exposure of the mouth
3. Nursing responsibilities
   a. Check mask for patency
   b. Adjust liter flow at 3 to 4 L. per minute as ordered
   c. Fit mask to patient's face to avoid oxygen leakage
   d. Provide skin care regularly to prevent irritation of skin
   e. Provide for humidification of oxygen

B. Oropharyngeal catheters
1. Purpose—the passage of an oropharyngeal catheter through the nasal passage to administer O_2 directly into the oropharynx in moderate concentrations of 35% to 50%
2. Nursing responsibilities
   a. Attach humidifier bottle to oxygen outlet
   b. Lubricate catheter with water or a water-soluble lubricant to promote ease of insertion and prevent aspiration pneumonia
   c. Adjust liter flow according to physician's order or at 3 to 4 L. per minute; maintain liter flow as ordered since an increase does not assure greater concentration but does increase drying of mucous membranes
   d. Pinch catheter and insert through nostril so that tip is visible at the uvula where oxygen is easily inspired; use the horizontal distance from nostril to ear lobe to determine length of catheter to be inserted
   e. Secure catheter after insertion
   f. Alternate nostril used frequently to prevent irritation and breakdown of skin and to facilitate cleaning and care of nares

C. Tents
1. Purpose—to administer a therapeutic concentration of up to 55% oxygen through a light, portable structure attached to a motor-driven unit that circulates and cools air high in oxygen and humidity
2. Nursing responsibilities
   a. Check efficiency and function of tent
   b. Connect unit to oxygen source and adjust liter flow at 15 L. per minute for 2 to 5 minutes to flood the tent
   c. Apply tent over patient and tuck in canopy securely under mattress
   d. Maintain liter flow of oxygen at 10 to 12 L. per minute unless otherwise ordered
   e. Allay patient's fears to increase patient comfort and enhance the treatment approach
   f. Provide safe environment for delivery of oxygen
   g. Protect patients from drafts and excessive cooling while air circulates in the tent
   h. Maintain tent temperature at a

level comfortable for the patient (usually 70°F. or 21°C.)

  i. Regularly communicate with patient who may feel totally isolated while in the tent

D. Postural drainage

  1. Purpose—a treatment approach in which position of the patient is used to promote drainage of fluid and/or mucus from the lungs by gravity with choice of position being dependent on the patient's age, size, area of lung to be drained, health problem, degree of illness, and emotional state

  2. Common positions for postural drainage

    a. Lying on right side to drain left lower lung

    b. Lying on abdomen to drain portions of lower lobes

    c. Lying on back to drain anterior portions of lungs

    d. Lying on left side to drain right lung

    e. Lying across bed on abdomen with head and shoulders dependent to drain lower lung lobes

    f. Sitting up at 45° angle to drain upper lobes

  3. Nursing responsibilities

    a. Know position being used for postural drainage of the patient

    b. Provide support for dependent portions of the body

    c. Encourage patient to maintain position for maximum effectiveness

    d. Encourage breathing and coughing deeply to facilitate loosening and drainage of secretions

    e. Use clapping or cupping if necessary to vibrate and loosen secretions

    f. Remain with patient during entire procedure to ensure safety since dizziness may accompany postural drainage techniques

    g. Increase lengths of procedure as tolerated by the patient and as warranted by the health problem

    h. Perform draining procedures at other than meal times, providing psychologic support and oral hygiene during and after procedure

    i. Teach patient to position and protect self, care for drainage raised;

teach importance of timing procedure and need for oral hygiene

    j. Evaluate effectiveness of treatment approach by assessing amount of drainage produced and character of respirations after procedure

E. Positioning

  1. Purpose—to position the patient to enhance maximum oxygenation with or without supportive oxygen

  2. Nursing responsibilities

    a. Assess type and extent of oxygen want

    b. Place patient in upright, sitting position (full or semi-Fowler's) to facilitate lung and muscle expansion

    c. Utilize orthopneic position for extreme systemic oxygen want

    d. Change position of anoxic parts frequently and regularly

    e. Apply side rails that the patient may use to help change own position and that assure safety in situations of decreased alertness

F. Inhalation therapy

  1. Purpose—treatment approach used to administer warm and cold vapor with or without medications to

    a. Humidify the air to allow for easier breathing

    b. Soothe mucous membrane of irritated nose, throat, bronchial tubes, and larynx

    c. Reduce evaporation of water from mucous membranes by increasing humidity of inspired air thus thinning secretions for more easy expectoration

    d. Warm and moisten air following surgery on trachea

  2. Methods of administration

    a. Steam kettle

    b. Cold or warm vapor humidifier

    c. Hand aerosol nebulizer

    d. Warm humidifying mask

    e. Intermittent positive pressure breathing (IPPB)

  3. Nursing responsibilities

    a. Know type of inhalation therapy to be utilized

    b. Add medication to appropriate part of equipment, if ordered

    c. Place apparatus in position that assures safe and effective inhalation of vapor

d. Encourage patient to inhale vapors deeply
e. Evaluate effectiveness of treatment approach by assessing amount of secretions expectorated, character of respirations, comfort of patient during breathing

NUTRITION

Introduction

A. A diet balanced in the essential nutrients, calories, and types of food commensurate with the individual's need is basic to an optimal degree of wellness
B. The nurse's responsibilities are many and varied

Basic concepts

A. General concepts and information related to nutrition, nutrients, and diet therapy are presented in the chapter on Nutrition
B. An individual's size, age, physical activity, and physiologic function affect nutritional need
C. Optimal nutrition is influenced by physiologic and psychosocial factors
1. Correct balance of essential nutrients (proteins, fats, carbohydrates, vitamins, minerals, and water) and calories that are required to maintain vital capacity
2. Ability to ingest, masticate, and swallow food
3. Capacity to digest, absorb, transport, and assimilate the nutrients
4. Patterns and habits of eating associated with
   a. Geographic location, economic status, and cultural orientation (national, familial, and individual)
   b. Choice of what, where, when, how, and with whom one eats (many times socially or developmentally determined)
   c. Deliberate exclusion of essential nutrients from diet; e.g., food fads, indiscriminate dieting, lack of appetite, etc.
   d. Inclusion of unnecessary quantities of nutrients or calories; e.g., predilection for certain foods or excess quantities of all foods, using food to fill psychologic need, etc.
5. Poverty of society, community, family, individual related to
   a. Money, unemployment, low income, high cost of living, etc.
   b. Knowledge or ignorance related to sources of nutrients that are both available and inexpensive
   c. Unavailability of certain foods
6. Affluence and culture in a society
   a. Mass media molds nutritional practices with high-pressure advertising
      (1) Attributes status and desirability to foods that may be nutritionally deficient
      (2) Encourages compulsive buying of foods calorically rich and nutritionally poor
   b. National and regional dietary patterns may be imbalanced in quality and quantity of nutrients and seasonings
D. Food habits and practices are difficult to change
1. Foods introduced in childhood are usually preferred
2. Patterns of eating or not eating may satisfy psychologic needs
3. Attitudes about food and its meaning to the individual are motivating forces
4. Knowledge about nutrition is usually insufficient to effect change
E. Malnutrition and obesity are 2 prevalent conditions that predispose the individual to many other major health problems
F. Health problems that interfere with ingestion, mastication, digestion, absorption, transportation, or assimilation of food may
1. Impair nutritional status
2. Threaten life
3. Require both internal and external adaptations relative to supplying nutrients

Nursing responsibilities

A. Knowledge about essential nutrients, their uses in the body, and their sources
B. Awareness of the psychosocial significance of food and eating habits to the individual
C. Assessment of the individual's nutritional needs related to
1. Physical status; e.g., weight gain or loss, allergies, skin color, tone and turgor, ability to ingest, masticate, swallow, etc.
2. Critical times; e.g., growth, development, pregnancy, disease, injury, etc.

3. Appetite (psychologic desire); e.g., likes, preferences, and dislikes
4. Hunger; its presence or absence (anorexia)
5. Encouragement or curtailment of specific nutrients; e.g., water, salt, potassium, carbohydrates, fats, etc.

D. Assurance of an adequate and satisfactory intake
   1. Provision for individual food preferences when possible
   2. Arrangement of the individual as comfortably as possible when eating; e.g., accessibility of food, utensils, position, etc.
   3. Creation of an environment conducive to eating; e.g., eliminate noxious stimuli, provide for sociability if desired, etc.
   4. Provision of assistance acceptable to the patient when unable to meet nutritional needs alone
   5. Observation and communication of actual nutritional intake (what is as well as what is not eaten)

E. Scheduling activities so that therapy and procedures do not coincide with mealtime except in an emergency

F. Administration of medications related to dietary patterns on time; e.g., insulin, antacids, antispasmodics, and other medications given before and after meals

G. Recognition that the majority of health problems may require diet therapy or modification of nutritional intake regarding
   1. Quantity—low calorie, high calorie, supplementary feedings, etc.
   2. Quality—restrictions in sodium, protein, fats, carbohydrates, seasonings, increases in protein, carbohydrates, etc.
   3. Consistency—fluid, chopped, pureed, blended, soft, etc.
   4. Frequency—6 small feedings, ulcer regime, every 2 hours, etc.

H. Teaching the individual what is necessary related to the diet and its modifications
   1. Ascertaining understanding by feedback
   2. Including key family members to facilitate adherence

I. Knowledge that there are alternate methods available to supply nutrients and maintain the highest level of nutrition possible when
   1. The gastrointestinal tract requires rest or has its integrity interrupted
   2. The individual is unable to ingest, masticate, swallow, or metabolize food as a result of physiologic or psychologic factors; e.g., coma, debilitation, anorexia, sutures, radical surgery
   3. Additional or rapid supplementation is necessary because of
      a. Excessive abnormal loss; e.g., vomiting, diarrhea, hemorrhage, suction, etc.
      b. Excess loss by over secretion and/or excretion

J. Knowledge of supplemental or extraoral procedures that support nutrition
   1. Nasogastric feeding or gavage—introduction of a liquefied powder or blender diet through a syringe or funnel attached to a nasogastric tube
   2. Gastrostomy feeding or gastrogavage—introduction of a liquefied powder or blender diet through a syringe attached to a tube that has been surgically inserted into the stomach through the abdominal wall
   3. Supplements—either oral or parenteral of nutrient elements
      a. Oral—vitamins, minerals, protein hydrolysates
      b. Intramuscular and subcutaneous injections—vitamins, hematinics, minerals, etc.
      c. Intravenous infusion—glucose, saline, potassium, calcium, vitamins, water, plasma, whole blood, etc.
      d. Hyperalimentation—high percentage glucose, amino acids, electrolytes, minerals, and vitamins infused into vena cava to avoid danger of thrombosis in peripheral veins
      e. Hypodermoclysis—administration of fluids, electrolytes into subcutaneous tissue

K. Assistance with procedures that support nutrition
   1. Assembling specific equipment required; e.g., tubes, syringes, needles, Intercaths, etc.
   2. Explanation of what to expect and what is expected
   3. Positioning patient appropriately for

insertion of tubing; e.g., high Fowler's position for insertion of gavage tubing

4. Ascertaining the patency and correct locations of tubes and needles; e.g., in stomach, in muscle, in vein, etc.
5. Storing and administering solution at correct temperature; e.g., heating gavage feeding to room temperature after removal from refrigerator
6. Administering the correct type, concentration, and amount of solution at the correct time; e.g., 200 to 350 ml. of tube feeding every 3 to 4 hours (on the first day each feeding is usually limited to 250 ml.)
7. Regulation of the rate of flow to avoid complications
   a. Intravenous—drops per minute, regulated according to need and condition of patient as well as the type of fluid
   b. Gavage—slowly by continuous drip or at specific intervals as ordered
   c. Hypodermocylsis—slowly with the aid of an enzyme preparation
   d. Hyperalimentation—slowly at a constant rate as ordered (should not be speeded up)
8. Avoiding the accumulation of air in or administration of air via tubing
9. Adherence to aseptic factors
   a. Tube feedings and oral supplements require medical asepsis with utensils clean and solutions free from contamination
   b. Parenteral infusions and injections require surgical asepsis with all equipment; preparations and solutions should be sterile and skin disinfected at point of insertion
10. Recognition of inherent dangers
    a. Aspiration if tube is not correctly placed or if regurgitation occurs; gavage feeding is terminated when there is back flow into the tube
    b. Phlebitis may result if needle displaced or nutrient is irritating to tissues
    c. Hyperglycemia may result with the highly concentrated solutions used in hyperalimentation; fractional urines are necessary and insulin coverage may be ordered

ELIMINATION
Introduction

A. Continuous or regular excretion of waste products is necessary to maintain the balance of body temperature, chemical composition, and osmotic pressure within the narrow limits required for life
B. Physiologic dysfunction, physical limitation, dietary deficiencies, and psychosocial maladjustments commonly interfere with natural elimination
C. Supportive assistance to maintain or restore function is then required

Basic concepts

A. A balance between intake of food and excretion of wastes and toxic substances is essential for life
   1. The individual requires an adequate intake of essential nutritive substances to maintain vital processes
   2. The body must effectively metabolize these elements
   3. There must be a capacity to transport products to the organs of disposal for excretion
B. Excretion or output is accomplished not only by the urinary system and gastrointestinal tract but by other means such as the integumentary and respiratory systems
C. A variety of wastes and toxic or other substances is eliminated from the body daily
   1. Sweat glands secrete approximately 1000 ml. of water, minerals, and sodium chloride
   2. Lungs through alveolar exchange remove water and carbon dioxide
   3. Kidneys secrete approximately 1200 to 2000 ml. of yellow fluid with a specific gravity of 1.010 to 1.030 that contains water, minerals, salts, nitrogenous wastes, hormones, etc. for excretion by bladder
   4. Colon propels indigestible material, intestinal secretions, bacteria, pigments, gases, salts, and some water to rectum for expulsion regularly (not necessarily daily)
D. Alteration in one avenue of elimination will cause deviation in the others; e.g., diaphoresis and diarrhea will affect urinary output
E. Usual patterns of elimination vary among

individuals but within defined limits of normalcy; for example

1. Voiding or micturition depends on fluid intake, capacity of bladder, integrity of stretch receptors, socially acceptable opportunity, etc.
2. The number of bowel movements or stools vary from person to person and within the same person at different age levels

F. A variety of cultural and psychosocial factors affect patterns and practices related to elimination
1. Emotional tension is produced by highly private and personal nature of elimination
2. Cultural values related to diet and elimination; e.g., bowel and bladder consciousness of culture, improper balance of foods, etc.
3. Injudicious use of or dependency on drugs such as laxatives and purgatives

G. Social and stress-laden situations prevalent in our institutions are not conducive to normal functioning
1. Environment itself leads to lack of privacy
2. Illness and anticipation of diagnostic tests
3. Attitudes of staff regarding process and products of elimination and its importance
4. Change in diet and usual routine
5. Confinement to bed decreasing mobility and altering usual positions for elimination
6. Use of medications such as sedatives and barbiturates

H. The extent of physiologic and psychosocial distress that is experienced when usual patterns of elimination are altered depends on the degree of deviation
1. Irregularities in any of the methods of elimination require intervention
2. Alterations not caused by pathologic change in the excretory systems may affect level of wellness and degree of resistance to superimposed problems
   a. Fluid and electrolyte imbalances caused by diaphoresis, diarrhea, vomiting, or anorexia
   b. Retention and distention following surgery
   c. Constipation caused by dietary change and limitations

d. Incontinence or impaction following cerebrovascular accident
3. Alterations resulting from pathologic change within the individual or excretory system constitute serious health problems that may be life threatening
   a. Renal failure
   b. Intestinal obstruction
   c. Respiratory failure with acid base alteration
   d. Extensive burns
   e. Congestive heart failure

I. Deviations in patterns of elimination can be broadly classified into 6 categories
1. Excesses in quantity such as polyuria and diaphoresis or deficiencies such as anuria, oliguria, obstipation
2. Excesses or deficiencies in quality (consistency, appearance, or composition) such as concentrated or diluted urine and diarrhea, clay-colored or constipated stools, tympanitis or intestinal distention
3. Presence of abnormal constituents either directly observable or determined by laboratory analysis such as parasites and frank or occult blood in stool, glycosuria, hematuria, bilirubinuria, pus in urine or feces, uremic frost on skin, or fruity odor to breath, etc.
4. Difficulty, discomfort, or pain at any point along the body's elimination systems up to and including the moment of excretion may indicate inflammation, infection, or obstruction
5. Impairment of control—incontinence of urine, feces, or flatus on a continual basis or periodically as in overflow incontinence, nocturia
6. Inability of terminal organs to properly expel waste materials; e.g., urinary retention, retention with overflow, constipation, impaction, etc.

Nursing responsibilities

A. Observation
1. Critical observation related to the nature of elimination; e.g., pattern, amount, color, odor, frequency, etc.
2. Knowledge of the significant deviations or changes in the nature of elimination; e.g., anuria, burning, tenesmus,

melena, unusual odor, change in shape or consistency, etc.

3. Interpretation of the observations in relation to the patient and the health problem
4. Collection of necessary specimens using correct methods
5. Preparation of the patient for diagnostic and therapeutic procedures so the patient knows what to expect and what is expected

B. Maintaining accurate records on all aspects of elimination
1. Individual elimination history, including usual patterns, habits, and preferences
2. Usual characteristics of products of elimination and any deviations
3. Reporting significant deviations promptly
4. Intake and output relationships
   a. Output—visible and insensible, normal and abnormal; e.g., vomitus, hemorrhage, diaphoresis, etc.
   b. Intake—oral and parenteral fluids
5. Recording results of tests; e.g., fractional urines, specific gravity, occult blood, etc.

C. Nursing measures to maintain optimal function
1. Sensitivity to cultural, social, and individual values that affect attitudes toward elimination
   a. Help patient feel comfortable and free to divulge elimination difficulties
   b. Prevent disturbances and stresses that may interfere
   c. Provide maximum privacy
   d. Recognize that complaints related to elimination may indicate other problems
2. Reduce possibility of embarrassment to patient
   a. Anticipate and answer calls for assistance promptly
   b. Adjust fluid schedule
   c. Position patient correctly on bedpan or toilet
   d. Place bedpans, urinals, or commodes where readily accessible
3. Promote natural elimination by positioning, fluid regulation, provision of excercise, privacy, and opportunity and provision of skin care
4. Instruct the patient concerning

a. Health practices related to elimination; e.g., diet, fluids, regularity, hand washing, use of laxatives, etc.
b. Responsibilities that the patient can assume while in the hospital; e.g., recording intake and output, saving of specimens, etc.
c. Measures of intervention that may be used to maintain elimination; e.g., catheter and gravity drainage, colostomy, etc.
d. Refer to sections on urinary and intestinal retraining and on teaching principles in Chapter 12, Rehabilitation
5. Administration of medications such as laxatives, stool softeners, suppositories, etc.

D. Assistance with procedures that support elimination
1. Knowledge of the variety of procedures used to support elimination; e.g., catheterization, enema, irrigation, instillation, Harris flush, rectal tube, etc.
2. Knowledge of the purposes for the intervention
   a. Assist the patient to eliminate retained wastes; e.g., urine, stool, or gas
   b. Secure specimens for laboratory analysis
   c. Relieve symptoms of inflammation and infection or prevent their occurrence; e.g., instillation of antibiotics or irrigation with antiseptic solutions
   d. Remove interference with elimination; e.g., blood clots, mucous shreds, or impactions
   e. Keep accurate record of all output
   f. Prepare patient for surgery or diagnostic procedures
3. Applications of common physiologic factors underlying irrigations or instillations
   a. Use appropriate equipment to ensure patient safety, comfort, and effectiveness of results
   b. Insert tubes safely and precisely into body cavities
      (1) Use lubrication when necessary
      (2) Use appropriate techniques; e.g., medical or surgical asepsis

(3) Insert appropriate distance to reach the area being irrigated and avoid injury; e.g., insert rectal tube for enemas approximately 4 inches

c. Position the patient anatomically and comfortably

d. Ensure an adequate return flow of solution introduced into body cavities (bladder, intestines) or through abnormal openings (cystostomy, colostomy)

e. Have temperature of solution conducive to physiologic function
(1) Room temperature for bladder treatments and commercially prepared enemas
(2) Other irrigations approximately 100° to 105°F. (37° to 40°C.)

f. Amount and type of solution must be appropriate for the structure being irrigated

g. Report any undue distress experienced by patient as well as characteristics of return flow

4. Important points related to specific procedures

a. Catheterization—insertion of a pliable tube into the urinary bladder to drain urine
(1) Sterile equipment and technique used
(2) Area of insertion at urinary meatus scrupulously cleansed
(3) Catheter selected depends on purpose
(a) Single or stat catheterization—plain, French whistle-tip, or round catheter
(b) Continuous gravity drainage—indwelling, retention, Foley catheter (clamping at intervals will permit intermittent drainage)
(c) Continuous or intermittent irrigation—three-way retention catheter
(4) Collection system may be
(a) Open in which disconnection of catheter, tubing, and collection container is possible
(b) Closed, which is not

disconnected and has a special air filter permitting escape of air but preventing bacterial entrance
(5) Once inserted, tubing must always be positioned to permit unimpeded flow from the bladder by gravity

b. Enemas—introduction of solutions rectally to facilitate expulsion of stool
(1) Clean equipment and techniques used
(2) Amount and type of solution varies according to
(a) Individual capacity
(b) Purpose of enemas; e.g., oil retention to soften feces, saline or tap water to cleanse
(c) Method of action; e.g., distention by 1000 ml. of tap water, chemical irritations with soapsuds, or a combination of distention and irritation by 120 ml. of prepared hypertonic enema
(3) Be aware of possible complications such as hyperirritation of colon or water intoxication when large or repeated quantities of hypotonic solution are used
(4) Request the patient to retain fluid for the appropriate time if possible; e.g., 2 to 7 minutes for prepared enemas, 30 minutes for oil retention enemas

c. Instillations and irrigations may be used to evacuate cavities, maintain potency of drainage tubing, or instilling medication
(1) Prophylactic or therapeutic irrigation of bladder
(a) At intervals inserting 30 to 50 ml. sterile solution or medication several times and permitting return flow by gravity
(b) Continuously by three-way catheter
(2) Rectal irrigations in addition to enemas

(a) Harris flush to relieve distention

(b) High colonic

(3) Ostomy irrigations

(a) Ascertain whether the opening should be irrigated or not; e.g., an ileal conduit or ileostomy is not irrigated while a colostomy or cecostomy is

(b) An ostomy may be permanent or temporary; e.g., double or single lumen colostomy, permanent or temporary cystostomy

5. Explanation to the patient prior to the start of any of these procedures

POSTURE, ACTIVITY, AND REST

Introduction

A. Mobility is one means an individual has to measure well-being, while fatigue serves as a protective mechanism

B. A relative balance between energy expenditure and the restoration that occurs during relaxation, rest, and sleep is necessary to maintain optimal well-being or restore it when injury or disease exists or threatens

Basic concepts

A. All physical, mental, and mechanical functions of the body are directly affected by posture, activity, and rest

1. Correct body posture and efficient body mechanics contribute significantly to the emotional security of individuals in a society that highly values the body beautiful

2. Correct body posture, whether standing, sitting, or lying, maintains alignment of articulating body parts

3. Correct body posture when standing, sitting, or lying supports adequate functions of vital organs such as lungs, heart, intestines, etc.

4. Routine activities of daily living (ADL) such as bathing, eating, working, walking, talking, dressing, reading, and thinking maintain mechanical efficiency in moveable body parts and articulations, thus promoting both mental and physical function

B. Mobility is a modality used in self-expression and definition

1. Movement is an expression of self (walking, dancing, nonverbal communication, use of hands)

2. Motor activity is a means of discharging emotions

C. A wide variety of physical, mental, and cultural activities provides emotional outlets for the individual

D. Regular periods of decreased or altered physical and mental activity refresh the human body

1. Rest, relaxation, and diversion, adjusted to individual need, support optimal physical, mental, and emotional stability

2. Sleep, regulated by individual need, is necessary to sustain satisfactory mental hygiene, intellectual productivity, and energy expenditure

E. Rest and sleep are promoted when stress is minimized (physiologic, psychologic, environmental)

F. Sleep is cyclic in nature

1. Individual patterns vary

2. It consists of 2 states that are repeated

a. Nonrapid eye movement sleep (NREM), stages I to IV

(1) Deep sleep occurs during stages III and IV

(2) Deep sleep is longer during early hours of sleep

b. Rapid eye movement sleep (REM) is when dreaming occurs

c. Sleep medications may influence both states of sleep

G. Both quantity and quality of sleep affect well-being

1. Need and patterns of sleep vary

a. Among individuals as a result of habit, stage of development, etc.

b. In the same individual as a result of activity, stress, etc.

2. Symptoms of physical, biochemical, or mental fatigue vary depending on the degree of sleep deprivation (can move from lapses of attention and irritability to confusion and hallucinations)

H. Impaired ability to maintain posture, activity, and rest results when disease or injury is present

1. Debilitation resulting from acute and chronic illnesses (cardiac disease, chronic obstructive lung disease, acute

colitis) causes weakness, lethargy, apathy, and depression

2. Physiologic and psychosocial stress (pain, fever, anxiety, fear) induced by illness and injury diminish the capacity to maintain a satisfactory level of rest, sleep, and diversional activity

3. Congenital defects often inhibit growth and development, thus affecting body mechanics, posture, and psychosocial activities

4. Enforced inactivity such as treatment for disease or injury (acute myocardial infarct, fracture of the extremities) inhibits physiologic and psychosocial function

5. Disrupted motor function tends to predispose the individual to permanent deformity, loss of mechanical function, and emotional distress

Nursing responsibilities

A. Consistent provision of emotional support and realistic encouragement in accordance with the needs, priorities, and wishes of the patient as a person
   1. Stressing abilities and not disabilities
   2. Helping the individual to acquire a sense of independence and control by providing opportunities for patient involvement

B. Critical observation of limitations or deviations of position or motion

C. Recognition that the effects of any prolonged rest or immobilization are varied and preventable; complications include
   1. Decreased circulatory efficiency
      a. Pooling of blood in the extremities contributing to edema and thrombus formation
      b. Orthostatic hypotension upon assuming the upright position (sitting or standing)
   2. Decreased respiratory efficiency
      a. Inability to aerate lungs, cough, or produce secretion
      b. Hypostatic pneumonia and atelectasis
   3. Generalized muscle weakness, disuse atrophy, and atony
   4. Loss of bone density and strength
   5. Contractures such as hip and knee flexures or foot drop
      a. Shortening of opposing muscle groups

b. Decrease in functional range of motion

6. Loss of skin integrity with formation of decubiti over bony prominences

7. Urinary stasis contributing to infection and calculi

8. Decreased mobility of gastrointestinal tract contributing to anorexia, constipation, and fecal impaction

9. Disturbances in psychologic status such as anxiety, depression, withdrawal, etc.

D. Consistent and regular alteration of position at least every 2 hours as an adjunct to minimal physical activity and for prevention of complications
   1. Utilize all positions in sequence unless contraindicated
   2. Maintain body alignment

E. Maintenance of functional range of motion (ROM) by regular exercise performed by the nurse or patient or both according to patient needs
   1. Passive—nurse does exercise for patient
   2. Assistive—patient assists the nurse in doing exercises
   3. Active—patient independently carries out exercise after being instructed
   4. Move all joints through full range twice daily
   5. Incorporate exercises with other activities such as bathing
   6. Maintain firm support under joints while handling extremities
   7. Exercise slowly and smoothly and not beyond the point of pain

F. Provision for optimal level of correct body posture whether lying, sitting, or walking to reduce the hazards of permanent deformity
   1. Using assistive devices such as pillows, hand rolls, footboards, slings, braces, frames, trochanter rolls, sandbags, etc.
   2. Frequent observation to see that alignment is maintained

G. Provision of an optimal level of hygienic care (cleanliness, nutrition, and elimination) including maintenance of integumentary integrity
   1. Adjustment of the frequency of skin care according to individual need
      a. Noting signs of pressure such as reddened or depressed areas
      b. Checking bony prominences such

as sacrum, vertebrae, scapula, heels, occiput, iliac crest, elbows, humerus, wrists, and ears

2. Lightly massaging areas of the body that are subject to pressure
3. Teaching able patients the techniques of self-inspection
4. Use of medications and treatments such as antiseptics, drying agents, or heat lamps as required
5. Use of assistive devices such as a turning sheet, frame, or lift to turn or move a patient when necessary
6. Securing even distribution of body weight and/or change of pressure points by the use of
   a. Assistive devices such as a trapeze
   b. Specialized equipment such as the Stryker frame or Circ-O-Lectric bed
   c. Specialized pads and mattresses such as silicone flotation pads, alternating pressure mattresses, water mattresses, and sheepskins
H. Teaching the patient to do assistive muscle setting (isometric contraction and relaxation of muscle without joint motion) when indicated, especially of the quadriceps, gluteal, and abdominal muscles
I. Providing opportunities and encouraging the patient to perform activities that are within functional capabilities
J. Continuous critical evaluation of all corrective or supportive devices to ascertain their efficiency and ensure that
   1. Their purpose is achieved
   2. Circulation is not diminished
   3. Motion is not unnecessarily limited
   4. Undue discomfort or pain does not result
K. Provision for optimal physical and diversional activity
L. Provision of an optimal level of physical, environmental, and psychosocial comfort as a prerequisite for rest and sleep based on
   1. A knowledge of the patient's sleep patterns
   2. The nature of sleep itself
M. Adjustment of nursing activities so they do not interfere with those states of sleep that provide the most rest
N. Ensuring continuity of care in the plans for activities necessary to maintain or restore sensorimotor function and to prevent or correct deformity

1. Communicate to other health team personnel significant information concerning the individual patient's needs, priorities, and wishes related to activity and rest
2. Request assistance from physical and/or occupational therapists in planning and implementing exercise programs
3. Follow through on activities initiated and practiced in therapy
O. See Chapter 12, Rehabilitation, for additional information on mobility, supportive devices, teaching and motivation, transfer of patients, bowel and bladder retraining, etc.

ADMINISTRATION OF MEDICATIONS
Introduction
A. The scientific age has introduced an increasing number of pharmaceuticals appropriate for relief of stress and symptoms, support of defense systems, and adjuncts to other supplemental and curative therapies
B. Increasingly, as part of the nursing care, the nurse assumes the dependent function of administering these medications, either singly or in combinations
C. In the interest of patient welfare and safety, it is imperative that the independent and collaborative responsibilities inherent in this function be understood and practiced

Basic concepts
A. Legally, the administration of medications is a dependent function requiring a physician's written order and knowledge of cause and effect
B. Legally, morally, and ethically, independent judgment is required before prescribed medications are administered
C. Certain chemical agents alter, inactivate, or potentiate other medications when mixed either prior to or after administration
D. Medications may be given for local or systemic effects
E. Pharmacologic actions of drugs tend to stimulate or depress physiologic activity
F. Medications may be given in a variety of ways, depending on factors such as the effect desired, rapidity of action desired, or the effect of the chemical on the tissues

Nursing responsibilities

A. Ascertain the presence and correctness of a physician's order
B. Know the common symbols and equivalents in the apothecary and metric systems
C. Know the common abbreviations denoting frequency and route of administration
D. Know the usual dosage of a drug, the usual route of administration, and the expected, unusual, untoward, or toxic effects of a drug
E. Use independent judgment before administering a medication by assessing
   1. The patient's need relative to such factors as p.r.n. medications and expected effects of the medication; e.g., diuresis or sleep, etc.
   2. Untoward or toxic manifestations of prior doses; e.g., pruritus following an antibiotic, bradycardia below 60 or visionary disturbances with digoxin
   3. Compatibility of medications administered at the same time; e.g.,
      a. The presence of clouding or a precipitate when mixing injectables; e.g., Luminal Sodium and Demerol
      b. Inhibition of medication; e.g., antacids or milk given with tetracycline interfere with absorption, resulting in decreased serum levels of the antibiotic
      c. Potentiation of another medication; e.g., A.S.A. given when a patient is on anticoagulants intensifies the anticoagulant effect
   4. Effects on living tissues; e.g.,
      a. Iron can discolor tissue and must be given through a straw in liquid form or by the Z-track method intramuscularly
      b. Abscess formation can occur when the same area is used too frequently for intramuscular administration, thus, rotation of site is necessary
      c. Pain, irritation, or inflammation can occur during intravenous administration and may necessitate adjustments such as greater dilution or slower flow rate
F. Assist the patient to accept ordered medications by independent actions such as
   1. Crushing tablets that cannot be swallowed
   2. Disguising unpalatable tastes with fruit juices
   3. Reinforcing the need for medication
G. Assure that the right medication is given to the right patient at the right time in the right dose and by the right route
   1. Verify orders
   2. Read labels
   3. Calculate the dosage accurately when prescribed dose is not available
   4. Pour or draw up correct amounts
   5. Identify the patient correctly by checking the arm band
   6. Prepare the patient psychologically by providing explanations as indicated
   7. Prepare the patient physically by
      a. Positioning appropriately for oral and parenteral medications
      b. Disinfecting the skin when it is to be punctured
   8. Use clean or sterile technique as indicated by route of administration
   9. Use the route specified as appropriate for the ordered medication and dosage
H. For assistance with calculation of solutions and dosages refer to a programmed text (see Bibliography)
I. Use the appropriate technique for administration
   1. Preparations such as tablets, capsules, pills, powders, or liquids may be swallowed orally; in addition
      a. Tablets; e.g., nitroglycerine may be held sublingually
      b. Powders may be inhaled with a Medihaler; e.g., Cromalyn Sodium
      c. Liquids may be nebulized and inhaled or they may be swabbed, sprayed, or instilled
   2. Parenteral preparations such as ampules or vials containing dosage in solution or powder to which sterile water or saline must be added may be given in several ways
      a. Subcutaneously or hypodermically in small volume (0.5 to 2 ml.)
         (1) Pinch the tissue on the outer surface of the upper arm or the anterior aspect of the thigh or the abdomen
         (2) Insert a 25 to 26-gauge needle ⅝ to 1 inch in length at a 45° to 60° angle and inject the medication
         (3) Massage to increase absorp-

tion (contraindicated when giving heparin)

b. Intramuscularly in slightly larger volume (up to 5 ml.)
  (1) Spread the tissue taut or pinch if necessary
  (2) Use the upper outer quadrant of the buttock or ventral gluteal muscle, the lateral aspect of the thigh, or the deltoid area of the arm
  (3) When using the gluteal muscle, promote relaxation of the muscle whenever possible by placing the patient in a prone position with toes pointing inward or on the side with the leg flexed
  (4) Insert a 19- to 22-gauge needle 1 to 2 inches in length at a 90° angle quickly and smoothly
  (5) Depth of insertion depends on factors such as the weight of the patient and the size of the muscle used
  (6) Aspirate when the needle is in place and tissue is released (unless giving a substance such as Inferon, where it is contraindicated)
    (a) If no blood returns, continue injection
    (b) If blood is aspirated, withdraw and prepare a fresh dose
  (7) Apply pressure or massage area after injection as required (unless contraindicated; e.g., Z-track technique)

c. Intradermally with very small volume for local effect
  (1) Use syringe with appropriate calibrations; e.g., tuberculin
  (2) Inject at a 15° angle using a 26-gauge needle, ⅜ to ½ inch in length with the bevel up

d. Piggy-back administration using intravenous tubing in place
  (1) Dilute medication according to directions—usually with 50 to 150 ml. of fluid
  (2) Remove air from tubing of piggy-back
  (3) Cleanse diaphragm on intra-

venous tubing already in place with alcohol
  (4) Insert needle in rubber diaphragm on tubing leading from the infusion that is keeping the vein open
  (5) Stop flow of solution
  (6) Adjust rate of flow on piggy-back medication to complete absorption in time designated —usually about 30 minutes
  (7) Remove the piggy-back and readjust flow rate

J. Clearly and accurately record and report the administration of medications and the patient's response

REVIEW QUESTIONS FOR FUNDAMENTALS OF NURSING

1. One of the stresses of hospitalization is the strangeness of the environment and activity. A nurse can best limit extension of this stress by
   1. Listening to the patient
   2. Calling the patient by first name
   3. Visiting the patient frequently
   4. Explaining what the patient can expect

2. An environment conducive to reducing emotional stress and providing psychologic safety is one in which
   1. Needs are a primary concern
   2. All the patient's needs are met
   3. Realistic limits and controls are set
   4. Physical environment is kept in order

3. During what stage of the nursing process is the interpretation of body language most useful?
   1. Assessment
   2. Planning
   3. Intervention
   4. Evaluation

4. Communications are promoted in an interview by
   1. Asking questions that are answered by a "yes" or "no"
   2. Telling the patient there is no cause for alarm
   3. Asking "why" and "how"
   4. Using broad, opening statements

5. The effectiveness of nurse-patient communication is validated by
   1. Health team conferences
   2. Medical assessments
   3. Patient feedback
   4. Patient's physiologic adaptations

6. A nurse can determine the extent of a patient's self-sufficiency by
   1. Taking a nursing history
   2. Encouraging ADL (activities of daily living)
   3. Teaching principles of body mechanics
   4. Recording subjective as well as objective assessments

7. An independent nursing action to prevent thrombus formation is the use of
   1. Gentle massage
   2. Passive range of motion exercises
   3. Encouraging fluids
   4. Elastic stockings
8. A nursing hypothesis is a nurse's
   1. Actual intervention
   2. Prescription for care
   3. Evaluation of data
   4. Evaluation of care
9. Where primary nursing is practiced, the nurse who plans for and delegates care with full authority to see that the plan is followed is the
   1. Clinical specialist
   2. Head nurse
   3. Nurse clinician
   4. Primary nurse
10. The following is an example of primary health care by the nurse
    1. Correction of dietary deficiencies
    2. Assisting in immunization programs
    3. Prevention of disabilities
    4. Rehabilitation
11. An objective method for data collection includes the
    1. Direct observation of the patient
    2. Speaking with the patient's family
    3. Listening to the patient's description of the illness
    4. Collection of specimens
12. What action is part of the assessment stage of the nursing process?
    1. Taking a nursing history
    2. Formulating a care plan
    3. Establishing priorities
    4. Determining approaches to care
13. An appropriate time for the nurse to collect a sputum specimen from the patient is
    1. Upon awakening
    2. Before meals
    3. Before an IPPB treatment
    4. After activity
14. Which of the following is an involuntary reaction to pain?
    1. Perspiration
    2. Crying
    3. Pulling knees up to abdomen
    4. Grimacing
15. The most important aspect of handwashing is
    1. Water
    2. Soap
    3. Friction
    4. Time
16. Sink faucets are considered contaminated because
    1. They are not in sterile areas
    2. Water encourages bacterial growth
    3. They are opened with dirty hands
    4. Large numbers of people utilize them
17. Foot drop can best be prevented in the bed patient by the use of
    1. Boards
    2. Blocks
    3. Cradles
    4. Sandbags
18. Sleep consists of cyclic patterns of light and deep stages. The frequency of these cycles is approximately every
    1. ½ hour
    2. 1 hour
    3. 1½ hours
    4. 2 hours
19. The temperature range for a tepid application is
    1. 80°F. to 93°F.
    2. 70°F. to 78°F.
    3. 60°F. to 68°F.
    4. 55°F. to 65°F.
20. A sprain accompanied by edema is treated with the application of compresses. What is the appropriate temperature range?
    1. 65°F. to 80°F.
    2. 80°F. to 93°F.
    3. 93°F. to 98°F.
    4. 98°F. to 105°F.
21. Short, cold applications produce
    1. Depression of vital signs
    2. Peripheral vasodilation
    3. Decreased viscosity of blood
    4. Local anesthesia
22. Local hot and cold applications transfer temperature to and from the body by
    1. Radiation
    2. Convection
    3. Insulation
    4. Conduction
23. Diastolic pressure is the point on the manometer scale where the pulse beat is heard
    1. Loudest
    2. First
    3. Muted
    4. Last
24. What must a nurse do to avoid an error of parallax when taking a patient's blood pressure?
    1. Use a narrow cuff
    2. Stand close to the manometer
    3. Elevate the patient's arm on a pillow
    4. Read at eye level
25. Pulse pressure is the
    1. Difference between the apical and radial rates
    2. Force exerted against an arterial wall
    3. Degree of ventricular contraction in relation to output
    4. Difference between systolic and diastolic readings
26. Stethoscope placement in apical pulse measurement should be
    1. At the xiphoid process
    2. Between the third and fourth ribs and to the left of the sternum
    3. Slightly below the left nipple
    4. Just to the left of the median point of the sternum
27. A correct central venous pressure reading is obtained when the water level in the manometer
    1. Drops and then rises
    2. Synchronizes with the blood pressure
    3. Rises and stops at a specific plateau
    4. Fluctuates with respirations
28. In what position should a patient be when

a central venous pressure reading is performed?
1. Horizontal
2. Low Fowler's
3. Side lying, on affected side
4. Side lying, opposite to manometer

29. A patient who complains of tinnitus is describing a symptom that is
1. Functional
2. Prodromal
3. Objective
4. Subjective

30. A patient with pyrexia will be expected to have
1. Dyspnea
2. Elevated blood pressure
3. Increased pulse rate
4. Precordial pain

31. If a routine urine specimen cannot be sent immediately to the laboratory, the nurse should
1. Discard and collect a new specimen later
2. Store on "dirty" side of utility room
3. Refrigerate the specimen
4. Take no special action

32. How should a fractional urine specimen be removed from a retention catheter?
1. Cleanse drainage valve and remove from collection bag
2. Disconnect and drain into clean catheter
3. Wipe catheter with alcohol and drain into sterile test tube
4. Use a sterile syringe to remove from a clamped, cleansed catheter

33. Which of the following nursing actions is most needed when collecting a 24-hour urine specimen?
1. Weighing the patient before starting
2. Checking if any "preservatives" are needed
3. Placing collection jar in ice
4. Checking intake and output

34. Which of the following methods used in a hospital setting is the most useful in encouraging patients to void?
1. Listening to the sound of running water
2. Warming a bedpan
3. Placing hands in warm water
4. Providing privacy

35. The nurse can best prevent the contamination from retention catheters by
1. Forcing fluids
2. Cleansing around the meatus periodically
3. Perineal cleansing
4. Irrigating the catheter

36. The nurse, when caring for a patient with a continuous bladder irrigation, should
1. Measure urinary specific gravity
2. Record hourly outputs
3. Include irrigating solution on intake and output
4. Exclude irrigating solution from any 24-hour urine tests ordered

37. Comprehension of which of the following principles is most beneficial in establishing routine patterns of defecation?
1. Gastrocolic reflex
2. Inactivity produces muscle atonia

3. Increased fluid promotes ease of evacuation
4. Increased potassium is needed for normal neuromuscular irritability

38. A rectal tube is sometimes inserted for the relief of distention. What is the minimal time it should remain in place to be effective?
1. 15 minutes
2. 30 minutes
3. 45 minutes
4. 60 minutes

39. How far into the rectum should a rectal catheter be inserted?
1. 2 inches
2. 4 inches
3. 6 inches
4. 8 inches

40. In what position should a patient be when receiving an enema?
1. Sims
2. Knee chest
3. Mid Fowler's
4. Back lying

41. What is the maximum safe height at which an enema can be held?
1. 12 inches
2. 15 inches
3. 18 inches
4. 24 inches

42. What should a nurse initially do when a patient complains of intestinal cramps while being given an enema?
1. Give at a slower rate
2. Lower the height of the container
3. Stop until cramps are gone
4. Discontinue the procedure

43. What comment by the patient is most indicative of the presence of a fecal impaction?
1. "I don't have much of an appetite."
2. "I have a lot of gas pains."
3. "I feel like I have to go and just can't."
4. "I haven't had a bowel movement for 2 days."

44. What assessment indicates the probable presence of a fecal impaction?
1. Tympanites
2. Decreased number of bowel movements
3. Fecal liquid seepage
4. Bright red blood in stool

45. A patient drank 7½ oz. of orange juice, 6 oz. of tea, and 8 oz. of eggnog. The calculated intake is
1. 515 ml.
2. 645 ml.
3. 625 ml.
4. 585 ml.

46. Calculate the intake-output of the following patient for an 8-hour period.
8:00 A.M.—I.V. with 5% D/W running and 900 ml. left in bottle
8:30 A.M.—150 ml. urine voided
9 A.M. to 3 P.M.—q.3h. intervals, 200 ml. gastric tube formula and 50 ml. H₂O. No aspirate obtained until final feeding. 25 ml. at this time. Vitamin sol., 10 ml. q.4h. from 8 A.M. to 4 P.M.

1:00 P.M.—220 ml. voided
3:15 P.M.—235 ml. voided
4:00 P.M.—I.V. with 550 ml. left in bottle
1. Intake—930 ml.; Output—650 ml.
2. Intake—1050 ml.; Output—680 ml.
3. Intake—1080 ml.; Output 595 ml.
4. Intake—1130 ml.; Output—630 ml.

47. A nurse can best assess the degree of edema in an extremity by
1. Checking for pitting
2. Weighing the patient
3. Measuring the affected area
4. Observing intake and output

48. A nursing measure to relieve edema is
1. Restricting fluids
2. Elevating affected area
3. Applying elastic bandages
4. Doing ROM exercises

49. Which of the following is most likely to occur in a patient with unresolved edema?
1. Thrombi formation
2. Tissue ischemia
3. Proteinemia
4. Contractures

50. Digitalis is effective because it
1. Slows and strengthens cardiac contraction
2. Lengthens refractory phase of cardiac cycle
3. Reduces edema in extracellular spaces
4. Increases ventricular contraction

51. A patient is to receive 0.2 mg. of Digoxin I.M. The ampule is labelled 0.5 mg. = 2 ml. How many milliliters should be administered?
1. 8 ml.
2. 0.8 ml.
3. 1 ml.
4. 1.2 ml.

52. When a patient is on anticoagulant therapy, the nurse should observe for
1. Headache
2. Epistaxis
3. Nausea
4. Chest pain

53. What should a nurse initially do when a patient complains of pain postoperatively?
1. Have the patient rest
2. Take vital signs
3. Administer p.r.n. analgesic
4. Check time of patient's last medication

54. When teaching a patient about an oral hypoglycemic medication, emphasis must be placed on the significance of
1. Manifestations of toxicity
2. Untoward reactions
3. Taking it regularly on time
4. Increasing dosage when necessary

55. What should the nurse initially do when an I.V. infusion infiltrates?
1. Attempt to flush the tube
2. Elevate the I.V. site
3. Discontinue the infusion
4. Apply warm, moist soaks

56. What is the longest possible period of time that 1 bottle of 1000 ml. 5% D/W to keep vein open can be infused without producing untoward effects?
1. 6 hours
2. 12 hours
3. 18 hours
4. 24 hours

57. The rationale for weight loss in a patient on I.V. feedings is
1. Insufficient carbohydrate intake
2. Lack of protein supplementation
3. Insufficient intake of water-soluble vitamins
4. Increased concentration of electrolytes in cells

58. A patient is on 24-hour I.V. feedings. The current fluid orders read: Bottle #1: 1000 ml. 5% D/W; bottle #2: 1000 ml. 5% D/0.9% NaCl; bottle #3: 1000 ml 5% D/0.33% NaCl. What is the approximate flow rate in gtts./minute? (I.V. tubing = 20 gtts./ml.)
1. 20
2. 25
3. 35
4. 40

59. Nursing care of patients receiving parenteral hyperalimentation must include
1. Doing urinary specific gravity
2. Vital signs every 2 hours
3. Fractional urines
4. Checking for muscular cramps

60. The nurse can prevent a major reaction to hyperalimentation infusions by
1. The slow administration of the fluid
2. Checking vital signs every 4 hours
3. Changing site every 24 hours
4. Recording of intake and output

61. The correct patient position for the insertion of a gavage tube is
1. High Fowler's
2. Mid Fowler's
3. Low Fowler's
4. Supine

62. Prior to insertion, a clear, polyethylene plastic gavage tube should be
1. Warmed
2. Used at room temperature
3. Placed in tepid saline
4. Iced

63. Which of the following would be an appropriate temperature for a gastric feeding?
1. 50°F. to 60°F.
2. 70°F. to 75°F.
3. 90°F. to 100°F.
4. 100°F. to 115°F.

64. What nursing observation should tell the nurse that the patient is unable to tolerate further tube feeding?
1. Passage of flatus
2. Rapid flow of feeding
3. Epigastric tenderness
4. Rise of formula in tube

65. At what angle should the head of the bed be to prevent the effects of "shearing force"?
1. 30°
2. 45°
3. 60°
4. 90°

66. In formulating a teaching care plan for a patient who has had a tracheostomy, the nurse emphasizes
1. Maintenance of sterile conditions
2. Suctioning on a regular schedule
3. Using a gauze cover when bathing
4. Constant cleanliness at the site

67. When is the least appropriate time of day to receive an intermittent positive pressure breathing (IPPB) treatment?
    1. Upon awakening
    2. Before a meal
    3. At bedtime
    4. After a meal
68. Independent nursing care of the acutely ill patient who has a large amount of respiratory secretions includes
    1. Turning and positioning
    2. Cupping
    3. Clapping
    4. Postural drainage
69. In creating a therapeutic environment for a patient who has had a myocardial infarct, the nurse should provide for
    1. Daily papers in the morning
    2. Telephone communication
    3. Short family visits
    4. Television for short periods
70. Your patient with pneumonia is dyspneic. An assistive position would be
    1. Trendelenburg
    2. Sims
    3. Orthopneic
    4. Supine
71. What determines the method of oxygen administration for a specific patient?
    1. Facial anatomy
    2. Pathology
    3. Age
    4. Degree of patient's activity
72. Which of the following activities are permissible when a patient is in an oxygen tent?
    1. Use of grounded electric equipment
    2. Combing a patient's hair
    3. Using lanolin cream for skin care
    4. Using a wool blanket
73. A preventive measure to be taken regarding the untoward effects of oxygen therapy is
    1. Padding elastic bands of face masks
    2. Humidification of the gas
    3. Taking apical pulse before starting therapy
    4. Placing patient in orthopneic position
74. Characteristic behavior in the initial stage of a patient's coping with dying includes
    1. Asking for an additional medical consultation
    2. Ringing a call light as soon as the nurse has left the room
    3. Criticism of medical care
    4. Sleep for long periods
75. The nurse can best help a patient in the stage of acceptance by
    1. Allowing unrestricted visiting
    2. Being around and not necessarily speaking
    3. Explaining all that is being done
    4. Allowing the patient to cry
76. The family rather than the patient is likely to require more understanding during which stage of dying?
    1. Denial
    2. Anger
    3. Depression
    4. Acceptance
77. The determining factor in the revision of a nursing care plan is the

1. Correctness of the original hypothesis
2. Method for providing care
3. Available time
4. Effectiveness of implementation

Mr. Rogers, with a long history of emphysema, is now terminally ill with cancer of the esophagus. His plan of care includes a soft diet, modified postural drainage and IPPB treatments b.i.d. Mr. Rogers is weak, dyspneic, emaciated, and apathetic. Questions 78 through 87 refer to this situation.

78. Nursing care plans for Mr. Rogers should give priority to
    1. Diet and nutrition
    2. Hygiene and comfort
    3. Body mechanics and posture
    4. Intake and output
79. Mr. Rogers expresses aversion to his meals and eats only small amounts. Nursing care that may alleviate this is to provide
    1. Only foods he likes in small portions
    2. Supplementary vitamins to stimulate appetite
    3. Nourishment between meals
    4. Small portions more frequently
80. The term used to describe Mr. Rogers' response to food most accurately is
    1. Anorexia
    2. Anoxia
    3. Apathy
    4. Dysphagia
81. After postural drainage, in order to obtain maximum benefits, the patient should be
    1. Placed in a sitting position to provide drainage
    2. Encouraged to cough deeply
    3. Replaced on an IPPB machine
    4. Encouraged to rest for 30 minutes before coughing

Mr. Rogers' pain and dyspnea are increasing in severity. The doctor has order 100 mg. meperidine p.r.n. and oxygen p.r.n.

82. In preparing Mr. Rogers' medication the nurse should know that meperidine is commonly available for dispensation as
    1. Darvon
    2. Doriden
    3. Demerol
    4. Narcan
83. You administer nasal oxygen at 2 L./minute. You would observe Mr. Rogers closely for
    1. Hyperemia and increased respirations
    2. Cyanosis and lethargy
    3. Anxiety and tachycardia
    4. Drowsiness and decreased respirations

Mr. Rogers has a 44-year-old wife, a 16-year-old daughter in high school, and a 20-year-old son in college. They visit him frequently.

84. In view of Mr. Rogers' extreme weakness and dyspnea, nursing care plans should include
    1. Limiting family visiting hours to the evening before sleep
    2. Allowing self-activity whenever possible
    3. Encouraging family to feed and assist him
    4. Planning all necessary care at one time with long rests in between

85. On one occasion Mr. Rogers says to you, "If I could just be free of pain for a few days, I might be able to eat more and regain strength." In reference to the stages of dying, the patient indicates
    1. Rationalization
    2. Frustration
    3. Bargaining
    4. Depression
86. The best nursing approach when a patient utilizes denial as a defense is to
    1. Ignore the patient's behavior
    2. Point out the reality of the situation
    3. Join him since denial is his only defense
    4. Recognize and accept the behavior at this point
87. When Mr. Rogers reaches the point of acceptance in the stages of dying, it may be manifested in his behavior by
    1. Euphoria
    2. Detachment
    3. Apathy
    4. Emotionalism

Miss Fleming, a 35-year-old executive secretary, is hospitalized for treatment of hypertension. Her orders include bedrest with bathroom privileges, low-sodium diet, Serpasil, Librium. She has been active in both her business and social life, usually having a cocktail before dinner and smoking a pack of cigarettes daily. Miss Fleming expresses disgust for her regimen and dissatisfaction with the nursing care. Questions 88 through 94 refer to this situation.

88. Miss Fleming's behavior is probably a manifestation of her
    1. Denial of illness
    2. Response to cerebral anoxia
    3. Reaction to hypertensive medications
    4. Fear of the health problem
89. Librium is primarily indicated for Miss Fleming because it
    1. Promotes rest
    2. Induces sleep
    3. Produces hypotension
    4. Reduces hostility
90. Miss Fleming has been receiving Librium 10 mg. q.i.d. for the past 5 days. You would question giving the medication if she exhibits
    1. Muscle twitching
    2. Blurred vision
    3. Hypotension
    4. Extreme drowsiness
91. Miss Fleming is receiving Serpasil (reserpine) because it is an effective
    1. Diuretic
    2. Hypnotic
    3. Antihypertensive
    4. Tranquilizer

Miss Fleming has been told she must stop smoking and eliminate her predinner cocktail.

92. You discover a pack of cigarettes in Miss Fleming's bathrobe. The best course of action to take at this time is to
    1. Report the situation to the head nurse
    2. Let the patient know you found them
    3. Discard them and say nothing to her
    4. Call the physician and request direction
93. Miss Fleming complains about everything and anything in the hospital. It is important to recognize that
    1. The complaints have some basis
    2. The patient is denying illness
    3. The behavior has meaning for the patient
    4. The patient must be helped to see reality
94. When Miss Fleming is being overtly verbally hostile, the most appropriate nursing response is
    1. Reasonable exploration of situations
    2. Complete withdrawal from her behavior
    3. Silent acceptance of her behavior
    4. Verbal defense of your position

Mr. Davis is a 55-year-old man who has suffered a cerebrovascular accident. He has right sided paralysis and is dysphagic and dysphasic. His nursing care includes frequent monitoring of vital signs. Questions 95 through 101 refer to this situation.

95. Mr. Davis' temperature should be taken
    1. Orally
    2. In the groin
    3. Rectally
    4. In the axilla
96. Mr. Davis is experiencing difficulty in
    1. Swallowing
    2. Focusing
    3. Writing
    4. Understanding
97. Blood pressure should not be taken on Mr. Davis' right arm because circulatory impairment may
    1. Precipitate the formation of a thrombus
    2. Hinder restoration of function
    3. Produce inaccurate readings
    4. Cause excessive pressure on the brachial artery
98. Mr. Davis' dysphasia requires initial provision for
    1. Routine hygienic needs
    2. Prevention of aspiration
    3. Effective communication
    4. Liquid formula diet
99. Three days after admission Mr. Davis has a nasogastric tube inserted and is prescribed liquid formula diet 6 times daily. For the first day the amount of liquid administered at one time should not exceed
    1. 150 ml.
    2. 350 ml.
    3. 450 ml.
    4. 250 ml.
100. The formula temperature most compatible for administration is
    1. Chilled
    2. Body
    3. Room
    4. 108° F.
101. Tube feeding diets are administered slowly to reduce the hazard of
    1. Indigestion
    2. Regurgitation
    3. Flatulence
    4. Distention

Mr. McNabb, a 65-year-old self-employed grocer, is admitted to the hospital with congestive failure and pulmonary edema. His treatment includes oxygen by mask, digoxin, Diuril, and a low-sodium diet. He is dyspneic, apprehensive, and restless. Questions 102 through 110 refer to this situation.

102. Mr. McNabb would be most comfortable with the oxygen set at
    1. 12 to 14 liters
    2. 6 to 8 liters
    3. 2 to 4 liters
    4. 16 to 18 liters
103. Safety precautions are especially important in Mr. McNabb's room because oxygen
    1. Is flammable
    2. Has unstable properties
    3. Increases apprehension
    4. Supports combustion
104. Mr. McNabb's restlessness is dangerous because it
    1. Decreases the amount of oxygen available
    2. Interferes with normal respiration
    3. Increases the cardiac workload
    4. Produces elevation in temperature
105. The method of oxygen administration least likely to increase apprehension in the patient is
    1. Catheter
    2. Cannula
    3. Tent
    4. Mask
106. After receiving a sedative, Mr. McNabb says to the nurse, "I guess you are too busy to

stay with me." The best response in this circumstance is
    1. "I have to see other patients."
    2. "The medication will help you rest soon."
    3. "I have to go now but I will come back in 10 minutes."
    4. "You will feel better; I will adjust your oxygen mask."
107. Bloody sputum is described as
    1. Hematuria
    2. Hematemesis
    3. Hematoma
    4. Hemoptysis
108. To relieve the patient with congestive heart failure complicated by pulmonary edema, the nurse should
    1. Elevate the lower extremities
    2. Place the patient in orthopneic position
    3. Encourage frequent coughing
    4. Prepare for modified postural drainage
109. Before giving Mr. McNabb digoxin, it is necessary to measure the
    1. Radial pulse in one arm
    2. Apical heart rate
    3. Radial pulse in both arms
    4. Difference between apical and radial pulse
110. Nursing care of Mr. McNabb includes observation for symptoms of electrolyte depletion caused by
    1. Sodium restriction
    2. Inadequate oral intake
    3. Continuous dyspnea
    4. Diuretic therapy

CHAPTER 9

Family-centered nursing

Birth, life, and death are phenomena common to every human being. The lives of most people throughout the world are influenced by a group of human beings called the family. The family may be nuclear, extended, one-parent, adoptive, or communal. Because these processes and the family are so closely related, much of the traditional maternal-child nursing content can be presented within the concept of the family. However, some of the knowledge needed to more fully understand the complexities of pregnancy, birth, and childhood cannot be wholly integrated. Therefore, the following sections, which are usually called obstetric and pediatric nursing, are divided into three areas: parent-child nursing, maternal nursing and reproductive problems, and pediatric nursing.

The first section, Parent-child nursing, discusses the newborn in light of the family, the role of the parents and development of mothering, the care of the newborn and growing infant, and the physical and psychosocial growth of the infant until 1 year of age. This section emphasizes the general principles of growth and development.

The second section, Maternal nursing and reproductive problems, emphasizes the pubertal changes of adolescence; the normal processes of conception, embryologic development, pregnancy, labor, delivery, and postpartum; and family planning. In addition, the newborn and the mother are discussed in relation to prematurity, birth injuries, and complications of labor and delivery. Current topics such as abortion, infant narcotic addiction, venereal disease, and sterility are included.

In the third section, Pediatric nursing, the normal growth and development of children over 1 year of age, the preventive aspects of health in children, and the major health problems from birth through adolescence are presented.

It is believed that this method of presenting the concepts encompassing maternal-child nursing will more fully emphasize the family, normal growth and development, and the nursing process in terms of preventive care and health problems while eliminating areas of repetition.

Childbirth is a family experience. Humanity's basic needs for survival are centered in the family because without continuous love, physical contact, food, and stimulation of the senses, the infant would never survive. As each new member becomes a part of the family unit, interactions with the environment and other human beings become a part of early physical and emotional development. What is learned is determined by the kinds of stimulation received from the interactions occurring within the family. It is through this reciprocal give-and-take between the newborn and the family that each person becomes an individual, unique self.

Although childbearing patterns differ the world over, there are constants. In order of priority, they are: immediate physical contact between the infant and the parents; ability of the parents to give the infant love, food, and protection from the environment; the biologic need in men and women to reproduce; and the maturation and growth process that occurs in male and female in their changing roles as parents.

The unique and changing responsibilities in the life cycle event of parenthood can be a real crisis. The changes occurring in society, be they social, economic, technical, or political, directly affect the patterns of childbearing and childrearing. Parenthood today is given serious thought since it concerns both the family and society with the emphasis on quality rather than quantity.

One of the most moving and significant moments in observing parents is when they participate in the birth of their baby. The birth is the culmination of much preparation and interaction with the baby from the moment of conception. Even in utero there is much biologic and psychologic interaction. In fact, the way parents react to the pregnancy relates to how they viewed childbirth within their own family units.

The parents' initial contact with the infant is the most significant factor in the beginning relationship within the family unit. By a process of touching, holding, comparing, talking to, feeding, and caring, the infant becomes an individual. Nurtured and guided through infancy, childhood, adolescence, and young adulthood, the individual is made ready for the responsibilities of parenthood. It is obvious then that the quality of care received greatly influences the ability to care for one's own children. Therefore, patterns of childbearing and childrearing are transmitted and culturally learned from generation to generation.

PARENT-CHILD NURSING

THE FAMILY

A. Structure of family
1. The basic unit of a society
2. Composition varies although one member is usually recognized as head
3. Usually share common goals and beliefs
4. Roles change within the group and reflect both the individual's and the group's needs
5. Status of members determined by position in family in conjunction with views of society

B. Family functions
1. Reproduction—group developed to reproduce and rear members of a society
2. Maintenance to provide
   a. Clothing, housing, food, and medical care
   b. Social, psychologic, and emotional support for family members
   c. Protection, since immaturity of young children necessitates that care be given by adults
   d. Status—child is a member of a family that is also a part of the larger community
3. Socialization
   a. Child is "humanized" by introduction to social situations and instruction in appropriate social behaviors
   b. Self-identity develops through relationships with other family members

C. Disturbances in parent-child relationships can be viewed in terms of disturbed role theory
1. Parental child abuse
2. Maternal deprivation

PARENT-CHILD RELATIONSHIPS

A. Infant
1. Before birth
   a. First 8 weeks is a period of rapid growth and development for fetus
   b. Any interference with maternal physiology may cause irreparable damage to fetus
   c. Increased maternal hormonal action is necessary for continued implantation of fetus in the uterus

2. Following birth, baby has need for
   a. Contact with one person on a consistent basis
   b. Food, fondling, caressing, rocking, speaking, clothing, bathing, comfort, and protection from environment
B. Mothering and fathering are
   1. Based on a biologic inborn desire to reproduce
   2. Role concepts that begin with own childhood experiences
   3. Primitive emotional relationships
   4. Maturing processes
   5. Conceptualizations of the physiologic and psychologic processes following infant's birth
   6. Fostered by the parent-infant interaction that constantly reinforces gratification as needs are met and security develops
   7. Abilities that are learned rather than innate
C. Parent-child relationships are affected by
   1. Readiness for pregnancy
      a. Planned or unplanned
      b. Health status prior to pregnancy
      c. Financial status
      d. Determinants such as age, cultural backgrounds, number in family unit, etc.
      e. Political forces
   2. Nature of pregnancy
      a. Health status during pregnancy
      b. Preparation for parenthood
      c. Support from family members and members of health team
   3. Character of labor and delivery
      a. Length and pattern of labor
      b. Type and amount of analgesia received
      c. Support from family and health team
      d. Anesthesia during delivery
      e. Type of delivery
   4. Period immediately after birth
      a. Early parent-infant contact
         (1) Allow mother to touch, fondle, and hold
         (2) Give mother ample time to inspect and begin to identify
         (3) Early give-and-take between parents and infant—rooming-in arrangement
         (4) Supportive nursing care in these beginning relationships

         (5) Identification of beginning disturbed relationships with nursing intervention
      b. Significant phases
         (1) Taking-in phase—mother's needs have to be met before she can meet baby's; behavior—talks about self rather than baby, doesn't seem too interested in baby, doesn't touch infant, cries easily
         (2) Transition phase—characterized by mother starting to take hold, looking at and reaching for baby, touching with fingertips, talking about baby, etc.
         (3) Taking-hold phase—kisses, embraces, gives care to infant, eye to eye contact, uses whole hand to make contact, calls baby by name, etc.

THE NEWBORN
Family history

A. Chronic illness in mother's or father's family
B. Previous medical-surgical illnesses of mother and father
C. Age and present health status of mother and father
D. History of previous pregnancies
E. Prenatal history
   1. Medical supervision during pregnancy
   2. Nutrition during pregnancy
   3. Course of pregnancy—illnesses, medications taken or treatments required
   4. Duration of gestation
   5. Course and amount of sedation and anesthesia required
   6. Type of delivery and significant events during immediate period following delivery
   7. Immediate response of newborn (Apgar score at 1 and 5 minutes following birth)

Adaptation to extrauterine life

A. Immediate needs at time of delivery
   1. Aspiration of mucus to provide an open airway
   2. Evaluation by use of Apgar score 1 minute and 5 minutes following birth (see Table 9-1)
   3. Maintenance of body temperature to prevent acidosis

Table 9-1. Apgar score chart*

Adaptation	0	1	2
Heart rate	Absent	Slow, below 100	Over 100
Respiratory effort	Absent	Weak cry	Strong cry
Muscle tone	Limp	Some flexion of extremities	Active motion
Reflex irritability	No response	Grimace	Cry
Color	Cyanotic, pale	Body pink, extremities cyanotic	Completely pink

*Scores: 7-10 good condition; 3-6 moderately depressed; 0-2 severely depressed.

4. Constant observation of physical condition
5. Eye care—prophylactic instillation of silver nitrate or other medication in each eye to prevent ophthalmia neonatorum

3. Appraisal of newborn after delivery
   1. Skin
      a. Body is normally pink with slight cyanosis of hands and feet for 24 hours (jaundice is abnormal during the first 24 to 48 hours of life)
      b. Check for abrasions, rashes, crackling, and elasticity, which indicates status of tissue hydration; at times, milia (white pinpoint spots over nose caused by retained sebaceous secretions), birthmarks, forceps marks, ecchymosis, or papules are present
   2. Respirations are abdominal and irregular, with a rate of 30 to 50 per minute (retractions—depression of sternum—are abnormal)
   3. Head and sensory organs
      a. Head and chest circumference nearly equal to the crown-rump length; chest slightly smaller than head
      b. Symmetry of face—as baby cries sides of face move equally
      c. Check head for molding, abrasions, or skin breakdowns; observe for caput succedaneum—edema of soft tissue of the scalp; cephalohematoma—edema of scalp caused by effusion of blood between the bone and periosteum; extend head fully in all directions for adequacy in range of motion
      d. Observe eyes for discharge or irritation, check pupils for reaction to light, equality of eye movements (normally there is some ocular incoordination); check sclera for clarity, jaundice, or hemorrhages
      e. Nose—observe for patency of both nostrils
      f. Mouth—observe gums and hard and soft palates for any openings—mucosa of mouth normally clear (white patches that bleed on rubbing indicate thrush, a monilial infection)
      g. Ears—auricles open; vernix covers tympanic membrane making otoscopic examination useless (ring bell close to ear—baby should stir); both eyes should be same level as ears; upper earlobes normally curved (flatness indicative of kidney anomaly)
   4. Chest and abdomen
      a. Chest auscultation—only respiratory sounds should be audible (noisy crackling sounds abnormal); heart rate—regular 120 to 160 per minute (rubbing or unusual sounds abnormal)
      b. Abdomen
         (1) Listen to bowel sounds over abdomen
         (2) Palpate spleen with fingertips under left costal margin—tip should be palpable
         (3) Palpate liver on right side—normally 1 cm. below costal margin
         (4) Observe umbilical cord for redness, odor, or discharge
         (5) Palpate femoral pulses gently at inner aspect of groin, which indicates intact circulation to extremities

5. Genitalia
   a. Boy
      (1) Palpate scrotum for testes, at times undescended at birth, which is normal (must descend by puberty or sperm destroyed by high temperature within the abdominal cavity)
      (2) Enlargement of scrotum indicates hydrocele (diagnosis affirmed by transparent appearance of scrotum when flashlight is held close to scrotal sac)
      (3) Observe tip of penis for urinary meatus (ventral opening—epispadias, dorsal opening—hypospadias)
   b. Girl—observe genitalia for labia and vaginal opening; edema of labia and bloody mucoid discharge normal, resulting from transfer of maternal hormones
6. Extremities
   a. Hands and arms—thumbs clenched in fist
      (1) Check for number and variation of fingers
      (2) Check clavicle and scapula while putting arm through normal range of motion (clicking or resistance indicates dislocation or fracture)
      (3) Palpate for fractures (crepitation is indicative)
   b. Feet and legs
      (1) Check toes, pattern, and number
      (2) Adduct and abduct feet through range of motion, there should be no resistance or tightness
      (3) Flex both legs onto lower abdomen, there should be no resistance or tightness
      (4) Place both feet on flat surface and bend knees—both knees should be at same height (when unequal, hip dislocation is present)
7. Back—turn baby on abdomen, run finger along vertebral column (any separations or swellings indicative of a spina bifida)
8. Anus—patency confirmed with passage of meconium (inability to insert rectal thermometer may be indicative of imperforate anus)
9. Neuromuscular development—check reflexes
   a. Rooting—touch baby's cheek, baby should root for finger
   b. Sucking—place an object close to baby's mouth, baby should make an attempt to suck
   c. Grasp—place fingers in palm of baby's hand and encircle palm with your hand; lift infant off a firm surface, baby will grasp; infant's head will lag as baby is raised up
   d. Babinski—run thumb up middle undersurface of infant's foot, toe will separate and flare out
   e. Plantar—run thumb up lateral undersurface of infant's foot and toe will curl downward
   f. Moro—making a loud, sharp noise close to the baby will result in the baby bringing both arms and legs close to the body as if in an embrace (disappears by 4 months of age)
   g. Crawl—when the baby is on a firm surface and turned on the abdomen crawling movements will follow
   h. Step or dance—by supporting the infant under both arms, stepping movements will occur when feet are placed on a firm surface
C. Changes in newborn during the first week of life
   1. Circulatory
      a. Tying of cord at birth brings changes in fetal circulation—closure of foramen ovale and ductus arteriosus and obliteration of umbilical arteries produce an adult-like circulation within 1 hour following birth
      b. Heart rate regular—120 to 180, but variable depending upon infant's activity—soft heart murmur common for first month of life
      c. Clotting mechanism poor because of low prothrombin concentration
      d. Liver immature (although large) cannot destroy excessive red cells in newborn resulting in physiologic jaundice by third day

e. Hemoglobin level high—14 to 20 g. per 100 ml. of blood

f. White blood count high—6000 to 22,000

2. Respiratory—respirations diaphragmatic, irregular, abdominal—30 to 50 per minute, quiet with periods of apnea

3. Excretory
   a. Kidneys immature—newborn should void during first 24 hours (2 weeks of age voids 20 times daily), albumin and urates (brick red staining on diaper) common during first week because of dehydration
   b. Stools—first stool, black-green and tenacious, called *meconium*, by third day, becomes mixed with light yellow, called *transitional*

4. Integumentary
   a. Lanugo—fine downy hair growth over entire body
   b. Milia—small, whitish, pinpoint spots over nose caused by retained sebaceous secretions
   c. Mongolian spots—blue-black discolorations on back, buttocks, and sacral region that disappear by first year

5. Digestive
   a. Has stores of nutrients from intrauterine existence, therefore needs very little nourishment first few days
   b. Roots and sucks when anything is brought to mouth
   c. Digests simple carbohydrates, fats, and proteins readily
   d. Cardiac sphincter of stomach not well developed, therefore regurgitates if stomach is overfull
   e. Needs to be bubbled frequently to get rid of air bubbles in stomach

6. Endocrine
   a. Metabolic—all newborns normally lose 10% of their body weight by first week of life
   b. Hormonal—enlargement of breasts in boys and girls is normal as a result of hormones transmitted to baby by mother

7. Neural
   a. Central nervous system and brain not well developed—infant needs constant supply of oxygen

b. Breathing, sucking, and crying are early neural activities necessary for the infant's survival

D. Needs of newborn
   1. Air for survival
      a. Suctioning of mucus as needed to maintain an open airway
      b. Positioning—side lying to facilitate drainage of mucus
      c. Observing any signs of air hunger such as cyanosis, flaring of nostrils, noisy respirations, sternal retractions would warrant aspiration and administration of oxygen by inhalation
   2. Warmth, comfort, and protection from the environment
      a. Keep in heated crib until body temperature is stabilized to prevent chilling
      b. Clothing should be loose, soft
      c. Crib should be firm and provide protection
      d. Skin should be kept clean and dry to maintain integrity
   3. Human contact—body contact with another human person is paramount for the newborn's survival, ministrations in giving care should be carried out with purpose and awareness of the importance of these early beginning relationships (talking, rocking, singing are an essential part of body contact with a newborn)
   4. Food
      a. Newborn needs to ingest simple proteins, carbohydrates, and fats for continued cell growth
      b. Caloric intake requirement—see Nutrition requirements, pp. 171-172
      c. Breast milk is ideal since it is readily accessible and easily digested
         (1) Infant's sucking at breast stimulates the maternal posterior pituitary to produce pitocin whose properties in the blood system constrict the lactiferous sinuses to move the milk down through the nipple ducts— known as the let-down reflex
         (2) Emotional stress in the mother and a poor sucking reflex will inhibit the let-down of milk
      d. A feeding of cow's milk, carbohydrate, and water to fulfill necessary

calorie requirements may also be used if breast feeding is not desired by the mother

e. Feeding should be offered on demand to meet the infant's needs

5. Sleep—since sleep lowers body metabolism it helps restore energy and assimilate nutriments for growth

HUMAN GROWTH AND DEVELOPMENT
Principles of growth

A. Traditional definition of growth is limited to physical maturation
B. Integrated definition includes functional maturation
C. Growth is complex with all aspects closely related
D. Growth is measured both quantitatively and qualitatively over a period of time
E. Although the rate is not even, growth is a continuous and orderly process
  1. Infancy—most rapid period of growth
  2. Preschool to puberty—slow and uniform rate of growth
  3. Puberty—growth spurt
  4. After puberty—decline in growth rate till death
F. There are regular patterns in the direction of growth and development, such as the cephalocaudal law and proximodistal law
G. Different parts of body grow at different rates; e.g.,
  1. Prenatally—head grows the fastest
  2. During first year—elongation of trunk dominates
H. Both rate and pattern of growth can be modified, most obviously by nutrition
I. There are critical periods in growth and development, such as brain growth during uterine life and infancy
J. Although there are specified sequences for achieving growth and development, each individual proceeds at own rate
K. Development is closely related to the maturation of the nervous system; as some primitive reflexes disappear they are replaced by a voluntary activity (such as grasp)

Characteristics of growth

A. Circulatory system
  1. Heart rate decreases with increasing age
    a. Infancy—130 beats per minute
    b. One year—100 to 110
    c. Childhood—70 to 80
    d. Adolescence to adulthood—60 to 70 (after maturity, women have slightly higher pulse rate than men)
  2. Blood pressure increases with age
    a. Base 60 to 90 mm. Hg systolic to 20 to 60 mm. Hg diastolic
    b. Increase of about 2 to 3 mm. Hg per year
    c. Systolic pressure in adolescence—higher in males than in females
  3. Hemoglobin
    a. Highest at birth, 17 g., then decreases to 11.5 to 12 g. per 100 ml. of blood by 1 year
    b. Fetal hemoglobin (60% to 90%) gradually decreases during first year to less than 5% of total hemoglobin
    c. Gradual increase in hemoglobin level to 14.5 g. between 1 and 12 years of age
    d. Hemoglobin level higher in males than in females
    e. Red blood cells in children contain less hemoglobin than in adults, but the hemoglobin has greater affinity for oxygen
B. Respiratory system
  1. Rate decreases with increase in age
    a. Infancy—30 to 40 per minute
    b. Childhood—20 to 24 per minute
    c. Adolescence and adulthood—16 to 20 per minute
  2. Vital capacity
    a. Gradual increase throughout childhood and adolescence with a decrease in later life
    b. Capacity in males exceeds that of females
  3. Basal metabolism
    a. Highest rate found in newborn
    b. Rate declines with increase in age, higher in males than females
C. Urinary system
  1. Premature and full-term neonates have some inability to concentrate urine
  2. Glomerular filtration rate greatly increased by 6 months of age
  3. Glomerular filtration rate decreases after 20 years of age
D. Digestive system
  1. Stomach size small at birth, rapidly increases during infancy and childhood

2. Peristaltic activity decreases with advancing age
3. Blood sugar levels gradually rise from 75 to 80 mg. per 100 ml. of blood in infancy to 95 to 100 mg. during adolescence
4. Premature infants have lower blood sugar levels than full-term infants
5. Enzymes are present at birth to digest proteins and a moderate amount of fat, but only simple sugars (amylase is produced as starch is introduced)
6. Secretion of hydrochloric acid and salivary enzymes increases with age until adolescence, then decreases with advancing age

E. Nervous system
1. Brain reaches 90% of total size by 2 years of age
2. All brain cells are present by end of first year, although size and complexity will increase
3. Maturation of brainstem and spinal cord follows cephalocaudal and proximodistal laws

GROWTH AND DEVELOPMENT TO 1 YEAR OF AGE

Erikson's stage of trust; Piaget's cognitive sensorimotor phase

A. One month
1. Physical
   a. Weight—gains about 150 to 210 g. (5 to 7 oz.) weekly during first 6 months of life
   b. Height—gains about 2.5 cm. (1 inch) a month for first 6 months of life
2. Motor
   a. Head sags, must be supported, may lift head temporarily
   b. Holds head parallel with body when placed prone
   c. Can turn head from side to side when prone or supine
   d. Asymmetric posture dominates, such as tonic neck reflex
   e. Primitive reflexes still present
3. Sensory
   a. Follows light to midline
   b. Eye movements coordinated most of time
4. Socialization and vocalization
   a. Smiles indiscriminately
   b. Utters small throaty sounds

B. Two to 3 months
1. Physical—posterior fontanel closed
2. Motor
   a. Holds head erect for short period of time, can raise chest, supported on forearms
   b. Can carry hand or object to mouth at will
   c. Reaches for attractive object, but misjudges distances
   d. Grasp, tonic neck, and Moro reflexes are fading
   e. Can sit when back is supported, knees will be flexed and back rounded
   f. Step or dance reflex disappears
   g. Plays with fingers and hands
3. Sensory
   a. Follows light to periphery
   b. Has binocular coordination (vertical and horizontal vision)
   c. Listens to sounds
4. Socialization and vocalization
   a. Smiles in response to a person or object
   b. Laughs aloud and shows pleasure in making sounds
   c. Cries less

C. Four to 5 months
1. Physical—drools because salivary glands are functioning and child has not learned to swallow saliva
2. Motor
   a. No head lag; balances head well in sitting position
   b. Sits with little support; holds back straight when pulled to sitting position
   c. Symmetrical body position predominates
   d. Can sustain portion of own weight when held in a standing position
   e. Reaches and grasps object with whole hand
   f. Can roll over from back to side
   g. Lifts head and shoulders at a 90° angle when prone
   h. Primitive reflexes such as grasp, Moro, and tonic neck have disappeared
3. Sensory
   a. Recognizes familiar objects and people
   b. Has coupled eye movements, accommodation is developing
   c. Visual acuity about 20/200

4. Socialization and vocalization
   a. Coos and gurgles when talked to
   b. Definitely enjoys social interaction with people
   c. Vocalizes displeasure when an object is taken away

D. Six to 7 months
   1. Physical
      a. Weight—gains about 90 to 150 g. (3 to 5 oz.) weekly during second 6 months of life
      b. Height—gains about 1.25 cm. (½ inch) a month
      c. Teething may begin with eruption of 2 lower central incisors, followed by upper incisors
   2. Motor
      a. Can turn over equally well from stomach or back
      b. Sits fairly well unsupported, especially if placed in a forward leaning position
      c. Hitches or moves backward when in a sitting position
      d. Can transfer a toy from one hand to the other
      e. Can approach a toy and grasp it with one hand
      f. Plays with feet and puts them in mouth
      g. When lying down, lifts head as if trying to sit up
      h. Transfers everything from hand to mouth
   3. Sensory
      a. Has taste preferences
      b. Will spit out disliked food
   4. Socialization and vocalization
      a. Begins to differentiate between strange and familiar faces and shows "stranger anxiety"
      b. Makes polysyllabic vowel sounds
      c. Vocalizes *m-m-m* when crying
      d. Cries easily on slightest provocation but laughs just as quickly

E. Eight to 9 months
   1. Motor
      a. Sits steadily alone
      b. Has good hand to mouth coordination
      c. Developing pincer grasp, with preference for use of one hand over the other
      d. Crawls, then creeps (creeping is more advanced because abdomen is supported off the floor)
      e. Can raise self to a sitting position but may require help to pull self to feet
   2. Sensory
      a. Depth perception is beginning to develop
      b. Displays interest in small objects
   3. Socialization and vocalization
      a. Shows anxiety with strangers by turning or pushing away and crying
      b. Definite social attachment is evident—stretches out arms to loved ones
      c. Is voluntarily separating self from mother by desire to act on own
      d. Reacts to adult anger—cries when scolded
      e. Has imitative and repetitive speech, using vowels and consonants such as *Dada*
      f. No true words as yet, but comprehends words such as *bye bye*

F. Ten to 12 months
   1. Physical
      a. Has tripled birth weight
      b. Upper and lower lateral incisors usually have erupted, for total of 6 to 8 teeth
      c. Head and chest circumferences are equal
   2. Motor
      a. Stands alone for short periods of time
      b. Walks with help—moves around by holding onto furniture
      c. Can sit down from standing position without help
      d. Can eat from a spoon and a cup but needs help, prefers using fingers
      e. Can play pat-a-cake and peek-a-boo
      f. Can hold crayon to make a mark on paper
      g. Helps in dressing, such as putting arm through sleeve
   3. Sensory
      a. Visual acuity 20/100
      b. Amblyopia may develop with lack of binocularity
      c. Discriminates simple geometric forms
   4. Socialization and vocalization
      a. Shows emotions such as jealousy, affection, anger

b. Enjoys familiar surroundings and will explore away from mother
c. Fearful in strange situation or with strangers; clings to mother
d. May develop habit of "security" blanket
e. Can say 2 words besides *Dada* or *Mama*
f. Understands simple verbal requests, such as "Give it to me."
g. Knows own name

PLAY DURING INFANCY (SOLITARY)

A. Mostly used for physical development
B. Toys need to be simple because of short attention span
C. Safety is chief determinant in choosing toys (aspirating small objects is one cause of accidental death)
D. Visual and audio stimulation is important
E. Suggested toys
   1. Rattles
   2. Soft stuffed toys
   3. Mobiles
   4. Push-pull toys
   5. Simple musical toys
   6. Strings of big beads and large snap toys

NURSING RESPONSIBILITIES FOR PARENTAL GUIDANCE DURING INFANT'S FIRST YEAR

A. Birth
   1. Understand each parent's adjustment to newborn, especially mother's post-partal emotional needs
   2. Teach care of infant and assist parents to understand that the infant expresses needs through crying
   3. Encourage parents to establish flexible schedule to meet needs of child and themselves
B. First 6 months
   1. Help parents understand infant's need for stimulation in environment
   2. Support parents' pleasure in seeing child's growing friendliness and social response, especially smiling
C. Second 6 months
   1. Prepare parents for child's "stranger anxiety"
   2. Encourage parents to allow child to cling to mother or father and avoid long separation from either
   3. Guide parents concerning discipline because of infant's increasing mobility
   4. Teach accident prevention because of child's motor skills and curiosity
   5. Encourage parents to leave child with suitable mother substitute to allow some free time

INFANT FEEDING
Developmental milestones associated with feeding

A. At birth full-term infant has sucking, rooting, and swallowing reflexes
B. Newborn feels hunger and indicates desire for food by crying
C. By 1 month of age is able to take food from a spoon
D. By 5 to 6 months of age can use fingers in eating zwieback or toast
E. By 6 to 7 months of age is developmentally ready to chew solids
F. By 8 to 9 months of age can hold a spoon and play with it during feeding
G. By 9 months of age can hold own bottle
H. By 12 months of age usually can drink from a cup although fluid may spill and bottle may be preferred at times

Self-regulation schedule

A. Each infant born with different degree of maturity and rhythm of needs
B. Superior to rigid schedule, but should be modified to meet needs of infant and parents
C. Usually fed every 4 hours, with a night-time feeding for first month, although schedule and amount are highly variable
D. Feeding behavior and degree of satisfaction reflect psychologic development of child
E. Close mother-infant relationship in feeding process meets basic need of trust (Erikson's stage of trust)

Self-selection of food

A. Bottle-fed babies tend to consume more than breast-fed babies because those that are breast-fed complete their feeding when satisfied rather than when the formula is consumed
B. Definite food preferences are evident and change periodically (usually beginning with bland foods that are slightly sweet, sour, or salty, rather than bitter or strongly spiced)

Nutritional requirements

A. Nutrition as it affects growth
1. Initial weight loss of 10% of birth weight is normal and usually regained by tenth day of life
2. Infant feeding usually delayed immediately after birth because of
   a. General weakness and danger of aspiration
   b. Reduced caloric requirement because of inactivity and low heat production of infant
3. Birth weight usually doubled by 6 months of age and tripled by 1 year of age (small babies may gain more weight in a shorter period)
4. Growth during first year should be charted to observe for comparable gain in length, weight, and head circumference
5. Generally, growth charts demonstrate the percentile of the child's growth rate (below the third and above the ninety-seventh percentile are considered abnormal)
6. Percentiles of growth curves must be seen in relation to
   a. Deviation from a steady rate of growth
   b. Hereditary factors of parents (size and body shape)
   c. Comparison of height and weight
7. Satisfactory rate of growth judged by
   a. Weight and length (overweight and underweight constitute malnutrition)
   b. Muscular development
   c. Tissue tone and turgor
   d. General appearance and activity level of child
   e. Amount of crying and needed sleep
   f. Presence or absence of illness
   g. Mental status and behavior in relation to norms for age
B. Proper feeding essential to growth and development of child
1. General good nutrition that promotes growth but prevents overweight
2. Prevention of nutritional deficiencies
3. Prevention of gastrointestinal disturbances, such as vomiting or constipation
4. Establishment of good eating habits later in life
5. Consistency of feedings should progress from liquid to semi-soft to soft to solids as dentition and jaw develop

Breast-feeding

A. Advantages
1. Psychologic value of closeness and satisfaction in beginning mother-child relationship
2. Optimum nutritional value for infant
3. Economical and readily accessible
4. Greater immunity to infection
5. Infant is less likely to be allergic to mother's milk
6. Develops facial muscles, jaw, and nasal passages of infant since stronger sucking is necessary
7. Assists in involution of uterus
B. Prerequisites
1. Psychologic readiness of mother is a major factor in successful breast-feeding
2. Adequate diet must be available prenatally and postnatally to ensure high-quality milk
3. Suitable rest, exercise, and freedom from tension for mother will provide increased satisfaction for both her and the infant
C. Length of nursing period
1. Self-demand schedule is desirable
2. Length of feeding time is usually 20 minutes with greatest quantity of milk consumed in first 5 to 10 minutes
D. Feeding techniques
1. Mother and infant in comfortable position, such as semi-reclining or in rocking chair
2. Initiate feeding by stimulating rooting reflex (stroking cheek toward breast, being careful not to stroke other cheek since this will confuse infant)
3. Burp or bubble baby during and after feeding to allow for escape of air by
   a. Placing baby over shoulder
   b. Sitting baby on lap, flexed forward
   c. Rubbing or patting back (avoiding jarring baby)
4. Breast milk intake similar to formula intake
   a. 130 to 200 ml. of milk per kg. (2 to 3 oz. of milk per pound) of body weight
   b. From ⅙ to ⅐ of baby's weight per day
5. After lactation has been established,

occasional bottle-feeding can be substituted

6. Length of time for continuing breast-feeding is variable (may be discontinued when teeth erupt since this can be uncomfortable for mother)

E. Care of breasts
   1. Cleanse with plain water once daily (soap or alcohol can cause irritation and dryness)
   2. Support breasts day and night with proper fitting brassiere
   3. Nursing pads should be placed inside bra cup to absorb any milk leaking between feedings
   4. Plastic bra liners should be avoided because they increase heat and perspiration and decrease air circulation necessary for drying of the nipple area

F. Contraindications
   1. In mother
      a. Active tuberculosis
      b. Acute contagious disease
      c. Chronic disease such as cancer, advanced nephritis, cardiac disease
      d. Extensive surgery
      e. Mastitis (temporary cessation)
      f. Narcotic addiction
   2. In infant—cleft lip or palate or any other condition that interferes or prevents grasp of the nipple is the only real contraindication

Bottle-feeding

Often referred to as artificial feeding

A. Factors affecting success
   1. Pasteurization of milk
   2. Tuberculin testing of cows
   3. Sanitation in milk handling
   4. Adequate refrigeration and storage
   5. Increased understanding of infant's nutritional needs
      a. Easy digestibility
      b. Proper amounts of
         (1) Protein
         (2) Fats
         (3) Carbohydrates
         (4) Vitamins and minerals
         (5) Fluid (130 to 200 ml. per kg. or 2 to 3 oz. fluid per pound of body weight)
         (6) Calories (110 to 130 calories per kg. or 50 to 60 calories per pound of body weight)
         (7) For exact requirements see Nutrition requirements, pp. 171-172

B. Types of formulas
   1. Fresh whole or skimmed milk
   2. Evaporated milk
   3. Dried milks (whole or skimmed)
   4. Commercial formulas

C. Preparation for bottle-feeding
   1. Calculation of formula to yield 110 to 130 calories and 130 to 200 ml. of fluid per kg. of body weight
   2. Proper preparation of formula by terminal heat method and feeding utensils (full 25 minutes of boiling)
   3. Proper refrigeration of formula
   4. Warming of formula before feeding by immersing bottle into warm water until approximately equal to body temperature (keep level of water in warmer below cap)

D. Feeding techniques
   1. Always hold infant during feeding to provide warm body contact (bottle propping may contribute to aspiration of formula)
   2. Hold bottle so nipple is always filled with milk to prevent excessive air ingestion
   3. Adjust size of nipple hole to needs of baby (a premature infant needs a larger hole that requires less sucking)
   4. After feeding and burping infant, place child on abdomen or side to aid digestion and prevent aspiration

Introduction of solid foods

A. Milk contains all needed nutrients for early growth except iron, vitamin C, larger amounts of vitamin D, and fluoride

B. Two principles guiding introduction of new foods
   1. Necessary nutrients should be stressed rather than any type of food
   2. Eating is a medium for learning good eating habits as well as cultural and social mores

C. Addition of new foods
   1. Highly variable; based on needs of growing child
   2. Second to third month—cereal (usually rice, because of easier digestibility) and fruit twice a day
   3. Third to fourth month—egg yolk (hard-boiled and sieved), vegetables, and meats (strained)
   4. About sixth month—zwieback or hard toast
   5. Seventh to ninth months—finely chopped table foods such as meat

(beef, lamb, or liver), mashed potato, and soft vegetables
6. One year—selected table foods, egg white
D. Method
1. When baby is hungry, after a few sucks of breast-milk or formula
2. Introduce 1 food at a time, usually at intervals of 4 to 7 days to allow for identification of food allergies
3. Begin spoon feeding by pushing food to back of tongue, because of infant's natural tendency to thrust tongue forward
4. Use small spoon with straight handle, begin with 1 or 2 teaspoons of food—gradually increase to a couple of tablespoons per feeding
5. As the amount of solid food increases, the quantity of milk may need to be decreased to prevent overfeeding
6. Never introduce foods by mixing them with the formula in the bottle
E. Weaning
1. Giving up the bottle or breast for a cup is psychologically significant since it requires the relinquishing of a major source of pleasure
2. Usually, readiness develops during second half of first year because of
   a. Pleasure from receiving food by a spoon
   b. Increasing desire for more freedom
   c. Acquiring more control over body and environment
3. Weaning should be gradual, replacing only 1 bottle at a time with a cup and finally ending with the nighttime bottle
4. If breast-feeding needs to be terminated before 5 or 6 months of age, then a bottle should be used to allow for the infant's continued sucking needs; after about 6 months weaning can be directly to a cup

MATERNAL NURSING AND REPRODUCTIVE PROBLEMS

PUBERTY

A period during which the organs of reproduction mature and are prepared for their reproductive function
A. Physical and physiologic changes
1. In male
   a. Occurs between 10 and 14 years of age—less dramatic than female
   b. Heralded by deepening of voice, growth of body hair on face, axillae, and genitalia
   c. Second year after onset—increased activity of sweat glands, spermatogenesis occurs with periodic erections and emissions of mature sperm
   d. Dramatic body growth spurt
   e. Ejaculation is beginning of fertility and end of puberty
2. In female
   a. Occurs between 9 and 13 years of age
   b. Sudden enlargement of breasts, growth of body hair on axillae and genitalia—changes in size and vascularity of internal reproductive organs
   c. Heralded by first menstrual flow called *menarche* (unlike male many first menstrual cycles are anovulatory and infertile)
   d. Dramatic body growth more evident than in male
B. Psychologic changes
1. Age differences in maturation
2. Heterosexual interests—girls earlier than boys, girls interested in older boys
3. Emancipation struggles with parents—independence versus dependence
4. Need for belonging to a peer group
C. Menstrual cycle
1. A rhythmic, cyclic pattern that occurs monthly in women
2. One ovum matures and is made ready for fertilization
3. The process begins at puberty and ends with menopause
4. The pituitary gland controls the hormonal function of the menstrual cycle
   a. Follicular phase—follicle-stimulating hormone (FSH) produced by anterior pituitary, interacts with the ovarian hormone, estrogen, to produce changes in the graafian follicle of the ovary and also causes thickening of the endometrial lining of the uterus
   b. Ovulatory phase—rise in estrogen levels stimulates the pituitary to produce luteinizing hormone (LH) which causes ovulation (rupture of follicle and release of the ovum) and a rise in basal body tempera-

ture as titers of progesterone increase

   c. Luteal phase
     (1) Cavity of ruptured follicle becomes filled with tissue known as corpus luteum, which secretes estrogen and progesterone for 8 days
     (2) Endometrial lining is succulent and in optimal condition for implantation of fertilized ovum
   d. Menstrual phase—should ovum not meet a sperm, progesterone level decreases, endometrial lining sheds, and menstrual flow occurs

MATERNITY CYCLE
Anteparal period

A. Maturation, fertilization, and implantation
  1. Maturation of ovum and sperm by mitosis and meiosis; reduction in chromosomes from 46 to 23
  2. Fertilization occurs when ovum and sperm unite in distal portion of fallopian tube
  3. Rapid division by cleavage without increase in cell cluster in 6 days (morula stage)
  4. Implantation within 6 to 9 days in upper fundal portion of uterus
  5. Blastocytic stage—rearrangement of cells into 3 layers: ectoderm, mesoderm, entoderm
  6. Trophoblastic stage—projection of villi into maternal tissue, later to become placenta, vehicle for exchange of nutriments and wastes

B. Growth and development of baby (cephalocaudal)
  1. 14 days—heart begins to beat, brain, early spinal cord, and muscle segments present
  2. 26 days—tiny buds for arms appear
  3. 28 days—tiny buds for legs appear
  4. 30 days—embryo ¼ to ½ inch in length, definite form, beginning of umbilical cord is visible
  5. 31 days—arm buds develop into hands, arms, and shoulders
  6. 33 days—finger outlines present
  7. 46 to 48 days—cartilage in upper arms replaced by first bone cells, amniotic fluid surrounds fetus (amniotic fluid is a protective cushion, equalizes pres-

sures, and facilitates baby's movements for adequate growth and development)
  8. 3 months (12 weeks)—fetus moves body parts, swallows, practices inhaling and exhaling, weighs 1 oz.
  9. 4 to 5 months (16 to 20 weeks)—fetal movements felt by mother (known as quickening), weighs 6 oz., is 8 to 10 inches in length
  10. 5 to 6 months (20 to 24 weeks)—hair growth on head, eyelashes and brow, skeleton hardens, eyelids closed, weighs 1 lb., is 12 inches in length, fetal heart audible with fetoscope
  11. 6 to 7 months (24 to 28 weeks)—eyelids open, amniotic fluid increases to 1 quart with a daily exchange of 6 gallons, weighs 1¼ pounds
  12. 7 to 8 months (28 to 32 weeks)—many fat deposits, weighs 1 to 1½ pounds
  13. 8 to 9 months (32 to 36 weeks)—stores protein for extrauterine life, gains 4 pounds in weight

C. Fetal circulation—differs from adult because of following accessory structures
  1. Placenta
    a. Adherent organ attached to maternal decidua
    b. A vehicle through which nutriments and wastes are exchanged by diffusion between mother and fetus
    c. Placenta functions as kidney, lung, and endocrine gland
    d. By 12 weeks, produces female sex steroids (estrogen, progresterone, and chorionic gonadotropin)
  2. Umbilical cord
    a. Inserted close to the central portion of the placenta and attached to fetus
    b. Umbilical cord has 1 vein (transports nourishment) and 2 arteries (transports wastes) between mother and baby
    c. Wharton's jelly is a protective covering surrounding the entire cord
  3. Foramen ovale is an opening between the right and left atria during fetal life
  4. Ductus arteriosus is a connection between pulmonary arteries and aorta
  5. Ductus venosus is a connection between umbilical vein and ascending vena cava

6. As a result of above structures all blood in fetal heart is mixed blood
7. Only oxygenated blood in the fetus is at the immediate entrance of the umbilical vessel on entering the liver

D. Physical and physiologic changes in mother during pregnancy (pregnancy is a normal physiologic process that affects all body systems and results in both objective and subjective changes)
1. Endocrine and reproductive systems
   a. Fatigue is a result of increased hormonal levels causing sodium and water retention and relaxation of smooth muscles
   b. Amenorrhea occurs since the corpus luteum persists and ovulation is inhibited
   c. Breast changes such as fullness, tingling, soreness, darkening of areola and nipple occur along with an increase in hormonal levels
   d. Leukorrhea is increased as hormonal levels rise and the increased acidity is a protection from bacterial invasion
   e. Changes in uterus are circulatory, hormonal, and related to fetal growth
      (1) Softening of cervix—Goodell's sign
      (2) Softening of lower uterine segment—Hegar's sign
      (3) Purplish hue to vaginal mucosa—Chadwick's sign
      (4) Changes in position of uterus—first trimester uterus is in pelvic cavity, second and third trimester uterus is in abdominal cavity before lightening occurs
2. Digestive system
   a. Reduction in hydrochloric acid interferes with gastric motility causing nausea and vomiting
   b. Pressure of the enlarged uterus against the internal organs in early and late pregnancy may cause constipation
3. Excretory system
   a. Proximity of uterus and bladder in early and late pregnancy causes urinary frequency
   b. Increased urinary output results in lowered specific gravity

c. Increased excretion of sugar caused by lowered renal threshold
d. Presence of gonadotropin hormone in the urine
4. Circulatory system
   a. Physiologic anemia is a result of increased blood volume as the maternal system excretes baby's wastes
   b. Cardiac output increases at end of second month, reaches a peak at seventh to eighth months, and falls abruptly to nonpregnant levels at term
   c. Heart rate increases 10 beats per minute in the latter half of pregnancy—approximately 14,000 extra beats in 24 hours
   d. Edema of extremities common in last 6 weeks of pregnancy because of stasis of blood
   e. Leg cramps are a result of calcium deficiency or increased phosphorus intake
5. Respiratory system
   a. At 36 to 38 weeks, pressure of enlarged uterus on diaphragm and lungs may cause dyspnea that subsides when lightening occurs
   b. More air is inspired during pregnancy although there is no change in vital capacity
6. Integumentary system
   a. Excretion of wastes through skin causes diaphoresis
   b. Skin changes—darkening of areola of breasts, darkening patches on face (chloasma), linea alba becomes nigra on abdomen, striae on abdomen and legs caused by skin stretching as pregnancy advances, erythematous changes on palms of hands and face in some women
7. Skeletal system—a softening of all ligaments and joints caused by increased hormonal action
8. Nervous system—no specific changes unless related to nonpregnant state

E. Course, signs, and diagnosis of pregnancy
1. Estimated date of delivery—Nagele's Rule—count back 3 months from the first day of the last normal menstrual period and add 7 days (9 calendar months, 270 days) or (10 lunar months, 290 days)

2. Positive signs of pregnancy are hearing fetal heart tones with fetoscope, palpating fetal parts, and visualization of bony skeleton of fetus on x-ray films
3. Diagnostic pregnancy tests—urine of pregnant women used to detect chorionic gonadotropin
   a. Animal tests—Friedman's, Aschheim-Zondek
   b. Chemical—Pregnosticon, Gravindex, radioimmunoassay for chorionic gonadotropin

Prenatal period

A. Medical supervision during pregnancy
   1. History, including medical, surgical, gynecologic and obstetric data; family history of hereditary and transmittable diseases such as diabetes, tuberculosis, heart disease, etc.
   2. Physical examination of skin, thyroid, teeth, lungs, heart, and breasts, abdominal palpation, auscultation, height of fundus, vaginal examination, and pelvic evaluation (prior to last 4 weeks of pregnancy)
   3. Smears taken for monilial and trichomonal infections, Papanicolaou test done for cancer
   4. Blood pressure; weight; and urinalysis for acetone, albumin, and sugar done at intervals
   5. Blood determination for typing, cross-matching, Rh factor, serologic test for syphilis, and a sickle-cell test for black women are done
B. Nutritional needs during pregnancy
   1. Consideration of preconceptional nutritional status; age and parity of mother; biologic interactions between mother, fetus, and placenta; and individual needs such as in times of stress
   2. Weight gain should be evaluated with regard to quality of gain (Is weight gain caused by edema or fat deposition?)
   3. Severe caloric restriction during pregnancy is contraindicated since it is a potential hazard to mother and fetus
   4. Weight reduction should never be started as a regimen during pregnancy
   5. Restriction of sodium and administration of diuretics are potentially dangerous to mother and fetus during pregnancy
   6. Consideration of the demands of pregnancy related to growth and development of the fetus during the various trimesters (see Nutrition requirements, p. 173 for recommendations of the National Research Council)
   7. The lactating mother needs additional caloric requirements (see Nutrition requirements, pp. 170-171)
   8. Dietary assessment should be an integral part of prenatal care for every pregnant woman
   9. Changes in dietary regimen should consider cultural, economic, and psychologic implications of food habits
C. Nursing goals to prepare parents for childbirth
   1. Assist parents to understand the anatomy and physiology of pregnancy, labor, and delivery
   2. Help parents to discuss and explore feelings related to childbearing and childrearing in attempting to alleviate fears
   3. Prepare the mother for the physical work of labor through the use of muscle and breathing exercises for the various phases of labor
   4. Prepare the father for coaching and supporting role during pregnancy, labor, and delivery
   5. Introduce families to health facilities available for continued health care of the family

Intrapartal period

A. Labor—a physiologic and mechanical process in which the baby, placenta, and fetal membranes are expelled through the pelvis and birth canal
B. Anatomy of bony pelvis
   1. Parts—ischium, ilium, sacrum, coccyx
   2. Joints—sacroiliacs, sacrococcygeal, symphysis pubis (all soften during pregnancy)
   3. Divisions—false pelvis supports the enlarged uterus in the abdominal cavity; true pelvis is the bony inner pelvis through which the baby must pass
   4. Diameters at inlet—true conjugate (anteroposterior diameter), transverse (widest diameter at inlet), right and left oblique diameters; at outlet—conjugate diagonal (anteroposterior is

widest diameter), transverse (one ischial tuberosity to other)
  5. Classification of pelvis—gynecoid (normal female pelvis), android (male pelvis), anthropoid, and platypelloid
  6. Normal female pelvis has an ample pubic arch, curved sacrum, curved side walls, blunt ischial spines, and a movable coccyx
C. Attitude—relationship of fetal parts to each other
D. Presentation—baby's body part that engages into true pelvis
  1. Cephalic (head)—vertex, brow, or face
  2. Breech—frank, complete, single, or double footling
  3. Shoulder—must be turned for delivery
E. Position—relationship of presenting part to 4 quadrants of mother's pelvis (the letters L. and R. are used for left or right; the letters A. and P. are used for anterior or posterior; the letter O. signifies occiput; the letter M. signifies mentum or face; the letter S. signifies sacrum)
  1. Vertex—occiput, L.O.A., L.O.P., R.O.A., R.O.P.
  2. Face—chin (mentum) L.M.A., L.M.P., R.M.A., R.M.P.
  3. Breech—sacrum, L.S.A., L.S.P., R.S.A., R.S.P.
F. Station—relationship of presenting part to false and true pelvis
  1. Floating—presenting part movable above true pelvic inlet
  2. Engaged—suboccipitobregmatic diameter fixed into pelvic inlet
  3. Station O—presenting part at level of ischial spines—levels below spines +1, +2, +3, levels above spines −1, −2, −3
G. Signs and symptoms prior to true labor
  1. Lightening—baby drops down into true pelvis
  2. Mother experiences Braxton Hicks contractions—painless tryout contractions in preparation for true labor
  3. Increased vaginal secretions
  4. Softening of cervix
H. Signs and symptoms of true labor
  1. Uterine contractions that increase in frequency, strength, and duration
  2. Bloody show—pressure of presenting part on the cervix causes effacement and dilatation of the cervix
  3. Rupture of the membranes

I. Mechanisms of labor—rotation of vertex presentation through true pelvis
  1. Engagement, descent with flexion—at onset of labor, head descends and chin flexes on chest
  2. Internal rotation—as labor contractions and uterine forces move baby downward, head internally rotates to pass through ischial spines
  3. Extension—occiput emerges under symphysis pubis and head is delivered by extension
  4. External rotation—to allow for rotation of shoulders to anteroposterior position
  5. Lateral flexion—allows for delivery of shoulders and body
J. Stages of labor
  1. First stage—encompasses period from onset of true labor to complete effacement and dilatation of cervix
  2. Second stage—from complete effacement and dilatation of cervix to birth of the baby
  3. Third stage—from birth of the baby through expulsion of the placenta
  4. Fourth stage—first hour following delivery
K. Changes in mother during labor
  1. First stage
    a. Latent phase—irregular contractions, cervix dilated 0 to 2 cm., mother excited and happy labor has started, some apprehension
    b. Relaxation phase—moderate to strong contractions 5 to 8 minutes apart, cervix dilates from 2 to 6 cm., bloody show, membranes may rupture, breathing techniques help in relaxing, medication may be necessary for discomfort, supportive measures by husband or nurse (such as encouragement, praise, reassurance, keeping mother informed of progress, providing rest between contractions, and presence of a supporting person)
    c. Transition phase—strong contractions 1 to 2 minutes apart, bloody show, mother becomes irritable, restless, agitated, highly emotional, belches, has leg tremors, perspires, pale white ring around mouth (circumoral pallor), flushed face, sudden nausea, and vomiting
  2. Second stage—beginning with full di-

latation of cervix and ending with birth of baby, perineum bulges, pushing with contractions, grunting sounds, behavior changes from great irritability to great involvement and work, sleep and relaxation occur between contractions, leg cramps are common

L. Nursing care during labor and delivery
1. Emotional support by husband, nurse, or significant others
2. Maintenance of asepsis
3. Timing frequency, duration, and strength of contractions
4. Auscultation or monitoring of fetal heart sounds as to rate, regularity, and tone
5. Frequent observation of perineum for show, rupture of membranes, and presenting part
6. Check vital signs at frequent intervals
7. Emergency equipment available for safe care of mother and baby such as oxygen, blood, drugs
8. Assessment of basic needs such as body fluids, bladder and bowel function
9. Assist mother with breathing techniques throughout labor

M. Danger signs and symptoms during labor
1. Tonic, strong, continuous contractions with sharp abdominal pain and, on palpation, abdomen taut and boardlike
2. Variations in rate, regularity, and tone of fetal heart sounds
3. Meconium-stained or excessive amount of amniotic fluid
4. Elevation or drop in blood pressure
5. Increase in pulse or temperature
6. Sudden excessive fetal movements
7. Bleeding, protrusion of umbilical cord or placenta

N. Nursing care immediately following delivery
1. Mother
a. Palpate fundus frequently for firmness and height in relation to umbilicus
b. Keep airway open if inhalation anesthesia has been given
c. Monitor blood pressure and pulse —report fluctuations
d. Check perineum for vaginal and suture line bleeding
e. Allow parents time for examining and holding infant

2. Baby
a. Clear airway of mucus
b. Observe frequently
c. Use Apgar scoring to determine respiratory effort
d. Maintain body heat
e. Assess the newborn for visible anomalies
f. Instill silver nitrate or other medication into each eye to prevent ophthalmia neonatorum
g. Identify mother and baby prior to leaving delivery room by use of prints and application of bands

Postpartal period

Puerperium—a 6-week period following delivery in which the reproductive organs undergo physical and physiologic changes, a process called *involution*
A. Systemic changes during puerperium
1. Reproductive system
a. Uterus—intermittent contractions bring about involution, after-contractions may cause discomfort necessitating analgesics
b. Lochia—vaginal flow following delivery, changes from rubra to serosa in 1 week then becomes alba (uterine lining regenerates with new epithelium in 2 or 3 days)
c. Vagina practically returns to its prepregnant state through a healing of soft tissue and cicatrization
d. Abdominal wall soft and flabby but eventually regains tone
e. Breasts
(1) As placenta is delivered, there is activation of luteinizing hormone in the anterior pituitary—secretion of prolactin also stimulates milk production
(2) Posterior pituitary secretes pitocin, an oxytocic that initiates the let-down reflex with milk ejection as the baby suckles
(3) Breast engorgement occurs on second or third day because of vasodilation prior to lactation
2. Digestive system
a. Added proteins and calories to replenish those lost with the process of involution

b. Lactating mother needs added calories and fluids

c. Roughage and exercise relieve constipation and distention

3. Circulatory system

a. Slight rise in blood volume and blood plasma

b. Blood fibrinogen levels increase during first week

c. Increase in leukocytes especially if labor was lengthy

d. Drop in hemoglobin and red blood count on fourth postpartal day

4. Excretory system

a. Increased urinary output second to fifth postpartal day

b. Bladder capacity increased during pregnancy—retention with overflow may occur

c. Activation of lactogenic hormone may result in lactose in urine

d. Excretion of nitrogen as involution occurs

5. Integumentary system—profuse diaphoresis as wastes are being excreted

B. Nursing care during puerperium—the nurse should

1. Use aseptic techniques in giving perineal care

2. Inspect breasts for tissue and nipple breakdown, palpate to rule out growths (teach self-breast examination for continued health), support breasts with well-fitted brassiere

3. Teach importance of handwashing in caring for self and baby (important for personnel in order to avoid cross-contamination)

4. Observe vital signs—temperature of 100.4°F. or above for 2 consecutive days (excluding first 24 hours after delivery) considered sign of beginning puerperal infection—bradycardia is a normal phenomenon following delivery

5. Palpate fundus for firmness and descent below umbilical level (involution normally follows a 1-finger breadth descent daily, by fifth or sixth day fundus cannot be felt)—a fundus that is boggy indicates poor contractile power of uterus and results in bleeding

6. Check lochia for color, amount, odor (foul odor indicates beginning infection); observe suture line for redness, ecchymosis, edema, or gapping

7. Promote bladder and bowel function

8. Provide diet high in proteins and calories to restore body tissues

9. Ambulate early to prevent blood stasis

10. Observe for postpartal blues that may be caused by a drop in hormonal levels on fourth or fifth day

11. Meet mother's needs to enable her to meet the baby's needs

12. Assist mother with self-care and care of baby as need arises

13. Provide for group discussions on breast-feeding, infant care, etc.

C. Concepts basic to mother-infant relationships

1. Early and frequent mother-infant contact is essential for survival

2. Mothering abilities can be fostered and developed

3. Biologic changes that occur at puberty and during pregnancy influence the development of nurturance

4. Interaction between mother and child begins from the moment of conception

5. Love for the infant grows as the mother interacts and cares for her infant

6. As the mother gives to the infant and the infant receives, the mother in turn receives satisfaction from her mothering tasks

7. Any disturbance in the give-and-take cycle sets up frustrations in both the mother and the infant

8. Maternal behavior is learned and frequent mother-infant contact enhances the development of motherliness

Deviations from the normal maternity cycle in the mother

Toxemias of pregnancy

Characterized by a triad of symptoms: edema, elevation of blood pressure, and proteinuria

A. Classification (American Committee on Maternal Welfare)

1. Acute toxemia of pregnancy—onset after twenty-fourth week

a. Preeclampsia—mild, severe

b. Eclampsia—convulsions and/or coma associated with hypertension, proteinuria, and edema

2. Chronic hypertensive vascular disease with pregnancy

a. Without superimposed acute toxemia (no exacerbation of hyper-

tension or development of proteinuria occurs)
  (1) Hypertension known to have antedated pregnancy
  (2) Hypertension discovered in pregnancy (before the twenty-fourth week and with postpartal persistence)
  b. With superimposed acute toxemia
  3. Unclassified toxemia (data insufficient to differentiate the diagnosis)
B. Guidelines for prevention of toxemia
  1. Sound nutrition counselling during pregnancy and lactation—vitamins and minerals should not substitute for a nutritious diet
  2. An additional 30 to 60 mg. of supplemental iron daily in the second and third trimester (continue for 2 to 3 months postpartally in breast-feeding mother)
  3. Severe caloric restriction is harmful during pregnancy—caloric intake should be increased 10% during pregnancy
  4. Restriction of sodium is harmful during pregnancy and can result in electrolyte imbalance and the elimination of essential nutritional components
  5. Diuretics are contraindicated during pregnancy since they cause a hypovolemia and deplete essential nutrients for mother and fetus
C. Treatment and nursing care in preeclampsia
  1. High protein diet
  2. Ambulatory care—frequent visits to obstetrician
  3. Instructions to report headaches, dizziness, blurring of vision, and scotoma
  4. Small doses of barbiturates 3 times daily
  5. Blood chemistry—rise in hematocrit, uric acid, blood urea nitrogen, and decrease in CO_2 combining power indicates worsening of toxemia
  6. Qualitative urinalysis—increase in albumin output and/or decrease in urinary output indicates worsening of toxemia
  7. Administration of albumin concentrate increases renal flow by correcting the hypovolemia
D. Treatment and nursing care for eclampsia
  1. Hospitalization and complete bed rest

  2. Check vital signs, fetal heart, irritability, restlessness, signs of labor
  3. When patient is receiving magnesium sulfate therapy, check frequently for depression of patellar reflexes and respirations (these side effects can be treated with the administration of calcium gluconate to the mother and levallorphan [Lorfan] to the newborn if respiratory depression occurs); magnesium sulfate also causes dizziness, diaphoresis, and vomiting
  4. Emergency equipment for possible convulsion, equipment to maintain an open airway, suction and oxygen, sedatives such as morphine sulfate, sodium luminal etc., tracheotomy set readily available on unit
  5. Once symptoms are under control labor may be induced or emergency cesarean section performed
  6. Insertion of Foley catheter assures accurate record of urinary output
  7. Limitation of visitors and reduction of environmental stimuli
  8. Daily blood chemistry

Bleeding during the maternity cycle

Bleeding is an abnormal sign indicating a possible interruption of pregnancy
A. First trimester bleeding
  1. Abortion
    a. Interruption of pregnancy in which there is complete expulsion or partial expulsion (incomplete) of the products of conception
    b. May be sudden, spontaneous, or induced by some external mechanical force
    c. Treatment consists of bed rest, immediate blood count, blood typing, Rh incompatibility, and cross-matching with availability of blood
    d. Vital signs and observing for signs of labor will indicate course
    e. Complete abortion—24 to 48 hours observation for bleeding is imperative
    f. Incomplete abortion—a dilatation and curettage is performed to empty the uterus of retained products of conception; same observation as with complete abortion
  2. Ectopic pregnancy
    a. Pregnancy in which implantation occurs outside the uterus (most frequent site is middle portion of

fallopian tube, other sites are abdomen, ovaries, or cervix)

b. Early signs and symptoms are usually concealed

c. Pattern in tubal pregnancy is usually one in which spotting may occur after 1 or 2 missed menstrual periods, sharp lower right or left abdominal pain radiating to shoulder develops, concealed bleeding from site of rupture leads to sudden shock

d. Treatment is immediate blood replacement and surgical removal of ruptured fallopian tube

3. Hydatidiform mole

a. An abnormal pregnancy in which there is a benign growth of the chorion

b. Spontaneous expulsion usually occurs between the sixteenth and eighteenth weeks of pregnancy

c. Toxemia symptoms are common

d. Diagnosis—suspected when uterus is excessively large for period of gestation and fetal parts are not palpable

e. Treatment—if spontaneous evacuation does not occur, evacuation by delicate curettage or hysterotomy is performed

f. Dangers include uterine perforation, hemorrhage, and infection

g. Continued follow-up of serum gonadotropin levels are imperative for 1 year to rule out metastasis from chorionic carcinoma (increased gonadotropin levels warrant immediate hysterectomy)

h. Preventing a new pregnancy is essential for follow-up

B. Third trimester bleeding

1. Placenta previa

a. Implantation of the embryo in the lower uterine segment

b. Three types: marginal (placental edge is close to internal os), partial (placenta partially covers internal os), and central (placenta completely covers internal os)

c. Painless bleeding in the latter part of pregnancy is only symptom

d. Treatment is to control bleeding—cesarean section is usually performed

2. Abruptio placentae

a. Premature separation of a normally implanted placenta

b. Symptoms—with partially detached placenta there is external vaginal bleeding; with totally detached placenta, there is concealed bleeding, excruciating abdominal pain, and a board-like abdominal wall

c. Common in individuals with toxemia, essential hypertension, and an abnormally short umbilical cord

d. Treatment
(1) Replacement of blood loss
(2) With fetal distress—emergency cesarean section
(3) Without fetal distress and in the presence of some cervical effacement and dilatation—induction of labor may be attempted

C. Postpartum hemorrhage

1. Bleeding in excess of 500 ml. within the first 24 hours following delivery

2. Frequent causes are uterine atony, vaginal and cervical lacerations, and retained placental fragments (bleeding occurring after 24 hours is usually caused by retained placental fragments)

3. Treatment for atony—massage fundal portion of uterus, administer oxytocics, and, with severe blood loss, blood replacement

4. Bleeding caused by retained placental fragments necessitates manual removal

5. Vaginal and cervical lacerations require surgical repair

D. Nursing care of mother with bleeding during maternity cycle—the nurse should

1. Institute measures to alleviate fear and anxiety

2. Check vital signs frequently

3. Observe for signs of labor and imminent delivery

4. Monitor fetal heart if pregnancy is beyond twentieth week

5. Explain the need for and maintain parenteral therapy

6. Maintain asepsis to prevent infection

7. Consider and provide for patient's spiritual needs

Dystocia

Abnormal labor

A. Dystocia or difficult labor may be mechanical (contracted pelvis, obstruction in pelvis, malpresentation or position of the fetus) or functional (caused by faulty uterine contractions)

1. Treatment for mechanical dystocia is cesarean section
2. Treatment for functional dystocia is oxytocics to stimulate labor or cesarean section—deciding factors are: length of labor, condition of mother and fetus, amount of cervical effacement and dilatation, presentation, position, and station of presenting part
3. Nursing care of mother in prolonged labor—the nurse should
   a. Observe for signs of maternal exhaustion such as elevation of body temperature, fruity odor to breath, diminished urinary output with positive acetone reaction
   b. Observe for signs of fetal distress
   c. Have oxygen suction and resuscitation equipment readily available
   d. Constantly monitor contractions, fetal heart, and vital signs when patient is receiving oxytocic stimulation

B. Precipitate labor—a rapid labor and delivery of less than 2-hour duration
1. Hazards to mother are perineal laceration and postpartum hemorrhage
2. Hazards to baby are anoxia and intracranial hemorrhage
3. At times, a safe anesthesia may help slow down labor process

C. Labor induction—initiation of labor contractions by medical (oxytocic drugs) or mechanical means (artificial rupture of membranes)
1. Elective induction may be done for medical or obstetric reasons: medical —diabetes, pyelonephritis; obstetric —toxemia, Rh incompatibility, polyhydramnios, abruptio placentae, premature rupture of membranes at term without onset of labor
2. Medical methods of induction
   a. Sparteine sulfate (Tocosamine)— 75 to 150 mg. I.M. (series given every ½ hour, every hour, or every 2 hours)
   b. Oxytocin (Pitocin)—5 units in 1000 ml. of 5% glucose in Ringer's lactate I.V. at 5 to 10 drops per

minute or buccal pitocin, 200 unit tablets, given in an hourly series
   c. Prostaglandins given orally, intravenously, or vaginally
   d. Breast pumping can be used but is the least effective method
3. Nursing care of mother undergoing induction of labor—the nurse should
   a. Prepare mother with explanation of treatment
   b. Vigilantly time contractions and monitor vital signs and fetal heart
   c. Constantly monitor intravenous flow rate
   d. Remain with patient at all times during induction
   e. Provide for blood typing, Rh incompatibility, cross-matching, and availability of blood
   f. Have oxygen, suction, and resuscitation equipment readily available
   g. Prepare for emergency cesarean section if necessary

D. Abdominal delivery (cesarean section) —delivery of baby via abdominal incision
1. Indicated in cephalopelvic disproportion, dystocia, placenta previa and abruptio placentae, postmaturity, growths impeding birth canal, diabetes, toxemia, Rh incompatibility, malpresentation, fetal distress
2. Nursing care following cesarean section—the nurse should
   a. Encourage early ambulation to prevent blood stasis
   b. Check vital signs
   c. Observe abdominal dressing for drainage
   d. Encourage eating of solids to promote peristalsis (prevents distention)
   e. Record intake and output
   f. Give analgesics as ordered

Childbirth injuries

A. Episiotomy is an incision into the perineum to facilitate delivery and prevent lacerations and overstretching of the pelvic floor
1. Routine procedure—closed surgically
2. Nursing care
   a. Keep area clean and dry
   b. Analgesics as ordered for comfort
   c. Heat and local spray medications
   d. Perineal exercise

B. Lacerations are tears of the perineum or vulva resulting from a difficult or precipitate delivery—characterized as first, second, third, or fourth degree depending on the amount of involvement
1. Treatment—surgical repair
2. Nursing care—same as above; however, healing is slower following repair of a laceration
C. Relaxations of the vaginal outlet—an overstretching of the perineal supporting tissues resulting from childbirth
1. Cystocele—a herniation of anterior vaginal wall with the descent and protrusion of the bladder
2. Rectocele—a herniation of the para-rectal fascia into the vagina
   a. Signs and symptoms—backache, feeling of heaviness and bearing down in the lower abdomen, urinary stress incontinence, and constipation
   b. Treatment—Kegal's exercises for stress incontinence (after childbearing period is completed, vaginoplasty is done)
   c. Nursing care with vaginoplasty consists of keeping perineal area clean and dry with insertion of Foley catheter or suprapubic catheter; warm sitz baths once healing has begun; analgesics for discomfort; antibiotics to prevent infection; high protein diet to promote tissue repair; ambulation may be delayed to promote healing but leg motion and deep breathing are essential
D. Uterine prolapse—a condition in which the uterus is found in a lower position than normal resulting from stretching and tearing of tissues during childbirth
1. Signs and symptoms—bearing-down sensation and a feeling of a dropping of the pelvic organs, leukorrhea with marked congestion of cervix or lacerations of exposed vaginal walls, frequency with retention, and eventually cystitis
2. Treatment—dependent on age, desirability for more children, and severity of symptoms; pessaries may be used as temporary measure; surgical intervention is usually a vaginal hysterectomy

E. Displacement of uterus—results from lesions of the pelvic organs or stretching and relaxation of the ligaments supporting the uterus (may be congenital or result from the trauma of childbirth)
1. Signs and symptoms—backache, excessive bleeding during menstruation, sense of pressure or fullness
2. Treatment—insertion of a pessary to relieve symptoms; severe symptoms warrant surgical intervention
F. Rupture of uterus usually occurs after period of viability of the fetus
1. Causes—perforation during attempted abortion, rupture of a previous uterine scar, spontaneous rupture of an intact uterus with abdominal overdistention, labor induction
2. Treatment—relieve symptoms of shock from hemorrhage and surgical intervention (the extent of surgical intervention depends on degree of rupture)

Medical diseases during pregnancy

A. Heart disease—90% of rheumatic origin, 10% congenital lesions or syphilis
1. Normal hemodynamics of pregnancy that adversely affect the pregnant woman with heart disease
   a. Growing fetus needs increase in oxygen supply
   b. Accelerated heart rate of mother in latter half of pregnancy puts extra workload on her heart
   c. Steady increase in mother's blood volume during the 36 weeks of pregnancy
   d. Rise in cardiac output from the tenth week through the twenty-eighth week of pregnancy
   e. The increase in oxygen consumption with contractions during labor makes length of labor a significant factor
   f. The sudden tachycardia during delivery or the sudden bradycardia and the normal increase in cardiac output following delivery may cause cardiac arrest
2. Review functional and therapeutic classification of heart disease in a medical-surgical nursing text
3. Management of mother with heart disease during pregnancy
   a. Extra rest and protection from infection

b. Medical supervision by cardiologist

c. Obstetric supervision by obstetrician

d. Low sodium, high protein diet

e. Immediate reporting of fatigue, dyspnea, hemoptysis, or edema

f. Hospitalization for any cardiac embarrassment

g. Minimal analgesia and anesthesia during labor and delivery

h. Forceps should be used to limit pushing efforts of mother since this increases cardiac workload

i. Scopolamine is contraindicated since it is a vasodilator that will affect hemodynamics

j. Oxytocics are administered cautiously if needed in intravenous solutions

k. Observation of vital signs during labor, delivery, and immediately following delivery

l. Prophylactic antibiotics are administered to prevent infection

m. Digitalis and diuretic therapy are instituted to prevent heart failure and pulmonary edema

n. Longer hospital stay to provide continued health supervision

4. Nursing care of the mother with heart disease

a. Prenatal—health teaching, rest and diet counseling, referral to community agencies for family care, avoidance of stress, preparation for the stress of labor and delivery, teaching importance of preventing infection

b. Intrapartal—early admission prior to start of labor, vital signs, observation for signs of heart failure and pulmonary edema, maintenance of Fowler's position, availability of oxygen, added support during labor, delivery in bed if necessary

c. Postpartal—observation for respiratory distress since there is an increase in cardiac output with tachycardia, monitoring of vital signs, rest and sedation to decrease heart action, referral to various agencies for family aid on discharge

B. Diabetes mellitus

1. Normal physiology of pregnancy that affects the pregnant woman with diabetes

a. Vomiting during pregnancy, especially in first trimester, decreases carbohydrate intake with resulting acidosis

b. Increased activity of anterior pituitary decreases the tolerance for sugar

c. Elevated basal metabolic rate and decrease in CO_2-combining power increases tendency toward acidosis

d. Normal lowered renal threshold for glucose may result in glucosuria that may confuse diabetic picture

e. Muscular activity during labor depletes glycogen, therefore, carbohydrate intake must be increased

f. During puerperium, hypoglycemia is common as involution and lactation occur

2. Hazards of diabetes during pregnancy

a. Often there is a history of repeated stillbirths and fetal deaths

b. Babies are excessively large, weighing over 4000 g.

c. Neonatal deaths occur as a result of hypoxia, hypoglycemia, congenital anomalies, and premature labor

d. Toxemia and hydramnios are common

3. Nursing care of the mother with diabetes

a. Early medical and prenatal supervision

b. Prevention of acidosis

c. Effective dietary regimen

d. Awareness of signs and symptoms of acidosis and hypoglycemia

e. Personal hygiene and avoidance of stress

f. Referral to public health nurse for continuity in care

g. Identification card on person

4. Nursing care of baby of a diabetic mother

a. Keep infant warm because of poor temperature control mechanisms

b. Observe respiration (stomach aspiration imperative at time of delivery since hydramnios in utero inflates stomach, which pushes up and interferes with diaphragm)

c. Observe for signs of hypoglycemia

such as lethargy, poor sucking reflex, cyanosis, or muscular twitching

d. Provide glucose water feeding to
prevent acidosis (with poor sucking reflex, glucose should be given
parenterally)

C. Acute and chronic pyelonephritis
1. Acute pyelonephritis is a diffuse inflammatory process of interstitial connective tissue of kidney (nephron involved when infection is extreme)
2. Most common organism is *Escherichia
coli;* occasionally *Staphylococcus* and
Streptococcus
3. Signs and symptoms are chills, fever,
severe backache, tenderness over kidney region, rise in nonprotein nitrogen, decrease in phenolsulfonphthalein excretion and dye excretion on
pyelography
4. Nursing care of mother with pyelonephritis
a. Adequate diet and rest
b. Force fluids
c. Sulfamides and antibiotics
d. Intake and output
e. Sims' position relieves pressure on
uterus
f. Teaching importance of health
supervision and follow-up care
after delivery
g. Family planning avoids risk of
early recurrence of pregnancy

**Deviations from the normal maternity
cycle in the newborn**

Neonatal respiratory distress

A. Asphyxia neonatorum occurs when respirations are not well established within
60 seconds after birth as a result of
anoxia, cerebral damage, or narcosis
1. Prevention—early prenatal care, prenatal education, early management
of deviations from the normal pregnancy, adequate medical management
during labor and delivery
2. Signs and symptoms—asphyxia livida:
persistent generalized cyanosis, good
muscle tone; asphyxia pallida: marked
pallor, poor muscle tone
3. Treatment—after initial resuscitation
keep baby under very close observation for first 24 hours, keep equipment for intubation and oxygen administration readily available

B. Atelectasis—an incomplete expansion of
the lung or a partial or total collapse of
the lung following initial expansion; common in prematurity, oversedation, damage to the respiratory center, or results
from inhalation of mucus or amniotic
fluid
1. Signs and symptoms—cyanosis, rapid
irregular respirations, flaring of the
nostrils, intercostal or suprasternal
retraction, grunting on expirations
2. Treatment—maintain an open airway, administer oxygen with high
humidity, stimulate respirations by
frequently changing baby's position,
administer antibiotics as ordered to
prevent infection

C. Hyaline membrane disease—a condition
in which protein material in the alveoli
prevents lung aeration; common following cesarean section and in low birth
weight infants
1. Symptoms—cyanosis, dyspnea, and
sternal retraction
2. Treatment—keep airway patent, keep
in Isolette with oxygen and high humidity, administer antibiotics as ordered

Birth injuries

A. Caput succedaneum—edema with extravasation of serum into scalp tissues
caused by molding during the birth
process; no treatment is necessary since
it subsides in a few days

B. Cephalohematoma—edema of the scalp
with effusion of blood between the bone
and periosteum; reabsorption usually occurs in a few days

C. Intracranial hemorrhage—bleeding into
cerebellum, pons, and medulla ob-
longata caused by a tearing of the ten-
torium cerebelli; occurs following prolonged labor, difficult forceps delivery,
precipitate delivery, version or breech
extraction
1. Symptoms—abnormal respirations; cyanosis; sharp, shrill, or weak cry;
flaccidity or spasticity; restlessness;
wakefulness; convulsions; poor sucking reflex
2. Treatment—keep in Isolette with oxygen, humidity, and minimal handling;
place in high Fowler's position, administer vitamins C and K to control
and prevent further hemorrhage;

with impaired sucking reflex, gavage feeding is necessary; support of parents is vital because of guarded prognosis

D. Facial paralysis—asymmetry of face caused by damage to facial nerves from a difficult forceps delivery; temporary paralysis disappears in a few days

E. Erb-Duchenne paralysis (brachial palsy) —caused by a difficult forceps or breech extraction delivery; treatment depends on severity of paralysis; massage and exercise prevent contractures; when severe, splints and casts are applied

F. Dislocations and fractures are diagnosed by crepitation, immobility, and variations in range of motion; treatment depends on the site of fracture, therefore swaddling, positioning, splints, slings, or casts may be used; referral to a public health agency assures continuity of care; if necessary, refer to Crippled Children's Commission

Infections

A. Thrush is a mouth infection caused by *Candida albicans;* it may be transmitted as the baby passes through the mother's vaginal canal, by unclean feeding utensils, or improper handwashing techniques by staff or mother
   1. Symptoms are white patches on tongue, palate, and inner cheek surfaces that bleed on examination, and difficulty with sucking
   2. Treatment—oral administration of nystatin (Mycostatin), application of 1% gentian violet, isolation of baby and equipment to prevent cross-contamination

B. Impetigo is an infectious skin eruption characterized by vesicles or pustules caused by *Staphylococcus* or *Streptococcus;* treatment consists of isolating infant, pHisoHex baths daily, breaking pustules with alcohol wipe, local application of gentian violet, neomycin, or bacitracin, and administration of antibiotics

C. Ophthalmia neonatorum is an eye infection caused by the *Neisseria gonorrhoeae* transmitted from the genital tract during delivery or by infected hands of personnel; prophylactic eye care is administered to all infants at birth; treatment for the eye infection consists of prompt antibiotic therapy to prevent eye damage; isolation of the infant, sterilization of all equipment, and strict handwashing are imperative

D. *Staphylococcus*—prevented by reduction of transient personnel in nurseries, adequate crib spacing, and medical asepsis

E. Epidemic diarrhea is caused by *Escherichia coli;* organism in stool characterized by forceful, watery, yellow-green stool; dry skin; rapid weight loss and acidosis; treatment—oral antibiotics, replacement of fluids parenterally, isolation to prevent cross-contamination

F. Syphilis—a spirochetal infection characterized by maculopapular lesions of the palms of the hands and soles of the feet, restlessness, rhinitis, hoarse cry, enlargement of the spleen and palpable lymph nodes, enlarged ends of long bones on x-ray examination; penicillin is a specific treatment for syphilis with a 1- to 2-year follow-up
   1. Prenatal syphilis is transmitted to fetus by the mother
   2. Incidence of fetal infection varies with stage of the disease in the mother at the time of pregnancy
   3. Fetus is seldom infected prior to fourth month of pregnancy; Langhan's cells in chorion are protective barrier
   4. Pregnant women treated immediately with penicillin (prior to fourth month, fetus not infected; after fourth month of pregnancy the longer the infection goes untreated, the greater the damage to the fetus)

Drug addiction in the newborn

A. Fifty percent of infants born of addicted mothers are of low birth weight and are delivered prior to term

B. Withdrawal signs usually visible within first 2 days following birth but may occur as late as 4 to 10 days

C. Signs of narcotic withdrawal in the newborn in order of frequency and occurrence are: irritability, tremors, vomiting, high pitched cry, sneezing, hypertonicity and hyperactivity, respiratory distress, fever, diarrhea, excessive mucus, diaphoresis, convulsions, yawning, scratching the face, poor feeding, salivation, stuffy nose, hiccoughs, dehydration and low basal body temperature, constantly sucking fists, fingers, or anything available in crib, exaggerated reflexes, stand-

ing rigidly on legs when held upright, absence of normal head lag
D. Treatment—administration of phenobarbital, Thorazine, or paregoric to control withdrawal symptoms (gradually smaller and smaller doses are given until no withdrawal symptoms are present); holding and cuddling aggravates tremors, therefore, the less handling, the better; bottle-feeding preferred to breast milk since breast milk contains narcotics; pacifier given to satisfy sucking urge; follow-up by child welfare agency and visiting nurse assures continuity in care
E. Although heroin addiction during pregnancy is serious, recent studies have shown that the pregnant woman should not be placed on methadone since withdrawal symptoms from methadone are more severe in the newborn

Congenital malformations

Birth defects present at birth are structural or metabolic (birth injuries are not included); they may be genetically determined or a result of environmental interference during intrauterine life (the congenital malformations are simply listed in this section; the treatment and nursing care appears in Pediatric nursing, pp. 372-384)
A. Prevention
  1. Professional genetic counseling—new methods of testing genetic carriers
  2. Early prenatal care and supervision
  3. National Foundation (March of Dimes)—research and study of birth defects, sponsor educational materials, programs, and treatment centers
B. Birth defects of digestive system
  1. Cleft lip and palate—embryonic cleavage of lip or palate may be unilateral or bilateral
  2. Galactosemia is a genetically determined biochemical disorder in which there is a lack of the enzyme necessary for proper metabolism of galactose; characterized by abdominal distention, vomiting, diarrhea, enlargement of liver, and mental retardation
  3. Phenylketonuria is a congenital disease caused by a defect in the metabolism of the amino acid phenylalanine; characterized by tremors, poor muscular coordination, excessive perspiration, and eventually convulsions and mental retardation; a simple blood test (Guthrie) done shortly after birth is now required by law in many states
  4. Atresia of esophagus—abnormal opening between esophagus and trachea, or the esophagus ends in a blind pouch; symptoms are excessive salivation with drooling, coughing, gagging, dyspnea, and cyanosis during feeding
  5. Obstructions of duodenum and small intestine
  6. Imperforate anus—complete or partial closure of the anus
C. Birth defects of circulatory system
  1. Hemolytic disease—an ABO or Rh incompatibility where there is a destruction of red cells and resulting anemia; caused by a transfer of incompatible blood from the fetal to the maternal circulation with antibody formation in mother; the antibodies are then transferred through the placental barrier to the fetus with a resulting agglutination and destruction of red cells
    a. Symptoms are jaundice within the first 24 hours of birth, anemia, enlargement of the liver and spleen, lethargy, poor feeding pattern, vomiting, tremors and convulsions indicative of kernicterus (signs of kernicterus are absence of Moro reflex, severe lethargy, apnea, high-pitched cry, and assuming an opisthotonos position)
    b. Treatment—during pregnancy amniotic fluid determinations are done by chemical and spectrophotometric analysis; elevated readings warrant either intrauterine transfusion or induction of labor depending on the weeks of gestation; following delivery exchange transfusion is done on the infant to decrease the antibody level and increase red blood cells and hemoglobin levels
    c. Prevention—RhoGAM, a preparation of Rho (D antigen) immune globulin is now given intramuscularly to the mother 72 hours after delivery or after abortion to prevent erythroblastosis fetalis in future pregnancies; mother must be negative for Rh antibodies to receive RhoGAM
  2. Patent ductus arteriosus—abnormal

connection between the pulmonary artery and aorta

3. Tetralogy of Fallot—congenital defect combining 4 structural anomalies: pulmonary stenosis (narrowing of the pulmonary artery), ventricular septal defect (abnormal opening between right and left ventricles), dextroposition of the aorta, and right ventricular hypertrophy

D. Birth defects of musculoskeletal system
1. Clubbed foot—foot twisted out of normal position
2. Dislocation of hip—femur dislocated from acetabulum

E. Birth defects of central nervous system
1. Spina bifida—a defect of the vertebral column caused by imperfect union of the paired vertebral arches at the midline
2. Hydrocephalus is characterized by enlargement of the cranium caused by an abnormal accumulation of fluid from overproduction or blockage

F. Birth defects of urinary system
1. Hypospadias—a developmental anomaly in the male in which the urethra opens on the underside of penis or on the perineum
2. Epispadias—a congenital malformation with absence of the upper wall of the urethra usually on the dorsum of the penis
3. Exstrophy of bladder—an exposure of the bladder that occurs during embryonic development as a result of failure in the uniting of the abdominal rectus muscles

G. Chromosomal aberrations
1. Down's syndrome—a congenital condition in which there is a trisomy defect in the twenty-first chromosome; characterized by physical malformations and some degree of mental retardation
2. Turner's syndrome—an absence or structural deformity of the second sex chromosome; characterized by retarded growth and sexual development, webbing of the neck, low posterior hair line margin, and other deformities
3. Klinefelter's syndrome—an abnormality of the sex chromosomes; characterized by the presence of small testes, with fibrosis and hyalinization of the seminiferous tubules without involvement of the interstitial cells of the testes, and an increase in urinary gonadotropins

H. Support of family when infant has a birth defect
1. All parents wish for perfect child during pregnancy
2. Image of the expected infant and the degree of abnormality reflect how the parents will react
3. Initial reaction for most parents is one in which they blame themselves for the defect
4. Other reactions are: "Why me?," "Will it happen with another pregnancy?"
5. The parents' reaction to a defective child is influenced by the type and degree of defect and their past experiences with their own family
6. Parents may experience feelings of loss, anger, and guilt
7. The interaction between parents and baby can either delay or expedite the grieving process depending on the amount of give-and-take between them
8. Parents need to verbalize their fears and anxieties, which is essential for acceptance of the infant
9. Support of the parents in any decision they make for the child is essential for maintenance of family equilibrium
10. Support and verbalization are also important for the nursing staff working with parents of defective infants (see Parents' reaction to a defective child in Pediatric nursing, p. 389)

The low birth weight infant

Prematurity

A. Prevention
1. Education of teenagers (prior to planning a family) in nutrition and general hygiene
2. Education of teenagers to the hazards of drug use and smoking
3. Adequate and early prenatal health supervision
4. Provisions for adequate housing and financial aid to persons of lower socioeconomic means
5. Adequate community agencies to facilitate available services to persons in need

B. Definitions
1. Classification of newborn infants is now made on the basis of gestational age as well as birth weight
2. An infant born at term (37 weeks or over) is called full size; an infant born before term (36 weeks or less) is called premature
3. A low birth weight infant is one who weighs 2500 g. (5½ pounds) or less
4. A full term infant may be a low birth weight infant; a premature infant need not be a low birth weight infant

C. Management of mother in premature labor (before thirty-seventh week of pregnancy)
1. Preanesthetic medications should be minimal to prevent depression of the fetus (barbiturates and opiates are especially contraindicated since they depress respirations, depleting oxygen to the fetus)
2. Regional anesthesias are safer than general anesthesias
3. Added support to the mother since she is concerned with the baby's welfare
4. Adequate preparation for the infant at birth; a heated Isolette and equipment for aspiration and resuscitation should be available
5. The pediatrician should be present at the time of delivery to care for the infant

D. Management of the low birth weight infant immediately following delivery
1. Aspiration of mucus to maintain an open airway is vital
2. Absence of respirations necessitates direct laryngoscopy, tracheal aspiration, intubation, and mouth-to-tube insufflation
3. Maintenance of body temperature is difficult because of heat loss by skin evaporation; heated Isolette is needed
4. Aspiration of stomach contents at birth facilitates respirations and is often indicated for the low birth weight infant
5. Infant should be moved to the nursery in the heated unit with oxygen and resuscitation equipment available

E. Differences in premature and full-size newborn
1. Premature infant has less subcutaneous fat, therefore the skin is wrinkled, blood vessels and bony structures are visible, lanugo present on face, eyebrows are absent, and ears are poorly supported by cartilage
2. The circumference of the head of the premature infant is quite large in comparison to the chest; the fontanels are small and bones are soft
3. Skin color changes when premature infant is moved; upper half of body pale and lower half red, known as harlequin color change
4. The premature infant's posture is one of complete relaxation with marked flexion and abduction of the thighs, random movements are common with slightest stimulus
5. Heat regulation poorly developed in the premature infant because of poor development of central nervous system; heat loss caused by large skin surface area; poorly developed respiratory center with diminished oxygen combustion causing asphyxia; weak heart action, therefore slower circulation and poor oxygenation; insufficient heat production caused by inadequate metabolism
6. Respirations are not efficient in the premature infant because of muscular weakness of lung and rib cage; retraction at xiphoid is evidence of air hunger; infant should be stimulated if apnea occurs
7. Greater tendency toward capillary fragility and intracranial hemorrhage in the premature infant; red and white blood cell counts are low with resulting anemia during first few months of life
8. Nutrition is difficult to maintain in the premature infant because of weak sucking and swallowing reflexes, small capacity of stomach, low gastric acidity, and slow emptying time of the stomach; the usual caloric intake of 110 to 130 calories per kg. (50 to 60 calories per pound) of body weight may need to be increased to 200 to 220 calories per kg. (100 calories per pound) for adequate growth and development

F. Nursing care of low birth weight and premature infants
1. Observe for changes in respirations, color, and vital signs
2. Check efficacy of Isolette—heat, humidity, and oxygen concentration

3. Maintain aseptic technique to prevent infection
4. Adhere to the techniques of gavage feeding for safety of infant
5. Determine blood gases frequently to prevent acidosis
6. Institute phototherapy should hyperbilirubinemia occur
7. Support parents by letting them verbalize and ask questions to relieve anxieties
8. Arrange follow-up before and after discharge by a visiting nurse
9. Provide flexible and liberal visiting hours for parents as soon as possible
10. Allow parents to do as much as possible for the infant after appropriate teaching

INFECTIONS OF THE FEMALE ORGANS OF REPRODUCTION

A. *Candida albicans* (Monilia)
  1. Yeastlike fungus that invades the vaginal canal causing vaginitis
  2. Symptoms—pruritus, redness, thick cheesy discharge
  3. Treatment—gentian violet tampons or nystatin (Mycostatin), a broad-spectrum, oral antibiotic
B. *Trichomonas vaginalis*
  1. Protozoal parasite commonly found in the vaginal canal
  2. Symptoms—pruritus, frothy white or yellow vaginal discharge, small hemorrhagic areas on the vaginal walls
  3. Treatment—increase the vaginal pH with vinegar douches; metronidazole (Flagyl), an antiprotozoal medication, is given orally to husband and wife (drug is contraindicated during pregnancy)
C. Streptococcal infection
  1. Organisms invade pelvic cavity through skin breakdown and are perpetuated when aseptic technique is not maintained; entrance into blood stream and lymphatics causes rapid invasion of the uterine lining, fallopian tubes, ovaries, and organs in the peritoneal cavity
  2. Symptoms—basal temperature, pulse rate, and white count are elevated; peritoneal invasion causes abdominal pain, distention, nausea, and vomiting
  3. Treatment—bed rest, intravenous fluid, analgesics for pain, antibiotics

specific for *Streptococcus* organism; when abscess formation and localization to a specific organ occurs, surgical intervention is often attempted
  4. Prevention of cross-contamination by handwashing after handling dressings and linens is important
D. Gonococcal infection (gonorrhea)
  1. The *Gonococcus,* a gram-negative diplococci, is transmitted through sexual contact; usually invades Skene's glands, Bartholin's glands, cervix, urethra, fallopian tubes, and peritoneal cavity
  2. Symptoms—profuse purulent leukorrhea, redness, irritation, and edema of vulva
  3. Treatment—penicillin therapy (in women allergic to penicillin, tetracycline is given)
E. Spirochetal infection (syphilis)
  1. Caused by the *Treponema pallidum,* a spirochete that invades the blood system through sexual contact
  2. Stages of syphilis
    a. Primary stage—7 weeks after exposure, a hard indurated painless ulcer called a chanchre may be visible on the vulva, cervix, or vaginal canal; this lesion may go unnoticed but there may be malaise, headache, and slight elevation in basal body temperature
    b. Secondary stage—a maculopapular rash with headache, malaise, and swelling of the inguinal lymph nodes; occasionally hypertrophic growths are seen on vulva (known as condylomata lata)
    c. Tertiary stage—chanchre becomes a gumma, a weeping lesion containing active spirochetes; gumma later becomes an indurated area
  3. Treatment
    a. Massive doses of penicillin
    b. Tetracycline for women allergic to pencillin
    c. Case-finding and treating all known contacts

INFERTILITY AND STERILITY

A. Definitions
  1. Sterility—the presence of an absolute factor that makes a person unable to produce offspring
  2. Infertility—the inability on the part of

a couple to reproduce after consistent attempts for a 1-year period
B. Male genital factors
   1. Disturbance in spermatogenesis
   2. Obstruction of seminiferous tubules
   3. Changes in amount and quality of seminal fluid
   4. Anomalies concerned with the ejaculatory process
   5. Emotional factors
C. Female genital factors
   1. Congenital anomalies of vagina and vulva
   2. Bacterial invasion of vagina
   3. Developmental anomalies of reproductive organs
   4. Blockage of cervical os or fallopian tubes
   5. Endocrine dysfunction
   6. Emotional factors
   7. Cervical factors such as position of uterus, patency of external os, quality and quantity of cervical secretions
D. Diagnostic measures
   1. Male—history, physical, semen analysis
   2. Female—history, physical, CBC, sedimentation rate, serology, urinalysis, serum protein-bound iodine, x-ray films of the chest, basal metabolic rate, Sims or Huhner tests, endometrial biopsy, tubal insufflation, hysterosalpingography, culdoscopy
E. Treatment depends on causative factor
F. Nursing care
   1. Apply principles of human relations and psychology
   2. Listen to and discuss couple's particular problems, giving necessary support
   3. Explain diagnostic procedure to alleviate anxiety and fear
   4. Refer to visiting nurse service for continuity in care

FAMILY PLANNING
A. Goals
   1. Maintain optimum emotional and physical health of the family
   2. Involve both partners in planning family size
   3. Inform parents of available methods of birth control and give them the freedom of choice
B. Contraceptive methods
   1. Oral contraceptives—combined progestins and estrogens, which suppress ovulation, when taken as prescribed

extremely effective; contraindicated in women with thromboembolic disease or those of premenopausal age with diagnosed breast cancer
   2. Intrauterine devices (I.U.D.)—mechanical device inserted into isthmus of uterus, prevents pregnancy by increasing tubal motility so that ovum gets to uterus before lining is optimum for implantation; not as effective as oral contraceptives since pregnancy may occur with device in place
   3. Diaphragm—mechanical device that fits over cervix and prevents sperm from entering cervical os
   4. Condom—a rubber sheath that covers penis, prevents semen from entering cervical os
   5. Creams, jellies, foam tablets, and vaginal suppositories—spermicidal preparations inserted into vaginal canal by applicator immediately prior to coitus (used in conjunction with the diaphragm and condom for added protection)
   6. Coitus interruptus—the withdrawal of the penis during sexual intercourse prior to ejaculation; least effective method
   7. Rhythm—the plotting of the basal body temperature to determine fertile period, with abstinence from coitus during that time
C. Sterilization
   1. Male—accomplished by surgical severance and suturing of the vas deferens preventing ejaculation of sperm (vasectomy); following vasectomy sperm are still produced, however after 3 azoospermic specimens, sterility is achieved
   2. Female—accomplished by abdominal laparotomy, laparoscopy, or culdoscopy; the fallopian tubes are severed and tied so there is no way the mature ovum can be impregnated by a mature sperm
D. Nursing implications
   1. Method of contraception used should be acceptable to couple since acceptability increases effectiveness
   2. Ideal contraceptive is one that is completely safe, free of side effects, reversible, easily obtainable, and inexpensive
   3. Periodic physical examination of all women using oral or mechanical de-

vices should include pelvic examination and Pap smear
4. Discussion groups help couples expand their knowledge related to the anatomy and physiology of the reproductive systems
5. Assess couples individually and together prior to sterilization since consideration of the physiologic and psychologic reactions to such procedures is vital

ABORTION

A. Methods of induced abortion
1. Vacuum aspiration—done under local paracervical, epidural, or general anesthesia in the first 12 weeks of pregnancy; the cervix is dilated and the products of conception are suctioned by a small hollow tube; the uterus is then curettaged to remove all fetal tissue
2. Dilatation and curettage is performed during the first 12 to 14 weeks of pregnancy under local paracervical or general anesthesia; the cervix is dilated and uterus is curettaged
3. Saline injection—labor is induced when a pregnancy is 14 to 24 weeks in duration by injecting a sterile saline solution into the uterus by amniocentesis; labor usually begins within 20 to 36 hours after instillation of saline
4. Hysterotomy—performed after 16 weeks of pregnancy by surgically removing the fetus and placenta abdominally
B. Nursing considerations
1. Be aware of own feelings about abortion—essential if nurse is to therapeutically intervene with women having abortions
2. Since the nurse is concerned with the maintenance of life, elective abortion may be in conflict with basic beliefs
3. Nurse needs to encourage patient's expression of frustration, fear, and anger
4. Nurse needs to be objective and support the woman's decision about abortion
5. Complete history and physical, complete laboratory work-up, pelvic examination and Pap test, and a pregnancy test are essential for safe care prior to induced abortion
6. Postabortion counselling in contraceptive methods should be available

7. If prone to Rh sensitization, RhoGAM is given when patient's blood is negative for antibodies
C. Prerequisites for choosing abortion (recommended by the College of Obstetricians and Gynecologists)
1. Verification of the diagnosis and duration of pregnancy
2. Preoperative instructions and counselling
3. Recorded preoperative history and physical examination
4. Laboratory procedures usually required for hospitalization, such as blood typing, Rh factor, etc.
5. Prevention of Rh sensitization
6. A receiving facility where client is prepared and may receive necessary preoperative medication and be observed prior to treatment
7. A recovery facility for care and observation following surgery, with a qualified anesthetist in attendance
8. Postoperative instructions and follow-up, including family planning
9. Adequate permanent records

MENOPAUSE

A period in a woman's life when there is gradual cessation of ovarian function and menstruation
A. Physiologic changes
1. Ovary loses ability to respond to gonadotropic hormones
2. Loss of progesterone as ovulation ceases with irregularity of menses
3. Increase in gonadotropin level in blood since it is not utilized by ovaries (false positive pregnancy test may occur)
B. Symptoms
1. Somatic—atrophic changes in reproductive organs resulting in dyspareunia, weight gain, facial hair growth, cardiac palpitations, hot flashes, profuse diaphoresis, constipation, pruritus, faintness
2. Psychic—headache, irritability, anxiety over loss of reproductive function, sexual feelings, and feelings of womanliness
C. Treatment
1. Hormonal therapy if necessary (when no history of malignancy is present)
2. For dyspareunia—vaginal estrogen creams

3. Tranquilizers and phenobarbital if necessary
D. Nursing care
 1. Prepare women for the changes that may occur with menopause
 2. Let women ventilate feelings
 3. Refer for medical supervision

AGENCIES PROVIDING MATERNAL-CHILD HEALTH SERVICES

A. Government
 1. World Health Organization—founded in 1948 by United Nations; 100 or more countries exchange knowledge and collaborate on elevating level of health throughout the world
 2. Children's Bureau—founded in 1972 under Department of Health, Education and Welfare; its purpose is to improve services for maintenance of health in mothers and children through research, care, and teaching
 3. Department of Family and Children's Services (HEW)—federal monies for food, shelter, and medical services for dependent children
 4. Women's Bureau—under Department of Labor, provides supervision of places of employment for pregnant women
 5. National Institutes of Health—monies provided for research on child health and human development
B. Private organizations
 1. La Leche League—international, organized in 1956 by mothers interested in fostering breast-feeding
 2. International Childbirth Education Association—federation of groups and individuals interested in fostering family-centered maternity and infant care, and to create an interest in education for childbirth
 3. American Society Prophylaxis Organization (A.S.P.O.)—responsible for teaching Lamaze method in preparation for childbirth

PEDIATRIC NURSING

BASIC CONCEPTS

A. Children are individuals, not little adults, who must be seen as part of a family
B. Family-centered care is the objective in the care of children to provide total health maintenance

C. Children are influenced by genetic factors, home and environment, and parental attitudes
D. Chronologic and developmental ages of children are the most important contributing factors influencing their care
E. Prevention of illness and maintenance of health are the main thrusts in health care of children
F. Play is a natural medium for expression, communication, and growth in children

PLAY

A. Purposes
 1. Educational
 2. Recreational
 3. Physical development
 4. Social and emotional adjustment
  a. Learn moral values
  b. Develop idea of sharing
 5. Therapeutic
B. Types
 1. Active, physical
  a. Push-and-pull toys
  b. Riding toys
  c. Sports and gym equipment
 2. Manipulative, constructive, creative, or scientific
  a. Blocks
  b. Construction toys such as erector sets
  c. Drawing sets
  d. Microscope and chemistry sets
  e. Books
 3. Imitative, imaginative, and dramatic
  a. Dolls
  b. Dress-up costumes
  c. Puppets
 4. Competitive and social
  a. Games
  b. Role playing
C. Criteria for judging suitability of toys
 1. Safety
 2. Compatibility
  a. Child's age
  b. Level of development
  c. Experience
 3. Usefulness
  a. Challenge to development of child
  b. Enhancing social and personality development
  c. Increasing motor and sensory skills
  d. Developing creativity
  e. Expressing emotions
D. Criteria for judging nonsuitability of toys

1. Beyond child's level of growth and development
2. Unsafe
3. Overstimulating
4. Limited uses and transient value (see also play for each age group)

IMMUNIZATIONS

A. Recommended schedule for active immunization of normal infants and children (Committee on Infectious Diseases of the American Academy of Pediatrics, October 1971)

Age	Immunization
2 months	DTP,* TOPV†
4 months	DTP, TOPV
6 months	DTP, TOPV
1 year	Measles, rubella, mumps, and tuberculin test
1½ years	DTP, TOPV
4 to 6 years	DTP, TOPV
14 to 16 years	Td, and thereafter every 10 years‡

*DTP—diphtheria, tetanus toxoid, and pertussis vaccine
†TOPV—trivalent oral poliovirus vaccine
‡Td—combined adult type tetanus and diphtheria toxoid, which contains less diphtheria antigen

B. Specific characteristics of immunizations
1. Tetanus toxoid nearly 100% effective, induces prolonged immunity
2. Diphtheria toxoid about 80% effective, febrile reaction more commonly seen in older children, therefore, adult type Td given
3. Pertussis vaccine (vaccine of whole organism) is least effective of DTP and has most side effects
   a. Started early in life because no passive immunity from mother, as with diphtheria and tetanus
   b. Not given after child is 4 to 6 years old because of more severe reactions
4. Td, after 4 to 6 years of age, is given routinely every 10 years and at 5-year intervals in the event of a possibly contaminated wound
5. Measles vaccine (live attenuated vaccine) generally is not given before 12 months of age because of the presence of natural immunity from mother
   a. If given before 12 months of age, a second dose should be administered
   b. Tuberculin testing should be administered before the measles vac-

cine since the vaccine can alter the findings
6. Rubella given to children mainly to prevent occurrence of the disease in women during first trimester of pregnancy
   a. Not given if pregnancy is suspected in the mother because of potential infection of fetus
   ✓ b. Pregnancy must be prevented until 2 months after immunization of the child to eliminate danger to fetus
7. Smallpox no longer routinely recommended in nonendemic areas since occurrence of fatal and severe reactions to the vaccination outweigh the risk of contracting the disease

C. Primary immunization for children not immunized in infancy
1. One through 5 years of age

Age	Immunization
First visit	DTP, TOPV, TB test
1 month later	Measles, rubella, mumps
2 months later	DTP, TOPV
4 months later	DTP, TOPV
6 to 12 months later	DTP, TOPV
14 to 16 years of age	Td, and thereafter every 10 years

2. Six years of age and over—same schedule as above except DTP is replaced by Td

D. General contraindications for immunizations
1. Presence of maternal antibodies
2. Administration of blood transfusion or immune serum globulin within 6 weeks
3. High fever, serious illness
4. Diseases in which immunity is impaired
5. Immunosuppressive therapy
6. Generalized malignancy such as leukemia
7. Allergy to egg protein
8. Neurologic problems such as convulsions when administering pertussis vaccine

THE INFANT
Health problems
Accident prevention

A. Accidents are one of the leading causes of death during infancy
1. Mechanical suffocation causes most accidental deaths in children under 1 year of age

2. Aspiration of small objects and ingestion of poisonous substances occurs most often during second half of first year and into early childhood
3. Trauma from rolling off bed or falling down stairs can occur at any time
B. Teaching is an essential aspect—parents should never
   1. Leave plastic bags in crib
   2. Restrain infants with items that may choke them
   3. Leave infants alone on a high surface or near stairs without a proper gate to protect them from danger
   4. Give infant objects with sharp edges or detachable parts that can be swallowed
   5. Take infants in the automobile without restraining them in an infant seat or appropriate carrier
   6. Leave any poisons in a place that crawling infants can explore
   7. Leave burning cigarettes, candles, or incense within infants' reach
   8. Leave electric sockets uncovered without plastic plugs
   9. Place crib near window where infant can fall or pull on blind cords

Congenital abnormalities
A. Chromosomal aberrations
   1. Down's syndrome or mongolism
      a. Chromosomal causes
         (1) Trisomy 21—associated with advanced maternal age (2% risk over age of 40), can occur earlier
         (2) Translocation 15/21—translocated chromosome transmitted by mother who is a carrier, age is not a factor
         (3) Mosaicism—mixture of normal cells and cells trisomic for 21
      b. Resulting defects
         (1) Hypotonia
         (2) Congenital heart defects, particularly atrioventricular defects
         (3) Mental retardation—about 30% may have mild or borderline intelligence
      c. Nursing considerations
         (1) Emotional support of parents
         (2) Genetic counselling appropriate for type of defect
         (3) Assist parents to set realistic

expectations and goals for the child
         (4) Prevention of infection, especially respiratory
         (5) Activity consistent with defects
         (6) Physical supervision and habilitation
         (7) Careful testing of intellectual functioning for guidance
         (8) Same principles as care of child with mental retardation and birth of a defective child (pp. 389 and 396)
   2. Trisomy 18
      a. Several physical anomalies of head, ears, mandible, hands, feet, heart, and kidneys
      b. Failure to thrive and short survival; if survive, severe mental retardation
      c. Nursing considerations
         (1) Genetic counselling
         (2) Because of short survival, preparation of parents for loss of their child
   3. Turner's syndrome (gonadal dysgenesis)
      a. Chromosome monosomy (XO karyotype)
      b. Congenital malformations such as short stature, webbed neck, infantile genitalia, and developmental failure of secondary sexual characteristics at puberty
      c. Usually normal intelligence; problems in directional sense and space-form recognition
      d. Nursing considerations
         (1) Genetic counselling of parents
         (2) Preparation of child for lack of pubertal changes and need for hormonal replacement
         (3) Counselling with emphasis on adoption rather than person's inability to conceive
   4. Klinefelter's syndrome
      a. Sex-chromosomal abnormality of XXY
      b. Physical characteristics—tall, skinny, long legs and arms, small firm testes, gynecomastia, and poorly developed secondary sex characteristics at puberty
      c. Behavioral disorders and mental defects are often present

d. Nursing considerations
(1) Counselling with emphasis on positive aspects such as adoption or donor insemination
(2) May also be larger problem of psychopathology with need for counselling

B. Malformations (structural anomalies present at birth)
1. Facial malformations
   a. Failure of union of embryonic structure of face
      (1) Fusion of maxillary and premaxillary processes between 5 and 8 weeks of fetal life
      (2) Palatal structures fuse between 9 and 12 weeks
   b. Cause unknown, evidence of hereditary influence
      (1) Incidence in general population is 1 in 800 births
      (2) If one child is born with cleft lip or palate but no history of anomaly in family, next child's chances are 1 in 150
      (3) If history of either anomaly in family and one child was born with it, next sibling has chance of 1 in 4
2. Cleft lip
   a. Bilateral or unilateral; if unilateral, more common on left side
   b. More common in males
   c. Can be of several degrees; complete cleft is usually continuous with cleft palate
   d. Treatment is surgical repair, usually done soon after birth because of psychologic difficulties of parents associated with visual effects of defect and child's inability to meet sucking needs
   e. Nursing difficulties and interventions
      (1) Main difficulty is feeding
         (a) Child cannot form vacuum in mouth to suck
         (b) Should be fed with soft, large-holed nipple or rubber-tipped syringe placed on top and side of tongue, toward back of mouth
         (c) Should be bubbled frequently because of swallowed air
      (2) Problem of swallowed air (mouth breather)
         (a) Distended abdomen, pressure against diaphragm
         (b) Mucous membranes of oropharynx become dried and cracked, leading to infection
         (c) Mother should be taught to give water after each feeding to cleanse mouth
      (3) Problem of infection from irritation by infant
         (a) Infant's hands may need restraining
         (b) May need pacifier to increase sucking pleasure
   f. Postoperative nursing care
      (1) Maintain patent airway
         (a) Problem because of edema of nose, tongue, and lips combined with child's habit of breathing through the mouth
         (b) Proper equipment such as laryngoscope, endotracheal tube, and suction at or near bedside
      (2) Cleanse suture line to prevent crust formation and eventual scarring
      (3) Prevent crying because of pressure on suture line (encourage mother to stay with infant)
      (4) Place child in supine position with arm or elbow restraints
         (a) Change position to side or sitting up to prevent hypostatic pneumonia
         (b) Remove restraints only when supervised
      (5) Feeding (same as before surgery)
      (6) Support parents by accepting and treating child as normal
3. Cleft palate
   a. More common in girls
   b. May involve soft or hard palate and may extend into nose, forming oronasal passageway
   c. Age for repair is usually after child has grown, but before speech is well developed
   d. Nursing problems and interventions

(only differences from cleft lip will be discussed)

(1) Feeding
    (a) Feed upright to prevent aspiration
    (b) In severe cases, gavage feeding may be necessary
    (c) Encourage early use of spoon and cup

(2) Infection, especially aspiration pneumonia

(3) Speech
    (a) Palate is needed to trap air in mouth
    (b) Tonsils usually not removed because they provide an additional mechanism to trap air
    (c) Child will need speech appliance to help prevent guttural sounds if repair is delayed beyond speech development

(4) Dental development
    (a) Excessive dental caries
    (b) Malocclusion from displacement of maxillary arch
    (c) Need for proper dental hygiene and regular dental supervision

(5) Hearing problems caused by recurrent otitis media (eustachian tube connects the nasopharynx and middle ear and easily transports foreign material to ear)

e. Postoperative nursing care—same as for cleft lip except
  (1) In maintaining patent airway, try to avoid use of suction, which traumatizes operative site
  (2) Place child in prone Trendelenburg position to prevent aspiration and promote postural drainage
  (3) Avoid trauma to suture line by instructing child not to rub tongue on roof of mouth
  (4) Feeding
    (a) Liquid diet, no milk because of curd formation on suture line
    (b) Avoid use of straw or spoon

  (5) Need for emotional support of parents is greater, for recovery is longer and prognosis uncertain

4. Tracheoesophageal anomalies
  a. Absence of esophagus
  b. Atresia of the esophagus without a tracheal fistula
  c. Tracheoesophageal fistula
  d. The most common type of anomaly is proximal esophageal atresia combined with distal tracheoesophageal fistula
  e. Signs and symptoms
    (1) Excessive drooling
    (2) Excessive mucus in nasopharynx causing cyanosis, which is easily reversed by suctioning
    (3) Choking, sneezing, and coughing during feeding, with regurgitation of formula through mouth and nose
    (4) Inability to pass catheter into stomach
  f. Treatment—surgical correction
  g. Postoperative nursing care
    (1) Frequent suctioning of mouth and pharynx
    (2) Provision of high humidity to liquefy thick secretions
    (3) Stimulation of crying and change of position to prevent pneumonia
    (4) Proper care of chest tubes if used
    (5) Maintenance of nutrition by oral, parenteral, or gastrostomy method
    (6) Use of pacifier if oral feedings are contraindicated
    (7) Need for comfort and physical contact because hospitalization is usually long

5. Intestinal anomalies
  a. Intestinal obstruction
    (1) Signs alerting nurse to life threatening obstruction
      (a) Abdominal distention
      (b) Absence of stools, especially meconium in newborn
      (c) Vomiting of bile-stained material that may be projectile
      (d) Cyanosis and weak grunting respirations

from abdominal disten-
tion causing diaphragm
to compress lungs
- (e) Paroxysmal pain
- (f) Weak, thready pulse
b. Imperforate anus
- (1) Most common intestinal anomaly
- (2) Failure of membrane separating rectum from anus to absorb during eighth week of
fetal life
- (3) Fistulas within vagina, urinary
tract, or scrotum are common
- (4) Diagnosed by
  - (a) Failure to pass meconium
stool
  - (b) Inability to insert thermometer or small finger
into rectum
  - (c) Abdominal distention
- (5) Treatment—immediate surgical correction unless fistula
is present
- (6) Postoperative nursing care—
dependent on type of surgery
performed
  - (a) Keep operative sites
clean and dry, especially
after passage of stool
  - (b) If perineal sutures are
present, position infant
on side rather than ab-
domen to prevent pulling
legs up under chest
  - (c) Care of colostomy—prevent excoriation of skin
by frequent cleansing
and use of diaper held on
by belly binder
  - (d) Instruct mother about
colostomy care (include
avoidance of tight dia-
pers and clothes around
abdomen)
c. Diaphragmatic hernia
- (1) Protrusion of abdominal viscera through opening into
thoracic cavity
- (2) Symptoms alerting nurse
  - (a) Severe respiratory difficulty with cyanosis
  - (b) Relatively large chest,
especially on affected
side
  - (c) Failure of affected side
of chest to expand dur-

ing respiration and ab-
sence of breath sounds
  - (d) Relatively small abdomen
- (3) Treatment—immediate surgical repair
- (4) Nursing care
  - (a) Gastric suction is used to
remove secretions and
swallowed air from
stomach and intestine
before and after surgery
  - (b) Preoperatively, to allow
full expansion of unaf-
fected side, position in-
fant with head elevated
on affected side
  - (c) Postoperatively, to decrease chance of swallow-
ing air, infant may be
fed by gavage
6. Congenital laryngeal stridor (laryngo-
malacia)
a. A crowing sound during inspiration
caused by different factors, most
often it is related to flabbiness of
the epiglottis
b. May correct itself as infant grows,
or may necessitate tracheostomy to
sustain life
c. Nursing problems and interventions
- (1) Feeding
  - (a) Infant must be fed
slowly, stopping fre-
quently to allow breath-
ing and then bottle or
breast reoffered
  - (b) Proper nipple hole size
and position at breast
important to regulate
flow
  - (c) Mother needs help to
learn correct feeding
method
- (2) Breathing
  - (a) Mother should be encouraged to listen to
sound of stridor to detect
a change
  - (b) Needs to be protected
from respiratory infec-
tion, which increases
breathing difficulty
7. Choanal atresia
a. Embryonic membrane obstructs
posterior nares at junction with
nasopharynx

b. Bilateral obstruction causes mouth breathing and dyspnea that is relieved by crying and aggravated by sucking

c. Nursing problems and interventions are the same as for laryngeal stridor

8. Congenital heart defects
   a. Normal circulatory changes that occur at or shortly after birth
      (1) Pulmonary circulation rapidly increases
      (2) Increased pressure from left side of heart results in closure of foramen ovale, ductus arteriosus, and ductus venosus
   b. General signs and symptoms of congenital heart defects in children
      (1) Dyspnea, especially on exertion
      (2) Feeding difficulty and failure to thrive often first signs discovered by mother
      (3) Stridor or choking spells
      (4) Heart rate over 200, respiratory rate about 60 in infant
      (5) Recurrent respiratory infections
      (6) In older child, poor physical development, delayed milestones, and decreased exercise tolerance
      (7) Cyanosis, squatting, and clubbing of fingers and toes
      (8) Heart murmurs
      (9) Excessive perspiration
   c. Classification of cardiac lesions
      (1) Acyanotic—shunt from left to right side of heart
          (a) No abnormal communication between pulmonary and systemic circulation
          (b) If such a connection exists, pressure forces blood from arterial to venous side of heart, where it is reoxygenated
      (2) Cyanotic—shunt from right to left side of heart
          (a) Abnormal connection between pulmonary and systemic circulation
          (b) Venous or unoxygenated blood enters systemic circulation

          (c) Polycythemia (increase in number of red blood cells) occurs as body tries to compensate for inadequate supply of oxygen
          (d) Compensation and nature of defect causes clubbing of fingers and toes, retarded growth, increased viscosity of blood, and can lead to congestive heart failure
   d. Types of acyanotic defects
      (1) Ventricular septal defect (VSD)
          (a) Abnormal opening between the 2 ventricles
          (b) Severity of defect depends on size of opening
          (c) High pressure in right ventricle causes hypertrophy, with development of pulmonary hypertension
          (d) Blowing type murmur heard throughout systole
          (e) Treatment procedure—close opening in septum
      (2) Atrial septal defect (ASD)—3 types
          (a) Secundum defect—high on septum
          (b) Primum defect—low on septum, can be associated with mitral and/or tricuspid regurgitation
          (c) Foramen ovale—failure to close at birth
          (d) Murmur heard high on chest, with fixed splitting of second heart sound
          (e) Treatment procedure—close opening in septum
      (3) Patent ductus arteriosus (PDA)
          (a) Failure of closure of fetal connection between aorta and pulmonary artery
          (b) Blood shunted from aorta back to pulmonary artery, may progress to pulmonary hypertension and cardiomegaly

(c) Machinery type murmur heard throughout heart-beat in left second or third interspace

(d) Treatment procedure—close opening between aorta and pulmonary artery

(4) Coarctation of aorta

(a) In utero, failure of aorta to develop completely; stricture usually occurs below level of aortic arch

(b) Increased systemic circulation above stricture —bounding radial and carotid pulses, headache, dizziness, epistaxis

(c) Decreased systemic circulation below stricture —absent femoral pulses, cool lower extremities

(d) Increased pressure in aorta above defect causes left ventricular hypertrophy

(e) Usually no murmur heard

(f) Treatment procedure—resection of defect and anastomoses of the ends of the aorta

(5) Aortic stenosis

(a) Narrowing of aortic valve

(b) Causes increased workload on left ventricle and lowered pressure base of aorta reduces coronary artery flow

(c) Treatment procedures—divide the stenotic valves of the aorta or dilate the constricting ring

(6) Pulmonary stenosis

(a) Narrowing of pulmonary valve

(b) Causes decreased blood flow to lungs and increased pressure to right ventricle

(c) Treatment procedures—valvulotomy or mechanical dilatation

e. Types of cyanotic defects

(1) Tetralogy of Fallot—4 associated defects

(a) Pulmonary valve stenosis

(b) Ventricular septal defect, usually high on septum

(c) Overriding aorta, receiving blood from both ventricles, or an aorta arising from right ventricle

(d) Right ventricular hypertrophy

(e) Treatment procedures—Potts-Smith-Gibson procedure—aortic to pulmonary artery anastomosis, or Blalock-Taussig procedure—subclavian artery to pulmonary artery anastomosis

(2) Transposition of the great vessels

(a) Aorta arises from the right ventricle, and pulmonary artery arises from the left ventricle

(b) Incompatible with life unless there is a communication between the 2 sides of the heart, such as an atrial septal defect, ventricular septal defect, or a patent ductus arteriosus

(c) Treatment procedures—Rashkind procedure—nonsurgical creation of an atrial septal defect at the foramen ovale through the use of a cardiac catheterization balloon, Blalock-Hanlon procedure—surgical creation of an atrial septal defect, or Mustard procedure—complete surgical repair with reconstruction of aorta and pulmonary artery to correct ventricle

(3) Tricuspid atresia

(a) Absence of tricuspid valve

(b) Incompatible with life unless there is a communication between 2 sides of heart, such as atrial septal defect, ven-

tricular septal defect, or patent ductus arteriosus
- (c) Treatment procedures— Blalock, Potts, or Glen procedure—anastomosis of superior vena cava to right pulmonary artery
- (4) Truncus arteriosus
  - (a) Single great vessel arising from base of heart, serving as pulmonary artery and aorta
  - (b) Systolic murmur is heard, and single semilunar valve produces a loud second heart sound that is not split
- f. Preoperative preparation
  - (1) Main assessment factor in preparation of child is the developmental and chronologic age, for example
    - (a) Explanation of heart differs according to age of child
    - (b) Child 4 to 6 years of age, knows heart is in chest, describes it as valentine shaped, and characterizes its function by the sound of "tick-tock"
    - (c) Child 7 to 10 years of age, doesn't see heart as valentine shaped, knows it has veins, has idea of function such as "It makes you live," but doesn't understand concept of pumping
    - (d) Child over 10 years of age, has concept of veins, valves, circulation, and why death occurs when heart stops
  - (2) Based on principle that fear of unknown increases anxiety
  - (3) The same nurse should participate in preoperative and postoperative preparation as source of support for child
  - (4) Nurse must know what equipment is usual after open or closed heart surgery
  - (5) Let child play with equipment such as stethoscope, blood pressure machine, oxygen mask, suction, syringes
  - (6) For young child, especially preschooler, use dolls and puppets to describe procedures
  - (7) Preparation for cardiac catheterization prior to surgery is essential as well
  - (8) For young child, talk about size of bandage; for older child, discuss actual incision
  - (9) Familiarize child with postoperative environment such as recovery room and intensive care unit, stressing the strange noises such as the monitors
  - (10) Have child practice coughing, using blow bottles and breathing on intermittent positive pressure machine
  - (11) Explain to child why coughing and moving are necessary even though they will hurt
  - (12) Explain to child what tubes may be used and what they will look like
  - (13) For more specific discussion of above, see specific age groups under Pediatric nursing
- g. Preoperative assessment areas necessary for planning postoperative care
  - (1) Keep sleep record so care can be organized around child's usual rest pattern
  - (2) Constipation and straining after surgery must be avoided —this can be accomplished by
    - (a) Knowing child's elimination pattern
    - (b) Knowing words child uses
    - (c) Having child practice using bed pan
  - (3) Record level of activity and list favorite toys or games that require gradually increased exertion
  - (4) Determine child's fluid preferences for postoperative maintenance
  - (5) When recording vital signs al-

ways indicate child's activity at the time of measurement

(6) Observe child's verbal and nonverbal responses to pain

(7) Specifics of postoperative care are similar to any major surgery

h. Adjustment of child and family to correction of cardiac defect

(1) Improved physical status is often difficult for the child who has become accustomed to the sick role and its secondary gains

(2) Improved physical status of the child is also difficult for the parents since it reduces child's dependency

(3) Child may have difficulty learning to relate to peers and siblings on a competitive basis

(4) Child can no longer use disability as a crutch for educational and social shortcomings

(5) Parental expectations must be adjusted to accommodate child's new physical vigor and search for independence

9. Spina bifida

a. Malformation of the spine in which posterior portion of laminae of vertebrae fails to close, most common site is lumbosacral area

(1) Spina bifida occulta—defect only of vertebrae; spinal cord and meninges are intact

(2) Meningocele—meninges protrude through vertebral defect

(3) Meningomyelocele—meninges and spinal cord protrude through defect; most serious type

b. Associated defects include weakness or paralysis below defect, bowel and bladder dysfunction, clubfeet, dislocated hip, and hydrocephalus

c. Arnold-Chiari syndrome—defect of occipitocervical region with swelling and displacement of medulla into the spinal cord

d. Nursing problems and intervention (meningomyelocele)

(1) Infection because breakdown

of sac leaves spinal cord open to environment

(a) Area must be kept clean, especially from urine and feces

(b) Diaper is not used, but sterile gauze with antibiotic solution may be placed over sac

(2) Associated orthopedic defects

(a) Maintain function through proper position, which also decreases pressure on sac

(b) Clubfeet and dislocated hip—prone position, hips slightly flexed and abducted, feet hanging free of mattress and slight Trendelenburg slope to reduce spinal fluid pressure

(3) Feeding because of restriction in position

(a) Must be fed prone, nurse should establish eye contact and encourage mother to visit and feed child

(b) If solids need to be introduced while infant still prone, may be mixed with formula in bottle with large-hole nipple

(4) Elimination, especially of neurogenic bladder

(a) Credé or slight pressure against abdomen may be necessary to fully empty bladder

(b) While infant is prone, can apply pressure to abdomen above symphysis pubis with sides of fingers and counterpressure with thumbs against buttocks

e. Postoperative nursing care

(1) Surgical repair of the sac may be done soon after birth to prevent infection and maintain neurologic function

(2) Care is same as above, with emphasis on habilitation of child's abilities

(3) Head size should be measured

to determine whether hydrocephalus is occurring

10. Hydrocephalus
    a. Abnormal accumulation of cerebrospinal fluid within ventricular system
       (1) Noncommunicating—obstruction within the ventricles such as congenital malformation, neoplasm, or hematoma
       (2) Communicating—inadequate absorption of cerebrospinal fluid resulting from infection or trauma
    b. Clinical signs
       (1) Increasing head size in infant because of open sutures and bulging fontanels
       (2) Prominent scalp veins and taut shiny skin
       (3) Sunset eyes (sclera visible above iris), bulging eyes, and papilledema of retina
       (4) Head lag, especially important after 4 to 6 months
       (5) Increased intracranial pressure—projectile vomiting not associated with feeding, irritability, anorexia, high shrill cry, convulsions
       (6) Damage to brain because increased pressure decreases blood flow to cells causing necrosis
    c. Treatment
       (1) Removal of obstruction
       (2) Mechanical shunting of fluid to another area of body
          (a) Ventriculoatrial shunt—catheter from lateral ventricle to internal jugular vein to right atrium of heart
          (b) Ventriculoperitoneal shunt—catheter is passed subcutaneously to peritoneal cavity
    d. General nursing problems and intervention
       (1) Breakdown of scalp, infection, and damage to spinal cord
          (a) Proper positioning—placed in Fowler's position to facilitate draining of fluid, postoperatively positioned flat with no pressure on shunted side
          (b) When held, neck and head must be supported
          (c) Observing shunt site (abdominal site in peritoneal procedure) for infection
       (2) Increasing intracranial pressure
          (a) Careful observation, minimal use of sedatives or analgesics, which can mask signs
          (b) Frequent checking of valve for patency
          (c) Pumping valve per physician's orders to ensure proper functioning
       (3) Nutrition
          (a) Frequent vomiting, irritability, lethargy, and anorexia decrease intake of nutrients
          (b) All care should be done before feeding to prevent vomiting, infant should be held if possible
          (c) Observe for signs of dehydration
       (4) Irritation of eyes if eyelid incompletely covers cornea
    e. Specific postoperative nursing care —similar to above except
       (1) Child is usually kept in bed after surgery with minimal handling to prevent damage to shunt
       (2) Parents need much support
          (a) Continued shunt revisions are usually necessary as growth occurs
          (b) Usually very concerned about retardation
       (3) Observe for brain damage by recording milestones during infancy
       (4) Parental teaching must include
          (a) Pumping of shunt
          (b) Signs of increasing intracranial pressure
          (c) Evidence of dehydration
11. Exstrophy of the bladder
    a. Entire lower urinary tract from

bladder to external urethral meatus is outside abdominal cavity

b. May be accompanied by defects such as epispadias, undescended testes, or short penis in males and a cleft clitoris or absent vagina in females

c. Treatment
(1) Plastic surgery
(2) Sigmoid implantation of ureters—may be complicated by
(a) Ascending infection (pyelonephritis from colon bacilli)
(b) Hydronephrosis from backup of urine into kidneys
(c) Electrolyte imbalance

d. Nursing problems and intervention
(1) Parental teaching is vital but objectives can only be achieved after parents have accepted both the disorder and the long-term sequelae
(2) Infection and care of skin
(a) Scrupulous cleansing of area, application of sterile petroleum gauze, and care of skin around bladder
(b) Clothing should be light to avoid pressure over area
(c) Frequent change of clothing because of odor
(3) Control of urination in sigmoid implantation
(a) When old enough to control bowels, child can learn to tighten anal sphincter to prevent seepage of urine
(b) Parents need encouragement because accidents are common

12. Displacement of urethral opening
a. Hypospadias
(1) In male, urethra opens on lower surface of penis from just behind the glans to the perineum
(2) In female, urethra opens into the vagina
b. Epispadias
(1) Occurs only in males
(2) Urethra opens on dorsal surface of penis, often associated with exstrophy of bladder
c. Nursing considerations
(1) Repair is usually of concern to parents, who need explicit explanation of child's future functioning
(2) Repair may be in several stages for male, who needs preparation for surgery and help in coping with adjustment to voiding in a sitting position
(3) Defect can be sign of ambiguous genitalia
(4) Procreation may be interfered with in severe cases

13. Orthopedic deformities
a. Clubfoot
(1) Foot has been twisted out of position in utero
(2) Most common type—talipes equinovarus: foot is fixed in plantar flexion (downward) and deviates medially (inward)
(3) Treatment is most successful when started early since delay causes muscles and bones of legs to develop abnormally, with shortening of tendons
(4) Treatment and nursing measures in infancy
(a) Denis Browne splint (appliance of a crossbar with shoes attached)
(1) Encourage activity since success of appliance depends on alternate kicking and extention of baby's legs
(2) Watch for circulatory impairment caused by swelling around ankles
(3) Pick up child frequently to prevent respiratory and other problems from immobility
(b) Gentle repeated manipulation of foot or forcible correction under anesthesia and application of a wedge cast

(1) Observe toes for signs of circulatory impairment, make sure toes are visible at end of cast

(2) Watch for signs of weakness and wear of cast especially if child is allowed to walk on it

(3) For other areas of cast care, see treatment of dislocated hip

(4) Main nursing objective is teaching mother all of above, stressing need for follow-up care that may be prolonged

(5) Follow-up care of patient

   (a) Extended medical supervision is required since there is a tendency for this deformity to recur (considered cured when able to wear normal shoes and walk properly)

   (b) Care emphasizes muscle reeducation (by manipulation) and proper walking

   (c) Heels and soles of braces or shoes prescribed following correction must be kept in repair

   (d) Corrective shoes may have sole and heel lifts on lateral border to maintain proper position

b. Dislocated hip

(1) Trochanter (head of femur) does not lie deep enough inside the acetabulum and slips out on movement (may be caused by lack of embryonic development of joint)

(2) Main clinical signs

   (a) Limitation in abduction of leg on affected side

   (b) Asymmetry of gluteal, popliteal, and thigh folds

   (c) Ortolani's sign—an audible click when abducting the leg on the affected side

   (d) Apparent shortening of the femur—Galeazzi's sign

   (e) Waddling gait and lordosis when child begins to walk

(3) Treatment—directed toward enlarging and deepening the socket by placing the trochanter within the acetabulum and applying constant pressure

   (a) Proper positioning—legs slightly flexed and abducted

      (1) Frejka pillow—a pillow splint that maintains abduction of legs

      (2) Use of pillow or rolled diapers between legs

      (3) Bryant's traction

      (4) Spica cast—body cast from waist to below knee

   (b) Surgical intervention such as open reduction with casting

(4) Specific nursing problems and intervention when spica cast is applied

   (a) Respiratory problems—hypostatic pneumonia

      (1) Need to change position from back to stomach frequently

      (2) Teach parents postural drainage and exercises such as blowing bubbles to increase lung expansion

      (3) Encourage parents to seek immediate medical care if child develops congestion or cough

   (b) Infection and excoriation of skin

      (1) Observe for circulation of toes, pedal pulses, and blanching

      (2) Do not let child put small toys or food inside cast

(3) Gauze strips may be used inside cast as a scratcher

(4) Alert parents to signs of infection such as odor

(5) Protect cast edges with adhesive tape or waterproof material, especially around perineum

(6) Minimize soiling of cast by feces and urine by using diapers and plastic lining

(c) Constipation from immobility

(1) Parents should observe for straining on defecation and constipation

(2) Increase fluids and roughage to prevent constipation

(d) Nutrition

(1) Provide small, frequent meals because of inflexibility of cast around waist

(2) Adjust caloric intake since less energy expenditure can lead to obesity

(e) Transportation and positioning

(1) Use wagon or stroller with back flat

(2) Protect child from falling when positioned

(3) Child must not be picked up by bar between cast (use 2 people to provide adequate body support if necessary)

(f) Emotional needs

(1) Since child cannot be picked up and cuddled, touch should be used as much as possible

(2) Stimulate and provide for play activities appropriate to age

(g) Parents need help and support

(1) Directions should be written

(2) Home visits should be routine, with telephone counselling available

(3) Treatment may be prolonged so follow-up care must be stressed

(4) Prepare parents for the possible use of an abduction brace after the cast is removed

c. Developmental anomalies of the extremities

(1) Polydactyly—extra digits

(2) Syndactyly—partial or complete fusion of 2 or more digits

(3) Amelia—absence of a limb

(4) Treatment—if possible, early correction and preparation for use of prosthesis

(5) Nursing considerations

(a) Recognize own reaction to deformity

(b) Accept parents' reactions of guilt, anger, and hopelessness

(c) Assist parents to set realistic goals for child

(d) Prepare parents to answer child's questions about the deformity and what it will mean in the future

C. Inborn errors of metabolism

1. Phenylketonuria (PKU)

a. Lack of enzyme phenylalanine hydroxylase, which changes phenylalanine (essential amino acid) into tyrosine

b. Transmitted by autosomal recessive gene

c. Clinical symptoms

(1) Mental retardation, from damage to nervous system from build up of phenylalanine

(a) Usually noticed by 4 months of age

(b) IQ is usually below 50 and most frequently under 20

(2) Strong musty odor in urine from phenylacetic acid

(3) Absence of tyrosine reduces production of melanin and results in blond hair and blue eyes

(4) Fair skin is susceptible to eczema

d. Treatment
(1) Prevention—test for PKU at birth
(a) Guthrie blood test—effective in newborns
(b) Ferric chloride urine test —only effective when infant is over 6 weeks of age
(2) Dietary—low phenylalanine diet: use Lofenalac as a milk substitute and foods restricted to those low in this amino acid (usually continued until child is 6 years of age)

e. Nursing considerations
(1) Parents need help in understanding the disease and the role of the diet
(2) Genetic counselling

2. Galactosemia
a. Missing enzyme that converts galactose to glucose
b. Transmitted by autosomal recessive gene
c. Treatment—dietary, reduction of lactose: use Nutramigen as a milk substitute and foods restricted to those low in lactose (usually continued until child is 3 years of age)
d. Nursing considerations similar to phenylketonuria

Noncongenital conditions

A. Surgical problems
1. Pyloric stenosis
a. Congenital hypertrophy of muscular tissue of pyloric sphincter, which usually is asymptomatic until 2 to 4 weeks after birth
b. Clinical signs
(1) Vomiting, progressively projectile
(2) Nonbile stained vomitus
(3) Constipation
(4) Dehydration and weight loss
(5) Distention of epigastrium, visible peristalsis, and palpable olive-shaped mass in right upper quadrant
c. Treatment is usually surgical—the Fredet-Ramstedt procedure (longitudinal splitting of hypertrophied muscle)
d. Postoperative nursing care
(1) Same as for any abdominal surgery
(2) Teach mother specific feeding method
(a) Use thickened formula to facilitate passage through sphincter muscle
(b) Hold baby in high Fowler's position during feeding and place on right side after feeding with head of bed slightly elevated
(c) Bubble frequently during feeding and avoid unnecessary handling afterward

2. Intussusception
a. Telescoping of 1 portion of intestine into another, occurs most frequently at the ileocecal valve
b. Clinical signs
(1) Healthy, well-nourished infant who wakes up with severe paroxysmal abdominal pain, evidenced by kicking and drawing legs up to abdomen
(2) One or 2 normal stools, then bloody mucous stool ("currant jelly" stool)
(3) Palpation of sausage-shaped mass
(4) Other signs of intestinal obstruction are usually present
c. Treatment
(1) Medical—reduction by hydrostatic pressure (barium enema)
(2) Surgical reduction and, if necessary, intestinal resection
d. Nursing considerations
(1) Same as for any abdominal surgery
(2) Since problem usually occurs when child is 6 to 8 months of age, separation anxiety is acute and provision must be made for mother's frequent visits

3. Megacolon (Hirschsprung's disease)
   a. Absence of parasympathetic ganglion cells in a portion of bowel that causes enlargement of the bowel proximal to the defect
   b. Clinical signs may occur gradually
      (1) Constipation, or passage of ribbon or pellet-like stool
      (2) Intestinal obstruction
   c. Treatment
      (1) Medical
         (a) Use of laxatives, enemas
         (b) Dietary management—decrease bulk and residue
      (2) Surgical
         (a) Removal of aganglionic portion of bowel
         (b) Colostomy if necessary
   d. Nursing considerations
      (1) Teach mother correct procedure for enemas (point out danger of water intoxication)
      (2) General postoperative care
B. Medical problems
1. Failure to thrive syndrome (often associated with maternal deprivation syndrome)
   a. Children are usually below third percentile in growth
   b. Lack of physical growth may be secondary to decreased emotional and sensory stimulation from mother or mother substitute
   c. Development delayed and demonstrates signs of maternal understimulation
   d. Unpliable, stiff, uncomforted, and unyielding to cuddling
   e. Slow in smiling and responding to others
   f. History of difficult feeding, vomiting, sleep disturbance, and excessive irritability
   g. Characteristics of mothers
      (1) Difficulty perceiving and assessing infant's needs
      (2) Frustrated and angered at infant's dissatisfied response
      (3) Frequently under stress and in crisis with emotional, social, and financial problems
      (4) Often have marital disturbances, such as absent husband, or if present, one who gives little emotional support
      (5) Tend to lead lonely, solitary lives with few outside interests or friends
   h. Nursing considerations
      (1) Child needs consistent care giver, who can begin to satisfy child's routine needs
      (2) Increased stimulation, appropriate to child's present developmental level
      (3) Provide mother with opportunity to talk
      (4) When necessary, relieve mother of childrearing responsibilities until she is able and ready to emotionally support the child
      (5) Demonstrate proper infant care by example, not lecturing (allow mother to proceed at own pace)
      (6) Supply mother with emotional support without fostering dependency
      (7) Promote mother's self-respect and confidence by praising achievements with child
2. Sudden infant death syndrome—SIDS (crib death)
   a. A definite syndrome with cause unknown
   b. Number one cause of death in infants between 2 weeks and 1 year of age with an incidence of 1 in every 350 live births
   c. Peak age of occurrence—healthy infant 3 to 4 months of age
   d. Nursing considerations to assist parents
      (1) Know signs of sudden infant death to distinguish it from child neglect or abuse
      (2) Reassure parents that they could not have prevented the death or predicted its occurrence
      (3) An autopsy should be done on every child to confirm diagnosis
      (4) Visit parents at home to discuss cause of death and help them with their guilt and grief
      (5) Refer parents to National Sudden Infant Death Syndrome Parent Group

3. Diarrhea
a. Symptom of variety of conditions such as viral or bacterial infection or allergy
b. Metabolic acidosis from loss of water and electrolytes, which decreases available bicarbonate
c. Clinical manifestations
(1) Dehydration is severe when weight loss is greater than 10%
(2) Poor skin turgor and dry mucous membranes
(3) Depressed fontanels and sunken eyeballs
(4) Decreased urine output, increased specific gravity, and increased hematocrit
(5) Irritability, stupor, convulsions from loss of intracellular water and decreased plasma volume
d. Treatment and nursing considerations
(1) In severe diarrhea, medical treatment is necessary to correct fluid and electrolyte imbalance
(2) Isolate infant until stool culture results are reported
(3) Identify causative agent and institute proper therapy (antibiotics are used if bacterial agent is present)
(4) Explain to parents why antibiotics and an increase in food are ineffective in treating viral diarrhea
(5) Mother should be taught progressive increase in diet—alterations in diet may control mild diarrhea
(a) Clear fluids to decrease inflammation of mucosa
(b) If tolerated, half strength skim milk may be given
(c) Regular diet of bland foods
4. Vomiting
a. A symptom of many conditions, such as poor feeding technique, chalasia (abnormal relaxation of cardiac sphincter), or infections
b. Results in metabolic alkalosis from loss of hydrogen ion
c. Clinical signs

(1) Dehydration
(2) Tetany and convulsions in severe alkalosis, resulting from hypokalemia and hypocalcemia
d. Nursing considerations
(1) Care directed toward correction of underlying problem
(2) Chalasia
(a) Thickened feeding
(b) Feed in upright position
(c) Maintain upright position 20 to 30 minutes after feeding
5. Colic
a. Paroxysmal intestinal cramps caused by accumulation of excessive gas
b. May be caused by excessive air swallowing, feeding too fast or too much, excessive carbohydrate intake, or emotional tension
c. Treatment—directed toward correction of underlying cause
d. Nursing considerations
(1) Nurse should observe mother feed infant before attempting to counsel
(2) Teach mother to bubble the infant frequently and position on abdomen after feeding
6. Constipation
a. Usually occurs as a result of diet although there may be a psychologic component
b. Treatment should be dietary—enemas should be avoided
c. If mineral oil is used, it should not be given with foods since it decreases absorption of nutrients
7. Respiratory infections
a. Frequent cause of morbidity
b. Acute infection may be bacterial or viral (refer to Microbiology for specific causative agents)
(1) Acute nasopharyngitis (common cold)
(2) Pneumonia
(3) Bronchitis
(4) Tonsillitis
(5) Epiglottitis
(6) Croup
(7) Acute laryngotracheobronchitis
c. General nursing care for respiratory conditions

(1) Increase fluid intake
    (a) Prevents dehydration from fever and perspiration
    (b) Loosens thickened secretions
(2) Increase humidity and coolness
    (a) Liquefies secretions
    (b) Decreases febrile state and inflammation of the mucous membrane
    (c) Causes vasoconstriction and bronchiolar dilation
(3) Promote nasal and pulmonary drainage
    (a) Clean nares with bulb syringes
    (b) Suction oronasal pharynx
    (c) Postural drainage, clapping, and vibrating
(4) Provide rest by decreasing stimulation
(5) Increase oxygen
(6) Tracheotomy if necessary (see Medical-surgical nursing, pp. 476-477, for general nursing care of tracheotomy)

8. Otitis media
  a. Acute otitis media—infection of middle ear, causative organism usually *Hemophilus influenzae, Staphylococcus,* or *Streptococcus*
  b. Symptoms
    (1) Pain—infant frets and rubs ear or rolls head from side to side
    (2) Drum bulging, red, no light reflex, may rupture
  c. Serous otitis—accumulation of uninfected serous or mucoid matter in middle ear, cause unknown
  d. Symptoms
    (1) No pain or fever, but "fullness" in ear
    (2) Drum appears gray, bulging
    (3) May be loss of hearing from scarring of drum
  e. Nursing considerations
    (1) Proper instillation of ear drops
      (a) If child is under 3 years of age, auricle pulled down and back
      (b) Older child, auricle pulled up and back
    (2) Check for complications such

as chronic hearing loss, mastoiditis, or possible meningitis

9. Meningitis
  a. Causative agent may be viral or bacterial, such as *Hemophilus influenzae, Neisseria meningitidis,* or *Diplococcus pneumoniae*
  b. Clinical manifestations (more severe in bacterial)
    (1) Opisthotonos—rigidity and hyperextension of neck
    (2) Headache
    (3) Irritability and high-pitched cry
    (4) Signs of increased intracranial pressure (p. 380)
    (5) Fever, nausea, and vomiting
  c. Nursing considerations
    (1) Provide for rest
    (2) Decrease stimuli from environment (control light and noise)
    (3) Position on side with head gently supported in extension
    (4) Medical isolation is generally used
    (5) Decrease fluids because of meningeal edema
      (a) Carefully record intake and output
      (b) Monitor intravenous fluid
    (6) Provide emotional support for parents since child usually becomes ill very suddenly
    (7) Administer antibiotic therapy as prescribed

10. Eczema
  a. An atopic manifestation of a specific allergen that may have an emotional component
  b. Most common during first 2 years of life
  c. Clinical manifestations
    (1) Erythema and edema from dilation of capillaries
    (2) Papules, vesicles, and crusts
    (3) Itching that may precipitate infection from scratching
    (4) Periods of remission and exacerbation
    (5) Seen mostly on cheeks, scalp, neck, and flexor surfaces of arms and legs
  d. Nursing considerations
    (1) Support parents because this long-term problem is often discouraging since the infant is difficult to comfort

(2) Restrain hands to keep infant from scratching when unsupervised but provide supervised unrestrained play periods

(3) Pick up frequently, since infant is irritable, fretful, and anorexic

(4) Clothing or blankets of wool should be avoided

(5) Provide mother with a list of foods permitted and omitted on elimination or allergenic diet

(6) Instruct mother how to apply topical ointments prescribed

11. Febrile convulsions
    a. Caused by elevation of temperature
    b. Usually occur in children between 6 months and 3 years of age
    c. Nursing considerations
       (1) Reduce fever with antipyretic drugs and sponge baths
       (2) General seizure precautions
           (a) Protect child from injury, do not restrain, pad crib rails
           (b) Prevent tongue from blocking airway and protect it from injury
           (c) Record time of seizure, duration, and body parts involved
           (d) Suction nasopharynx, administer oxygen as required
           (e) Observe degree of consciousness and behavior after seizure
           (f) Provide rest after seizure
    g. For further discussion of convulsive disorders, see Medical-surgical nursing, pp. 559-560

Hospitalization during infancy

A. Reactions to maternal separation (greatest from 6 months to 2 years of age)
   1. Protest
      a. Prolonged loud crying, consoled by no one but mother or usual care giver
      b. Continually asks to go home
      c. Rejection of nurse or any other stranger
   2. Despair

a. Alteration in sleep pattern
b. Decreased appetite and weight loss
c. Diminished interest in environment and play
d. Relative immobility and listlessness
e. No facial expression or smile
f. Unresponsive to stimuli
   3. Detachment or denial
      a. Cheerful undiscriminating friendliness
      b. Lack of preference for parents
B. Prevention of separation anxiety
   1. Encourage mother to stay with child in hospital or visit as frequently as possible
   2. Provide consistent care giver
   3. Provide individual attention, physical touch, sensory stimulation, and affection
   4. Prepare mother for child's reaction to separation
   5. Involve mother in child's care as much as possible
   6. If mother is unable to visit, establish phone contact with her so that she is aware of child's progress and doesn't feel like a stranger
C. General problems in care of infant
   1. Small size of infant
      a. Body warmth and temperature control
      b. Maintenance of fluids—prone to edema, dehydration, and electrolyte imbalance
         (1) Infants have a higher percentage of extracellular fluid than adults, which can be quickly excreted
         (2) Infants' kidneys are unable to concentrate urine
   2. Immaturity of organ systems
      a. Primary defense mechanisms just developing—loss of antibodies from fetal life increases infant's susceptibility to infection
         (1) Antibody level lowest at 6 weeks to 2 months of age, then infant begins to develop own system
         (2) Problem subsides as child grows older
      b. Blood vessels are still developing; increased fragility causes hemorrhage
      c. Some essential enzymes such as glucuronyl transferase, which is

necessary for conjugation of bilirubin, are still developing—more chance for jaundice and brain damage

Reaction of parents to a defective child

A. Parents exhibit a variety of responses, such as grief and mourning, chronic grief, and excessive use of defense mechanisms
B. Chronic grief
1. Shock and disbelief—parents tend to
   a. Learn about the deformity, but deny the facts
   b. Feel inadequate and guilty
   c. Feel insecure in their ability to care for the child
   d. "Doctor shop" in hope of finding solutions
2. Awareness of the handicap—parents tend to
   a. Feel guilty, angry, and depressed
   b. Envy well children—closely related to bitterness and anger
   c. Search for clues or reasons why this happened to them
   d. Reject and feel ambivalent toward child
3. Restitution or recovery phase—parents tend to
   a. See child's defect in proper perspective
   b. Function more effectively and realistically
   c. Socially and emotionally accept the child
   d. Reintegrate family life without centering it around handicapped child
C. Implications for nursing
1. Helping parents gain awareness of child's defect
   a. Learning cannot take place until awareness of problem exists
   b. Help parents develop awareness through their own realization of problem rather than identifying problem for them
   c. Help parents see problem by drawing attention to certain manifestations of problem, such as failure to walk or talk
2. Help parents understand child's potential ability and assist them in setting realistic goals
   a. Help parents feel a sense of adequacy in parenting by emphasizing

good care, identifying small steps in learning process of child, and acquainting them with parents of children with similar problems
   b. Teach parents how to work with their handicapped child in simple childhood tasks of walking, talking, toileting, feeding, and dressing
   c. Teach parents how to stimulate child's learning of new skills
3. Encourage parents to treat child as normally as possible
   a. Avoid overprotection and use consistent, simple discipline
   b. Help parents become aware of the effects of this child on siblings who may resent excessive attention given to this child
4. Provide family with an outlet for own emotional tensions and needs
   a. Acquaint them with organizations, especially parent groups, who have children with similar problems
   b. Be a listener, not a preacher
   c. Assist siblings who may fear the possibility of giving birth to children with similar defects

THE TODDLER
Growth and development

Erikson's stage of autonomy; Piaget's cognitive sensorimotor phase
A. Fifteen months
1. Motor
   a. Walks alone well by 14 months, with wide-based gait
   b. Creeps upstairs
   c. Builds tower of 2 blocks
   d. Drinks from a cup and can use a spoon
   e. Enjoys throwing objects and picking them up
2. Vocalization and socialization
   a. Ten to 15 single words
   b. Has learned "No," which may be said while doing requested demand
   c. Indicates when diaper is wet
B. Eighteen months
1. Physical
   a. Growth has decreased and appetite lessened—"physiologic anorexia"
   b. Anterior fontanel is usually closed
   c. Abdomen protrudes, larger than chest circumference

2. Motor
    a. Walks sideways and backward, runs well
    b. Climbs stairs or up on furniture
    c. Scribbles vigorously, attempting straight line
    d. Drinks well from a cup, still spills with a spoon
    e. May begin to control bowel movements
3. Vocalization and socialization
    a. Uses phrases composed of adjectives and nouns
    b. Has new awareness of strangers
    c. Begins to have temper tantrums
    d. Very ritualistic, has favorite toy or blanket, thumb-sucking may be at peak

C. Two years
1. Physical
    a. Weight—about 11 to 12 kg. (26 to 28 pounds)
    b. Height—about 80 to 82 cm. (32 to 33 inches)
    c. Teeth—16 temporary
2. Motor
    a. Gross motor skill quite well refined
    b. Can walk up and down stairs, both feet on one step at a time, holding onto rail
    c. Builds tower of 5 cubes or will make cubes into a train
    d. Control of spoon well developed
    e. Toilet trained during daytime
3. Sensory
    a. Accommodation well developed
    b. Visual acuity 20/40
4. Vocalization and socialization
    a. Vocabulary of about 300 words
    b. Uses short 2- to 3-word phrases, using pronouns
    c. Obeys simple commands
    d. Still very ritualistic, especially at bedtime
    e. Can help undress self and pull on simple clothes
    f. Shows signs of increasing autonomy and individuality
    g. Does not share possessions, everything is "mine"

D. Two and one half years
1. Physical
    a. Full set of 20 temporary teeth
    b. Decreased need for naps
2. Motor
    a. Walks on tiptoe
    b. Stands on 1 foot
    c. Builds tower of 8 blocks
    d. Copies horizontal or vertical line
3. Vocalization and socialization
    a. Beginning to see self as separate individual from reflected appraisal of significant others
    b. Still sees other children as "objects"
    c. Increasingly independent, ritualistic, and negativistic

E. Toilet training—major task of toddler
1. Physical maturation must be reached before training is possible
    a. Sphincter control adequate when child can walk
    b. Able to retain urine for at least 2 hours
    c. Usual age for bowel training—18 months to 2 years of age
    d. Daytime bowel and bladder control —during second year
    e. Night control—by 3 or 4 years of age
2. Psychologic readiness
    a. Aware of the act of elimination
    b. Able to inform mother of need to urinate or defecate
    c. Desire to please parent
3. Process of training
    a. Usually begin with bowel, then bladder
    b. Accidents and regressions frequently occur
4. Parental response
    a. Choose specific word for act
    b. Have specific time and place
    c. Do not punish for accidents

F. Discipline—need for independence without overprotection
1. Should be consistent—set realistic limits
2. Reinforce desired behavior
3. Should be constructive, geared to teach self-control
4. Punishment should be given immediately after wrongdoing
5. Punishment should be appropriate

Play (parallel)

A. Child plays alongside other children but not with them
B. Mostly free and spontaneous, no rules or regulations
C. Attention span is still very short and change of toys occurs at frequent intervals

D. Safety is important
   1. Danger of breaking toy through exploration and ingesting small pieces
   2. Ingesting lead from lead-based paint on toys
   3. Danger of burns from potentially flammable toys
E. Imitation and make-believe play begins by end of second year
F. Suggested toys
   1. Play furniture, dishes, cooking utensils, dress-up clothes
   2. Telephone
   3. Puzzles with a few large pieces
   4. Pedal-propelled toys, such as tricycle
   5. Straddle toys and rocking horse
   6. Clay, sandbox toys, crayons, finger paints
   7. Pounding toys, blocks

Acute and chronic health problems
Hospitalization

A. Specific response of toddler is separation anxiety (see the section on Hospitalization during infancy, p. 388)
B. Toddler experiences basic fear of loss of love, fear of unknown, fear of punishment
C. Immobilization and isolation present additional crises to toddler
D. Nursing considerations in preparing parents and child for hospitalization
   1. Primary consideration is maintaining mother-child relationship by preventing separation
   2. Through assessment, establish routines and rituals that child is accustomed to in the areas of
      a. Toilet training
      b. Feeding
      c. Bathing
      d. Sleep patterns
      e. Recreational activities
   3. Prepare mother for regression of child to previous modes of behavior and loss of newly learned skills
   4. Hospitalization is usually not a time for teaching child new skills
   5. Allow child's release of tension, especially aggression, through play (banging a drum, knocking blocks over, or scribbling on paper)
   6. Only minimal advance preparation of child for hospitalization is possible since cognitive ability to grasp verbal explanation is limited

Accidents

A. Leading cause of death in children over 1 year of age
B. Children under 5 years of age account for over half of all accidental deaths during childhood
C. More than half of accidental child deaths are related to automobiles and fire
D. Accidents can be viewed in terms of child's growth and development, especially curiosity about the environment
   1. Motor vehicle
      a. Walking, running, especially after objects thrown into street
      b. Poor perception of speed, lack of experience to foresee danger
      c. Child often unseen because of small size, can be run over by car backing out of driveway, or when playing in leaves or snow
      d. Failure to restrain in car (sitting in person's lap, improper use of seat belts rather than appropriate car seat)
   2. Burns
      a. Investigating—pulls pots off stoves, plays with matches, inserts objects into wall sockets
      b. Climbing—reaches stove, oven, ironing board and iron, cigarettes on table
   3. Poisons
      a. Learning new tastes and textures, puts everything into mouth
      b. Developing fine motor skill—able to open bottles, cabinets, jars
      c. Climbing to previously unreachable shelves and cabinets
   4. Drowning
      a. Child and parents do not recognize the danger of water
      b. Child is unaware of inability to breathe under water
   5. Aspirating small objects and putting foreign bodies in ear or nose
      a. Puts everything in mouth
      b. Very interested in body and newly found openings
   6. Fractures
      a. Climbing, running, and jumping
      b. Still developing sense of balance
E. Prevention through parent education and child protection is goal

Burns

For specific details, see Medical-surgical nursing, pp. 504-506

A. Principles of treatment
  1. Stop the burning process
     a. Remove from source of danger
     b. Remove smouldering clothes
     c. For superficial burns, immerse affected area in cool water
  2. Administer prompt first aid
     a. Maintain patent airway
     b. For first degree burns, cleanse area, apply sterile dressing soaked in sterile saline if possible
     c. Do not apply creams, butter, or any household remedies
     d. For severe burns (more than 10% of body) oral fluids are not given
  3. Transport patient to proper care facility
     a. Children are hospitalized with burns of 5% to 12% of body surface or more
     b. Large body surface in proportion to weight results in greater potential for fluid loss
     c. Shock—primary cause of death in first 24 to 48 hours
     d. Infection—primary cause of death after initial period
B. Nursing problems and interventions
  1. Fluid and electrolyte loss
     a. Greatest in first 24 to 48 hours because of tissue damage
     b. Immediate replacement of both fluids and electrolytes is essential
     c. Accurate measurement of both intake and output is critical (daily weights, diaper count, and weight)
     d. Hematocrit, hemoglobin, and chemistries should be done daily to provide a guide for replacement
  2. Isolation
     a. Child has feelings of guilt and punishment
     b. Children under 5 years of age rarely understand reason for isolation
     c. Furthers separation between parents and child
     d. Encourage child to express feelings
     e. Allow child to play with gown, mask, and gloves so that they are less strange
  3. Touch deprivation
     a. Touch, a child's main means of comfort and security, is now painful
     b. Pleasurable touch must be reestablished (apply lotion to unaffected areas and let child apply it to a doll)
     c. Prepare child for baths and whirlpool treatments, which can be frightening and painful
  4. Nutrition
     a. High in protein, vitamins, and calories
     b. Child is frequently anorexic because of discomfort, isolation, emotional depression
     c. Provide child with food preferences when feasible, do not force eating or use it as a weapon, encourage parent participation
     d. Alter diet as needs change, especially when high calorie foods are no longer needed and can cause obesity
  5. Contractures
     a. Make moving a game, use play that utilizes affected part, such as throwing a ball for arm movement
     b. Provide for proper body alignment; place child so that attention is focused on an object that will keep body in specific position
     c. Do passive exercises during bath or whirlpool
  6. Body image
     a. For younger child, more of a concern to parents whose reactions are communicated to child
     b. For older child, especially adolescent, body damage is of great concern
     c. Emphasize what can be done to improve looks (plastic surgery, wigs, appropriate clothing, make-up)
  7. Pain
     a. Assessed by observing behavior of young child, rather than verbal complaints
     b. Distinguish pain from fear of dark, being left alone, or in strange surroundings
C. Main nursing consideration—prevention
  1. Parent education especially in regard to child's growth and development and specific dangers at each age level
  2. Child education regarding fire safety
     a. Tell child to leave house as soon as smoke is smelled or flames seen, without stopping to retrieve a pet or toy

b. Involve all members of the family in fire drills

c. Demonstrate rolling rather than running if their clothes are on fire

3. Fire and burn prevention in the house
   a. Intelligent use of heaters, barbecue, and fireplace
   b. Children should be supervised at all times
   c. Maintain integrity of electric system
   d. Escape route must be maintained

Poisoning

A. Principles of treatment
   1. Identify poison
      a. Bring empty container to hospital
      b. Save any urine or vomitus and bring to hospital
      c. Call hospital before arrival
   2. Avoid excessive manipulation of child
   3. Prompt treatment
      a. Call Poison Control Center if specific ingredients of ingested substance are unknown or for specific antidote
      b. Administer specific or universal antidote
      c. Induce vomiting unless
         (1) Substance is corrosive (lye or drain cleaners) or petroleum distillate (turpentine or gasoline)
         (2) Child is comatose
      d. Vomiting can be induced by
         (1) Syrup of ipecac, 15 ml. with a glass of water, may be repeated once within 20 to 30 minutes if necessary
         (2) Stimulate back of throat
         (3) Glass of milk or water with 1 tablespoon mustard

B. Common clinical symptoms
   1. Gastrointestinal—pain, vomiting, anorexia
   2. Respiratory and circulatory signs of shock
   3. Central nervous system—loss of consciousness, convulsions

C. Salicylate poisoning
   1. One of the most common drugs taken by children
   2. Toxic dose—$3\frac{1}{3}$ grains per kg. of body weight or 6 adult aspirins for a 2 year old
   3. Clinical signs
      a. Hyperventilation—confusion, coma
      b. Metabolic acidosis—anorexia, sweating, increased temperature
      c. Bleeding, especially if chronic ingestion
   4. Treatment
      a. Induce vomiting, gastric lavage
      b. Intravenous fluids
      c. Vitamin K if bleeding
      d. Peritoneal dialysis in severe cases
   5. Nursing considerations
      a. Parents need to explain to child that medicine is not candy
      b. All medication should be stored in locked cabinets
      c. Parents should have syrup of ipecac in house and know how to use it

D. Petroleum distillates—kerosene, gasoline, benzene
   1. Substance quickly absorbed
   2. Treatment—administer 1.5 ml. of mineral oil per kg. of body weight
   3. Vomiting is not induced—aspiration is a particular danger because of the nature of the substance

E. Corrosive chemicals—lye
   1. Symptoms—pain, dysphagia, prostration
   2. Treatment—neutralize substance with dilute vinegar or lemon juice
   3. Never induce vomiting, since regurgitation of the substance will cause further damage to the mucous membranes

F. Lead poisoning
   1. Most common between 18 months and 3 years of age because of ingestion of abnormal quantities of lead (usually from eating lead chips from peeling paint or sucking on objects painted with lead-based paint)
   2. Characteristics of child and parents
      a. About 50% of mothers had habit of pica (eating nonfood substances)
      b. High level of oral activity in child, such as use of pacifier, thumb-sucking
      c. Oral gratification used as method of relieving anxiety in child
      d. Maternal dependency, despair, passivity
         (1) Mother is absent from home
         (2) Mother present but unable to supervise child
   3. Clinical manifestations (chronic ingestion)

a. Loss of weight, anorexia
b. Abdominal pain, vomiting
c. Constipation
d. Anemia, pallor, listlessness, fatigue
e. Lead line on teeth and density of long bone
f. Behavior changes such as impulsiveness, irritability, hyperactivity, or lethargy
g. Headache, insomnia, joint pains
h. Brain damage, convulsions, death
i. Increased blood lead level
(1) Normal—below 40 μg. per 100 ml. of blood
(2) Borderline—below 60 μg. per 100 ml. of blood
(3) Treatment begun—usually 60 μg. or higher
(4) Convulsions and irreversible brain damage—about 80 μg.
4. Treatment
a. Objective—reduce concentration of lead in blood and soft tissue by promoting its excretion and deposition in bones
(1) Use of calcium disodium edathamil (EDTA) and dimercaprol (BAL) as chelating agents
(2) Use vitamin D, calcium, and phosphorus
b. Prevention of further ingestion
5. Nursing considerations
a. Prevention through education, proper housing, supervision of children
b. Screening for these children by recognizing signs, especially behavior changes
c. Careful planning for rotation of injection sites and preparation of child
d. Seizure precautions
e. Discharge planning and follow-up care of child
f. Teach parents to prevent further ingestion

Fractures

For general information on fractures, see Medical-surgical nursing, pp. 473-474
A. Greenstick fractures—an incomplete break and bending of a long bone occurring in young children because the bones are soft and not fully mineralized
B. Treatment of fractures—splint, traction, or cast

1. Bryant's traction—for fractured femur
a. Generally used for children under 2 years of age
b. Legs are suspended vertically with buttocks slightly off bed and upper body maintaining contertraction
2. Spica cast may be used for child any age (see pp. 382-383 for further details)
C. Nursing considerations
1. Child must be kept flat on back
2. A restraining jacket may be necessary to prevent moving
3. Provide activity to keep child occupied and entertained

Aspiration of foreign objects

A. Symptoms
1. Substernal retractions
2. Cough and inability to speak
3. Increased pulse and respiratory rate
4. Cyanosis
B. Treatment
1. Immediate first aid if object is in trachea
a. Try to pull object out
b. Turn small child upside down
c. Heimlich maneuver—grasp victim around upper abdomen and squeeze, forcing diaphragm up
d. Do not slap victim on back because object may be forced lower in respiratory tract
2. Medical removal by bronchoscopy
3. Surgical relief by a tracheotomy below level of object
C. Prevention
1. Keep small objects out of child's reach
2. Inspect large toys for removable objects
3. Teach child not to run or laugh with food or fluid in the mouth
4. Avoid giving young children foods easily aspirated, such as nuts
5. Teach child to chew food well before swallowing

Battered child syndrome

A. Refers to both physical abuse and emotional neglect
B. Majority of abused children are under 4 years of age
C. About 70% to 80% of abuse is by parents
D. One theory—role reversal: a reversal of dependency role in which parent turns to the child for nurturing and love

E. Characteristics of abusing parents
1. Their own childrearing included abuse
2. Have incorrect concept of what a small child is and can do
3. Plagued by deep sense of inferiority and lack of identity
4. Tend to be young, immature, and dependent
5. Frequently expect child to provide them with nurturing and love
6. Tend to be depressed, lonely people, yearning for love and understanding
7. Have no outside resources for emotional support or relief from responsibility, especially in time of crisis, thus they take out frustration on child

F. How to identify child neglect or abuse
1. Child has many unexplained injuries, scars, bruises
2. Parents offer inconsistent stories explaining child's injuries when questioned
3. Emotional response of parents is inconsistent with degree of child's injury
4. Parents may resist or fail to be present for questioning
5. Child exhibits physical signs of neglect—malnourished, dehydrated, unkempt
6. Child cringes when physically approached
7. Child responds in a manner that indicates avoiding punishment rather than gaining reward

G. Nursing considerations
1. Main objective—protect child from abusing environment (nurse must be aware of child abuse laws)
2. Be alert for clues that indicate child abuse
3. Focus on helping parents with their own dependency needs
   a. Group therapy
   b. Home visiting
   c. Foster grandparents
4. Help parents learn to control frustration through other outlets
5. Educate parents about child's normal needs and development, new modes of discipline, and realistic expectations
6. Provide emotional support and therapy for the child, since abused children frequently grow up to be abusing parents

Mental retardation

A. Usually defined as low intelligence quotient of 70 or below, which represents about 3% of population
B. American Association of Mental Deficiency defines subaverage IQ as 83 or 84 associated with impairment in adaptive behavior, which represents about 16% of population
C. Retardation can be further classified by the use of the following intelligence test scores; it should be noted that the numbers are approximate and should not be used in a fixed manner for diagnosis
1. Normal—90 to 110 IQ
2. Slow—71 to 89 IQ
3. Mildly retarded—50 to 70 IQ
   a. Educable, can achieve a mental age of 8 to 12 years
   b. Can learn to read, write, do arithmetic, achieve a vocational skill and function in society
4. Moderately retarded—36 to 49 IQ
   a. Trainable, can achieve a mental age of 3 to 7 years
   b. Can learn activities of daily living, social skills, and can be trained to work in a sheltered workshop
5. Severely retarded—below 35 IQ
   a. Barely trainable—can achieve a mental age of 0 to 2 years
   b. Totally dependent on others and in need of custodial care

D. Causes
1. Prenatal—heredity, PKU, Down's syndrome, severe malnutrition (relationship is under study), rubella
2. Natal—kernicterus (high bilirubin level), intracranial hemorrhage, anoxia
3. Postnatal—lead poisoning, meningitis, encephalitis, neoplasms, recurrent convulsions

E. Diagnosis
1. Delayed milestones
   a. Infant fails to suck
   b. Head lag after 4 to 6 months of age
   c. Slow in learning self-help; slow to respond to new stimuli
   d. Slow or absent speech development
2. Conditions that may lead to a false diagnosis of mental retardation
   a. Emotional disturbance, such as autism or maternal deprivation
   b. Sensory problems, such as deafness or blindness
   c. Cerebral dysfunctions, such as cere-

bral palsy, learning disorders, hyperkinesia, epilepsy
F. Characteristics of mentally retarded children
1. Mental abilities are concrete—abstract ability is limited
2. Lack power of self-appraisal
3. Do not learn from errors
4. Cannot carry out complex instructions
5. Do not relate with peers—more secure with adults
6. Comforted by physical touch
7. Learn rote responses and socially acceptable behavior
8. May repeat words—echolalia
9. Short attention span, but usually attracted to music
G. Nursing considerations
1. Always deal with child's developmental not chronologic age
   a. Educate mother regarding developmental age
   b. When child is nearing adolescence, sexual feelings accompany maturation and need to be explained according to child's mental capacity
2. Set realistic goals, teach by simple steps for habit formation rather than for understanding or transference of learning
   a. When teaching a skill, break process down into simple steps that can be easily achieved
   b. Each step must be learned completely before teaching child next step
   c. Behavior modification is a very effective method of teaching these children
   d. Praise for accomplishment must be given to develop child's self-esteem
3. Discipline must remain simple, geared toward learning acceptable behavior rather than developing judgment
4. Routines are foundation of child's life style, hospitalization should be based on child's normal schedule
5. See Parents' reaction to a defective child, p. 389

Cerebral palsy

A. Neuromuscular disability or difficulty in controlling voluntary muscles (caused by damage to some portion of brain, with associated sensory, intellectual, emotional, or convulsive disorders)
B. Characteristics of cerebral palsy
1. Affects young children, usually becoming evident before 3 years of age
2. Nonprogressive, but persists throughout life
3. Some motor dysfunction is always present
4. Mental deficiency may or may not be present
C. Major causes
1. Anoxia of brain caused by a variety of insults at or near the time of birth
2. Infection of central nervous system
D. Types—classified according to predominant clinical manifestation
1. Spasticity (65%)—hyperactivity of muscle stretch reflex, which becomes worse with rapid passive motion
2. Athetosis—slow, wormlike, involuntary purposeless movement
3. Rigidity—persistent stiffness of muscles on movement, which becomes less severe with rapid passive motion
4. Ataxia—disturbance in sense of balance
5. Tremor—rhythmic purposeless movement, which becomes worse with excitement or intentional movement
6. Flaccidity—decreased muscle tension
E. Clinical manifestations
1. Difficulty in feeding, especially sucking and swallowing
2. Asymmetry in motion or contour
3. Delayed motor development and speech
4. Excessive or feeble cry
5. Any of the muscular abnormalities listed under types (above)
F. Nursing problems and interventions
1. Feeding
   a. Drooling results from difficulty in swallowing
   b. Use spoon and blunt fork, with plate attached to table for easier self-feeding
   c. Require increased calories because of excessive energy expenditure, increased protein for muscle activity, and increased vitamins especially B_6 for amino acid metabolism
2. Relaxation
   a. Provide rest periods in area with little stimuli

b. Set limits and control activity level
3. Safety
   a. Protect from accidents resulting from poor balance and lack of muscle control
   b. Provide helmet for protection against head injuries
   c. Always restrain in chair, bed, etc.
   d. Institute seizure precautions
4. Play
   a. Keep safety as main objective
   b. Must not be overstimulating, should have educational value, appropriate to child's developmental level and ability
5. Elimination
   a. Difficulty in toilet training because of poor muscle control
   b. May need special bowel and bladder training
6. Speech
   a. Poor coordination of lips, tongue, cheeks, larynx, and poor control of diaphragm make formation of words difficult
   b. May need speech therapy
7. Breathing
   a. Poor control of intercostal muscles and diaphragm causes child to be prone to respiratory infection
   b. Need to protect child from exposure to infection as much as possible; be alert for symptoms of aspiration pneumonia
8. Dental problems
   a. Problems in muscular control affects development and alignment of teeth
   b. Frequent dental caries occur and there is a great need for dental supervision and care
   c. Parent may have to be taught to brush child's teeth because of muscular dysfunction
9. Vision
   a. Common ocular problems such as strabismus and refractive errors may be related to poor muscular control
   b. Must look for such disorders to prevent further problems such as amblyopia
10. Hearing problems may be present depending on the basic cause of the brain damage

Hearing disorders
A. Types
   1. Conductive—loss from damage to middle ear
      a. Accounts for about 80% of reduced hearing
      b. Conductive loss of 30 decibels or more may require a hearing aid
   2. Sensorineural—damage to inner ear structures or auditory nerve
      a. Distortion in clarity of words
      b. Problem in discrimination of sounds
   3. Mixed conductive—sensorineural
   4. Central auditory
      a. Not explained by other 3 causes
      b. Child hears but doesn't understand
B. Causes
   1. Maternal factors—rubella, syphilis
   2. Perinatal—anoxia, kernicterus, prematurity, excessive noise
   3. Postnatal—mumps, otitis media, head trauma, drugs such as streptomycin
C. Developmental and behavioral manifestations of hearing loss
   1. Lack of Moro reflex in response to sharp clap
   2. Failure to respond to loud noise
   3. Failure to localize a source of sound at 2 to 3 feet after 6 months of age
   4. Absence of babble by 7 months of age
   5. Inability to understand words or phrases by 12 months of age
   6. Use of gestures rather than verbalizations to establish wants
   7. History of frequent respiratory infections and otitis media
D. Nursing considerations
   1. Detection—can and should be identified within the first year of life
   2. Specific guidelines for working with a deaf child
      a. Face child to facilitate lipreading
      b. Do not walk back and forth while talking
      c. Have good light on speaker's face
      d. Be level with child's face and speak toward good ear
      e. Always enunciate and articulate carefully
      f. Do not talk too loudly, especially if the loss is sensorineural
      g. Use facial expressions since verbal intonations are not communicated
      h. Encourage active play to build self-confidence

Visual disorders

A. Strabismus—imbalance of extraocular muscles causing a physiologic incoordination of the eyes
1. A cause of blindness—amblyopia develops in the weak eye from disuse
2. Must be corrected before 4 years of age to prevent blindness
3. Treatment
a. To force weak eye to fixate—patch good eye and exercise weak eye
b. Surgery to lengthen or shorten extraocular structures
B. Functional definition of blindness—visual loss of acuity to read print, must use braille, may have light perception
C. Causes other than strabismus
1. Maternal—albinism, congenital cataracts, rubella, galactosemia
2. Perinatal—retrolental fibroplasia
3. Postnatal—trauma, diabetes, syphilis, tumor
D. Developmental and behavioral manifestations indicating a reduction in vision
1. Retarded motor development
2. Rocking for sensory stimulation
3. Squinting, rubbing eyes
4. Sitting close to television, holding book close to face
5. Clumsiness, bumping into objects
E. Nursing considerations
1. Early detection of loss
2. Specific nursing intervention when working with a blind child
a. Always talk so child can hear clearly
b. Use noise so child can locate your position
c. Help child learn through other senses, especially touch through play activities
d. Facilitate eating by
(1) Arranging food on plate at clock hours and teaching child location
(2) Providing finger foods when possible
(3) Providing light spoon and deep bowl so child can feel weight of food on spoon

Pinworms

Most common intestinal parasites
A. Children reinfect themselves by fingers to anus to mouth route
B. Can also be infected by breathing airborne ova
C. Symptoms
1. Severe pruritus of anal area
2. Vaginitis
3. Irritability and insomnia
4. Poor appetite and weight loss
5. Eosinophilia
D. Diagnosis—Scotch tape test to isolate eggs from anal area (must be done in morning before first bowel movement)
E. Nursing considerations
1. Prevent reinfestation
a. Child should not be allowed to scratch anus; may need to wear mittens
b. Fingernails should be kept short
c. Should wear a tight diaper or underpants
d. Wash anal area thoroughly at least once a day
e. Change clothes daily; wash in hot water
f. Air out bedroom, dust and vacuum house thoroughly
2. Teach parent administration of medication
a. Overdose will not produce a quicker recovery
b. Stools may turn bright red from medication

Anemia

A. Most prevalent nutritional disorder among children in the United States, caused by lack of adequate sources of dietary iron
1. Infant usually has iron reserve for 6 months
2. Premature infant lacks reserve
3. Children receiving only milk have no source of iron
B. Insidious onset, usually diagnosed because of an infection
C. Clinical manifestations
1. Pallor, weakness
2. Slow motor development
3. Poor muscle tone
4. Hemoglobin below 10 g.
D. Nursing considerations
1. Prevention
a. Teach pregnant women importance of their iron intake
b. Encourage feeding of fortified cereal
c. Introduce foods high in iron

2. Good nutrition and proper administration of supplemental iron
   a. Vitamin C aids absorption
   b. Hydrochloric acid aids absorption
   c. Oxalates, phosphate, and phytates decrease absorption
   d. Use a straw since some liquid preparations stain teeth
   e. Discolors stools; may cause gastric irritation or constipation

Celiac disease

A. Chronic intestinal malabsorption and inability to digest gluten, a protein found mostly in wheat and rye
B. Usually begins in infancy or toddler stage, but later in breast-fed infants
C. Clinical manifestations
   1. Progressive malnutrition—secondary deficiencies: anemia, rickets
      a. Stunted growth
      b. Wasting of extremities
      c. Distended abdomen
   2. Steatorrhea—fatty, foul, frothy, bulky stools
   3. Celiac crisis—severe episode of dehydration and acidosis from diarrhea
D. Treatment—dietary
   1. Low in glutens, eliminate wheat, rye, oats, and barley
   2. High calories and protein
   3. Low fat
   4. Smooth, soft foods with low roughage and residue
   5. Small, frequent feedings; adequate fluids
   6. Vitamin supplements, all in water miscible form
   7. Supplemental iron
E. Nursing considerations—parental education
   1. Protect child from infection
   2. Strict adherence to dietary regimen
   3. Need for frequent follow-up supervision, home visits

Cystic fibrosis of the pancreas

A. Autosomal recessive disorder affecting mucus-secreting glands
B. Pathology—defect in overproduction of mucus or an absence of normal mucus-removing mechanism
   1. Pancreas—becomes fibrotic with a decreased production of pancreatic enzymes
      a. Lipase—causes steatorrhea

   b. Trypsin—causes increased nitrogen in stool
   c. Amylase—inability to breakdown polysaccharides
   2. Intestines—increased mucus production preventing enzymes from reaching duodenum and resulting in an inability to absorb fat
   3. Sweat glands—high electrolyte content of soduim and chloride (3 to 5 times higher than normal)
   4. Respiratory system—increased viscous mucus in trachea, bronchi, and bronchioles resulting in
      a. Obstruction interfering with expiration (emphysema)
      b. Infection
   5. Liver—possible cirrhosis from biliary obstruction, malnutrition, or infection
C. Clinical manifestations
   1. Based on above pathophysiology
   2. Similar to celiac disease
   3. Some early manifestations during infancy
      a. Meconium ileus at birth (about 15%)
      b. Failure to regain normal 10% weight loss at birth
      c. Presence of cough or wheezing during first 6 months of age
   4. Because of respiratory involvement, there may be clubbing of fingers, barrel-shaped chest, cyanosis, distended neck veins
   5. Cardiac enlargement, particularly right ventricular hypertrophy (cor pulmonale)
D. Nursing problems and interventions
   1. Prevention of respiratory infection
      a. Postural drainage, percussion, vibrating
      b. Croupette at home with high humidity, additional oxygen as needed
      c. Use of expectorants and antibiotics
   2. Nutrition
      a. Replacement of pancreatic enzymes, given with cold food
      b. Replacement of fat-soluble vitamins in water miscible form
      c. High protein diet of easily digested food, normal fat, high calories
      d. Small frequent feedings
   3. Mobility and activity
      a. May have little tolerance for exertion

b. Help child regulate own tolerance
c. Provide frequent rest periods
4. Body image
   a. Barrel-shaped chest, poor weight gain, thin extremities, bluish coloring, smell of stools, poor posture
   b. Encourage good hygiene and select clothes that compensate for protuberant abdomen and emaciated extremities
5. Counselling
   a. Long-term problem causing financial and emotional stresses
   b. Illness can become a major controlling factor in family
      (1) Child begins to recognize that wheezing brings attention and uses this knowledge
      (2) Help parents deal with such behavior by recognizing false attacks and using consistent discipline
   c. Encourage family to join the Cystic Fibrosis Foundation

Sickle cell anemia

A. Autosomal recessive disorder affecting hemoglobin
B. Defective hemoglobin causes red blood cells to become sickle shaped and clump together under reduced oxygen tension
C. Clinical manifestations of a sickle cell crisis
   1. Severe pain in abdomen, legs, and flank area
   2. Fever
   3. Anemia, pallor, weakness
   4. Vomiting, anorexia
   5. Convulsion, stiff neck, coma
   6. Jaundice
   7. Enlarged spleen, liver, heart
D. Nursing problems and interventions
   1. Prevention of a crisis
      a. Avoid infection, dehydration, and other conditions causing strain on body, which precipitates crisis
      b. Avoid hypoxia
         (1) Avoid drugs that depress respiratory center
         (2) Treat respiratory infections immediately
         (3) Administer additional oxygen with high humidity
      c. Avoid dehydration

(1) May cause a rapid thrombus formation
(2) Daily fluid intake should be calculated according to body weight (130 to 200 ml. per kg.—2 to 3 oz. per pound)
(3) During crisis, fluid needs to be increased, especially if patient is febrile
   2. Care during crisis—provisions should be made for
      a. Adequate hydration (may need intravenous therapy)
      b. Proper positioning, careful handling
      c. Exercise as tolerated (immobility promotes thrombus formation and respiratory problems)
      d. Adequate ventilation
      e. Control of pain (avoid narcotics or barbiturates)
      f. Blood transfusions for severe anemia
   3. Genetic counselling
      a. Disorder mostly of black race
      b. Parents need to know risk of having other children with trait or disease
      c. Screen young children for disorder, since clinical manifestations usually don't appear until after 1 year of age

THE PRESCHOOL AGE CHILD
Growth and development

Erikson's stage of initiative; Piaget's cognitive preconceptual phase
A. Three years
   1. Motor
      a. Walks backward
      b. Rides a tricycle, using pedals
      c. Walks upstairs, alternating feet
      d. Begins to use scissors
      e. Imitates a 3-block bridge
      f. Can unbutton front or side button
      g. Usually toilet trained at night
   2. Sensory—visual acuity 20/30
   3. Vocalization and socialization
      a. Vocabulary of about 900 words, uses 8 to 9 word sentences
      b. May have normal hesitation in speech pattern
      c. Uses plurals
      d. Begins to understand ideas of sharing and taking turns
   4. Mental abilities

a. Little understanding of past, present, future, or aspect of time
b. Stage of magical thinking

B. Four years
1. Motor
   a. Climbs and jumps well
   b. Walks up and down stairs like an adult
   c. Can button buttons and lace shoes
   d. Throws ball overhand
2. Vocalization and socialization
   a. Vocabulary of 1500 words or more
   b. May have imaginary companion
   c. Tends to be selfish and impatient, but takes pride in accomplishments
   d. Exaggerates, boasts, and tattles on others
3. Mental abilities
   a. Reading readiness is present
   b. Can repeat 4 numbers and is learning number concept
   c. Knows which is longer of 2 lines
   d. Has poor space perception

C. Five years
1. Motor
   a. Gross motor is well developed
   b. Can balance on 1 foot for about 10 seconds
   c. Can jump rope, skip, and roller skate
   d. Can draw a picture of a person
   e. Prints first name and other words as learned
   f. Dresses and washes self
   g. May be able to tie shoelaces
2. Sensory
   a. Minimal potential for amblyopia to develop
   b. Color recognition is well established
3. Vocalization and socialization
   a. Vocabulary of about 2100 words
   b. Talks constantly
   c. Asks meaning of new words
   d. Generally cooperative and sympathetic toward others
   e. Basic personality structure is well established
4. Mental abilities (Piaget's phase of intuitive thought)
   a. Beginning understanding of time in terms of days as part of a week
   b. Can determine between difference in weights
   c. Has not mastered concept that

parts equal a whole regardless of their appearance

Play during preschool years (cooperative)

A. Loosely organized group play where membership changes readily and rules are absent
B. Through play, child deals with reality, learns control of feelings, and expresses emotions more through words than actions
C. Play is still physically oriented, but is also imitative and imaginary
D. There is increasing sharing and cooperation among preschool children, especially 5 year olds
E. Suggested toys (same principles as discussed before)
1. Puppets
2. Additional dress-up clothes, dolls, house, furniture, small trucks, animals, etc.
3. Painting sets, color books, paste, and cut-out sets
4. Illustrated books
5. Puzzles with large pieces and more shapes
6. Tricycle, swing, slide, and other playground equipment

Acute and chronic health problems
Hospitalization

A. Reaction of child
1. Fears about body image are now greater than fear of separation
2. The fears include
   a. Intrusive experiences—needles, thermometer, otoscope
   b. Punishment and rejection
   c. Pain
   d. Castration and mutilation
B. Preparation
1. Can prepare child beforehand since increased cognitive and verbal ability make explanations possible
2. General considerations for nursing intervention
   a. Should begin a few days before, but not too soon because of poor concept of time
   b. Clarify cause and effect because of child's phenomenalistic thinking (in child's mind proximity of 2 events relates them to each other)
   c. Explain routines of hospital admission, but not all procedures at

one time since this would be over-whelming

d. Play is an excellent medium for preparation (use dolls, puppets, make-believe equipment, dress-up doctor and nurse clothes)

e. Provide time for play as an outlet for fear, anger, and hostility, as well as a temporary escape from reality

f. Verbal explanation should be as simple as possible and always honest

g. Add details about procedures, drugs, surgery, and the like as child's cognitive level and personal experiences increase

Cancer

A. Second leading cause of death in children

B. Leukemia—principal type of cancer
1. Peak incidence—3 to 4 years of age
2. Malignant neoplasm of blood-forming organs
3. In children, overproduction of immature leukocytes—blast-cell or stem-cell leukemia
   a. Lymphocytic—about 85% of cases, better prognosis than myelogenous
   b. Myelogenous—about 10%, extremely poor prognosis
4. Symptoms—caused by overproduction of immature nonfunctional cells
   a. Anemia—pallor, weakness, irritability
   b. Infection—fever
   c. Tendency toward bleeding—petechiae and bleeding into joints
   d. Pain in joints caused by seepage of serous fluid
   e. Tendency toward easy fracture of bones
   f. Enlargement of spleen, liver, lymph glands
   g. Abdominal pain and anorexia resulting in weight loss
   h. Necrosis and bleeding of gums and other mucous membranes
   i. Later symptoms—central nervous system involvement and frank hemorrhage
5. Treatment objectives
   a. Induce remission by chemotherapy
      (1) Prednisone—steroid
      (2) Vincristine

(3) Methotrexate—folic acid antagonist
(4) 6-Mercaptopurine—purine antagonist
(5) Cyclophosphamide—alkylating agent
(6) Daunoribicin—cytoxic antibiotic
   b. Prevent CNS involvement by use of irradiation and intrathecal methotrexate because leukemic cells invade brain, but most antileukemic drugs do not pass blood-brain barrier
   c. Transfusions to replace and provide blood factors such as platelets, white cells, and clotting factors
6. Nursing considerations
   a. Prognosis—improving and not always immediately fatal
      (1) Adjustment of parents may be difficult because of potential long-term prognosis
      (2) Must deal with child's idea of death—discussion should be appropriate to level of understanding
         (a) Preschooler—concept that death is reversible; greatest fear is separation
         (b) Child 6 to 9 years of age —concept that death is personified; person actually comes and removes child
         (c) Child over 9 years of age —adult concept of death as irreversible and inevitable
   b. Palliative treatment
      (1) Be alert for and attempt to support the child experiencing side effects of drugs, for example
         (a) Cytoxan—severe nausea and vomiting
         (b) Vincristine—constipation, alopecia, neurotoxicity
      (2) Prevent infection with use of reverse isolation
      (3) Handle child carefully because of pain and hemorrhage
      (4) Provide gentle oral hygiene,

soft, bland foods, and increased liquids

    (5) Provide for frequent rest periods, quiet play

  c. See Behavioral sciences, pp. 201-202, for further details on behavioral changes that result from physical illness

Nephrosis or nephrotic syndrome

A. Pathology—abnormal, increased permeability of glomerular basement membrane to plasma albumin
B. Cause unknown—theories include
  1. Hypersensitivity
  2. Antigen-antibody response (rationale for use of glucocorticoids and other immunosuppressive drugs)
C. Peak incidence—2 to 5 years of age
D. Clinical manifestations
  1. Generalized edema, especially genital, periorbital, and ascites
  2. Proteinuria
  3. Hypoproteinemia—poor general health, loss of appetite
  4. Hyperlipemia
  5. May also see symptoms usually associated with nephritis
    a. Hematuria
    b. Hypertension
E. Nursing problems and interventions
  1. Infection—both disease state and drug therapy increase susceptibility
    a. Should be protected from others who are ill
    b. Teach parents signs of impending infection and encourage them to seek medical care
  2. Malnutrition caused by loss of protein and poor appetite
    a. Regular diet is usually allowed; added salt and salty foods discouraged
    b. Protein is usually not adjusted; encourage child to select food likes from high protein choices
    c. Fluids may be restricted, but this generally causes more discomfort than benefit
  3. Respiratory difficulty caused by ascites
    a. Proper positioning—place in Fowler's position to decrease pressure against diaphragm
    b. Frequent change of position is vital because of dependent edema

  4. Discomfort caused by edema, pressure areas
    a. Positioning and skin care provide some relief
    b. Support genitalia if edematous
  5. Change in body image caused by edema and steroids
    a. Of greater concern as child grows older
    b. Emphasize clothes, hairdo, and the like that make child attractive
    c. Stress that "diets" will not help weight loss
  6. Behavioral changes such as irritability and depression
    a. Parents need to understand that mood swings are influenced by physical condition
    b. Encourage child to participate in own care
    c. Encourage diversionary activities that provide satisfaction

Urinary tract infection

A. Very common in females because of anatomy of lower urinary tract—urethra is short and meatus is close to anus
B. Nursing considerations—teach prevention
  1. Proper cleansing of genitalia
  2. Voiding when necessary as opposed to holding urine in bladder
  3. Increased fluids, particularly those that acidify urine
  4. Identification of asymptomatic infections

Allergy

A. Altered tissue response to a substance, either inhaled, ingested, or contacted on skin
B. Most common types in children
  1. Eczema
  2. Allergic rhinitis
  3. Asthma
C. General nursing considerations
  1. Family history can be a significant factor
  2. A comprehensive study of child and environment is essential
    a. Prepare child for skin tests
    b. Study environment in terms of emotional stresses as well as physical allergens
  3. Teach parents to eliminate allergenic substances and to administer drugs properly

D. Asthma
   1. Pathology
      a. Bronchiolar spasm
      b. Bronchiolar constriction
      c. Increased secretions
      d. Respiratory acidosis from buildup of carbon dioxide
   2. Clinical manifestations
      a. Wheezing, especially on expiration
      b. Labored breathing, cough, increased secretions
      c. Flaring nares, distended neck veins
   3. Nursing considerations
      a. Treatment—use of antispasmodic drugs and bronchodilators; parents must know how to give medication and why it must be given even if child does not have an attack
      b. Good respiratory hygiene; teach parents postural drainage, need for increased fluids, and the use of a cool mist humidifier to provide high humidity in home
      c. Proper environment
         (1) Free of as many allergens as possible
         (2) Avoid exertion and exposure to cold air and people with infections
         (3) Avoid as much as possible emotional factors that precipitate attacks

Tonsillectomy and adenoidectomy

Not done routinely since lymphoid tissue helps prevent invasion of organisms
A. Indications for surgical removal
   1. Recurrent tonsillitis or otitis media
   2. Enlargement that interferes with breathing or swallowing
B. Contraindications for removal
   1. Occasional infections that clear up rapidly
   2. Cleft palate, hemophilia, or debilitating disease such as leukemia
C. Complications after surgery
   1. Hemorrhage—first 24 hours
      a. Frequent swallowing, bright red blood in vomitus
      b. Restlessness
      c. Increased pulse, pallor
   2. Hemorrhage from sloughing of tissue —5 to 10 days postoperatively
D. Nursing considerations
   1. Keep child on abdomen or side with head turned to side

   2. After surgery, child should have cool liquids, not red in color, and not thick or mucus-producing
   3. Ask child to talk; provide assurance that it is possible
   4. Ice collar to decrease edema
   5. Attempt to limit crying

THE SCHOOL AGE CHILD
Growth and development

Erikson's stage of industry; Piaget's cognitive phase of concrete operations
A. Physical growth
   1. Permanent dentition, beginning with 6-year molars and central incisors at 7 or 8 years of age
   2. Growth has decreased, about 1 inch in height a year
   3. Tends to look lanky because bone development precedes muscular development
B. Motor
   1. Refinement of coordination, balance and control is occurring
   2. Motor development necessary for competitive activity becomes important
C. Sensory—visual acuity of 20/20
D. Mental abilities
   1. Readiness for learning, especially in perceptual organization—names months of year, knows right from left, can tell time, can follow several directions at once
   2. Acquires use of reason and understanding of rules
   3. Trial and error problem solving becomes more conceptual rather than action oriented
   4. Reasoning ability allows greater understanding and use of language
   5. Quantity conservation (Piaget)— child knows that quantity remains the same even though appearance differs

Play

A. Number of play activities decreases while amount of time spent in one particular activity increases
B. Likes games with rules because of increased mental abilities
C. Likes games of athletic competition because of increased motor ability
D. Child should learn how to work as well as play, with a beginning appreciation for economics and finances
E. In beginning of school years, boys and

girls play together, but gradually separate into sex-oriented type of activities

F. Suggested play for 6 to 9 year olds
1. More housekeeping toys that work, doll accessories, paper doll sets, simple sewing machine, and needlework
2. Simple work and number games, games calling for increased skills
3. Physically active games such as hopscotch, jump rope, climbing trees
4. Stamp collecting and the like and building simple models
5. Bicycle riding

G. Suggested play for 9 to 12 year olds
1. Handicrafts of all kinds
2. Model kits, collections, hobbies
3. Archery, dart games, chess, jigsaw puzzles
4. Sculpturing materials such as pottery clay
5. Science toys, magic sets

Acute and chronic health problems
Diabetes mellitus

A. Symptoms—juvenile diabetes may be more severe and variable than diabetes in adults
1. Onset—rapid, obvious
2. Child usually thin, underweight; obesity does not appear to be a factor
3. Increased thirst, fluid intake, appetite, and urinary output
4. Hypoglycemia and ketoacidosis common

B. Differences between childhood and adult diabetes
1. Onset
   a. Rapid in child
   b. Insidious in adult
2. Obesity
   a. Does not appear to be a factor in child
   b. Predisposing factor in adult
3. Dietary treatment
   a. Rarely adequate for child
   b. Possible in one third of adults
4. Oral hypoglycemics
   a. Contraindicated for child
   b. Helpful in one third of adults
5. Insulin
   a. Almost universally necessary in children
   b. Necessary for only one third of adults
6. Hypoglycemia and ketoacidosis

    a. Quite frequent in children
    b. More uncommon in adults
7. Degenerative vascular changes
   a. Develop after adolescence in child
   b. May be present at time of diagnosis in adult

C. Hypoglycemia—insulin shock
1. Causes
   a. Overdose of insulin
   b. Decreased food intake
   c. Excessive physical exercise—increases muscle activity and movement of glucose into muscle cells
2. Signs
   a. Sweating, flushing, pallor
   b. Numbness, trembling, chilliness
   c. Unsteadiness, nervousness, irritability
   d. Hunger
   e. Hallucinations
   f. Late signs—convulsions, coma, death
3. Emergency treatment—immediate supply of readily available glucose

D. Hyperglycemia—ketoacidosis or diabetic coma
1. Causes
   a. Decreased insulin
   b. Emotional stress
   c. Fever
   d. Infection
   e. Increased food intake
2. Signs
   a. Weakness, drowsiness
   b. Lack of appetite, thirst
   c. Abdominal and/or generalized pain
   d. Acetone breath
   e. Late signs—Kussmaul breathing (deep, rapid respirations), cherry red lips, loss of consciousness, death
3. Treatment—hospitalization with administration of insulin

E. Hereditary influence
1. Inherited as a recessive characteristic
2. "Anticipation"—manifestation of disease occurs earlier in succeeding generations

F. Peak ages of incidence in the school age group
1. Six years of age
2. Twelve years of age

G. Nursing problems and interventions—main objective is control of diabetes and education of child and family

1. Explain differences between childhood and adult diabetes to parents who may think child is faking because their own illness doesn't cause serious problems
2. Teach factors that affect insulin requirements and signs of insulin overdose and diabetic coma
   a. Give family written list explaining symptoms
   b. Emphasize that sugar can be given if insulin shock is suspected, but insulin should not be increased if diabetic coma is developing
   c. Emphasize need for close medical supervision
3. Infection—teach need for
   a. Good skin care, frequent baths
   b. Properly fitting shoes
   c. Prompt treatment of any small cut
   d. Protection from undue exposure to illness
4. Diet—should be well balanced, with fairly equal quantities of food eaten frequently and regularly, usually unrestricted within reason
5. Urine testing—child should learn how to do this to increase independence
6. Administration of insulin
   a. Child should be taught as early as motor and mental ability allows, usually by 7 or 9 years of age
   b. Explanation should be simple; diagrams for rotating sites should be used
   c. Periodic observation by an adult should be routine to discover faulty or careless technique

Hemophilia

A. Defects in clotting mechanism of blood —3 most common deficiencies
   1. Factor VIII, classic hemophilia
   2. Factor IX, Christmas disease
   3. Factor XI
B. Hereditary influence—sex-linked recessive gene classically occurring in males
C. Clinical manifestations
   1. Prolonged bleeding from any wound
   2. Bleeding into the joints (hemarthrosis), resulting in pain, deformity, and retarded growth
   3. Anemia
   4. Intracranial hemorrhage
D. Nursing problems and interventions
   1. Bleeding
      a. Instruct child and parents on treatment of bleeding, especially of joints
         (1) Immobilization of area
         (2) Compression of area
         (3) Elevation of body part
         (4) Application of cool compresses
      b. Appropriate activity that lessens chance of trauma, which is often difficult since boys are so physically active
   2. Pain
      a. Avoid use of aspirin or phenylbutazone
      b. Control joint pain so child uses extremity to prevent muscle atrophy
   3. Repeated hospitalizations—objective now is to strive for home care, with self-administration of coagulation factors such as cryoprecipitate
   4. Guilt of parents
      a. Provide counselling since disease is genetic and parents need assistance
      b. Encourage parents to treat child as normally as possible, avoiding overprotection or overpermissiveness

Rheumatic fever

A. Collagen disease—characterized by damage to connective tissue and usually blood vessels
B. Cause unknown—frequently follows infection with group A *beta hemolytic streptococci*
C. One of chief causes of death in school age children, peak incidence between 6 and 8 years of age, with familial incidence
D. Predisposing factors—crowded living conditions, general lack of hygiene, temperate climate, poor nutrition
E. Clinical manifestations
   1. Carditis—possible damage to mitral valve
      a. Increased pulse, especially at night, poor pulse quality
      b. Low-grade fever in afternoon
      c. Anemia, pallor, weakness
      d. Anorexia, weight loss
      e. Increased respirations
   2. Arthritis
      a. Enlarged joints, with migratory pain
      b. Joint is red, hot, swollen, and tender, but deformity does not result

3. Sydenham's chorea (St. Vitus's dance)
   a. Gradual onset
   b. Involuntary, purposeless movements
   c. Facial grimaces
   d. Restlessness and inability to maintain same position
   e. Emotional instability
4. Subcutaneous nodules on extensor tendons of hands, feet, elbows, scapulae, patellae, vertebrae
   a. Nonpainful
   b. Skin moves freely over nodules
F. Laboratory findings
   1. Increased erythrocyte sedimentation rate
   2. Antistreptolysin-O titer
   3. Presence of C-reactive protein
   4. Aschoff bodies—in heart, arteries, nodules
   5. Leukocytosis
G. Nursing problems and interventions
   1. Bedrest—to reduce workload of heart
      a. Often difficult to maintain when child is feeling better
      b. Encourage child to do schoolwork and keep up with class
      c. Stimulate the development of quiet hobbies and collections
      d. Gradually increase activities over a period of weeks to months
   2. Pain
      a. Handle painful joints carefully
      b. Maintain proper body alignment to prevent deformities
      c. Monitor need for pain medication and administer when necessary
   3. Nutrition
      a. Increase fluids
      b. Provide small, frequent, nutritious meals
   4. Emotional support
      a. Prevent invalidism by emphasizing abilities rather than limitations
      b. Maintain child's status in home and school by keeping channels of communication open during illness
      c. Help mother with home problems that may have served as predisposing factors
   5. Public health prevention
      a. Proper and prompt treatment of streptococcal infections with antibiotics
      b. School screening and health promotion programs

c. Improvement of low socioeconomic housing
d. Teach proper standards of hygiene

Juvenile rheumatoid arthritis
A. Collagen disease, cause unknown, may occur in response to stress
B. Clinical manifestations
   1. Joint enlargement
      a. Stiffness, pain, and limited motion, especially in morning upon awakening
      b. Spindle-fingers—thick proximal joint with slender tip
   2. Low grade fever
   3. Erythematous rash on trunk and extremities
   4. Weight loss, fatigue, weakness
   5. Tachycardia
   6. Enlargement of spleen, liver, and lymph nodes
C. Treatment
   1. Large doses of aspirin
   2. Steroids
   3. Physical therapy
D. Nursing problems and interventions
   1. Joint deformity and pain
      a. Emphasize that aspirin must be taken regularly, even in period of remission, to decrease inflammation and pain
      b. Promote proper body alignment and provide passive range of motion
      c. Encourage warm bath in morning to decrease stiffness and increase mobility
      d. Encourage exercises such as swimming
   2. Acceptance of disease by family and child
      a. Encourage parents to accept the child's illness, but to limit the use of the disease to foster dependency or control relationships
      b. Teach family why aspirin is given in large dosages and why other medications are not used
   3. Aspirin toxicity—demonstrated by tinnitus, vertigo, nausea, vomiting, sweating, and other signs of salicylate poisoning

Skin infections
A. Pediculosis—lice
   1. May infest head, body, pubic area (also called crabs)

2. Eggs (greenish, translucent oval bodies) attach to hair
3. Severe itching may lead to secondary infection
4. Treatment—special shampoo, use of fine-toothed comb to remove nits or eggs
5. Prevention
   a. Cleanliness
      (1) Teach proper hair care
      (2) Encourage frequent bathing and change of clothes
   b. Screening in schools to identify source of infection
B. Scabies—produced by itch mite
1. Female burrows under skin to lay eggs (usually in folds of skin)
2. Intensely pruritic—scratching can lead to secondary infection with the development of papules and vesicles
3. Treatment—all members of the family must be treated since it is highly contagious
   a. Must wear clean clothes
   b. Must wash with sulfur or other special soap
C. Ringworm—fungus disease
1. Scalp (tinea capitis)
   a. Reddened, oval or round shaped areas of alopecia
   b. Treated topically or orally with an antifungal drug such as griseofulvin
   c. Head should be covered to prevent spread of infection
2. Feet (athlete's foot)
   a. Scaly fissures between toes, vesicles on sides of feet, pruritus
   b. Particularly common in summer; contacted in swimming areas and gymnasium locker rooms
   c. Prevention—do not walk barefooted, dry feet carefully, wear lightweight shoes to decrease heat, disinfect shoes and socks
   d. Treatment with antiseptic soaks and antifungal ointments and powders
D. Intertrigo—excoriation of any adjacent body surfaces caused by moisture and chafing (diaper rash)
1. Keep area clean and dry, rinse wastes from skin
2. Expose area to light and air
3. Apply bland ointment at night
4. Avoid strong alkalis such as bleach in clothes washing

E. Impetigo
1. Bacterial infection of skin by streptococci or staphylococci
2. Sequelae of streptococcal infection—rheumatic fever, glomerulonephritis
3. Highly contagious, other areas of body frequently become infected
4. Treatment—antibiotics systemically and locally, isolate child, keep from scratching other areas of the body

Minimal brain dysfunction (MBD)

A. A disturbance of central nervous system functioning in which specific motor, sensory, or intellectual impairment exists
B. Characteristics of children with minimal brain dysfunction
1. Difficulty in attention span
2. May be hyperkinetic or underactive but are awkward and clumsy
3. Impulsive acting out
4. Problems with remembering, language, conceptualization, and perception
5. Normal intellectual functioning
C. Nursing considerations—teach parents to
1. Avoid overstimulation, provide frequent rest periods throughout day
2. Structure situations to provide less frustration (play with only one other child rather than group)
3. Provide firm and consistent discipline, ignore temper tantrums
4. Learning is best done through play and use of concrete examples, such as 2 halves of an orange to teach fractions
5. Provide exercises in perceptual-motor coordination and balance
6. Structure learning experience to utilize child's ability
7. Provide opportunities so that child can experience success and satisfaction
8. Administration of drugs such as amphetamines to reduce hyperactivity

THE ADOLESCENT
Growth and development

Erikson's stage of identity; Piaget's cognitive phase of formal operations
A. Physical growth (see Maternal nursing, pp. 350-351, for physical changes during puberty)
B. Mental abilities
1. Abstract thinking

a. New level of social communication and understanding
  (1) Can comprehend satire and double meanings
  (2) Can say one thing and mean another
b. Can conceptualize thought, more interested in exploring ideas than facts
c. Can appreciate scientific thinking, problem solve, and theoretically explore alternatives

2. Perception
a. Can appreciate nonrepresentational art
b. Can understand that the whole is more than the sum of its parts

3. Learning
a. Much longer span of attention
b. Learns through process of inference, intuition, and surmise, rather than repetition and imitation
c. Enjoys regressing in terms of language development by using jargon to suit changing moods

C. Social patterns
1. Peer group identity
a. One of strongest motivating forces of behavior
b. Extremely important to be part of the group and like everyone else in every way
c. Clique formation; usually based on such common denominators as race, social class, ethnic group, or special interests

2. Interpersonal relationships
a. Major goal is learning to form close intimate relationship with opposite sex
b. Adolescents may develop many crushes and worship many idols
c. Time of sexual exploration and questioning of one's sexual role

3. Independence
a. By 15 or 16 years of age, adolescents feel they should be treated as adults
b. Ambivalence—adolescent wants freedom but is not happy about corresponding responsibilities and frequently yearns for more carefree days of childhood
c. Parental ambivalence and discipline problems are common as parents try to allow for increasing independence but continue to offer constructive guidance and enforce discipline

D. Problems of adolescence
1. Accidents—still number one cause of death, with motor vehicle accidents causing most fatalities
2. Suicide—one of chief causes of death among this age group
3. Drug abuse
4. Delinquency
5. Alcoholism
6. Many problems of adolescence similar to those of adults; see specific areas in Psychiatric and medical-surgical nursing for further discussion

REVIEW QUESTIONS FOR FAMILY-CENTERED NURSING
Maternal nursing and reproductive problems

1. Pregnancy and birth are called crises since
  1. They are periods of change and adjustment to change
  2. There are hormonal and physiologic changes in the mother
  3. There are mood changes during pregnancy
  4. Narcissism in the mother affects the husband-wife relationship

2. The nurse will alleviate crisis by
  1. Involving the mother in preparation classes
  2. Getting the mother to express her feelings
  3. Understanding the family interaction
  4. Involving the father in preparation classes

3. A pregnant woman is concerned about her "stretch marks," her "dark nipples," and the "dark line" from her navel to her pubis. The nurse explains that these adaptations are caused by hyperactivity of the
  1. Adrenal gland
  2. Thyroid gland
  3. Ovaries
  4. Pituitary gland

4. Mrs. Jackson, 5 months pregnant, asks the nurse whether smoking will affect the baby. Her answer reflects the following knowledge
  1. Fetal and maternal circulation are separated by the placental barrier
  2. The placenta is permeable to specific substances
  3. Smoking relieves tension and the fetus responds accordingly
  4. Vasoconstriction will affect both fetal and maternal blood vessels

5. The major concern for a pregnant out-of-wedlock teenager is that she is
  1. Socially ostracized
  2. Diabetogenic
  3. Financially dependent
  4. Prone to toxemia

6. A predisposing factor that causes morning sickness during the first trimester of pregnancy is the adaptation to increased levels of
  1. Estrogen

2. Progesterone
3. Luteinizing hormone
4. Chorionic gonadotropin
7. The nurse helps the pregnant woman overcome morning sickness by suggesting she
   1. Eat nothing until the nausea subsides
   2. Take an antacid before bedtime
   3. Request her doctor to prescribe an antiemetic
   4. Eat dry toast and some jam before arising
8. The presence of multiple gestation should be detected as early as possible and the pregnancy managed with high risk in mind because
   1. Perinatal mortality is 2 to 3 times greater than in single births
   2. Maternal mortality is much higher in multiple births
   3. The mother needs time to adjust psychologically and physiologically
   4. Postpartum hemorrhage is frequent
9. The nurse encourages continued medical supervision for the pregnant woman with pyelitis because
   1. Antibiotic therapy is given until the urine is sterile
   2. Toxemia frequently occurs following pyelitis
   3. Pelvic inflammatory disease occurs with untreated pyelitis
   4. A low protein diet is given until pregnancy is terminated
10. The most common type of ectopic pregnancy is tubal. Within a few weeks after conception the tube may rupture, causing
    1. Sudden knife-like lower quadrant abdominal pain
    2. Continuous dull lower quadrant adbominal pain
    3. Painless vaginal bleeding
    4. Intermittent abdominal contractions
11. If anemia is present with a hemoglobin of 8 g. or lower, a mother with cardiac disease probably will go into
    1. Cardiac failure
    2. Heart block
    3. Atrial fibrillation
    4. Cardiac compensation
12. The diabetic pregnant woman requires
    1. Increased dosage of insulin
    2. Administration of estrogenic hormones
    3. Decreased caloric intake
    4. Administration of pancreatic enzymes
13. Preeclampsia is first suspected in the pregnant woman when there is
    1. An excessive weight gain
    2. Fluctuation of the blood pressure
    3. Progressive ankle edema
    4. Presence of albuminuria
14. A pregnant woman with toxemia is being given magnesium sulfate. The nurse must be alert for the first sign of excessive blood levels, which is
    1. Development of cardiac arrhythmia
    2. Disappearance of the knee jerk reflex
    3. Depression of the respiratory rate
    4. Disturbance of the bearing ability
15. The first sign of a convulsion in a patient with preeclampsia is

1. Rolling of the eyes to one side with a fixed stare
2. Spots or flashes of light before the eyes
3. Persistent headache and blurred vision
4. Epigastric pain, nausea, and vomiting
16. Following a convulsion in a woman with eclampsia, an elevated temperature of 102° F. is noted. This is caused by
    1. Development of a systemic infection
    2. Dehydration caused by rapid fluid loss
    3. Disturbance of the cerebral thermal center
    4. Excessive muscular activity
17. The following care is essential for a patient with eclampsia
    1. Encourage ingestion of clear fluids
    2. Protect against extraneous stimuli
    3. Isolate in a dark room
    4. Maintain in a supine position
18. The danger of a convulsion in a woman with preeclampsia ends
    1. After labor begins
    2. After delivery occurs
    3. 24 hours postpartum
    4. 48 hours postpartum
19. The nurse knows a woman has begun the transitional phase of labor when she
    1. Complains of pains in the back
    2. States the pain has lessened
    3. Perspires and her face flushes
    4. Assumes the lithotomy position
20. The perception of pain for a woman in labor is influenced most by the
    1. Difficulty of the labor
    2. Tension of the patient
    3. Length of the labor
    4. Parity of the patient
21. When positioning a woman on the delivery table, both legs should be placed in the stirrups at the same time to prevent
    1. Excessive pull on the fascia
    2. Pressure on the perineum
    3. Trauma to the uterine ligaments
    4. Venous stasis in the legs
22. One hour following delivery the nurse finds that the patient's uterus has become boggy. The initial response would be to
    1. Notify the physician
    2. Check the blood pressure
    3. Massage it until firm
    4. Observe the amount of bleeding
23. Painless vaginal bleeding during the last trimester is usually caused by
    1. Abruptio placentae
    2. Frequent intercourse
    3. Placenta previa
    4. Excessive alcohol ingestion
24. Nursing care for the patient hospitalized for placenta previa includes
    1. Withholding food and fluids
    2. Encouraging ambulation with supervision
    3. Inspecting the bed for hemorrhage
    4. Avoiding all extraneous stimuli
25. If a vaginal examination is to be performed on a patient with placenta previa, the nurse must be prepared for an immediate
    1. Induction of labor
    2. Cesarean section

3. Forceps delivery
4. X-ray examination
26. A major complication of the second half of pregnancy is premature separation of the normally implanted placenta. Signs and symptoms include
    1. Decrease in size of uterus, cessation of contractions, visible or concealed hemorrhage
    2. Firm and tender uterus, concealed or external hemorrhage, shock
    3. Increase in size of uterus, visible bleeding, no associated pain
    4. Shock, decrease in size of uterus, absence of external bleeding
27. Abruptio placentae is most apt to occur in a woman with the following complication of pregnancy
    1. Toxemia
    2. Cardiac disease
    3. Hyperthyroidism
    4. Cephalopelvic disproportion
28. The abdominal pain associated with abruptio placentae is caused by
    1. Hemorrhagic shock
    2. Inflammatory reactions
    3. Blood in the uterine muscle
    4. Concealed hemorrhage
29. Bleeding following severe abruptio placentae is usually caused by
    1. Hypofibrinogenemia
    2. Hyperglobulinemia
    3. Thrombocytopenia
    4. Polycythemia
30. A predisposing factor in determining whether a woman will have a postpartum hemorrhage is the knowledge that
    1. Her uterus was overdistended
    2. She has had more than 5 pregnancies
    3. Her duration of labor was very short
    4. She is over 40 years of age
31. Postpartum hemorrhage may occur for all of the following reasons. The most common one is
    1. Retained secundines
    2. Lacerations of the cervix
    3. Atony of the uterus
    4. Secondary infections
32. The two most important predisposing causes of puerperal infection are
    1. Hemorrhage and trauma during labor
    2. Toxemia and retention of placenta
    3. Malnutrition and anemia during pregnancy
    4. *Streptococcus* organism present in birth canal and trauma during labor
33. The most effective position for the nurse to place the woman in labor when she notes a prolapsed cord is
    1. Sims
    2. Fowler's
    3. Trendelenburg
    4. Lithotomy
34. Which of the following fetal and neonatal hazards is *not* associated with breech delivery?
    1. Intracranial hemorrhage
    2. Cephalohematoma
    3. Compression of cord
    4. Separation of placenta prior to delivery of head

35. The most effective method of determining if there is cephalopelvic disproportion for the woman in labor is
    1. Pelvimetry
    2. X-ray examination
    3. Amniocentesis
    4. Duration of labor
36. After an Rh-negative mother delivers an Rh-positive baby, Rh₀ (D) is administered intramuscularly to
    1. Prevent antibody formation in the mother
    2. Expand the antibody pool of the mother
    3. Accelerate the mother's production of immune bodies
    4. Suppress the activity of Rh-negative antibodies
37. A postpartum patient has decided not to nurse her baby. The medication used to suppress lactation would include the following hormone
    1. Testosterone
    2. Cortisone
    3. Oxytocin
    4. Estrogen
38. A patient who is 2 days postpartum complains of pain in her right leg. The nurse's initial response would be to
    1. Encourage ambulation and exercise
    2. Massage the affected area
    3. Apply hot soaks
    4. Place on bed rest and notify the physician
39. The nurse, while checking the fundus of a patient who is 2 days postpartum, observes that it is at the umbilicus and displaced to the right. She recognizes that the patient probably has
    1. A full, overdistended bladder
    2. Overstretched uterine ligaments
    3. A slow rate of involution
    4. Retained placental fragments
40. The fetus is most likely to be damaged by the pregnant woman's ingestion of drugs during the
    1. First trimester
    2. Second trimester
    3. Third trimester
    4. Entire pregnancy
41. A medication given to a woman in labor that might cause respiratory depression of the newborn is
    1. Meperidine (Demerol)
    2. Scopolamine
    3. Promazine (Sparine)
    4. Promethazine (Phenergan)
42. The most important weak or absent reflex for the nurse to report in her initial evaluation of the newborn is
    1. Moro
    2. Tonic-neck
    3. Gag
    4. Babinski
43. An Apgar score of 4 in a newborn would most likely indicate one of the following
    1. Body pink, extremities blue
    2. Heart rate over 100
    3. Flaccid muscle tone
    4. Respirations of 35
44. In assessing a newborn, the nurse observes an

unequal Moro reflex on one side, flaccid arm in adduction. The nurse suspects
1. Brachial palsy
2. Supratentorial tear
3. Fracture of the clavicle
4. Crigler-Najjar syndrome

45. If the newborn has asymmetric gluteal folds, it most likely indicates
1. A dislocated hip
2. Peripheral nervous system damage
3. An inguinal hernia
4. Central nervous system damage

46. An important and useful early clinical sign in idiopathic respiratory distress syndrome in the newborn is
1. Sternal and subcostal retractions
2. Nasal flaring
3. Rapid respiration
4. Grunting

47. Mrs. Howard is examining her day-old newborn and asks if all babies have a "yellowish" color at first. The nurse realizes this is probably caused by
1. The expected destruction of fetal hemoglobin
2. Poor lighting giving the effect
3. An Rh or ABO incompatability
4. An obstruction of the common bile duct

48. If a newborn infant has muscle twitchings, convulsions, cyanosis, abnormal respirations, and a short shrill cry, the nurse should suspect that the infant has
1. Tetany
2. Intracranial hemorrhage
3. Spina bifida
4. Hyperkalemia

49. More than half of the neonatal deaths in the United States are caused by
1. Atelectasis
2. Prematurity
3. Respiratory distress syndrome
4. Congenital heart disease

50. Infants with risk conditions are frequently deprived of pleasurable comforting contacts with a specific person after birth. Which of the following behaviors would be an unusual response to this lack?
1. Lack or slowness of weight gain
2. Looking at ceiling lights rather than persons caring for them
3. Limited emotional response to stimuli
4. Excessive crying and clinging when approached

51. The nursery admission of a premature infant is often an emergency situation. The nurse will routinely do all of the following *except*
1. A rapid initial evaluation
2. Support of body temperature
3. O₂ administration
4. Recording of vital signs

52. The *most* common complication in the low birth weight infant is
1. Brain damage
2. Respiratory distress
3. Aspiration of mucus
4. Hemorrhage

53. Urinary function of the premature baby
1. Is the same as a full-term newborn

2. Causes the loss of large amounts of urine
3. Maintains stability of acid-base and electrolyte balance
4. Tends to overconcentrate the urine

54. The premature baby stabilizes temperature at
1. 97.5°F. to 98.6°F.
2. 97°F. to 99°F.
3. 95°F. to 97°F.
4. 94°F. to 96°F.

55. The new mother who exhibits postpartum blues is probably adapting to
1. A decrease in progesterone levels
2. Changes in body image
3. Psychologic letdown after labor
4. Rejection of her newborn

56. Experience has shown that parents are better able to cope with the birth of an abnormal child if informed
1. After the first 48 hours when the mother's strength has returned
2. When bringing the baby to the mother for the first time
3. After the birth while the mother is still in the delivery room
4. When the parents ask if something is wrong with their baby

57. Research indicates that the early mother-infant relationship is vital to future mental health. Which of the following statements is true?
1. Ambivalence and anxiety about mothering are common
2. A rejected pregnancy will result in a rejected infant
3. A good mother experiences neither ambivalence nor anxiety about mothering
4. Maternal love is fully developed within the first week after birth

58. Gerald Caplan, in his description of initial maternal behavior, has coined the term "maternal time-lag" to identify the span of time required
1. To develop mother love
2. To lose the strong emotional attachment to the fetus
3. For a new mother to feel that the baby really belongs to her
4. To endow the new baby with its own personality

59. Mrs. Jones is 36 weeks pregnant and you are caring for the family. On a home visit Mrs. Jones verbalizes, "I am sick and tired of wearing these same old clothes; how I wish all this would be done and over with." Your best response would be
1. "Is there something bothering you, you sound discouraged?"
2. "Most women feel the same way you do at this time."
3. "I understand how you feel, what do you know about labor?"
4. "Yes, this is the most uncomfortable time during pregnancy."

60. As you assess Mrs. Jones' legs for edema, you notice she is wearing round garters. Since you understand the physiology of circulation during pregnancy, you would ask
1. "Did you know round garters are bad for your circulation during pregnancy?"

2. "I see you are wearing round garters, did you know these should not be worn during pregnancy?"
3. "Do you find it necessary to wear round garters often?"
4. "Round garters are constricting and may cause varicose veins."

61. Mr. and Mrs. Jones attend a class in preparation for childbirth. The philosophy that prevails in these classes is that labor
1. Should be painless and uneventful
2. May be uncomfortable but medication is available when needed
3. Will be painful but you will be taught how to tolerate it
4. Will be uncomfortable, however, medication will not be needed

62. Mrs. Penny, a gravida VI, para 5 is admitted to the labor unit by ambulance and delivery is imminent. She keeps bearing down and with 2 contractions the baby's head is crowning. You would
1. Tell her to breathe through her mouth and pant during contractions
2. Tell her to breathe through her mouth and not to bear down
3. Transfer her immediately by stretcher to the delivery room
4. Tell her to pant, support the perineum with your hand to prevent tearing

63. With the next contraction Mrs. Penny delivers a large baby girl spontaneously. You are alone at the bedside; your initial action would be to
1. Ascertain the condition of the fundus
2. Establish an airway for the baby by milking the trachea
3. Quickly tie and cut the umbilical cord
4. Move mother and baby to delivery room

64. The physician arrives and cares for the baby and delivers the placenta. Pitocin, an oxytocic, is administered intramuscularly. Since Mrs. Penny had a precipitous delivery, it is important to observe for
1. Bleeding and infection
2. Sudden chilling
3. Elevation in blood pressure
4. Respiratory insufficiency in the baby

Mrs. Kim, a 22-year-old primigravida at term, is brought to the hospital by her husband. They have attended preparation for childbirth classes and plan to be together during labor. On admission Mrs. Kim is having 3 to 5 minute contractions, she has a bloody show, membranes intact. On vaginal examination the cervix is fully effaced and 4 cm. dilated, vertex presenting at a +1 station. Vital signs are T.P.R. 98.6-76-20, F.H. 140 L.L.Q., B.P. 118/74. Mr. Kim is coaching and supporting his wife well and Mrs. Kim appears to be quite relaxed. Questions 65 through 69 refer to this situation.

65. According to the above data, Mrs. Kim is in what stage of labor?
1. Early first stage
2. Latter part of relaxation
3. Transition phase of first stage
4. Second stage

66. Station +1 indicates that the presenting part is
1. Slightly below the ischial spines
2. Slightly above the ischial spines
3. High in the false pelvis
4. On the perineum

67. Mrs. Kim was uncomfortable and asked for medication. Demerol 50 mg. and Phenergan 50 mg. were ordered to be administered intramuscularly. This medication would
1. Induce sleep until the time of delivery
2. Increase her pain threshold resulting in relaxation
3. Act as an amnesic drug
4. Act as a preliminary to anesthesia

68. Suddenly Mrs. Kim's membranes rupture spontaneously. In order to give safe care the nurse would
1. Check frequency of contractions
2. Notify the doctor immediately
3. Give perineal care
4. Check fetal heart tones

69. A few hours later Mrs. Kim becomes very restless, her face is flushed, she is very irritable, she is perspiring profusely, and feels she is going to vomit. The above symptoms are indicative of
1. Second stage
2. Relaxation phase
3. Transition phase
4. Third stage

Mrs. Allen, a gravida III, para 2 had an uneventful labor and delivery. After a 7-hour labor she delivered an 8 lb. 2 oz. baby girl spontaneously. Questions 70 through 74 refer to this situation.

70. In checking Mrs. Allen you find the fundus firm, shifted to the right, and 2 fingers above the umbilicus. This would indicate
1. A normal process
2. An abnormal process
3. A full bladder
4. Impending bleeding

71. In checking Mrs. Allen's vital signs you would *normally* find
1. An elevated basal temperature, a decrease in respirations
2. A decided bradycardia, no change in respirations
3. A slight lowering of basal temperature, increase in respirations
4. A decided tachycardia, a decrease in respirations

72. Eight hours following delivery you notice that Mrs. Allen is voiding frequently in small amounts. Intake and output are important in the early postpartal period since small amounts
1. Are commonly voided and should cause no alarm
2. May be indicative of beginning glomerulonephritis
3. May indicate retention of urine with overflow
4. Common since less fluid is excreted following delivery

73. In helping Mrs. Allen develop motherliness you would
1. Do things for the baby in the mother's presence

2. Find out what she knows about babies and proceed from there
3. Demonstrate baby bath and baby care before discharge
4. Provide enough time for her and the baby to be together

74. Mrs. Allen asks you why sugar is added to the baby's formula. Your response would depend on the following understanding
   1. Cow's milk contains fewer calories than breast milk
   2. Sugar in cow's milk is not assimilated well
   3. Diluted cow's milk provides less sugar than the baby needs
   4. Sugar in cow's milk is a disaccharide

Mrs. Evans, a diabetic, suspects that she is pregnant because she is experiencing breast changes, missed 2 periods, has some early morning nausea and excessive fatigue. Despite the nausea and fatigue, her urine tests are consistently negative for sugar. Mrs. Evans seeks the advice of an obstetrician who confirms the diagnosis of pregnancy. Mrs. Evans is taking 30 units of NPH insulin daily at this time. Questions 75 through 78 refer to this situation.

75. The diabetic mother's homeodynamics are significantly altered during pregnancy as a result of
   1. The increased effect of insulin during pregnancy
   2. The effect of hormones and enzymes produced in pregnancy on carbohydrate and lipoid metabolism
   3. An increase in the glucose tolerance level of the blood
   4. The lower renal threshold for glucose
76. Regulation of usual insulin coverage in the pregnant diabetic woman is difficult since
   1. Sugar can normally be found in the urine of a pregnant woman
   2. Sugar is metabolized more rapidly during pregnancy
   3. The basal metabolic rate is altered during pregnancy
   4. As a result of increased blood volume, insulin is absorbed more rapidly
77. Mrs. Evans is referred to the clinic nutritionist for nutrition assessment and counselling. The dietary program worked out for her is
   1. A low carbohydrate, low calorie diet to stay within her present insulin coverage and avoid hyperglycemia
   2. A diet high in protein of good biologic value and decreased calories
   3. Adequate balance of carbohydrate and fat to meet energy demands and avoid ketosis
   4. Insulin adjusted as needed to balance increased dietary needs
78. The baby of a diabetic mother needs newborn care that requires
   1. Decreased glucose intake
   2. Care similar to all newborn
   3. Administration of insulin
   4. Care similar to a premature baby

Mrs. Greene, a 22-year-old primigravida, is attending prenatal clinic. She has misssed 2 menstrual periods. She relates that the first day of her last menstrual period was July 22. Questions 79 through 84 refer to this situation.

79. Mrs. Greene's estimated date of confinement would be
   1. May 5
   2. April 29
   3. April 15
   4. May 14
80. As you prepare Mrs. Greene for the pelvic examination, she complains of feeling very tired and sick to her stomach especially in the morning. The best response for the nurse to make would be
   1. "This is common during the early part of pregnancy. There is no need to worry."
   2. "This is a common occurrence during the early part of pregnancy because of all the changes going on in your body."
   3. "These are common occurrences during pregnancy with all the body changes; can you tell me how you feel in the morning?"
   4. "Perhaps you might ask the doctor when he arrives."
81. Mrs. Greene works as a secretary in a large office. Her job would have implications for her plan of care during pregnancy. The nurse would most likely recommend that Mrs. Greene
   1. Ask for a break in the morning and afternoon so she can elevate her legs
   2. Inform her employer that she cannot work beyond the second trimester
   3. Ask for a break in the morning and afternoon for added nourishment
   4. Try to walk about every few hours of her work day
82. The doctor proceeds to do a pelvic examination on Mrs. Greene. On pelvic examination Mrs. Greene had a normal female pelvis with
   1. Sacrum well hollowed, coccyx movable, spines not prominent, pubic arch wide
   2. Sacrum flat, coccyx movable, spines prominent, pubic arch wide
   3. Sacrum deeply hollowed, coccyx immovable, pubic arch narrow, spines not prominent
   4. Sacrum flat, coccyx movable, spines prominent, pubic arch narrow
83. Mrs. Greene is concerned since she read nutrition during pregnancy is important for proper growth and development of the baby. She wants to know something about the foods she should eat. The nurse would proceed by
   1. Giving her a list of foods so she can better plan her meals
   2. Assess what she eats by taking a diet history
   3. Emphasize the importance of limiting salt and highly-seasoned foods
   4. Instructing her to continue eating a normal diet
84. Mrs. Greene states, "I'm worried about gaining too much weight because I've heard it's bad for me." The nurse would respond
   1. "Yes, weight gain causes complications during pregnancy."
   2. "Don't worry about gaining weight. We

are more concerned if you don't gain
enough weight to ensure proper growth of
your baby."
3. "The quality of the weight gain is more
important than the amount that is gained
from eating enough of the foods you need."
4. "If you gain over 15 pounds, you'll have
to follow a low calorie diet."

Mrs. Joyce, a primigravida, had decided to breast-
feed her baby. However, she has some doubts as
to whether she will be successful since her breasts
are small. She is also concerned about putting on
weight since she is proud of her petite figure.
Questions 85 through 89 refer to this situation.

85. Considering Mrs. Joyce's statement concerning
the size of her breasts, your best response
would be
1. "The size of your breasts has nothing to
do with the production of milk."
2. "The amount of glandular tissue rather
than the size of your breasts determines the
amount of milk produced."
3. "The amount of glandular tissue and the
stimulation of the baby's sucking determine
the amount of milk."
4. "The amount of fat and glandular tissue
in the breasts determines the amount of
milk produced."

86. Mrs. Joyce is now 2 days postpartum and asks
you about cleansing the nipples. Your best
response would be
1. "Thoroughly scrub the nipples with soap
and water before each feeding."
2. "Cleanse the nipples with sterile water before each feeding."
3. "Cleanse the nipples with an alcohol sponge
before and after each feeding."
4. "Wash the breasts and nipples daily using
soap sparingly on nipples."

87. Mrs. Joyce is concerned since she heard that
her neighbor's breasts suddenly dried up when
she got home and had to discontinue nursing.
An appropriate comment for the nurse to make
is
1. "This commonly happens with the excitement of going home. Putting the baby to
breast more frequently will reestablish
lactation."
2. "This commonly happens, however, we will
give you a formula to take home so the
baby won't go hungry until your milk supply returns."
3. "This is not true, once lactation is established this rarely happens."
4. "You have little to worry about since you
already have a good milk supply."

88. Mrs. Joyce has heard of "demand" feeding
and wonders how anyone ever finds time to
do anything but feed the baby. Your best
response would be
1. "Most mothers find babies on breast do
better on demand feeding, since the amount
of milk ingested varies at each feeding."
2. "Perhaps a schedule might be better, since
the baby is already used to hospital
routine."
3. "Although the baby is on demand, he will

eventually set his own schedule, so there
will be time for your household chores."
4. "Most mothers find that feeding the baby
whenever he cries works out fine."

89. Mrs. Joyce wants to know whether or not it
is true that she will not have to use contraceptives while nursing. Your most appropriate response would be
1. "Since lactation suppresses ovulation, you
probably don't have to worry about becoming pregnant."
2. "As long as you have no menstrual period
you won't have to worry about using contraceptives."
3. "It is best to use contraceptive measures,
since ovulation may occur without a menstrual period."
4. "It is best to delay any sexual relations
until you have your first menstrual period."

90. Following an 8-hour uneventful labor, Mrs.
Knight, a gravida II, para 1 delivered a baby
boy spontaneously under epidural block anesthesia. As you place her baby in her arms
immediately following delivery she asks, "Is
he normal?" Your most appropriate answer
would be
1. "Of course he is, your pregnancy and labor
were so normal."
2. "Shall we unwrap him so you can look him
over for yourself?"
3. "He must be all right, he has such a good
strong cry."
4. "Most babies are normal, of course he is."

91. Shortly following delivery Mrs. Knight tells
you she feels as if she is bleeding. On checking the fundus there is a steady trickling of
blood from the vagina. Your first action would
be to
1. Call the physician immediately
2. Hold the fundus firmly and gently massage
it
3. Check Mrs. Knight's blood pressure and
pulse
4. Take no action since this is a common
occurrence

92. The newborn must be observed carefully for
the first 24 hours particularly for
1. Respiratory distress
2. Change in body temperature
3. Frequency in voiding
4. Duration of cry

93. Acute salpingitis is most commonly the result
of
1. Abortion
2. Gonorrhea
3. Hydatidiform mole
4. Syphilis

94. Hot flashes are caused by
1. Overstimulation of adrenal medulla
2. Accumulation of acetylcholine
3. Cessation of pituitary gonadotropins
4. Hormonal stimulation of sympathetic system

95. The basic idea on which rhythm practice rests
is that ovulation usually occurs
1. 7 days after the completion of the menstrual period

2. 14 days after the completion of the menstrual period
3. 7 days before the end of the menstrual cycle
4. 14 days before the end of the menstrual cycle

96. The most important complication associated with the use of IUDs in humans is
    1. Rupture of the uterus
    2. Excessive uterine hemorrhage
    3. Expulsion of the IUD
    4. Pain

97. What is the menopausal implication for women on oral contraceptives?
    1. Prolongs menses
    2. Intensifies menopausal symptoms
    3. Causes menorrhagia
    4. Has no effect on menopause

Pediatric nursing

1. Johnny Smith, 12 months of age, is brought to the Preventive Health Clinic for a regular physical assessment. In reviewing his immunizations for the past 10 months the nurse would expect him to have been immunized against
   1. Measles, rubella, polio, TB, and pertussis
   2. Polio, pertussis, tetanus, and diphtheria
   3. Measles, mumps, rubella, and TB
   4. Pertussis, tetanus, polio, and measles

2. Before a child receives the rubella vaccine, the nurse should check to see if
   1. He had received booster doses of measles vaccine recently
   2. The mother is pregnant
   3. There are younger siblings at home
   4. He has received the completed DPT series

3. In terms of preventive teaching for a 1 year old, the nurse would speak to the mother about
   1. Adequate nutrition
   2. Accidents
   3. Sexual development
   4. Toilet training

4. A toddler has swallowed a liquid drain cleaner containing lye. The immediate intervention is to administer
   1. Syrup of ipecac
   2. Two ounces of milk
   3. Dilute vinegar solution
   4. Sodium bicarbonate and water

5. Two-year-old Jimmy swallowed kerosene from a soda bottle stored in the garage. Immediate treatment for ingestion of petroleum distillates is to have the child swallow
   1. Milk of magnesia
   2. Strong tea
   3. Weak salt solution
   4. Mineral oil

6. John Lee, a 6-month-old infant, is admitted to the hospital with diarrhea for 2 days. The most important clinical manifestation of the degree of dehydration would be
   1. Sunken fontanel
   2. Weight loss
   3. Decreased urine output
   4. Dry skin

7. PKU is a treatable condition if diagnosed early in life. A test that can be done on a newborn before discharge from the nursery to detect PKU is a
   1. Guthrie blood test
   2. Ferric chloride urine test
   3. Phenistix test
   4. Clinitest serum phosphopyruvic acid

8. Treatment of PKU is dietary and consists of a
   1. Low phenylalanine diet
   2. Phenylalanine free diet
   3. Dietary supplement for the amino acid, phenylalanine
   4. Protein-free diet

9. In terms of dietary counselling, the parents need much help and support in adhering to specific regimes. A frequent question asked by parents is, "How long will my child have to be on this diet?" An appropriate response by the nurse might be
   1. "Unfortunately, this is a life-long problem and dietary management must always be maintained."
   2. "Usually, if the child does well for 1 year he then can gradually begin eating regular foods."
   3. "As of now, research shows that a child needs to be on this diet until he is about 6 to 8 years of age. Then he can gradually begin to eat other foods."
   4. "No one knows, but why don't you discuss it with your doctor."

Debbie Marsh was born with a unilateral cleft lip and palate. The lip defect extended through the floor of the nostril and communicated with the defect in the palate. The physician recommended that the lip be repaired as soon as possible after birth because the child was in good physical condition otherwise. Questions 10 through 15 refer to this situation.

10. Cleft lip is usually repaired early because of
    1. The emotional impact upon the parents
    2. Feeding difficulty
    3. Infection
    4. Obstruction in breathing

11. Mr. and Mrs. Marsh are very concerned about the defect and ask the nurse, "What caused our baby to be born deformed?" The nurse might reply
    1. "I don't know, but you don't need to worry because surgery can correct it."
    2. "I am glad that you are able to ask these kinds of questions."
    3. "Are you feeling guilty?"
    4. "It sounds as if you are wondering what you might have done to cause this situation."

12. In informing the parents about the significance and etiology about cleft lip and palate, the nurse would
    1. Assess the family history for presence of the defect in other siblings or relatives, since this would affect the chances of having other children with cleft lip or palate
    2. Emphasize that the 2 defects follow laws of Mendelian genetics
    3. Prepare the parents for the likelihood of mental and psychologic problems in the child

4. Stress that the defect is rare and will probably never happen in the same family twice

13. Before the baby's birth, Mrs. Marsh had wanted to breast feed Debbie. Now, feeding will probably be
    1. With a rubber tipped syringe or medicine dropper
    2. Too difficult because of breathing problems
    3. With a soft, large-holed nipple
    4. Intravenous fluids

14. Debbie's cleft lip predisposes her to infection primarily because
    1. Of poor nutrition from disturbed feeding
    2. Of poor circulation to the defective area
    3. Mouth breathing dries the mucous membranes of the oropharynx
    4. Of accumulation of waste products along the defect

15. Debbie's lip is repaired 4 days after birth. In caring for her postoperatively, the nurse would do all of the following *except*
    1. Observe for swelling of the tongue, lips, and mucous membranes
    2. Place her on her abdomen to prevent aspiration
    3. Keep the suture line clean and free of crusting
    4. Encourage the parents to visit as much as possible to prevent the infant from crying

Paul Tye, a 1-month-old male, has been having vomiting for 1 week. Mrs. Tye explains that the vomiting has been progressively more forceful and contains undigested formula. Presently, the child is dehydrated and has abdominal distention. A tentative diagnosis of pyloric stenosis has been made. Questions 16 through 21 refer to this situation.

16. Vomiting caused by pyloric stenosis is usually non–bile stained because
    1. The obstruction is above the opening of the common bile duct
    2. The bile duct is also obstructed
    3. The obstruction of the cardiac sphincter prevents bile from entering the esophagus
    4. The sphincter of the bile duct is connected to the hypertrophied pyloric muscle

17. During the physical assessment of the child, the nurse would particularly observe for visible peristaltic waves and
    1. An olive-shaped mass in the right upper quadrant
    2. Decreased bowel sounds
    3. Severe cramping movements in the lower intestine
    4. A board-like abdomen

18. Preoperatively, Paul was fed thickened formula through a gavage tube. During insertion of the tube, which signs or reactions of the child would be considered abnormal by the nurse?
    1. Choking
    2. Cyanosis
    3. Flushing
    4. Gagging

19. How should the nurse determine the distance needed to advance the gavage tube?
    1. Advance the tube until she feels resistance
    2. Measure the distance from the nose, to the

ear lobe, to the epigastric area of the abdomen
    3. Measure from the mouth to the umbilicus and add one half the distance
    4. Advance the tube as far as necessary to aspirate gastric content

20. A Fredet-Ramstedt procedure was performed and Mrs. Tye is to be taught how to feed Paul after the operation. The feeding regime after a pylorotomy is based on the principle that
    1. Clear liquids are tolerated best because they contain no large curds that would have difficulty passing through the pylorus
    2. Thickened feedings are avoided since they may put pressure on the surgically repaired pylorus
    3. Easily digested fluids are given in large amounts to prevent dehydration
    4. Thickened feedings mechanically aid in helping food pass through the pylorus muscle

21. The nurse also instructs Mrs. Tye concerning the proper feeding technique to prevent vomiting, such as
    1. Feed child in semi-Fowler's position and position him prone after feeding
    2. Hold child in as upright a position as possible during feeding and position him on right side with head elevated after feeding
    3. Hold the child after each feeding until he falls asleep
    4. Do not move the child during or after feeding because movement can induce vomiting

22. A mother asks about the introduction of new foods to her 2-month-old baby's diet. The nurse might suggest
    1. "Mix the pureed food with the formula and give through the bottle to help him learn new tastes."
    2. "Offer a new food every day until he likes one."
    3. "Offer a new food after he has had some milk when he is still hungry."
    4. "Offer a new food after he has had his regular feeding."

23. She also asks about what foods she should begin to introduce. A likely choice would be
    1. To start with rice cereal and fruit then add egg yolk
    2. To start with cereal and add a soft-boiled egg for breakfast
    3. To introduce fruit first, then add meat and vegetables
    4. To start with sweets, such as fruits and puddings

Frank Anvel, a 6-month-old male, is admitted to the hospital because of increasing head size and a possible diagnosis of hydrocephalus. Questions 24 through 29 refer to this situation.

24. In performing a developmental appraisal, what clue would be most important to the nurse in light of the diagnosis
    1. Absence of Moro, tonic-neck, and grasp reflex
    2. Presence of Babinski reflex

3. Head lag
4. Inability to sit unsupported
25. Because of the diagnosis the nurse is especially alert to signs of increased intracranial pressure such as
    1. Bulging fontanel, "sunset" eyes, projective vomiting not associated with feeding
    2. Depressed fontanel, bulging eyes, irritability
    3. Dilated scalp veins, depressed and sunken eyeballs, decreased blood pressure
    4. High, shrill cry, decreased skin turgor, elevated fontanels
26. Proper positioning of a child with hydrocephalus is essential to prevent breakdown of the scalp. A suitable position would be
    1. Prone, with legs elevated about 30°
    2. Prone or supine, with head elevated about 45°
    3. Positioned on either side and flat
    4. Supine and Trendelenburg
27. Hydrocephalus, if untreated, can cause mental retardation because
    1. Hypertonic, cerebrospinal fluid disturbs normal plasma concentration, depriving nerve cells of vital nutrients
    2. Cerebrospinal fluid dilutes blood supply causing cells to atrophy
    3. Increasing head size necessitates more oxygen and nutrients than normal blood flow can supply
    4. Gradually increasing size of ventricles depresses brain against bony cranium; anoxia and decreased blood supply result
28. After several tests have been performed the diagnosis of noncommunicating hydrocephalus is confirmed and a ventriculoperitoneal shunt is performed. Postoperative care of this child includes all of the following *except*
    1. Positioning the child flat for about 48 hours
    2. Administering sedatives and analgesics to keep the child quiet
    3. Encouraging the mother not to pick up the child even to prevent crying
    4. Checking the valve frequently and pumping it as ordered
29. Mr. and Mrs. Anvel have been very anxious during their child's admission and especially concerned about the prognosis. The nurse should explain that
    1. The prognosis is excellent and that the valve is permanent
    2. The shunt may need to be revised as the child grows older
    3. If any brain damage has occurred it is reversible during the first year of life
    4. Hydrocephalus usually is self-limiting by 2 years of age and then the shunt is removed
30. Infants with sickle cell anemia may not be diagnosed as having this disorder because of
    1. The presence of fetal hemoglobin during the first year of life
    2. Compensation of increased hematocrit and hemoglobin if well-fed
    3. Absence of respiratory disorders
    4. General good health and an excellent growth curve

31. The sickling process of the red blood cell occurs in conditions of
    1. Decreased fluids
    2. Decreased oxygen
    3. Poor iron intake
    4. Decreased calcium intake
32. To prevent thrombus formation in capillaries, as well as other problems from stasis and clotting of blood in the sickling process, the main nursing intervention is
    1. Administration of oxygen
    2. Increasing fluids by mouth and humidifier
    3. Complete bedrest
    4. Use of heparin or other anticoagulants

Julie Syms, a 12-month-old female, is admitted to the hospital with a diagnosis of failure to thrive. Her weight is below the third percentile, her development is retarded, and she shows signs of neglect. Questions 33 through 37 refer to this situation.

33. Based on this assessment, what behaviors might also support the possibility of maternal deprivation?
    1. Infant is cuddly, responsive to touch, and wants to be held
    2. Infant is stiff, unpliable, and uncomforted by touch
    3. Infant is a poor eater, sleeps soundly, and is easily satisfied
    4. Infant is responsive to adults, rarely cries but shows no interest in her environment
34. A plan of care that would best meet the needs of this child should include
    1. A vigorous schedule of stimulation geared to the infant's present level of development
    2. A plan to have all staff members pick her up and play with her whenever they can
    3. A schedule of care that allows the infant stimulation and physical contact by several staff members
    4. As consistent a care giver as possible, with stimulation that is moderate and purposeful
35. During the nurse's assessment of Julie, she observes that the child has good head control, can roll over, but cannot sit up without support or transfer an object from one hand to the other. Based on these facts, the nurse concludes that Julie is developmentally at age
    1. 2 to 3 months
    2. 3 to 4 months
    3. 4 to 6 months
    4. 6 to 8 months
36. Which toys would be *unsuited* for Julie based on her present developmental age?
    1. Brightly colored mobiles
    2. Soft stuffed animals that she can hold
    3. Small rattle that she can hold
    4. Snap toys, large snap beads
37. The nurse who has been caring for Julie decides on a plan of care for the mother as well. Her main objective is to
    1. Set up a schedule for teaching the mother how to care for her baby
    2. Discuss the matter with her in a nonthreatening manner
    3. Show by her example how to care for the infant and satisfy her needs

4. Supply emotional support to the mother and encourage her dependency

38. Roy Brown, an 18-month-old male, is admitted to the hospital with an upper respiratory infection. This is his first hospitalization and prolonged separation from his mother. Based on this information, the nurse may expect to see which type of behavior during the initial admission?
    1. Generally crying when people enter the room, but does respond with a smile after a few minutes
    2. Crying relentlessly, unconsoled by no one except his mother or father
    3. Withdrawn, sitting quietly, not interested in playing
    4. Initially unhappy and crying, but contented after meeting his roommates

39. After a prolonged period of hospitalization, Roy became depressed, withdrawn, and apathetic toward his mother. Eventually, he began playing with toys and relating to others, even strangers. The nurse should realize that
    1. He has accepted his hospitalization well and has matured because of this experience
    2. He has grown out of the stage of separation and realizes that he has to depend on others
    3. He has probably become a disturbed child because of this traumatic separation
    4. He has finally recognized that the staff is not out to hurt him

Mrs. Jones is sitting with her 18-month-old son, Ben, at the well-baby clinic. She tells the nurse that Ben has been "driving her crazy" by saying no to everything she suggests and that she needs help in handling him. Questions 40 through 43 refer to this situation.

40. The nurse explains to Mrs. Jones that Ben's negativism is normal for his age and that it is helping him meet his need for
    1. Discipline
    2. Independence
    3. Attention
    4. Trust

41. Mrs. Jones states, "This morning I gave Ben his juice and he said 'no.' He says 'no' and I get angry, but he needs his fluids. What shall I do?" The nurse suggests that she
    1. Be firm and hand him his glass
    2. Distract him with some food
    3. Let him see he's making her angry
    4. Offer him a choice of two things to drink

42. The nurse plans to talk to Mrs. Jones about toilet training Ben, knowing that the most important factor in the process of toilet training is the
    1. Child's desire to be dry
    2. Approach and attitude of the mother
    3. Ability of the child to sit still
    4. Mother's willingness to work at it

43. Before Mrs. Jones leaves the clinic, the nurse tells her that she can *best* help her son learn to control his own behavior by
    1. Rewarding him for good behavior
    2. Allowing him to learn by his mistakes

3. Punishing him when he deserves it
4. Setting limits and being consistent

Sue Green, a two-year-old female, is admitted to the pediatric unit with respiratory wheezing, dyspnea, and cyanosis. One of the tentative diagnoses is cystic fibrosis. Questions 44 through 48 refer to this situation.

44. Cystic fibrosis can predispose Sue to bronchitis mainly because
    1. Tenacious secretions obstruct the bronchioles and respiratory tract and provide a favorable medium for growth of bacteria
    2. Increased salt content in saliva can irritate and necrose mucous membranes in nasopharynx
    3. Neuromuscular irritability causes spasm and constriction of the bronchi
    4. The associated heart defects of cystic fibrosis cause congestive heart failure and respiratory depression

45. Sue is small and underdeveloped for her age primarily because she
    1. Ingested little food for several months because of poor appetite
    2. Failed to absorb nutrients because of a lack of pancreatic enzymes
    3. Secreted less than normal amounts of pituitary growth hormone
    4. Developed muscular and bony atrophy from lack of motor activity

46. The foul-smelling, frothy characteristic of the stool in cystic fibrosis results from the presence of large amounts of
    1. Sodium and chloride
    2. Semidigested carbohydrates
    3. Undigested fat
    4. Lipase, trypsin, and amylase

47. Medications that will probably be used for Sue in her therapeutic regimen will include
    1. A steroid and an antimetabolite
    2. Antibiotics, a multivitamin preparation, and cough drops
    3. Pancreatic enzymes and antibiotics
    4. Aerosol mists, decongestants, and fat soluble vitamins

48. In cystic fibrosis, frequent stools and lack of mucus often produce
    1. Intussusception
    2. Anal fissures
    3. Meconium ileus
    4. Rectal prolapse

Two-year-old Mike Cox was admitted to the hospital for the second surgical repair of his cleft palate. Mrs. Cox cannot stay overnight with her son since visiting hours are restricted. On the morning after admission, Mike is standing in his crib crying. He refuses to be comforted and calls for his mother. Questions 49 through 52 refer to this situation.

49. The nurse approaches Mike to bathe him and he screams louder. She recognizes this behavior as the stage of protest and
    1. Picks him up and walks with him around the room

2. Sits by his crib and bathes him later when his anxiety decreases
3. Decides he really does not need a bath when he's this upset
4. Fills the basin with water and proceeds to bathe him

50. On the third postoperative day Mike begins to regress and lies quietly in his crib with his blanket. The nurse recognizes that Mike is in a stage of
    1. Denial
    2. Mistrust
    3. Rejection
    4. Despair

51. During his second week of hospitalization, Mike smiles easily, goes to all the nurses happily, and no longer cries when his mother goes home. After leaving Mike's room, Mrs. Cox tells the nurse she is pleased that Mike is adjusting well. Before responding to Mrs. Cox, the nurse understands Mike's behavior and realizes that he
    1. Is repressing his feelings for his mother
    2. Has established a routine and feels safe
    3. Feels better physically so his behavior has improved
    4. Has given up fighting and accepts the separation

52. The nurse explains the meaning of Mike's behavior to Mrs. Cox and tells her that after he goes home she should expect that
    1. Mike will miss the nurses and hospital routine
    2. It will be easier for Mike to adjust to his home situation
    3. Mike will continue his happy, normal behavior
    4. It will take some time before the mother-child relationship is reestablished

In many states across the country, failure by the nurse to report a suspected case of child abuse is punishable by the law. Child abuse is one of the major causes of death in young children.

53. When a child is admitted to the hospital with traumatic injuries, a common clue that the child was battered is that he
    1. Cries for longer periods of time
    2. Ignores all offers of toys and favors
    3. Shows no expectation of being comforted
    4. Is more afraid than other children when admitted

54. There are many common reactions of parents who batter their children. One reaction the nurse should be aware of is that the parent
    1. Seldom touches or looks at the child
    2. Shows signs of guilt about the child's injury
    3. Is quick to inquire about the discharge date
    4. Is very concerned about his own physical health

The nurse in the outpatient Pediatric Clinic is talking to a group of parents whose children have been diagnosed as having minimal brain dysfunction.

55. One of the major behavioral characteristics of children with minimal brain dysfunction is their
    1. Inability to use abstract thought
    2. Overreaction to stimuli
    3. Continued use of rituals
    4. Retarded speech development

56. In helping the parents to cope with their children's behavior, the nurse suggests that one of their best approaches would be to
    1. Write a list of expectations to avoid confusion
    2. Be consistent and firm about established rules
    3. Avoid asking specific questions
    4. Allow the child to set up his own routines

57. The handicapped child has the same needs as the normal child although his means of satisfying these needs are limited. This limitation frequently causes
    1. Emotional disability
    2. Overcompensation
    3. Frustration
    4. Rejection

Three-year-old Mary is admitted with second and third degree burns over 60% of her body. She is placed in a warm isolation room with a humidifier and strict sterile technique is instituted. The doctor orders a Foley catheter to be inserted and I.V. therapy to begin immediately. One nurse is assigned to care for Mary each shift for the first 48 hours. Questions 58 through 61 refer to this situation.

58. Nursing observations in the first 48 hours of hospitalization are directed primarily toward preventing
    1. Pneumonia
    2. Contractures
    3. Dehydration
    4. Shock

59. Despite the child's physical distress and discomfort, the weight must be accurately taken because it
    1. Provides a baseline for future growth
    2. Provides a measure of the amount of burned surface area
    3. Provides a basis for calculating fluid replacement and medications
    4. Serves as a guideline for dietary and fluid management

60. On the second day of hospitalization, the nurse observes that Mary has decreased urinary output with edema. She recognizes this as one sign of toxicity that commonly occurs in the first 2 days. The nurse observes Mary for other signs of toxicity, which are
    1. Vomiting, bradycardia
    2. Subnormal temperature, slow pulse
    3. High fever, cyanosis
    4. Rapid pulse, low blood pressure

61. The nurse must accurately measure Mary's urinary output each hour to evaluate kidney function. The *minimum* safe output of urine per hour is
    1. 10 to 20 ml.
    2. 25 to 50 ml.
    3. 40 to 60 ml.
    4. 75 to 100 ml.

Three-year-old Roger was admitted to the Pediatric Unit with a diagnosis of nephrosis. Questions 62 through 64 refer to this situation.

62. The most important nursing intervention for Roger is
   1. Encouraging fluids
   2. Regulating his diet
   3. Maintaining bed rest
   4. Preventing infection
63. As Roger gets older and has repeated attacks of nephrosis, it is most important for the nurse to help him develop
   1. Fine muscle coordination
   2. Acceptance of possible sterility
   3. A positive body image
   4. The ability to test his own urine
64. During his nap, Roger wet the bed. The best approach by the nurse would be to
   1. Change his clothes and make no issue of it
   2. Explain that big boys should try to call the nurse
   3. Tell him to help you remake the bed
   4. Change his bed, putting a rubber sheet on it

Four-year-old Ann weighs 40 pounds and is in a private Pediatric room on "hand and linen precaution." She was admitted for weight loss, anorexia, vaginitis, and insomnia. A diagnosis of pinworm infestation was made. Questions 65 through 69 refer to this situation.

65. The most effective time for the nurse to do a Scotch Tape test for pinworms is
   1. At bedtime before bathing
   2. Just following a bowel movement
   3. Immediately after meals
   4. Early morning before arising
66. Pinworms cause a number of symptoms other than anal itching. One of the most common sequelae of pinworm infestation that the nurse would observe for is
   1. Pneumonitis
   2. Stomatitis
   3. Hepatitis
   4. Appendicitis
67. Pyrvinium pamoate (Antiminth) is an effective single dose drug to eliminate pinworms. How many mg. will you give Ann if it is ordered 5 mg. per kg. of body weight?
   1. 90 mg.
   2. 18 mg.
   3. 40 mg.
   4. 200 mg.
68. After administering pyrvinium pamoate (Antiminth) to Ann, it is important to alert the staff that a normal side effect of this drug is that it colors the stool or vomitus
   1. Dark brown
   2. Light green
   3. Bright red
   4. Gentian blue
69. The nurse's decision to alert the staff is based on her knowledge that
   1. Irritation by pinworms in the rectum may cause ulceration and bleeding
   2. The cyanine dye origin of the drug colors the stool

3. The stool contains hemoglobin-like metabolic products of disintegrating pinworms
4. The drug is irritating to the intestinal mucosa and may cause transient bleeding
70. Mary is admitted to the pediatric unit with an asthmatic attack, and an I.V. of D5% 1/2 NS is started. Aminophylline is to run in via Soluset, over 20 minutes every 8 hours. Before administering the drug, the nurse should
   1. Check temperature
   2. Monitor blood pressure
   3. Administer oxygen
   4. Take pulse

Four-year-old Sam has been hospitalized with acute glomerulonephritis. Questions 71 through 73 refer to this situation.

71. The nurse observes Sam primarily for
   1. Polyuria, high fever
   2. Dehydration, hematuria
   3. Hypertension, circumocular edema
   4. Oliguria, hypotension
72. When planning nursing care for Sam, the nurse realizes that he needs help in understanding his restrictions, one of which is
   1. Bedrest for at least 4 weeks
   2. A bland diet high in protein
   3. Daily doses of I.M. penicillin
   4. Isolation from other children with infections
73. Sam loves to ride his bike and his parents are very concerned about his activity when he returns home. You base your answer to them on the fact that after the urinary findings are nearly normal
   1. He must remain on bedrest for 2 weeks
   2. Activity doesn't affect the course of the disease
   3. He must not play active games
   4. Activity must be limited for 1 month
74. Karen Vale, a five-year-old female, was admitted to the hospital 1 week before surgery for tetralogy of Fallot. The defects associated with this heart anomaly include
   1. Right ventricular hypertrophy, atrial and ventricular defects, and mitral valve stenosis
   2. Right ventricular hypertrophy, ventricular septal defect, stenosis of pulmonary artery, and overriding aorta
   3. Origin of the aorta from the right ventricle and of the pulmonary artery from the left ventricle
   4. Abnormal connection between the pulmonary artery and the aorta, right ventricular hypertrophy, and atrial septal defects
75. Karen's laboratory analysis indicates a high red blood count. This polycythemia can best be understood as a compensatory mechanism for
   1. Cardiomegaly
   2. Low iron level
   3. Low blood pressure
   4. Tissue oxygen need
76. Karen has heart surgery to repair the anomaly. Postoperatively, it is essential that the nurse prevent which of the following?
   1. Constipation
   2. Unnecessary movement

3. Crying
4. Coughing

77. Eight-year-old John Kee is being discharged following treatment for sickle cell crisis. He is allowed to return to school and resume normal activities. The nurse explains to Mrs. Kee that a very important aspect of care for John at home should include
    1. At least 14 hours sleep per day
    2. Avoidance of all strenuous play and activities
    3. Ingestion of huge quantities of liquids
    4. Protection from emotional upsets

78. Common nursing care that helps prevent both sickle cell crisis and celiac crisis is
    1. Limitation of activity
    2. Protection from infection
    3. High iron, low fat, high protein diet
    4. Careful observation of all vital signs

Eight-year-old Kim is admitted to the hospital for the first time with a diagnosis of diabetes. Questions 79 through 82 refer to this situation.

79. Juvenile diabetes
    1. Has a more rapid onset than adult
    2. Occurs more often in obese children
    3. Does not always require insulin
    4. Involves early vascular changes

80. The nurse plans to include the entire family in Kim's care and is especially concerned that
    1. The parents receive immediate instruction about urine testing
    2. Kim is taught to give injections before being discharged
    3. The parents and child be helped to understand their feelings about diabetes
    4. Kim's activity be limited and the parents understand the need for this

81. The doctor orders 12 units of NPH insulin daily for Kim. The vial reads 1 ml. = 40 units of NPH. You do not have an insulin syringe so you use a regular syringe and give
    1. 6 minims
    2. 4.5 minims
    3. 4 minims
    4. 3.5 minims

82. Before Kim goes home, the nurse reviews with the family the importance of their knowing that Kim's insulin needs will be decreased when
    1. There is an emotional upset
    2. An infectious process is present
    3. She reaches puberty
    4. She participates in active exercise

Sally, age 8, is readmitted to the hospital for exacerbation of acute lymphatic leukemia after being in remission for a year. Sally is pale and weak, has multiple hematomas on her legs, and has an elevated temperature. The doctors have ordered vincristine and prednisone to be given every other day as her chemotherapeutic regime. Questions 83 through 85 refer to this situation.

83. A major objective of nursing care related to Sally's drug regime is to
    1. Maintain reverse isolation
    2. Reduce unnecessary stimuli

3. Check her vital signs every 2 hours
4. Prevent all physical activity

84. Understanding the side effects of vincristine, the nurse prepares a diet for Sally that is
    1. Low residue with increased fluids
    2. High in iron, decreased fluids
    3. High in both roughage and fluids
    4. Low fat, regular fluids

85. Because Sally's platelet count is very low, the nurse plans to observe her urine for the presence of
    1. Erythrocytes
    2. Leukocytes
    3. Casts
    4. Lymphocytes

86. Ten-year-old Jim Smith is admitted to the emergency room because of a car accident. However, normal measures to stop the bleeding are unsuccessful, and upon further study, Jim was found to have a mild case of classic hemophilia. Mr. and Mrs. Smith are very concerned about this and wonder how it happened. The nurse should explain that

    1. Hemophilia is a sex-linked recessive disorder in which the mother is usually the carrier of the illness but is not affected by it
    2. Hemophilia is a sex-linked dominant disorder in which the woman carries the trait
    3. Hemophilia follows regular laws of Mendelian inherited disorders such as sickle cell anemia
    4. This disorder can be carried by either male or female, but occurs in the opposite sex of the carrier

87. Jim's parents are very worried about their other children, two girls and another boy, and want to know what the chances are concerning their having the disorder or being a carrier. An appropriate answer to this question would be that
    1. All the girls will be normal and the other son a carrier
    2. Each son has a 50-50 chance of being a victim and each daughter a 50-50 chance of being a carrier
    3. All the girls will be carriers and one half of the boys will be victims
    4. Each son has a 50-50 chance of being either a victim or a carrier and the girls will all be carriers

88. The most common site of internal bleeding in hemophiliacs is
    1. Cerebrum
    2. Ends of long bones
    3. Intestines
    4. Joints

89. Maria Lory, a 15-year-old female, is admitted to the hospital with the diagnosis of acute lymphocytic leukemia. Which signs and symptoms would you consider unusual with this diagnosis?
    1. Multiple bruises, petechiae
    2. Marked fatigue, pallor
    3. Enlarged lymph nodes, spleen, and liver
    4. Marked jaundice and generalized edema

90. A pathophysiologic change underlying the production of symptoms in leukemia is

1. Progressive replacement of bone marrow with fibrous tissue
2. Destruction of red blood cells and platelets by overproduction of white blood cells
3. Proliferation and release of immature white blood cells into the circulating blood
4. Excessive destruction of blood cells in the liver and spleen

91. To induce a remission, Maria was placed on a drug regime including Cytoxan, prednisone, vincristine, and methotrexate. Considering the side effects of these drugs, which requires the greatest preparation of this patient?
    1. Constipation
    2. Generalized, short-term paralysis
    3. Retarded growth in height
    4. Alopecia

92. Besides preparing Maria for the drug therapy, it is also essential to discuss with her another treatment, irradiation of the spine and skull. This treatment is used *mainly* because
    1. Leukemia cells invade the nervous system slower, but the usual drugs are ineffective in the brain

    2. Radiation will retard growth of cells in bone marrow of the cranium
    3. Neoplastic drug therapy without radiation is effective in most cases, but this is a precautionary treatment
    4. Radiation will decrease cerebral edema and prevent increased intracranial pressure

93. One day Mr. Lory asks the nurse whether or not he should tell his son, who is 7 years old, the truth about Maria. The nurse might reply
    1. "A child of his age cannot comprehend the real meaning of death so don't tell him until the last moment."
    2. "Your son probably fears separation most and wants to know that you will care for him, rather than what will happen to his sister."
    3. "Your son probably doesn't understand death as we do, but fears it just the same. He should be told the truth to let him prepare for his sister's possible death."
    4. "Why don't you talk this over with your doctor who probably knows best what is happening in terms of Maria's prognosis."

CHAPTER 10

Psychiatric nursing

Psychiatric nursing is the care of patients with severe emotional problems. However, the principles utilized in the care of psychiatric patients are applicable to all patients regardless of their diagnosis. Nursing, concerned with total care, must provide for the individual's physical (soma) as well as emotional (psyche) needs.

The individual is continuously faced with emotional stress from the moment of birth until the moment of death. How people adapt to this stress and the problems resulting from the adaptations are the focus of psychiatric nursing.

In Chapter 5, Behavioral sciences, culture, society, and behavior was presented as an integral part of emotional development. This material should be reviewed before beginning this chapter, which is chiefly concerned with the patterns of behavioral responses commonly identified as manifestations of emotional problems.

BASIC PRINCIPLES OF PSYCHIATRIC NURSING

A. These principles
   1. Are by necessity general in nature
   2. Form the guidelines for the emotional care of all patients
B. In caring for patients, the nurse should attempt to
   1. Accept and respect people as individuals regardless of their behavior
   2. Limit or reject the individual's inappropriate behavior without rejecting the individual
   3. Recognize that all behavior has meaning and is meeting the needs of the performer regardless of how distorted or meaningless it appears to others
   4. Accept the dependency needs of individuals while supporting and encouraging moves toward independence
   5. Help individuals set appropriate limits for themselves or set limits for them when they are unable to do so
   6. Encourage individuals to express their feelings in an atmosphere free of reprisal or judgment
   7. Recognize that individuals need to use their defenses until other defenses can be substituted
   8. Recognize how feelings affect behavior and influence relationships
   9. Recognize that individuals frequently respond to the behavioral expectations of staff members
   10. Recognize that all individuals have a potential for movement toward emotional health

ANXIETY AND BEHAVIOR

A. Anxiety
   1. Is a state of apprehension, tension, or uneasiness
   2. Is an internal phenomenon aroused by impulses
   3. Occurs when the ego is threatened
   4. Frequently stems from an anticipation of danger
   5. May arise from known, unknown, or unrecognized sources
B. Levels of anxiety
   1. Alertness level—an automatic response of the central nervous system that
      a. Prepares the body for danger by regulating internal processes

b. Concentrates all energies for internal activity
2. Apprehension level—a response to anticipation of short-term danger that
   a. Prepares the individual for efficient performance
   b. Occurs when facing new situations
   c. Creates some conscious awareness of discomfort
3. Free-floating level—a response to generalized anxiety that
   a. Creates a feeling of impending doom
   b. Produces an acute feeling of discomfort
4. Panic level—a total response to anxiety characterized by uncontrolled, unrealistic behavior that
   a. Lessens perception of the environment to protect the ego from awareness
   b. Increases the danger to the entire system
C. Defenses
1. Conscious defenses—first line defenses against anxiety that are used by all people in times of stress; they comprise the individual's deliberate effort to maintain control, reduce tension, and limit anxiety (individual may be aware of behavior but is not always aware of underlying reason)
   a. Remove self from source of anxiety
   b. Escape through bodily satisfactions
   c. Focus psychic energy on other more pleasant activities
   d. Use of substitute gratifications
   e. Consciously avoid painful subjects
   f. Give socially acceptable reasons for behavior
   g. Release tensions by acting out impulsively
2. Unconscious defenses—include the second, third, and fourth line defenses against anxiety; these defenses may be used by all people in extremely stressful situations; however, if these defenses are used consistently, the individual is considered emotionally ill
   a. Second line defenses are the personality traits developed to handle interpersonal relationships and protect the ego
      (1) Exaggerated dependency and immaturity

      (2) Passive submission
      (3) Domination of others
      (4) Aggression toward others
      (5) Withdrawal from others
      (6) Compulsive ambition
      (7) Perfectionism and grandiosity
   b. Third line defenses are the neurotic traits developed to handle interpersonal relationships and protect the ego
      (1) Repudiation and opposition of inner drives by the use of reaction formation
      (2) Avoidance of emotional or feeling level by placing complete emphasis on intellectual reasoning
      (3) Inhibition of affective, autonomic, and visceral functions to deaden actual awareness of repressed impulses
      (4) Displacement of impulses to an external object, which is then feared and avoided
      (5) Use of compulsive rituals to magically neutralize inner impulses
   c. Fourth line defenses are the psychotic traits developed to handle interpersonal relationships and protect the ego
      (1) Regression to dependency level of development frequently accompanied by the attitudes and behavior of the child
      (2) Denial and withdrawal from others and reality
      (3) Internalization of hostility
      (4) Excited, uncontrolled acting out
3. As anxiety and the threat to the ego is increased or decreased, shifts in the lines of defense will occur; the individual's behavior is altered by these shifts

PERSONALITY DEFENSES
Defense mechanisms provide initial protection for the personality

A. The more commonly used normal defense mechanisms are presented in Chapter 5 (p. 197)
B. In addition to the normal defenses, all individuals may use compensatory type defenses in times of stress; these defenses,

although still considered normal, serve to further distort reality; if used to excess they frequently create greater emotional problems

1. Conversion—the emotional conflict is unconsciously changed into a physical symptom that can be expressed openly and without anxiety
2. Denial—the emotional conflict is blocked from the conscious mind and the individual refuses to recognize its existence
3. Displacement—the emotions related to an emotionally charged situation or object are shifted to a relatively safe substitute situation or object
4. Fantasy—the conscious distortion of unconscious wishes and needs to obtain gratification and satisfaction
5. Projection—the unconscious denial of unacceptable feelings and emotions in oneself while attributing them to others
6. Reaction formation—the individual unconsciously reverses unacceptable feelings and behaves in the exact opposite manner
7. Regression—the return to an earlier stage of behavior when stress creates problems at the present stage
8. Repression—the involuntary exclusion from consciousness of those ideas, feelings, and situations that are creating conflict and causing discomfort
9. Suppression—the voluntary exclusion from consciousness of those ideas, feelings, and situations that are creating conflict and causing discomfort
10. Transference—feelings and emotions that were previously present toward important figures are applied and attributed to another person in the present

C. As the use of the above compensatory defenses increases and encompasses more of the individual's life, contact with reality is interrupted and distortions begin
D. Identifiable patterns of response begin to form when individuals respond to most situations they encounter with the same type of behavior
E. These patterns of behavior are considered deviations and are usually looked upon as symptoms of emotional problems
F. Although all individuals may, in times of severe emotional stress, use many of the behaviors listed, it is their repetitive use in most situations that is indicative of problems

Deviate patterns of behavior
Withdrawn behavior

A. Definition—a pathologic retreat from or an avoidance of people and the world of reality
B. Developmental factors
1. Unhappy childhood caused by conflict, tension, and anxiety in the home
2. Inconsistent relationships with parents
   a. Lack of firm standards for reward or punishment
   b. Variations between verbal and nonverbal communications
3. Failure to develop a sense of security
4. Failure to develop positive self-image
5. Interpersonal relationships create a continuous source of anxiety
6. Chronic anxiety results in loss of interest in interpersonal relationships and reality testing
7. Extreme sensitivity, narcissism, and introversion develop
C. Compensatory mechanisms used to reduce and avoid stress include
1. Fixation
2. Rigidity and compulsiveness
3. Reaction formation
4. Sublimation
5. Rationalization
6. Regression
D. Effects of compensatory mechanisms on behavior
1. Isolation and failure to test reality result in greater distortions of reality situations
2. Behavior can progress until loss of contact with reality develops and individual retreats into the psychosis usually identified as schizophrenia (pp. 432-433)

Projective behavior

A. Definition—a pathologic denial of one's own feelings, faults, failures, and emotions while continually attributing them to others
B. Developmental factors
1. Parents set extremely high demands and continually raise expected standards of performance
2. Expectations of failure are fostered

creating feelings of inadequacy and feelings of inferiority

3. Childhood experiences continue to reinforce these feelings and chronic insecurity, suspiciousness, and extreme sensitivity develop
4. Feelings of hostility develop and cannot be expressed
5. Inability to establish interpersonal relationships with others interferes with reality testing
6. Individual develops a rigid, structured, narcissistic personality
7. Competitive society fosters and supports projective patterns of behavior

C. Compensatory mechanisms used to reduce and avoid stress include
   1. Displacement
   2. Projection
   3. Rigidity
   4. Denial
   5. Rationalization
   6. Delusions
   7. Ideas of reference

D. Effects of compensatory mechanisms on behavior
   1. Unable to tolerate suspense, prolonged anxiety, or tension
   2. Unacceptable impulses and wishes are denied and faults and failures are disclaimed for self and attributed to others
   3. Delusional ideas develop and begin to dominate behavior
   4. Ideas of reference result in continual misinterpretation of events
   5. Delusions become more systemized and spread out
   6. Behavior can progress until loss of contact with reality is complete and the individual retreats into the psychosis usually identified as paranoid schizophrenia (p. 433) or paranoid states (pp. 433-434)

Aggressive behavior

A. Definition—a pathologic anger and hostility that is turned outward on others or inward upon oneself
B. Developmental factors
   1. Security is chronically threatened, resulting in a continual struggle to maintain it
   2. Strong need for approval
   3. Failure to develop self-concept and self-esteem

4. Chronic anxiety and tension, which is often increased by the real or imagined loss of a love object
5. Demands and responsibilities are high

C. Compensatory mechanisms used to reduce and avoid stress include
   1. Displacement
   2. Rigidity
   3. Denial
   4. Rationalization
   5. Repression
   6. Hostility that can be directed on
      a. Self
      b. Environment

D. Effects of compensatory mechanisms on behavior
   1. Need for approval results in compliance to demands
   2. Necessary compliance creates resentment
   3. Hostility develops and fosters feeling of guilt
   4. Self-doubt increases anxiety and tension
   5. Increased anxiety and tension reduces interpersonal relationships and reality testing
   6. Behavior can progress until there is a complete loss of contact with reality and the individual retreats into the psychosis usually identified as an affective disorder (pp. 430-432)

Psychoneurotic behavior

Includes anxiety reactions, conversion reactions, phobic reactions, and obsessive-compulsive reactions

A. Definition—a maladjustive type of response, characterized by many fears, anxieties, and/or physical symptoms
B. Developmental factors
   1. Usually lack a stable family life and effective guidance
   2. Frequently overprotected and fail to acquire the necessary skills to cope with problems
   3. Experience chronic insecurity, anxiety, and tension
   4. Goals are set for them by the parents and acceptance depends on achieving the goals
   5. Constant struggle to gain reassurance and security
   6. Gains satisfaction from behavior and substitutes this satisfaction for the

satisfaction desired but not obtained through interpersonal relations
C. Compensatory mechanisms used to reduce anxiety and avoid stress include
   1. Displacement
   2. Rationalization
   3. Regression
   4. Rigidity and compulsiveness
   5. Conversion
   6. Denial
D. Effects of compensatory mechanisms on behavior
   1. Behavior is purposeful and is unconsciously resorted to when the person feels threatened
   2. Continued use of behavior can
      a. Create new problems for the individual
      b. Be out of proportion to the degree of stress, impair social effectiveness, and dominate the individual's total life
   3. When impairment of functioning occurs, the individual is usually considered to be deviating from the normal and is usually classified as psychoneurotic (pp. 434-435)

Socially aggressive behavior

A. Definition—a maladjustive response resulting from a defect in the development of the personality that is characterized by peculiar actions or misbehavior
B. Developmental factors
   1. Approval and disapproval do not appear sufficiently strong in childhood to influence the behavior along accepted patterns
   2. Long history of maladjustment that creates more problems as child matures and standards for acceptable behavior are increased
   3. May show a history of severe emotional trauma in early life that interferes with emotional development
   4. Parents frequently provide a cold, emotionally sterile environment
C. Compensatory mechanisms used to reduce anxiety and avoid stress include
   1. Displacement
   2. Repression
   3. Denial
   4. Regression
   5. Hostility
   6. Rejection

D. Effects of compensatory mechanisms on behavior
   1. Appear competent but are usually unreliable and lack a sense of responsibility
   2. Have the potential to succeed but show a history of repeated failure
   3. Lack perseverance, honesty, and sincerity
   4. Completely egocentric and incapable of emotional investment in others
   5. Experience no remorse or shame
   6. Explosive under pressure
   7. Unable to tolerate criticism
   8. Fail to profit from past experiences and care little about the consequences for present acts
   9. Impairment of judgment usually creates problems and brings individual into conflict with society; usually classified as personality disturbances (pp. 435-437)

Addictive behavior

A. Definition—the repeated or chronic use of alcohol or drugs with a resulting dependency on these substances
B. Developmental factors
   1. Feelings of loneliness and isolation develop
   2. Chronic anxiety, fears, and low tension tolerance develop as a result of early relationships
   3. Feelings of inadequacy in interpersonal relationships serve to increase anxiety
   4. Inability to delay satisfaction
   5. Struggles for independence yet unconsciously desires to be dependent
   6. Impulsiveness and resentment of responsibility
C. Compensatory mechanisms used to reduce anxiety and avoid stress include
   1. Denial
   2. Regression
   3. Rationalization
   4. Addiction
   5. Displacement
   6. Fantasy
   7. Repression
D. Effects of compensatory mechanisms on behavior
   1. Drug or alcohol reduces inhibitory self-control
   2. Drug or alcohol allows for expression

of inner feelings but increases the guilt and requires more of the substance to relieve the guilt

3. Alcohol and drugs decrease feelings of inferiority and reduce anxiety
4. Alcohol and drugs increase social isolation and cause deterioration of personal habits
5. Individual becomes increasingly less efficient and devotes less energy to goals and ambitions
6. Dependency and tolerance develop and the substances are needed in increasing amounts to achieve the same dulling of reality
7. Securing the alcohol or drug becomes the main objective in life and functioning is totally impaired; these individuals are then classified as drug addicts (p. 438) or alcoholics (pp. 437-438)

CLASSIFICATION OF MENTAL DISORDERS

The following is the Standard Nomenclature of Mental Disorders that has been adapted from the *Diagnostic and Statistical Manual of Mental Disorders,* ed. 2, published in 1968 by the American Psychiatric Association in Washington, D.C.

A. Organic brain syndromes
  1. Psychoses
    a. Senile and presenile dementia
    b. Alcoholic psychosis
    c. Psychosis associated with intercranial infection
    d. Psychosis associated with other cerebral conditions
    e. Psychosis associated with other physical conditions
  2. Nonpsychotic organic brain syndromes

B. Psychoses not attributed to physical condition
  1. Major affective disorders
  2. Schizophrenia
  3. Paranoid states
  4. Other psychoses

C. Neuroses

D. Personality disorders and certain other nonpsychotic mental disorders
  1. Personality disorders
  2. Sexual deviations
  3. Alcoholism
  4. Drug dependence

E. Psychophysiologic disorders

F. Special symptoms

G. Transient situational disturbances

H. Behavioral disorders of childhood and adolescence

I. Mental retardation

J. Conditions without manifest psychiatric disorders and nonspecific conditions
  1. Social maladjustment without manifest psychiatric disorder
  2. Nonspecific conditions

PATHOLOGY, SYMPTOMS, THERAPIES, AND NURSING APPROACHES FOR THE MAJOR DIAGNOSTIC ENTITIES IN PSYCHIATRY

Organic brain syndromes

Associated with actual changes in the tissue of the brain

Psychoses

A. Acute brain syndrome—syndromes from which patient usually recovers since the situation is often reversible and temporary
  1. Pathology
    a. Infection
      (1) Intracranial or nervous system; e.g., meningitis or encephalitis
      (2) Systemic or toxic; e.g., pneumonia or typhoid
    b. Trauma to the head
    c. Circulatory disturbances resulting in impairment of blood flow to the brain
    d. Metabolic disorders—electrolyte imbalance; e.g., dehydration, diarrhea, vomiting
    e. Drug intoxication or poisoning
    f. Alcoholic intoxication
  2. Symptoms
    a. Delirium and its accompanying confusion, hallucinations, and delusions
    b. Disorientation and confusion as to time, place, identity
    c. Memory defects for both recent and remote facts
    d. Slurring of speech may occur along with an indistinct pronunciation or use of words
    e. Tremors, incoordination, imbalance, and incontinence may develop
  3. Therapy
    a. Reduce causative agent such as fever, toxins, drugs, or alcohol
    b. Prevent further damage

    c. Provide diet high in calories, protein, and vitamins

    d. Provide mild sedative if necessary

  4. Nursing approach

    a. Provide quiet environment, reduce stimuli

    b. Provide assurance to patient and family

    c. Since lability of mood is common, plan care so that the staff approaches these patients when they appear receptive

    d. Ensure adequate intake and output

    e. Observe for changing physiologic and neurologic symptoms

B. Chronic brain syndrome—syndromes from which patient does not recover since the damage is irreversible and permanent; there may be some improvement with treatment of the underlying cause, but disturbances in memory and judgment will remain

  1. Pathology

    a. Prenatal injury or malformation; e.g., hydrocephalus, microcephalus, neurosyphilis

    b. Infections such as general paresis

    c. Alcohol; e.g., alcoholic encephalopathy, Korsakoff's syndrome

    d. Trauma where head injury results in permanent brain damage

    e. Circulatory disturbances causing anoxia and permanent brain damage; e.g., cerebral arteriosclerosis, cerebral vascular accidents

    f. Deterioration and death of brain cells; e.g., senile psychosis

    g. Loss of brain tissue in presenile psychosis; e.g., Alzheimer's disease and Pick's disease

    h. Nutritional deprivation of brain cells; e.g., pellagra

    i. Damage resulting from generalized diseases; e.g., multiple sclerosis, hepatolenticular disease, Huntington's chorea, Parkinson's disease

    j. Damage resulting from pressures of brain tumors

  2. Symptoms—same as those resulting from acute brain syndrome

  3. Therapy—same as those for acute brain syndrome with greater emphasis placed on preventing further damage

  4. Nursing approach

    a. Provide a safe environment

    b. Continually orient the patient to time, date, and place

    c. Keep schedule of activities flexible to utilize patient's lability of moods and easy distractability

    d. Provide adequate nutrition

    e. Provide exercise

    f. Provide diversional activities that the patient enjoys and can handle

Nonpsychotic organic brain syndromes

Included in this classification are all of the acute and chronic brain syndromes in which there is a demonstrable organic change in the brain, but where psychotic behavior is not a major problem

Psychoses not attributed to physical conditions

Classified as functional psychoses since there is no organic basis or change in the structure of the brain

Major affective disorders

A. Manic depressive psychosis

  1. Pathology

    a. Premorbid personality utilizes the compensatory mechanisms associated with the aggressive patterns of behavior

    b. Occurs between 20 and 49 years of age

  2. Symptoms

    a. Cyclic, periodic episodes of acute self-limiting mood swings; can be all manic, all depressed, or mixed manic and depressed; occurring before 40 years of age but after 20 years of age

    b. Individual is able to function at usual activity between episodes

    c. Obesity is a frequent precursor of attack and onset can be slowed or modified by dieting

    d. Depression most common form

      (1) Triad of symptoms are present: lowering of mood tone—dejection, slowing of thinking and speech, and decrease in psychomotor activity

      (2) Insomnia—difficulty in falling asleep and staying asleep, tend to wake early

      (3) Decreased appetite

      (4) Feelings of guilt and worthlessness

(5) Difficulty in performing daily tasks

(6) Tearful with a great deal of suicidal rumination

(7) Speaks slowly and uses monosyllabic words

(8) Orientation and logic are unaffected

(9) Sex drive is decreased

(10) Constipation and urinary retention may occur

e. Manic phase occurs less frequently

(1) Difficulty sleeping

(2) Extremely active—always in a hurry

(3) Humor good although remarks can be caustic

(4) Monopolizes conversations and irritability is only superficially covered

(5) Orientation is clear but judgment is poor

(6) Always planning and scheming

(7) Increased sex drive

3. Therapy

a. Electroconvulsive therapy is the treatment of choice

b. Lithium carbonate, mood elevating psychotherapeutic drugs, and sedatives are used

c. High protein, high carbohydrate diet is provided for energy especially in manic phase

d. Psychotherapy is useful between attacks

4. Nursing approach

a. Monitor patient's intake and output

b. Keep environment nonchallenging and nonstimulating

c. Avoid irritating routines as much as possible

d. Protect patient against suicide during the entire episode

e. Keep activities simple, uncomplicated, and repetitive in nature; they should be of short duration and require little concentration

f. Overactive manic patients should be

(1) Accepted by staff even though their behavior may be rejected

(2) Permitted to express hostility and ambivalence without reinforcement of guilt feelings

(3) Approached in a calm, collected manner by staff that have good self-control

(4) Given limits for their behavior

(5) Responded to in a nonargumentative manner, using their easy distractability

(6) Approached in a consistent manner by all staff

g. Depressed patient should

(1) Be allowed time for their slowness

(2) Be accepted even when they are unable to carry out daily routines

(3) Be given demands they can meet

(4) Be helped to express hostility and have their responses accepted without rejection

(5) Have their self-esteem realistically built up

(6) Be presented with simple rather than complex routines and activities

(7) Have their feelings of worthlessness accepted as real to them; their feelings should not be denied, condoned, or approved, just accepted

(8) Be protected against suicidal attacks especially when the depression begins to lift (suicide is a real and ever-present danger)

B. Psychotic depressive reactions

1. Pathology—similar to manic depressive psychosis except

a. Occurs before 20 years of age or after 60 years of age

b. Precipitating factor can always be identified

2. Symptoms

a. Severe depression

b. Absence of history of repeated episodes

c. Gross misinterpretations of reality

3. Therapy—same as manic depressive psychosis

4. Nursing approach—same as manic depressive psychosis

C. Involutional depressive psychosis

1. Pathology similar to manic depressive psychosis except

a. Depression is agitated rather than retarded

b. Depression occurs after 40 years of age and before 60 years of age
c. Precipitating factors such as the marriage of children, the loss of a job, the breakup of a marriage, the death of a partner can often be identified
d. Depression is closely related to the menopause or climacteric, and hormonal and endocrine changes are considered by many to play an important role in this disorder
e. Individual is usually rigid, inflexible, overassertive, overly meticulous, and worrisome

2. Symptoms
a. Wakes early after difficulty in falling asleep
b. Feelings of unreality and sinfulness
c. Complains of somatic delusions
d. Extremely jumpy and agitated
e. Pacing and wringing of hands as well as other increased motor activity
f. Triad of symptoms present—delusions of sin and/or poverty, obsession with death, somatic delusions especially related to the gastrointestinal tract

3. Therapy—same as manic depressive psychosis
4. Nursing approach—same as manic depressive psychosis

Schizophrenia

This syndrome constitutes the largest group of behavioral disorders in our society; at the present time 1 person in 100 will spend some time in a hospital with this disorder and this number is increasing

A. Pathology
1. Premorbid personality—individuals use the compensatory mechanism of the withdrawn pattern of behavior; in addition, the paranoid schizophrenic uses the compensatory mechanism of the projective pattern of behavior
2. Severe emotional problems, although unrecognized, begin early in life; however, the most common age for the break with reality is from 18 to 34 years of age
3. There is a chronic insecurity and almost a total failure in interpersonal relationships
4. Etiology is still unknown although some interesting findings in genetics, biochemistry, psychology, and sociology present hope for a breakthrough
5. Regardless of the ultimate etiology, there appears to be a close causal relationship with the environment
6. Course of the disease is either acute or chronic; although it can stop or retrogress at any point, it does not appear to ever permit a full restoration of integrity to the personality

B. Symptoms
1. Alterations in feeling, thinking, and relating to the external world are present
2. Association defects occur and associative links weaken; the individual appears incoherent, bizarre, and unpredictable
3. Distortions interfere with attention, perception, concentration, and memory
4. Affect and emotional expression are flattened
5. Ambivalence is common and frequently is so exaggerated that any action or decision becomes impossible
6. Detachment from reality results in autistic thinking and serves to further distort reality
7. Disturbance occurs in body image since the undeveloped ego has few strengths and no boundaries (frequently refer to self in the second or third person instead of using the first person)
8. Secondary symptoms such as hallucinations, delusions, confusion, stupor, and catatonia may or may not be present

C. Types of schizophrenia—although historically a great deal of time and effort were directed toward identifying types of schizophrenia, it should be recognized that the classification is not static; there is a great deal of overlapping symptomatology; individuals diagnosed as being in one classification frequently are diagnosed at a later time in another classification
1. Simple schizophrenia—rarely hospitalized since they are the unattached, withdrawn, affectively and intellectually diminished individuals who are

a part of the vagabond or transient groups of our society

2. Hebephrenic schizophrenia—picture of severe and pronounced mental incapacity; great mental and emotional deterioration occurs; behavior is retarded with sexual preoccupations, emotional dulling, infantile silliness; onset is usually between 12 and 25 years of age

3. Catatonic schizophrenia—picture of withdrawal and distortions in reality testing, accompanied by total ambivalence, which is frequently exhibited in rather unpredictable motor activity; the ambivalence makes movement and decision making impossible since the individual cannot decide how or where to move; they can be literally frozen in their tracks—akinetic (stuporous)—or forced into the aimless hyperkinetic fugue (excited) movements

4. Paranoid schizophrenia—these individuals use the withdrawn compensatory mechanisms to distort reality and then develop a rather intricate delusional system by using the projective pattern of behavior; they are secretive, suspicious, use ideas of references, and finally develop delusions of grandeur

5. Undifferentiated schizophrenia—these individuals demonstrate the primary thought, affect, and withdrawal defects of schizophrenia but cannot be classified under a specific type because of mixed symptoms

6. Schizoaffective schizophrenia—these individuals demonstrate a mixture of symptoms from both the schizophrenia and the affective reactions; the thought processes and bizarre behavior appears schizophrenic but there is usually marked elation or depression; such individuals usually prove to be basically schizophrenic in nature

7. Pseudoneurotic schizophrenia—these individuals appear neurotic but cannot function as a neurotic; they present the autism, ambivalence, and thought disturbances of the schizophrenic while also demonstrating the all-pervading anxiety of the neurotic; such individuals are difficult to diagnose but usually prove to be basically schizophrenic in nature

D. Therapy
1. Administration of chlorpromazine and other major tranquilizers
2. Psychotherapy—both individual and group
3. Motivation therapy
4. Occupational therapy
5. Electroconvulsive therapy may be useful in some instances to modify behavior

E. Nursing approach
1. Observe for adverse drug reactions in all patients receiving large doses of the major tranquilizers
2. Encourage patients to follow a plan of organized activity
3. Respect patients as human beings with both dignity and worth
4. Accept patients at their present level of functioning
5. Avoid trying to argue patients out of their delusions or hallucinations
6. Accept that the patients' hallucinations and delusions are real and frightening to them
7. Encourage the development of interpersonal relationships between patients and others
8. Point out reality to patients but do not force your reality upon them
9. Accept patients' misinterpretation of events

Paranoid states

Those individuals who demonstrate the suspiciousness and delusions common to paranoid conditions but who do not exhibit the thinking and behavioral disorganization or the personality disintegration found in the other psychoses

A. Pathology
1. The premorbid personality uses the compensatory mechanism of the projective pattern of behavior
2. Paranoid defenses are considered by some to be defenses against unconscious homosexuality or overt hostility
3. Exact etiology is unknown

B. Symptoms
1. Paranoia—these individuals exhibit a rather elaborate, highly organized paranoid delusional system while preserving the other functions of the personality; in spite of this system, think-

ing is not interfered with and personality function usually continues without interruption

2. Involutional paranoid state—these individuals experience an onset of delusions during the involutional period; the thought and emotional disorganization of schizophrenia is absent; the depressive overtones present lead many to believe that this state is a manifestation of the involutional psychosis

C. Therapy

1. Chemotherapy with tranquilizers is the most helpful in treating these individuals

2. Individual psychotherapy may provide some relief of symptoms

3. Electroconvulsive therapy may prove helpful for some patients

4. Paranoid patients are the most challenging to reach since none of the present therapies appear to be helpful in breaking down the delusional system

D. Nursing approach

1. Provide an environment with some intellectual challenge that does not threaten security

2. Avoid counter-aggression and retaliation against the patient

3. Accept and recognize patient's need for superior attitude

4. Meet sarcasm and ridicule in a matter of fact manner

5. Guard patient's self-esteem from attack by other patients

6. Accept patient's misinterpretations of events

7. Point out reality but don't directly challenge patient's delusions

Neuroses

Common responses to emotional problems that are rarely treated in psychiatric settings; they are disturbances in personality but there is no great defect in reality testing or severe antisocial behavior

A. Pathology

1. All six subgroups of the neuroses use the compensatory mechanisms of the psychoneurotic pattern of behavior

2. The development of the symptoms usually permits some measure of social adjustment

3. Usually begins in early 20s as a result of environmental factors in childhood

4. Early life is rigid and orderly

5. Pressures of decision making regarding life style that occur in the early adult years seem to act as precipitating factors

6. Individuals are usually of superior intellectual capacity

B. Symptoms

1. Anxiety reactions—anxiety is unconsciously expressed through physical means

a. Pervasive, continuous feeling of free-floating anxiety, tension, and apprehension

b. Episodes of dyspnea, palpitations, irritability, dizziness, insomnia, fainting, weakness, chest pain, trembling, and headaches

c. Symptoms usually appear in relation to stress situations such as crowded rooms, public gatherings, pregnancy, military service, etc.

d. Patient appears anxious and is often mildly depressed

2. Conversion reactions—anxiety is unconsciously converted to physical symptoms

a. Patient presents a history of loss of motor or sensory function without any adequate physical cause; e.g., paralysis, blindness, deafness

b. There is a noticeable lack of concern about the problem; this lack of concern has been labeled *la belle indifférence*

c. Impairment may vary over different episodes and does not follow anatomic structure; paralysis or numbness may circle the foot or arm instead of beginning at the joint and is known as stocking and glove anesthesia

d. Patient appears relieved by symptoms and demonstrates little anxiety when observed

3. Dissociative reactions—anxiety is unconsciously isolated from consciousness

a. Alterations in state of consciousness

b. Patient attempts to deal with anxiety by walling off certain areas of reality

c. Frequently expressed as amnesia or somnambulism (sleepwalking)

d. Patient escapes by isolating self from situation
e. In very rare instances multiple personalities may develop; they result from the splitting off of certain mental processes from the main body of consciousness; the multiple personalities may be two or more organized systems of behavior that take turns in controlling the individual; co-conscious personalities are usually aware of the conscious personality but the conscious personality is usually unaware of the co-conscious personalities

4. Phobic reactions—anxiety is unconsciously transferred to an inanimate object, which then symbolically represents the neurotic conflict and can be avoided
  a. Anxiety appears when patients find themselves in places that threaten their sense of security
  b. Patients attempt to avoid these distressing situations
  c. Depending on the phobic object, the individual's life style can be greatly limited
  d. Common phobias include
    (1) Acrophobia—high places
    (2) Astraphobia—thunder and lightning
    (3) Claustrophobia—closed places
    (4) Hydrophobia—water
    (5) Photophobia—strong lights

5. Obsessive-compulsive reactions—unconscious control of anxiety by the use of rituals and thoughts
  a. Patients complain about thoughts that persist and become repetitive and obsessive
  b. These thoughts may be turned into compulsions that are repetitive acts of irrational behavior that the individual is emotionally forced to carry out although they serve no rational purpose
  c. Patients are indecisive and demonstrate a striving for perfection and superiority
  d. Intellectual and verbal defenses are used
  e. Anxiety and depression may be present in various degrees particularly if rituals are prevented

6. Depressive reactions—guilt and depression are used unconsciously to relieve anxiety
  a. Symptoms of depression, insomnia, anorexia, decreased sexual drive, weight loss, constipation, fatigue; closely resembles manic-depressive psychosis but differs in depth and awareness of reality
  b. Depression is real and suicide can occur

C. Therapy
  1. Complete medical work-up to reassure patient and rule out medical problems
  2. Psychotherapy in the form of psychoanalysis
  3. Sedatives and minor tranquilizers may be used if necessary

D. Nursing approach
  1. Accept symptoms as real to patient
  2. Attempt to limit use of defenses, but do not stop them until patient is ready to give them up
  3. Encourage patient to develop a balance between work and play
  4. Help patient develop better ways of handling anxiety-producing situations
  5. Accept physical symptoms, but do not emphasize or call attention to them
  6. Reduce demands on the individual as much as possible

Personality disorders and certain other nonpsychotic mental disorders
Personality disorders

Borderline states falling between the neuroses and psychoses, characterized by defects in the development of the personality or by pathologic trends in its structure

A. Personality can be defined as
  1. The sum of all traits that differentiates one individual from another
  2. The total behavior pattern of an individual through which the inner interests are expressed
  3. The individual's unique and distinctive way of behaving and reacting to the environment
  4. The constellation of defense mechanisms for dealing with inner and outer pressures

B. Pathology
  1. Habitual attitudes and reaction patterns in human relationships develop early in life and form the character structure of the individual

2. In most instances these behaviors create little discomfort or stress
3. The personality disturbances are, in reality, the selection and utilization of specific defense mechanisms that are used so often that they form a lifelong pattern of action that, while not normal, is neither neurotic nor psychotic
4. The premorbid personality of individuals demonstrating any of the 10 classified personality disturbances resembles the compensatory mechanism associated with the psychotic or neurotic counterpart

C. Symptoms
1. Paranoid personality
   a. Frequent use of projective mechanisms
   b. Presence of suspiciousness, fear, irritability, and stubbornness
   c. Reality testing is not greatly impaired
2. Cyclothymic personality
   a. Alternating mood swings between elation and sadness, which seem unrelated to external environment
   b. Usually warm and friendly, approaching life with an obvious enthusiasm
   c. Mood swings do not demonstrate great emotional intensity
3. Schizoid personality
   a. Avoidance of meaningful interpersonal relationships
   b. Use of autistic thinking, emotional detachment, and daydreaming
   c. Although introverted since childhood, maintain fair contact with reality
4. Explosive personality
   a. Periodic outbursts of rage with verbal and/or physical acting out
   b. These outbursts are intense and unable to be controlled
   c. Outbursts are easily stimulated by environmental stresses
5. Obsessive-compulsive personality
   a. Characterized by rigidity, overconscientiousness, and an inordinate capacity for work
   b. Individuals are driven by obsessive concerns
   c. Behavior contains many rituals
6. Hysterical personality
   a. Characterized by emotional instability and great excitability

b. Behavior is extroverted and directed toward gaining attention
   c. These individuals are vain and deliberately manipulative
7. Asthenic personality
   a. Characterized by lack of enthusiasm
   b. Overwhelmed by physical and emotional stress
   c. Appear unable to experience enjoyment
8. Antisocial personality (sociopathic personality disturbances)
   a. Chronic lifelong disturbances that conflict with society's laws and customs
   b. Unable to postpone gratification
   c. Randomly act out their aggressive egocentric impulses on society
   d. Do not profit from past experience or punishment and live only for the moment
   e. Have the ability to ingratiate themselves but they "do not wear well"
   f. Are in contact with reality but do not seem to care about it
9. Passive-aggressive personality
   a. Rather helpless and indecisive demonstrating passive obstructionism while clinging and pouting
   b. Frequent outbursts and temper tantrums when frustrated
   c. Frequently create many problems for others
10. Inadequate personality
    a. Limited intellectual, emotional, social, and physical response
    b. Appear to be mentally deficient but are not
    c. Demonstrate poor judgment and social ineptness

D. Therapy
1. Difficult to get into treatment
2. Considered sane and responsible for their actions
3. Pose severe problems in rehabilitation
4. Because of their personality makeup, these individuals are hesitant to invest the necessary energies and emotions in therapy

E. Nursing approach
1. Maintain consistency in approach
2. Accept patients as they are and do not retaliate against the obvious flaws in behavior

3. Protect them from other patients and other patients from them
4. Place realistic limits on behavior and let individual know what the limits are

Sexual deviations

Changing social and cultural mores have resulted in removing many of the sexual behaviors that were previously considered deviations from the list; sexual deviations today are considered those sexual activities directed toward objects other than people of the opposite sex and toward sexual acts not considered "normal" or not performed under usual circumstances

A. Pathology—may be symptomatic of other personality or psychiatric disorders or may occur as a behavior aberration of a disordered personality
B. Symptoms
1. Homosexuality—sexual relations between members of the same sex as the preferred method of gratification; when this relationship occurs between 2 consenting adults, some no longer consider it a sexual deviation
2. Fetishism—substitution of an inanimate object for the genitals
3. Transvestism—individual wears clothing of the opposite sex to achieve sexual pleasure
4. Exhibitionism—sexual pleasure is obtained by exposing the genitals
5. Pedophilia—attraction to children as sex objects
6. Voyeurism—sexual gratification obtained by watching the sexual play of others
7. Sadism—cruelty to others is substituted for or must accompany the sex act
8. Masochism—self-suffering is substituted for or must accompany the sex act
C. Therapy—rather unsuccessful with these individuals unless they really want to change; if change is desired, psychoanalysis is most effective
D. Nursing approach
1. Accept patients even though their sexual behavior may be repulsive
2. Avoid punitive remarks or responses
3. Protect patient from others
4. Set limits on patient's sexual acting out
5. Provide diversional activities

Alcoholism

Alcohol intake that interferes with normal functioning or is necessary as a prerequisite to normal functioning

A. Pathology—premorbid personality utilizes the compensatory mechanisms of the addictive pattern of behavior
B. Patterns of drinking and symptoms
1. Intoxication—a state in which coordination or speech is impaired and behavior is altered
2. Episodic excessive drinking—individual becomes intoxicated as infrequently as 4 times a year; episodes may vary in length from hours to days or weeks
3. Habitual excessive drinking—individual becomes intoxicated more than 12 times a year or is recognizably under the influence of alcohol more than once a week even though not considered intoxicated
4. Alcohol addiction—direct or strong presumptive evidence that individual is dependent on alcohol; evidence may be demonstrated by withdrawal symptoms or by the inability to go for a day without drinking; when there is a history of heavy drinking for 3 or more months the individual is considered addicted to alcohol
5. Early symptoms of alcoholism include frequent drinking sprees, increase in intake, drinking alone or in the early morning, occurrence of blackouts
C. Therapy
1. Should be multifaceted social and medical; involves psychotherapy, both individual and group, especially Alcoholics Anonymous
2. Negative conditioning with the use of disulfiram (Antabuse) appears to help
3. Patients can only be assisted when they admit they need help
4. Physical needs must be cared for since dietary needs have often been ignored for long periods
D. Nursing approach
1. Provide well-controlled, alcohol-free environment
2. Plan a full program of activities but provide adequate rest periods
3. Meet patient's need for a great deal of support without criticism or judgment

4. Avoid trying to talk patient out of problem
5. Accept individual's smooth facade while approaching the lonely and fearful individual behind it
6. Accept failures without judgment or punishment
7. Accept hostility without criticism or retaliation
8. Recognize ambivalence and limit need for decision making
9. Maintain patient's interest in therapy program

Drug dependence

The misuse of drugs usually by self-administration
A. Pathology—premorbid personality utilizes the compensatory mechanisms of the addictive pattern of behavior
B. Definitions
1. Addiction—the condition of habituation and tolerance to drugs other than alcohol, tobacco, and ordinary caffeine-containing beverages; medically prescribed drugs are excluded if they are taken under medical direction; addiction can occur simultaneously to 2 or more drugs or to alcohol and drugs; lately combined addiction to a multiplicity of drugs has become more common
2. Habituation—no physical dependency exists but the individual desires and becomes psychologically accustomed to a drug
3. Tolerance—the condition of physical dependency to a drug in which the presence of the drug in increasingly higher dosage is needed to achieve the same effect; tolerance can exceed the usual lethal limits of a drug
C. Symptoms
1. Needle marks on limbs along path of veins
2. Addicted individuals tend to wear long sleeve shirts even in warm weather
3. Yawning, lacrimation, rhinorrhea, and perspiration appear 10 to 15 hours after last opiate injection
4. Severe abdominal cramps will develop if too much time elapses between injections
5. Physical examination usually reveals an underweight, malnourished individual with multiple dental caries and depressed central nervous system functioning
D. Therapy
1. Treatment is far from satisfactory and costly
2. Methadone maintenance programs do not treat addiction but change the addiction from an illegal drug to a legal drug, which is administered under supervision; has only proved successful in individuals with long-standing addictions
3. High caloric, high protein, high vitamin diet because of poor eating habits
4. Treatment in groups run by ex-addicts appears to be achieving the most success for abstinence
5. Psychotherapy should be provided if mental problems are present
6. If patient is to be withdrawn from drugs, decreasing amounts of methadone and/or tranquilizers must be administered to reduce physiologic and psychologic discomfort
D. Nursing approach
1. Set firm controls and keep area drug free
2. Do not permit patients to leave the hospital impulsively
3. Keep atmosphere pleasant and cheerful but not overly stimulating
4. Contribute to patient's self-confidence, self-respect, and security in a realistic manner
5. Walk the fine line between a relatively permissive but firm attitude
6. Expect and accept evasion, escape, and negativism, but require the patient to shoulder certain standards of responsibility
7. Accept the patient without approving the behavior
8. Do not permit patients to isolate themselves
9. Introduce patient to group activities as soon as possible
10. Protect patients from themselves and others

Psychophysiologic disorders

A. Physical illnesses where psychogenic factors are the predominant causative agents
B. Anxiety stimulates the autonomic nervous system and the nervous and endo-

crine impulses appear to center on one particular organ, creating actual physical illness and changes in the tissue structure

C. The reason a certain organ is involved with one patient and a different organ with another is still undetermined
  1. Pathology—premorbid personality appears to be one of unexpressed aggression resulting from the unresolved struggle between dependent need and independent striving
  2. Symptoms
     a. Skin
        (1) In neurodermatitis, dermatitis factitia, pruritus, and trichotillomania, psychic factors appear to dominate
        (2) There appears to be a relationship between endocrine imbalance and disturbances in the autonomic regulation of skin physiology
        (3) Stress seems to lead to rash, itching, and discomfort
     b. Musculoskeletal
        (1) Anxiety and fear often create a tightening of muscles
        (2) This becomes an aggravating factor in arthritis, backache, tension headache, or any other musculoskeletal disorder in which increased tension and spasm are involved
     c. Respiratory
        (1) Hyperventilation syndrome
           (a) Panting occurs with tension and excitment and this forced respiration can produce biochemical changes in the blood
           (b) These changes can alter the cerebral circulation and cause a reduction in consciousness and syncope
        (2) Bronchial asthma
           (a) Stress and tension appear to create increased secretions and changes in the bronchi
           (b) Individuals with asthma tend to exhibit a strong desire for protection and dependency yet fear rejection

           (c) The wheeze associated with asthma is considered by some to be a suppressed cry for this protection
     d. Cardiovascular
        (1) Essential hypertension
           (a) Anxiety and other stresses are believed to play a role in releasing a pressor from the kidney, which causes chronic vasoconstriction of the vessels
           (b) All other primary causes for hypertension must be ruled out before this cause can be diagnosed
           (c) Individuals with hypertension have difficulty handling hostile feelings, are less assertive, and have more obsessive-compulsive traits than nonhypertensive ones
           (d) Hypertension may be considered a state of chronically unexpressed rage that arises from conflicts between passive-dependent longings and the struggle for independence
        (2) Coronary occlusion and angina
           (a) Coronary attacks frequently occur following periods of fatigue and anxiety
           (b) These individuals place a high value on work and success; they become depressed when inactive
     e. Hemolymphatic
        (1) Certain blood dyscrasias and responses can be linked to emotional stress
        (2) In some individuals the neutrophil count drops, the clotting time is decreased, both blood viscosity and erythrocyte sedimentation rate rise
        (3) Nature of this response to stress is still controversial
     f. Gastrointestinal
        (1) Peptic ulcer
           (a) Anxiety and other stress

appear to create a condition of hyperactivity, hypersecretion, hyperacidity, and engorgement of the mucosa

(b) Related to stresses in life, particularly those concerned with conflicts between passivity and aggression

(c) Use reaction formation to cover the strong, somewhat irrational need to achieve security from others

(2) Ulcerative colitis

(a) Parasympathetic stimulation of the lower bowel produces an enzyme that interferes with the protective coating of the bowel

(b) May occur as a reaction to a variety of stresses but most often in situations that demand accomplishment and arouse fear of not succeeding

(c) Many patients are immature and have not gained any feelings of independence

g. Genitourinary

(1) Disturbances in genital and urinary problems may occur under stress

(2) Enuresis, amenorrhea, frigidity, and impotence appear to be related to psychologic factors

(3) Depression and feelings of helplessness may be related to urinary retention

(4) Fear may be related to urgency and frequency

h. Endocrine

(1) Eating patterns and dependency on food for satisfaction and reduction of stress appears related to both diabetes mellitus and obesity

(2) Feelings of insecurity and an unusual sense of responsibility appear associated with onset of hyperthyroidism

i. Organs of special sense—some evidence that certain neurologic disturbances, such as atypical facial neuralgia, are related to emotional conflict

3. Therapy—must be directed toward both the physical and emotional problems

4. Nursing approach

a. Reduce emotional stimulation when possible

b. Explain all procedures carefully and allow patient time for questions

c. Provide patient with talking time

d. Avoid material that appears to stimulate conflict for the patient

e. Accept patient's behavior and encourage expression of feelings

f. Remember patient is really physically ill and the symptoms have a physiologic basis

Special symptoms

Primary symptoms of emotional conflict rather than symptoms of other emotional disorders

A. Pathology—mainly unknown, does seem to relate to unresolved conflicts

B. Symptoms

1. Learning disturbances—appear in children of normal intelligence

2. Speech disturbances—stuttering and stammering

3. Somnambulism—sleepwalking

4. Enuresis that is not related to genitourinary problems

C. Therapy—determine the underlying cause of the conflict and work toward resolution

D. Nursing approach

1. Recognize and accept that a problem exists

2. Help the patient and/or parents identify the problem

3. Support and avoid humiliation of the patient

Transient situational disturbances

Acute reactions to overwhelming environmental stress

A. Pathology

1. No apparent underlying mental disorder in these individuals although present behavior may be extremely disturbed

2. The individual seems to have the ca-

pacity to adapt to the overwhelming stress when given the time to do so

3. Problems with distortions or interruptions in thinking process and decision making tend to resolve themselves

B. Symptoms

1. Adjustment reaction of infancy—the infant is upset and demonstrates grief when separated from the mother

2. Adjustment reaction of childhood—the child regresses to an earlier level of development when a new sibling arrives or experiences intense anxiety on entering school

3. Adjustment reaction of adolescence—the adolescent's struggle for independence leads to hypersensitivity and frequent episodes of heightened anxiety

4. Adjustment reactions of adult life—the adult experiences heightened anxiety in response to the stresses associated with marriage, pregnancy, divorce, change of employment, purchase of a house, etc.

5. Adjustment reaction of later life—the menopause and climacteric, the plan for retirement, the "loss" of children to marriage, and the death of a mate all serve to produce extreme stress situations

Behavioral disorders of childhood and adolescence

A. Diagnosis is difficult since pathology must be separated from the normal disturbances that occur during this period of life

B. The most common problems found in children are the personality disorders and the psychophysiologic disorders; the neuroses and the psychoses are less common

C. The American Psychiatric Association has classified these disorders under the behavior exhibited

1. Hyperkinetic reaction
2. Withdrawal reaction
3. Overanxious reaction
4. Run away reaction
5. Unsocialized aggressive reaction
6. Group delinquent reaction

D. The symptoms exhibited by children so classified can arise from organic or environmental pathology

E. Behavioral disorders can occur as a response to illness

1. Pathology
   a. Can be responses to alterations in the central nervous system cells such as those created by
      (1) Infectious disorders such as high fevers
      (2) Communicable diseases such as viral, toxic, or postinfectious encephalitis
      (3) Anemias and blood dyscrasias
      (4) Brain lesions or tumors
   b. Can be responses to organic changes in other body tissues and cells such as those created by
      (1) Thyroid, adrenal, and pituitary glands
      (2) Any change in any part of the endocrine or autonomic nervous system
   c. Can be responses to the stress of being ill
      (1) Regression to earlier levels of development occurs with any illness
      (2) Restriction in activities, pain, and separation

2. Symptoms—the symptoms of these disorders depend on the cells affected as well as the child's ability to contain or integrate the experience

3. Therapy—therapy is directed at reducing the underlying cause of the problem

4. Nursing approach—since the nursing approach for children and adolescents is similar for all types of behavioral disorders it will be summarized at the end of this area

F. Behavioral disorders can occur as symptoms of neuroses

1. To be classified as neurotic behavior, disorders should meet the following criteria; the behavior
   a. Is destructive to the child's own general aims
   b. Is repeated despite rational arguments to the contrary and despite punishment
   c. Involves the discharge of affects stemming from unconscious conflicts
   d. Leads to getting caught and punished

2. Pathology—the same developmental

factors listed under the psychoneurotic pattern of behavior are involved

3. Symptoms—the more common types of neuroses found in childhood are
   a. Sleeping difficulties—somnambulism and insomnia
   b. Stealing—truancy and running away
   c. Learning difficulties—severe reading problems, underachievement, school phobias, reverse or backward reading (the reading from right to left rather than left to right)
   d. Enuresis—bedwetting
   e. Regressive reaction
   f. Physiologic disturbances
      (1) Eating problems—nausea and vomiting
      (2) Excretion problems—constipation or diarrhea
      (3) Respiratory and circulatory problems—asthma and tachycardia
      (4) Allergies—skin rashes and hives
   g. Excessive rebelliousness
   h. Excessive conformity

4. Therapy
   a. Psychotherapy—in children, usually in the form of play therapy
   b. Medications—amphetamines and mild tranquilizers are quite effective with children

5. Nursing approach—since the nursing approach for children and adolescents is similar for all types of behavioral disorders it will be summarized at the end of this area

G. Behavioral disorders can occur as symptoms of psychoses
1. The psychoses of children have 2 basic features
   a. An alienation or withdrawal from reality
   b. A severe disturbance in the child's feeling of self-identity

2. Pathology
   a. As with adult psychoses, many theories are being studied as causes of child psychoses; however, no definitive cause has as yet been established
   b. Failure to develop satisfactory relationships with the significant adults regardless of the cause, appears to be an underlying problem with all of these children

3. Symptoms
   a. General symptoms
      (1) Inability to differentiate between self and environment
      (2) Confusion in self-boundaries frequently characterized by speaking of self only in the third person
      (3) A defect in ego formation or an inadequate functioning ego system
      (4) A conflict between self and reality
      (5) A defect in the adaptive, inhibitory, and steering mechanisms of the personality
      (6) Interference with intellect may be so profound, child appears to be mentally retarded
   b. Autistic psychosis
      (1) Lack of meaningful relationships with outside world
      (2) Use of autistic fantasy resulting in communication defects
      (3) Turning to inanimate objects and self-centered activity for security
   c. Symbiotic psychosis
      (1) Intense though morbid relationship between mother and child
      (2) Child unable to separate identity from that of mother
      (3) Lacks adequate concept of reality
      (4) Inability to relate to peers or adults
   d. Childhood schizophrenia
      (1) Profound apathy
      (2) Looseness of association
      (3) Autistic thinking
      (4) Ambivalence
      (5) Absence of communication skills
      (6) Poor grasp of reality
      (7) Bizarre, unpredictable, uncontrolled behavior
      (8) Inability to relate to others
      (9) Total interference with intellectual functioning

4. Therapy
   a. Psychotherapy directed toward the developmental level of the child—play, group, or individual therapy

b. Medications—tranquilizers and amphetamines provide some reduction of symptoms

c. Removal from the home situation may be necessary although day school type situations frequently provide enough relief so that hospitalization can be avoided

5. Nursing approach—these approaches are general and provide a guide that can be used for the care of all children with emotional problems; care should be directed toward helping the child grow up emotionally by

a. Establishing a favorable environment in which the child can gain or regain a favorable equilibrium

b. Establishing a constructive relationship

c. Helping child to see self as a worthwhile person

d. Recognizing that the behavior has meaning for the child

e. Being as realistic and as truthful as possible in dealing with the child

f. Attempting to establish trust

g. Setting limits that are as realistic as possible but as firm as necessary

h. Pointing out reality but accepting the child's views of it while pointing it out

i. Being consistent both in approach and in rules and regulations

j. Making all explanations as clear as possible

k. Supporting and encouraging the child's moves toward independence but allowing dependency when necessary

Mental retardation

The area of mental retardation is covered in Pediatric nursing (pp. 395-396)

Conditions without manifest psychiatric disorders and nonspecific conditions

A. Individuals without diagnosable psychosis or other psychiatric illness who have problems that are severe enough to interfere with their usual level of functioning are included in this category

B. This category includes social maladjustment, marital maladjustment, occupational maladjustment, and the dissocial behavioral group

C. These individuals usually benefit from brief psychotherapy but can progress to the other psychiatric disorders if help is not received

Community mental health services

A. Purposes
   1. To provide prevention, treatment, and rehabilitation services for individuals and families with emotional problems
   2. To maintain these individuals and families in the community
   3. To provide hospital care within the community in those instances when the individual cannot be maintained on an outpatient basis

B. Types of settings in which services are provided
   1. Outpatient services
      a. Storefront clinics
      b. Walk-in clinics in hospitals
      c. Emergency rooms
      d. Crisis intervention centers including hot-line phone centers
      e. Day-care centers
      f. Private offices
   2. Inpatient services
      a. Specialized psychiatric hospitals
      b. General hospital psychiatric units
   3. After-care services
      a. Foster homes
      b. Halfway houses
      c. Sheltered workshops
      d. Day-care services

C. Types of services
   1. Observation and diagnosis
   2. Assessment of patient's needs
   3. Provide direct care services to patients including
      a. Individual and/or group therapy
      b. Medications
      c. Electroconvulsive therapy
      d. Occupational therapy
      e. Recreational therapy
   4. Provide a therapeutic milieu that
      a. Supports the individual during the period of crisis
      b. Helps the individual learn new ways of coping with problems
   5. Referral to proper community agencies for necessary services
   6. Provide educational setting for key professional groups in mental health concepts

D. The nurse's role includes
   1. Case finding
   2. Assessment of patient's needs

3. Establishment of the therapeutic milieu
4. Consultation with other professionals; e.g., physicians, psychologists, social workers, school teachers, clergy, etc.
5. Active participation with the health team including the patient and family
6. Active involvement in individual and group therapy
7. Coordination of health services for the patient and family
8. Education of groups within the community

REVIEW QUESTIONS FOR PSYCHIATRIC NURSING

1. During the oedipal stage of growth and development, the child
   1. Loves the parent of the same sex and hates the parent of the opposite sex
   2. Loves the parent of the same sex and the opposite sex
   3. Has ambivalence toward both parents
   4. Loves the parent of the opposite sex and hates the parent of the same sex
2. Which stage of growth and development is basically concerned with role identification?
   1. Oral
   2. Oedipal
   3. Latency
   4. Genital
3. Autism can usually be diagnosed when the child is about
   1. 6 months of age
   2. 1 to 3 months of age
   3. 2 years of age
   4. 6 years of age
4. The autistic child responds to
   1. Loud cheerful music
   2. Own self-stimulating acts
   3. Individuals in small groups
   4. Large group activity
5. The autistic child is often obsessed with
   1. Brightly colored toys and blocks
   2. Mechanical and inanimate objects
   3. Dancing and music
   4. Faces and hands
6. An observable symptom of the autistic child is
   1. Sad blank facial expressions
   2. Flapping of hands, rocking
   3. Smiling, flat personality
   4. Lack of response to any stimulus
7. Which one of the following is most characteristic of the emotionally disturbed child?
   1. Responds to any stimulus
   2. Totally involved with the environment
   3. Responds to little external stimulus
   4. Seems unresponsive to the environment
8. Given a choice, the emotionally disturbed child would usually enjoy playing with a
   1. Cuddly toy
   2. Large red block
   3. Small yellow block
   4. Playground merry-go-round

9. When there is nothing organically wrong with the organs of communication and yet the individual is unable to communicate, the condition is referred to as
   1. Organic psychosis
   2. Mental deficiency
   3. Chronic brain pathology
   4. Functional psychosis
10. Functional mental illnesses are mainly the result of
    1. Genetic endowment
    2. Deterioration of brain tissue
    3. Infection and inflammation
    4. Social environment
11. Schizophrenia is classified as a functional psychosis. This means that the
    1. Genes of the child may carry the schizophrenic factor
    2. Brain itself undergoes actual physical change that produces the symptoms of schizophrenia
    3. Brain itself undergoes no actual physical change, but the operation of the organ is disturbed, producing the symptoms of schizophrenia
    4. Individual is predisposed to schizophrenia because of poor housing and living conditions during childhood
12. The nurse can minimize psychologic stress by
    1. Learning what is of particular importance to the patient
    2. Explaining in fine detail all procedures and therapies
    3. Confidently advising the patient that the nurse is in charge of the situation
    4. Avoiding the discussion of any areas that may be emotionally charged
13. A phobic reaction will rarely occur unless the person
    1. Thinks about the feared object
    2. Absolves the guilt of the feared object
    3. Introjects the feared object into the body
    4. Comes into contact with the feared object
14. Anxiety can be recognized as
    1. Fears that are related to the total environment
    2. A behavior pattern observable in ourselves and others
    3. A totally unique experience and feeling
    4. Consciously motivated thoughts and wishes
15. The patient who makes up stories to fill in the blank spaces of the memory is said to be
    1. Denying
    2. Confabulating
    3. Lying
    4. Rationalizing
16. Which personality factor is the main problem for patients who need props to blur reality?
    1. Dependency
    2. Mistrust
    3. Role blurring
    4. Ego ideal
17. Projection, rationalization, denial, and distortion of reality by hallucinations and delusions are examples of a disturbance in
    1. Thought processes
    2. Associations

3. Logic
4. Reality testing
18. If prevented from performing an intense compulsion, a person would most likely react with
 1. Aggression
 2. Anxiety
 3. Withdrawal
 4. Hostility
19. A compulsive act is one that
 1. A person performs willingly
 2. Is performed after long urging
 3. Is purposeful but useless
 4. Seems absurd but is necessary to the person
20. A person, seeing a design on the wallpaper, perceives it as an animal. This is an example of a
 1. Delusion
 2. Hallucination
 3. Illusion
 4. Idea of reference
21. A patient expresses the belief that the F.B.I. is out to kill him. This is an example of
 1. Hallucinations
 2. Self-accusatory delusions
 3. Delusions of persecution
 4. Errors in judgment
22. The affect most commonly found in the schizophrenic patient is one of
 1. Happiness and elation
 2. Sadness and depression
 3. Apathy and flatness
 4. Anger and hostility
23. The neurotic personality is characterized by
 1. Marked emotional maturity
 2. Elaborate delusional system
 3. Doubts, fears, and indecisiveness
 4. Rapid, frequent mood swings
24. In a patient with a conversion reaction, anxiety is
 1. Diffuse and free floating
 2. Localized and relieved by the symptom
 3. Consciously felt by the patient
 4. Projected onto the environment
25. An individual with a psychoneurotic disorder may handle the anxiety *in all but one* of the following ways
 1. Converting anxiety into a physical symptom
 2. Acting out the anxiety with antisocial behavior
 3. Displacing anxiety onto less threatening objects
 4. Regressing to earlier levels of adjustment
26. Peptic ulcer is considered to be a psychosomatic disorder in which it is believed that
 1. Structural changes have occurred as a result of psychologic conflicts
 2. Illness is a defense against psychologic conflicts
 3. Structural changes have occurred as a result of physiologic changes caused by psychologic conflict
 4. Physiologic changes stimulated psychologic changes
27. The basic difference between psychosomatic illness and hypochondria is that in psychosomatic illness there is
 1. An emotional cause
 2. A feeling of illness

3. An actual tissue change
4. A restriction of activities
28. The patient with a sociopathic personali order
 1. Is generally unable to postpone gratification
 2. Suffers from a great deal of anxiety
 3. Has a great sense of responsibility toward others
 4. Rapidly learns by experience and punishment
29. The sociopath has difficulty in relating to others because of never having learned to
 1. Count on others
 2. Be dependent on others
 3. Communicate with others socially
 4. Empathize with others
30. Which of the following statements regarding the danger of suicide in depressed patients is true?
 1. Patients with simple depressions rarely attempt suicide
 2. Once the severe depression begins to lift the danger of suicide is no longer a problem
 3. Depressed patients are potentially suicidal during the entire course of their illness
 4. Opportunities to attempt suicide are practically absent on a locked psychiatric ward
31. The preferred treatment for a patient with a diagnosis of severe depression would be
 1. High doses of mood elevators
 2. Psychoanalysis
 3. Electrostimulation therapy
 4. Nondirective psychotherapy
32. Patients with organic brain damage frequently demonstrate a lability of mood and can switch from being pleasant and happy to being hostile and sad without external cause. The nurse can best care for these patients by
 1. Avoiding them when they are angry and sad
 2. Attempting to give nursing care when they are in a pleasant mood
 3. Encouraging them to talk about their feelings
 4. Trying to point out reality to them
33. Activities for the overactive patient would include
 1. Carving figures out of wood
 2. Sanding and varnishing wooden bookends
 3. Stenciling designs on copper sheeting
 4. Lacing tooled leather wallets
34. In planning nursing care for the neurotic patient, the nurse recognizes that
 1. It is best to ignore the patient's complaints
 2. The patient's behavior indicates a lack of will power
 3. The patient's symptoms are evidence of a disturbed personality
 4. If additional stress is added the patient will become psychotic
35. The patient who has a chronic brain syndrome needs an environment that is
 1. Stimulating
 2. Nonstimulating
 3. Unfamiliar
 4. Familiar
36. The best approach in helping a very with-

drawn patient is to provide an environment with
1. A large variety of activities
2. A specific routine
3. A trusting relationship
4. Group involvement

37. One day while you are staying with a patient who is shaving, he states: "I have hidden a razor blade and tonight I am going to kill myself." You could best reply
1. "You're going to kill yourself?"
2. "You better finish shaving since it's time for lunch."
3. "I'm sure you don't really mean that."
4. "Things can't really be that bad."

38. A patient, Mrs. S., appears to be responding to voices. She cries out at intervals, "No, no, I didn't kill him!" After one of these episodes she turns to you and states, "You know the truth, tell that policeman. Please help me!" You would
1. Respond by saying, "Mrs. S., I want to help you and I realize you must be very frightened."
2. Sit there quietly and don't respond at all to her statements
3. Respond by saying, "Who are they saying you killed Mrs. S.?"
4. Respond by saying, "Mrs. S., do not become so upset. No one is talking to you; we are alone. This is part of your illness."

39. It is important for the team, working with the mentally ill, to accept a common approach of care because the patient needs
1. A protective environment
2. To act out feelings
3. To learn acceptable behavior
4. To know what is expected

40. The patient who has obsessive-compulsive behavior can best be treated by
1. Calling attention to the behavior
2. Restricting his movements
3. Supporting but limiting the behavior
4. Keeping him busy to distract him

41. Group therapy can best help those who
1. Are emotionally ill
2. Are dependent on others
3. Feel they have a problem
4. Have no one to listen to them

42. Which of the following type activities would be *least* helpful to the severely depressed patient?
1. Allowing the patient to plan own project
2. Specific simple instructions to be followed
3. Simple, easily completed, short-term projects
4. Monotonous, repetitive type projects and activities

43. Mrs. Somers is an elderly patient who has been taking chlorpromazine hydrochloride (Thorazine) for several months. After observing that the patient sits rigidly in the chair, the nurse observes her closely for other evidence of adverse effects occurring during long-term therapy with the drug. She will look for
1. Inability to concentrate, excess salivation
2. Minimal use of nonverbal expression, rambling speech
3. Incoordinate movement of extremities, tremor

4. Reluctance to converse, nonverbal clues indicating fear

44. A patient on a high dosage of Thorazine has developed tremors of the hands. The appropriate action of the nurse would be
1. Report the symptoms to the physician
2. Withhold the medication
3. Tell the patient it is transitory
4. Give the patient finger exercises

Gail, 17, has had a history of being a loner. She made excellent grades in school but often her thinking was highly symbolic. During her senior year in high school she refused to get out of bed, there was a loss of appetite and disorganized speech. She was hospitalized at one of the community hospitals. Questions 45 through 52 refer to this situation.

45. One of the primary goals in providing a therapeutic environment is to
1. Get her involved in a group with her peers
2. Remove her from the home
3. Foster a trusting relationship
4. Give her medication on time

46. Gail feels that "a man on television" is responsible for her being sick. This is an example of
1. Autistic thinking
2. An illusion
3. A hallucination
4. A delusion

47. While in the hospital Gail still refused to get out of bed and became very hostile with the staff when approached. The most immediate therapeutic nursing approach would be
1. Require that Gail get out of bed at once
2. Stay with her until she calms down
3. Give her the p.r.n. tranquilizer that is ordered
4. Allow her to stay in bed for now but leave her alone

48. Gail starts to repeat phrases that others have just said. This type of speech is known as
1. Autism
2. Echopraxia
3. Echolalia
4. Neologism

49. Gail is on chlorpromazine (Thorazine) 2000 mg. every day. She comes to the nurse complaining of her "fingers twitching." The best reply would be
1. "This is a temporary thing until your body adjusts to the medication."
2. "I will get the doctor to order a medication that will help overcome the side effects of the drug you need."
3. "You need the medication that we are giving you. You will soon get used to the side effects."
4. "Let's wait a few days and see whether the side effects of the drug you are taking go away."

50. Which of the following symptoms would cause the nurse to stop giving Thorazine to Gail until further lab work was done?
1. Photosensitivity
2. Shuffling gait
3. Yellow sclera
4. Grimacing

51. Whenever Gail became upset she would become suspicious of others. Her delusions centered on the thought that "others" controlled her. This type of behavior is known as
    1. Catatonic
    2. Withdrawn
    3. Projective
    4. Ritualistic
52. On being discharged Gail should be encouraged to
    1. Go back to her regular activities
    2. Continue in the after-care clinic
    3. Call the unit whenever upset
    4. Find a group who have similar problems

Mr. Smith, 55, has had difficulty in sleeping and eating. He has lost a great deal of time from work because he "wasn't feeling well." Lately he has just sat in his room staring at the floor with a sad look on his face. His one wish is that he would die. Questions 53 through 57 refer to this situation.

53. Mr. Smith was brought to the general hospital after taking an overdose of phenobarbital. After a gavage, Mr. Smith states "Let me die, I'm no good." The nurse's most appropriate response would be
    1. "Of course you're good, we'll take care of you."
    2. "You must have been upset to try and take your life."
    3. "Do you feel like telling me why you did that?"
    4. "You have been through a rough time, let me take care of you."
54. Mr. Smith has been placed on suicidal precautions. A therapeutic community would provide this precaution by
    1. Removing all "cutting" objects
    2. Not allowing him to leave his room
    3. Giving him an opportunity to ventilate his feelings
    4. Assigning a staff member to be with him at all times
55. Mr. Smith is to receive a series of electrostimulating therapy. The nurse, in explaining this procedure to the patient, should emphasize that
    1. He will have amnesia afterward
    2. The treatments will make him better
    3. Someone will be with him all the time
    4. He should not be afraid, it won't hurt
56. Mr. Smith was given a muscle relaxant just before the electrostimulating therapy. The major disadvantage of this drug is that it inhibits which muscles?
    1. Intercostal and diaphragmatic
    2. Biceps and triceps
    3. Facial and thoracic
    4. Sternocleidomastoid and abdominal
57. A treatment program was planned for Mr. Smith. The staff made specific goals directed toward having the patient
    1. Develop trust in others
    2. Express his hostile feelings
    3. Set realistic life goals
    4. Get involved in activities

Mr. Brown was admitted to the hospital with delirium tremens. He was placed on bedrest, paraldehyde, thiamine chloride, and nicotinic acid. Questions 58 through 67 refer to this situation.

58. Mr. Brown, on admission, should be given which room?
    1. One-bed room next to the bathroom
    2. Two-bed room at the quiet end of the unit
    3. One-bed room next to the nurses' station
    4. Two-bed room next to the nurses' station
59. The nurse understands that paraldehyde is given to combat which of Mr. Brown's problems?
    1. Fluid and electrolyte
    2. Detoxification from alcohol
    3. Emotional
    4. Motor and sensory
60. Mr. Brown is suspicious of others and blames others for his difficulty. The nurse understands that the patient uses this behavior because he has problems
    1. In identifying who bothers him
    2. With dependency and independency
    3. In telling the truth
    4. With meeting his ego ideal
61. When Mr. Brown was able to eat, the diet ordered for him was
    1. High protein, low carbohydrate, low fat
    2. Protein to tolerance, moderate fat, high calorie, high vitamin, soft
    3. High carbohydrate, low saturated fat, 1800 calories
    4. Low protein, high carbohydrate, high fat, soft
62. Mr. Brown requires thiamine chloride and nicotinic acid because these vitamins are needed for the maintenance of
    1. Good circulation
    2. The nervous system
    3. Prothrombin formation
    4. Elimination
63. A high caloric diet fortified with vitamins will prevent damage to which organ that detoxifies alcohol?
    1. Kidneys
    2. Liver
    3. Pancreas
    4. Adrenals
64. Mr. Brown asks if you, the nurse, can see the bugs that are crawling on his bed. Your best reply would be
    1. "I will get rid of them for you."
    2. "No, I don't see any bugs."
    3. "I will stay with you until you are calmer."
    4. "Those bugs are a part of your sickness."
65. As Mr. Brown begins to feel better he denies excessive use of alcohol. The nurse understands that denial is meeting which of Mr. Brown's needs? To
    1. Make him look better in the eyes of others
    2. Live up to other's expectations
    3. Make him seem more independent
    4. Reduce his feelings of guilt
66. Mr. Brown asks if it is required that he attend Alcoholics Anonymous. Your best reply would be
    1. "No, it is best to wait until you feel you really need them."
    2. "Yes, because you will learn how to cope with your problem."

3. "Do you have feelings about going to these meetings?"
4. "You'll find you'll need their support."
67. Groups such as Alcoholics Anonymous help people like Mr. Brown because in a group the person learns that
   1. He does not need a crutch
   2. His problems are not unique
   3. His problems are caused by alcohol
   4. People stand stronger together

Mrs. Cox, a 33-year-old housewife, is admitted with a diagnosis of manic-depressive psychosis, manic phase. She has been eating and sleeping very little and has charged hundreds of dollars worth of purchases to her husband. Questions 68 and 69 refer to this situation.

68. The symptoms that Mrs. Cox would probably exhibit in the hospital would include
   1. Decreased psychomotor activity
   2. Increased interest in the environment
   3. Depressed mood and crying
   4. Increased insight into her behavior
69. While the nurse is talking with Mrs. Cox in her room, the patient's conversation becomes embarrassingly vulgar. The nurse would best respond to her behavior by
   1. Restricting Mrs. Cox's contact with staff until this symptom passes
   2. Tactfully teasing her about the use of such vulgarity
   3. Asking her to limit her vulgarity and continuing the conversation with her
   4. Discreetly refusing to talk to her when she is speaking in this manner
70. James Cote is a narcotic addict who had surgery to repair a laceration of his heart caused by a bullet. Postoperatively he is receiving methadone hydrochloride orally. The drug
   1. Provides postoperative pain control without causing narcotic dependency
   2. Counteracts the depressive effects of long-

term opiate usage on cardiac and thoracic muscles
   3. Allows symptom free termination of narcotic addiction
   4. Converts narcotic use from an illicit to a legally controlled drug
71. Hard drugs easily cause dependency because of their ability to
   1. Ease pain
   2. Clear sensorium
   3. Blur reality
   4. Decrease motor activity
72. How many hours after the last dose would the nurse expect the heroin addict's withdrawal symptoms to reach a peak?
   1. 8 to 24
   2. 24 to 48
   3. 48 to 72
   4. 72 to 96
73. The basic personality of the drug addict is marked by insecurity and
   1. Infantile passion for self-gratification
   2. The need to delay gratification
   3. The use of psychosomatic mechanisms
   4. Weak id drives
74. When methadone hydrochloride dosage is lowered, James must be observed closely for evidence of
   1. Agitation, attempts to escape from the hospital
   2. Piloerection, lack of interest in surroundings
   3. Skin dryness, scratching under incisional dressing
   4. Lethargy, refusal to participate in therapeutic exercise
75. The medication used to combat an overdose of methadone is
   1. Phenobarbital
   2. Narcon
   3. Dexedrine
   4. Caffeine

CHAPTER 11

Medical-surgical nursing

Medical-surgical nursing is concerned with those aspects of nursing care that are related to the physical and emotional needs of patients with specific types of health problems. The concepts, principles, and skills included here have evolved as a logical sequence to the more general concepts, principles, and skills presented in the chapter on Fundamentals of nursing.

Medical-surgical content has been developed by combining the framework of patients with problems and a modified systems approach. The areas covered include preoperative, postoperative, and emergency care, immunologic responses, neurohormonal regulation, sensorimotor functioning, cardiopulmonary functioning, nutrition and elimination, fluid and electrolyte balance, and reproductive organs. The format for each section follows a similar pattern, beginning with basic concepts and moving into the etiology and pathophysiology of the area. A commonly encountered disease entity has been selected as an example of a specific pathophysiology. The clinical manifestations and diagnostic procedures used in the assessment of the patient precede the usual medical therapies. Nursing diagnoses related to the unique needs of patients with the specific disease are developed and the interventions predicated by the needs are presented.

No attempt has been made to cover all the common medical entities, and supplemental medical-surgical nursing texts must be used when depth of material is desired or questions arise.

GENERAL PREOPERATIVE, POSTOPERATIVE, AND EMERGENCY NURSING INTERVENTION

PREOPERATIVE NURSING CARE

A. Preparation period before surgery—all patients going for surgery, regardless of the operative procedure, have many similar needs that require similar nursing intervention
B. General needs
1. Patient needs to be informed about treatment
   a. Allow patient time to ask questions about procedures and surgery
   b. Explain all procedures to the patient and give reasons and objectives for them

   c. Determine patient's level of understanding of operative procedure to ascertain that signature on permit represents informed consent
2. Patient needs emotional support
   a. Allow and encourage patient to ventilate feelings about diagnosis and surgery
   b. Answer patient's questions as honestly as possible
   c. Use open-ended reflective techniques but don't raise questions patient doesn't ask
   d. Tell patient what to expect in the operating room, recovery and/or intensive care units
   e. Inform patients if plan is to return them to other than the present room

f. Provide spiritual counselor if desired by patient or family
g. Consider needs of the family on day of surgery
3. Patient needs health teaching
a. Teach patient the activities that will be instituted after surgery; e.g., deep breathing, coughing, turning
b. Teach patient physical exercises that will be used to promote circulation after surgery; e.g., isometric leg exercises, ambulation routines
c. Inform patient to expect some discomfort after surgery and teach the importance of requesting medication for pain
4. Patient has specific preoperative safety needs
a. Ascertain that history and physical have been completed
b. Make certain that all routine and ordered laboratory tests have been done and reports are available
c. Inform all members of the medical team, especially the anesthesiologist, of patient's allergies and other health problems and prominently mark the chart
d. Carry out ordered preoperative preparation; e.g., shave, Betadine, pHisoHex washes, enemas, douches, etc.
e. Remove nail polish from fingers and toes
f. Administer prescribed sleeping medication
g. Inform patient not to take anything by mouth after midnight, remove fluid, and place obvious signs at bedside
h. In the morning, check patient's vital signs and assess overall physical status; record and report any deviations to physician
i. Have patient void
j. See that any drainage tubes (catheter or Levin tube) that are ordered are inserted
k. Make certain that name identification band is on patient's wrist
l. Have patient remove dentures and other prosthetic devices and store valuables
m. Administer prescribed preoperative medication
n. Put side rails up after administering medications
o. Transfer patient to stretcher when operating room calls and fasten stretcher strap in place before transporting

POSTOPERATIVE NURSING CARE

A. Period following surgery—the surgical patient experiences many stresses regardless of the type of surgery performed, including depression of the central nervous system from general or regional anesthesia, an interruption in the integrity of the skin, depressed respiratory functioning, alterations in circulation and fluid and electrolyte balance, depression of gastrointestinal and urinary functioning, and emotional trauma
B. General needs
1. Patient has specific postoperative safety needs
a. Maintain patent airway by keeping artificial airway in place until gag reflex returns, suctioning trachea as needed, keeping head extended and turned to the side, observing rate and character of respirations
b. Assess patient's physical status—note and record level of consciousness, vital signs, color and temperature of skin, condition of surgical site, presence and functioning of intravenous and drainage tubes, return of sensorimotor functioning; report significant changes
c. Protect patient from injury by keeping patient under close observation, keeping side rails in place, positioning patient to prevent excessive pressure on body parts or on tubing, controlling restlessness and preventing patient from pulling on tubes or dressing, making certain all equipment is in safe working condition and that it is properly used
2. Patient needs to be protected from the immediate and delayed complications of surgery
a. Turn patient frequently and encourage deep breathing and coughing to prevent the development of atelectasis or hypostatic pneumonia
b. Perform or encourage range of motion and isometric exercises and

early ambulation to prevent phlebitis, paralytic ileus, and circulatory stasis

c. Maintain patency of tubing (catheter, gastric tubes, T-tube, chest tubes, etc.) to promote drainage and maintain decompression to reduce pressure on suture line

d. Monitor patient's overall physical status, vital signs, dressing, and drainage to observe for early signs of hemorrhage and prevent excessive blood loss and shock

e. Use surgically aseptic technique when changing dressings or as necessary when irrigating tubing to prevent infection

f. Monitor intake and output to prevent dehydration, fluid and electrolyte imbalance, and urinary suppression or retention

g. Observe for abdominal distention to prevent discomfort and intestinal obstruction

h. Give medication for pain as ordered to prevent discomfort and restlessness

i. Regulate intravenous therapy to prevent circulatory overload

j. Support or encourage patient to support and splint incisional site when coughing, moving, or turning to prevent tension on suture line

k. Position patient as required by type of surgery to prevent misalignment and prevent the accumulation of fluid or the blocking of drainage tubes

3. Patient needs emotional support

a. Reorient patient to time, place, and situation

b. Call patient by name

c. Answer questions as honestly and as simply as possible avoiding complicated, involved explanations

d. Medicate for pain and restlessness

e. Expect and accept repetitious questions and give patient necessary reassurance

EMERGENCY NURSING CARE

A. Life threatening emergencies—although many emergencies arise in day-to-day situations, there are times when patient needs require immediate independent nursing actions to prevent loss of life

B. Types of emergency situations

1. Cardiac arrest—the sudden and unexpected cessation of the heart and effective circulation; the patient needs to reestablish cardiac function within a 3-minute period to avoid irreversible brain damage and death

a. External cardiopulmonary resuscitation

(1) In witnessed arrest

(a) Check for loss of consciousness

(b) Place patient on firm surface

(c) Administer a sharp blow to the lower sternum

(d) Hyperextend the neck and clear airway

(e) Ventilate patient's lungs 4 times

(f) Check for carotid pulse

(g) If carotid pulse is absent, begin cardiac compression over lower third of sternum

(h) Maintain a pattern of 15 compressions to 2 breaths if alone or a ratio of 5 compressions to 1 breath if 2 people are available

(i) Maintain a compression rate of approximately 60 per minute

(j) Once established do not interrupt pattern

(k) Maintain efforts until patient responds or help arrives

(2) In unwitnessed arrest where patient is found unconscious

(a) Omit the sharp blow to the sternum

(b) Hyperextend the neck and begin resuscitation

b. Cardiac monitoring—if cardiac monitor is available, patient should be placed on monitor to direct intervention; type of intervention depends on whether patient is in ventricular fibrillation or asystole

c. Ventricular fibrillation—a defibrillator is used to shock the heart in an attempt to change ventricular fibrillation to normal sinus rhythm

d. Asystole—defibrillation is not used and the nurse maintains cardiac resuscitation until the physician arrives to administer intracardiac epinephrine and/or insert a pacemaker

2. Foreign body in larynx or trachea—sudden onset of respiratory difficulty following the inhalation of a foreign object that completely or partially blocks air from entering the trachea

 a. 80% of incidence occurs in children under 15 years of age
 b. In adults, foreign bodies are usually large boluses of food
 c. Symptoms include hoarseness, cough, and gagging; may progress to dyspnea, stridor, cyanosis, and unconsciousness
 d. If permitted to continue, death will result from anoxia so immediate intervention must be instituted
 e. Intervention is directed toward removing the object
  (1) In child, turn upside down and deliver a flat hand slap to the area between the shoulder blades; in adult, deliver a strong slap to the area between the shoulder blades in an attempt to dislodge object
  (2) Use forceps or Choke-Saver to manually remove the object
  (3) Use Heimlich maneuver (bear hug above beltline with sharp abrupt compression) in an attempt to force the diaphragm against the lungs and use the trapped air to propel the object out
  (4) If object cannot be removed and breathing stops, an emergency incision into the trachea (cricothyroidotomy) must be done to create a temporary airway until object can be surgically removed

3. Hemorrhage—a large volume of blood is lost either internally or externally in a short period of time

 a. Symptoms are related to hypovolemic shock and include rapid thready pulse, thirst, cold clammy skin, sighing respirations, dizziness, syncope, pallor, apprehension, restlessness, and hypotension
 b. Obvious bleeding may be evident from wounds or body cavities; substantial blood loss can occur without external evidence
 c. Intervention is directed toward stopping the flow of blood
  (1) Apply pressure directly to the wound or to pressure points
  (2) Elevate the involved part to reduce blood flow
  (3) Apply ice if possible to constrict vessels
  (4) Treat shock by maintaining body temperature and keeping individual flat
  (5) If bleeding in an extremity is extreme, cannot be controlled, and presents an immediate threat to the patient's life, a tourniquet may be applied; a tourniquet is used only after the decision is made to sacrifice the limb; once applied the tourniquet should not be released until surgical help is available
  (6) Internal hemorrhage requires medical therapy and there is little emergency nursing intervention

4. Fractures—see section on Patients with problems in sensorimotor functioning, pp. 473-474

5. Anaphylactic shock—see section on Patients with problems with immunologic response, pp. 453-454

6. Drug overdose
 a. If drug was taken orally, induce vomiting
 b. Support respiratory functioning by positioning, loosening clothing, etc
 c. Treat respiratory failure if it develops (cardiopulmonary resuscitation)
 d. Get medical attention as soon as possible

7. Pediatric emergencies; e.g., poisoning—see Pediatric nursing, pp. 393-394

PATIENTS WITH PROBLEMS WITH IMMUNOLOGIC RESPONSE

TYPES OF IMMUNOLOGIC PROBLEMS

A. Inappropriate or abnormal response of antibodies to external antigens (hypersensitivity)

3. Insufficient amount of antibodies available (hyposensitivity)
   1. Deficiency in production
   2. Failure or inadequacy to respond to antigens
C. Inappropriate or abnormal response of antibodies to internal antigens (autoimmunity)

BASIC CONCEPTS

A. A variety of antigens enter the body via the skin, respiratory, or digestive tract; e.g., bacteria, pollens, chemicals, tissues
B. A person's response to antigens is influenced by
   1. Heredity
   2. Congenital factors
   3. Emotional factors
   4. Exposure to antigens
   5. Physical status
C. Immunologic responses can be beneficial or detrimental
D. Reticuloendothelial system is stimulated to produce antibodies against these antigens; these antibodies are carried by gamma globulin or fixed in the tissues
E. Antibodies are selective of specific antigens and are ineffective against others
F. Antigen-antibody reactions cause cells to release mediators; e.g., histamine, acetylcholine, leukotaxine, bradykinin, and heparin
G. These mediators cause both localized and systemic reactions; e.g., sneezing, localized edema, generalized urticaria, bronchial constriction, and anaphylaxis

HYPERSENSITIVE RESPONSE TO ANTIGENS

A. Etiology and pathophysiologic processes
   1. Inflammation develops as an adaptation directed toward localizing and reducing stress
   2. Repeated contact with an antigen produces a more immediate and increased response by the reticuloendothelial system
   3. Continued exposure produces a hypersensitivity to the specific antigen involved
   4. Allergies (hypersensitive reactions) may be mild or severe, immediate or delayed, localized or systemic
B. Assessment of patient
   1. Clinical manifestations depend on the type of antigen and the organ or tissues involved
      a. Localized responses
         (1) Skin—pruritus, redness, burning, localized skin lesions, angioneurotic edema; usually associated with poison ivy, contact dermatitis, and eczema
         (2) Mucous membrane—swelling, redness, congestion and pressure, increased secretions, itching; usually associated with conjunctivitis, sinusitis, hay fever, and vaginitis
         (3) Respiratory tract—edema of bronchial mucosa, mucoid secretions, spasm of smooth muscles, wheeze, dyspnea, cough; usually associated with asthma
         (4) Gastrointestinal tract—increased secretions, spasm of smooth muscle, nausea, increased peristalsis, diarrhea; usually associated with reactions to foods, drugs, and bacteria
      b. Systemic responses
         (1) Skin—generalized urticaria, rash, pruritus, redness, edema, purpura; usually associated with reactions to foods, drugs, toxins, chemicals, serums, vaccines, and ultraviolet rays
         (2) Vascular and neuromuscular —headache, muscle spasm, joint pains, lymphadenopathy, fever, malaise, anorexia; usually associated with reactions to foods, drugs, toxins, chemicals, sera, and vaccines
         (3) Anaphylactic shock—sneezing, smooth muscle spasm, choking, apprehension, dyspnea, cyanosis, vascular collapse, loss of consciousness, dilated pupils, convulsions; usually associated with reactions to drugs, toxins, chemicals, insect and animal bites, sera, vaccines, blood transfusions, and certain foods such as shellfish; these symptoms usually have a very sudden onset, are serious and pro-

found, and the patient progresses rapidly toward death unless process is interrupted

2. Diagnostic measures
   a. Health history—including family, personal, and environmental background
   b. Skin tests to determine hypersensitivity to specific antigens
      (1) Patch tests—airtight patches containing suspected antigens are applied to skin surface and localized responses are noted in 2 to 5 days
      (2) Scratch tests—suspected antigens induced into skin by means of epidermal scratches and localized responses are noted in 15 to 30 minutes
      (3) Intracutaneous tests—suspected antigens are diluted and injected intradermally to form a wheal and localized responses are noted in 10 to 20 minutes
   c. Food elimination tests—food diary is kept and patient is then instructed to remove 1 food at a time for a designated period; this test may be carried out by removing all foods and adding 1 food at a time for a designated period
   d. Laboratory tests
      (1) Differential white count to detect eosinophilia
      (2) Agglutination test to detect presence and titer of specific or nonspecific agglutinins
C. Medical therapy—the physician may
   1. Attempt to identify the specific antigen and if possible have patient reduce contact; e.g., environmental alterations, elimination diet
   2. Prescribe drug therapy to
      a. Reduce localized response; e.g., caladryl lotion, cortisone ointment, eye drops, nose drops, bronchodilators
      b. Reduce systemic response; e.g., antihistamines, epinephrine, ACTH, cortisone, sedatives, tranquilizers
   3. Promote desensitization by the administration of small amount of specific antigen at designated intervals until exposure to the antigen causes no reaction

4. Encourage patient to reduce emotional stress
D. Nursing diagnosis and intervention
   1. Patient needs protection from recurrence of hypersensitive reactions
      a. Identify all known allergies in both patient and family
      b. Eliminate or reduce specific antigens where possible; e.g., dust from room, plastic covers on pillows, encourage adherence to dietary regimen
      c. Administer medications as ordered
      d. Teach patient how to prevent attacks and reduce complications
   2. Patient needs additional safety precautions
      a. Observe carefully for hypersensitive reactions especially when introducing additional drugs or foods
      b. Keep epinephrine available at all times
      c. Instruct patient to report early symptoms
      d. Have patient purchase and wear a medical alert tag or bracelet
      e. Share information about patient's allergies with entire staff and label patient's record
      f. Institute immediate emergency measures if necessary; e.g., anaphylactic shock, laryngeal edema, or status asthmaticus
   3. Patient needs emotional support
      a. Keep patient and family informed about progress and procedures
      b. Encourage patient to verbalize feelings
      c. Allow patient to be dependent but foster independence
      d. Encourage patient and family to participate in planning care
      e. Let patient know you are aware of discomfort
      f. Realistically support patient's body image and ego strengths

HYPOSENSITIVE RESPONSE TO ANTIGENS

A. Etiology and pathophysiologic processes
   1. Hypogammaglobulinemia or hyposensitive responses may be genetic (sexlinked) or acquired (chronic disorders causing protein loss, lymphatic malignancy, or resulting from immunosuppressant therapy)

2. Reticuloendothelial system is depressed and the production of gamma globulin is limited although some antibodies exist at the cellular level
3. The individual has only a limited ability to respond to any infection-causing antigen
4. Failure to develop immunologic responses is always dangerous; therapeutically, it must be used with caution even when deliberately induced to limit tissue rejection in transplant surgery

3. Assessment of patient
   1. Clinical manifestations depend on the the type of antigen but chronic or acute systemic responses are common
      a. Symptoms of chronic infections such as a low-grade fever, malaise, diarrhea, pneumonitis
      b. Recurrent severe infections that differ from those in the normal individual by their frequency and severity
   2. Diagnostic measures
      a. Health history—including family, personal, and environmental background
      b. Skin tests—to determine quality of immunologic response to a battery of antigens
      c. Laboratory tests—to determine serum levels of immunoglobulins

C. Medical therapy—the physician may
   1. Administer human gamma globulin at designated intervals to maintain acceptable serum levels to increase resistance to infection
   2. Prescribe antibiotics at the first sign of infection to maintain high serum levels
   3. Treat primary cause of hyposensitivity where possible
   4. Control environment to reduce possibility of infection

D. Nursing diagnosis and intervention
   1. Patient needs protection from infection
      a. Isolate from other people
      b. Use barrier techniques when entering patient's room
      c. Control environmental temperature to prevent chilling or overheating
      d. Observe for and promptly report any signs of infection or illness
      e. Provide health teaching in the areas of rest, diet, hygiene, clothing, medication
      f. Instruct patient to report the signs and symptoms of even the most minor infections immediately
   2. Patient needs emotional support
      a. Keep patient and family informed about progress and procedures especially need for gown, mask, etc.
      b. Encourage patient to verbalize feelings
      c. Provide contact with patient on a regularly planned basis
      d. Allow patient to be dependent but foster independence
      e. Encourage patient and family to participate in planning and implementating care
      f. Provide patient with means of communicating with others; e.g., letters, telephone, intercom
      g. Provide patient with realistic diversional activities

AUTOIMMUNE RESPONSES

A. Etiology and pathophysiologic processes
   1. The antigens normally present in the internal cells stimulate the development of antibodies
   2. Antibodies are unable to distinguish antigens of the internal cells from external antigens
   3. The antibodies act against the internal cell to cause both localized and systemic reactions
   4. The reactions affect the epithelial and connective tissue of the body to create a variety of diseases
   5. These diseases can be divided into 2 general categories
      a. Collagen diseases—systemic lupus erythematosus, dermatomyositis, periarteritis nodosa, scleroderma, rheumatoid arthritis
      b. Autoimmune hemolytic disorders—idiopathic thrombocytopenic purpura, acquired hemolytic anemia, autoimmune leukopenia
   6. The exact pathophysiologic process involved in these diseases is still unknown and remains under study

B. Assessment of patient
   1. Clinical manifestations depend on the organs or systems affected
      a. Systemic lupus erythematosus—a

disease of the connective tissue involving the vascular, dermal, serous, and synovial membranes

  (1) Symptoms include fever, sun sensitivity, anorexia, weight loss, malaise, erythema, and rash on exposed body surfaces and upper chest frequently accompanied by classic butterfly rash on face, joint pains, tachycardia, other general symptoms of autoimmune hemolytic disorders

  (2) Remissions and exacerbations occur and death may result from kidney shutdown

b. Rheumatoid arthritis—a chronic systemic disease with inflammatory changes throughout the body's connective tissue

  (1) Symptoms include fatigue, muscle stiffness especially after periods of inactivity, anemia, weight loss, malaise, joint pain and swelling with progressive deformity of the joints, paresthesias, subcutaneous nodules

  (2) Remissions and exacerbations are common but interference with function of involved joints is irreversible

c. Idiopathic thrombocytopenic purpura—a chronic hemolytic disorder with decreased formation and premature destruction of platelets

  (1) Symptoms include petechiae, ecchymosis, epistaxis, bleeding from gums, disturbances in menstruation, pallor, fatigue, malaise, fever

  (2) Death may result from hemorrhage

2. Diagnostic measures

a. Systemic lupus erythematosus

  (1) L.E. prep—blood smear is microscopically examined for the presence of lupus erythematosus cells

  (2) Sedimentation rate is elevated

  (3) Tissue biopsy to test for the presence of lupus erythematosus cells

  (4) Serum proteins to test for increase in serum gamma globulin

  (5) Complete blood count to test for anemia, leukopenia, and thrombocytopenia

b. Rheumatoid arthritis

  (1) Examination of synovial fluid for color, viscosity, and chemical analysis

  (2) C-reactive protein to test for inflammatory response

  (3) Sedimentation rate is elevated

  (4) Latex fixation test to determine presence of "rheumatoid factors"

  (5) Blood studies to determine presence of anemia and leukopenia

  (6) X-ray films to identify change in the joints

c. Idiopathic thrombocytopenic purpura

  (1) Blood studies to determine platelet count, bleeding time, coagulation time

  (2) Tourniquet test to determine capillary fragility

  (3) Bone marrow study to examine platelets

C. Medical therapy—the physician may

  1. Prescribe corticosteroids, anti-inflammatory, or immunosuppressive drugs

  2. Treat additional symptoms as they develop; e.g., transfusions for hemorrhage; analgesics for pain; physiotherapy to prevent deformities

  3. Regulate diet according to need; e.g., increased iron in idiopathic thrombocytopenic purpura; reducing diet in rheumatoid arthritis

  4. Intervene surgically for corrective and preventive purposes as necessary; e.g., hip replacement, splenectomy

D. Nursing diagnosis and intervention

  1. Patient needs release from pain and prevention of deformities

    a. Administer analgesics and other medications as ordered

    b. Teach patient to take medications as ordered

    c. Apply heat and cold as ordered

    d. Promote rest and position to ease joint pains

    e. Provide for range of motion exercises up to the point of pain, recognizing that some discomfort is always present

    f. Prevent pressure by encouraging

patient to turn or by turning patient frequently

g. Support patient in a functionally aligned position

2. Patient needs additional safety precautions

a. Observe for signs of hemorrhage

b. Support while ambulating since balance is poor (make certain shoes offer proper support)

c. If necessary provide side rails or overhead trapeze for turning in bed

d. Protect from infection

e. Prevent chilling or overheating

f. Observe for signs and symptoms of complications; e.g., renal involvement in lupus; hemorrhage in purpura; contractures in arthritis

g. Observe for and teach patient to be aware of the signs and symptoms of side effects of medications; e.g., gastric ulcers from steroids; bleeding and tinnitus from salicylates

3. Patient needs emotional support

a. Encourage patient to verbalize feelings

b. Help patient to understand the disease process

c. Help patient to recognize limitations but focus on strengths

d. Refer patient and family to community based agencies concerned with the specific illness

e. Help patient set realistic goals

f. Accept patient's anger and discouragements while tempering false hopes

PATIENTS WITH PROBLEMS WITH NEUROHORMONAL REGULATION

NEURAL REGULATION

A. Types of neural problems

1. Hyperfunction of neural regulators—excessive stimulation and/or transmission of neural impulses

2. Hypofunction of neural regulators

a. Impaired neural reception of stimuli

b. Interrupted transmission of neural impulses

B. General etiology and physiologic processes in neural regulation

1. The nervous system imposes control on all parts of the body as well as on itself

2. Structures within the central and peripheral divisions of the nervous system serve as a closely interrelated communication network that receives stimuli and either voluntarily or involuntarily responds

3. Interference with the reception, interpretation, and transmission of stimuli may directly or indirectly affect the function of other parts of the body

4. The nature of the effect is directly related to the cause, location, and size of the interference

5. Since there is a hierarchy of control in the nervous system, the higher the interference within the central nervous system the greater the systemic involvement

6. Interference with reception, interpretation, and transmission can result from inflammation, neoplasms, chemical changes, degenerative changes, infection, or trauma

7. There is a direct relationship between hormonal and neural regulation

Hyperfunction of neural regulators

Etiology and pathophysiologic processes

A. Localized or systemic chemical, microbiologic, developmental, and physical stresses can result in various types of hyperfunction of neural regulators

B. These types of hyperfunction include an increase in reception, a hyperirritability of the nerves to stimuli, an increase in the rate of neural transmission

C. Localized stress can result in localized symptoms of hyperfunction (tic douloureaux) or generalized symptoms of hyperfunction (poliomyelitis)

D. Generalized stress can result in localized symptoms of hyperfunction (neuritis resulting from alcoholism) or generalized symptoms of hyperfunction (convulsions resulting from fever)

Hyperfunction of a peripheral nerve

Example: herpes zoster or shingles, an acute viral infection of nerve structures characterized by inflammation along the path-

ways of one or more peripheral sensory nerves
A. Assessment of patient
   1. Clinical manifestations depend on the location of the involved nerve and the extent of the involvement
      a. Symptoms include severe pain and paresthesia; malaise, headache, and fever; painful, pruritic vesicles arranged along the pathway of the involved nerves
      b. May frequently occur in patients with other debilitating illness; e.g., tuberculosis, Hodgkin's disease
      c. Caused by the same virus that causes chicken pox
      d. Occurs more frequently in the elderly
   2. Diagnostic measures
      a. Diagnosis is made on the basis of clinical manifestations
      b. Stains may be made from lesion exudate to isolate organism
B. Medical therapy—the physician may
   1. Prescribe medications for pain, relaxation, itching, and preventing secondary infection
   2. Control pain by blocking the nerve by injecting drugs such as lidocaine or applying medication such as triamcinolone (Kenalog)
   3. Prescribe anti-inflammatory drugs such as systemic steroids or Kenalog ointment to decrease inflammation
C. Nursing diagnosis and intervention
   1. Patient has need for comfort and relief from pain
      a. Administer analgesics and other medications as ordered
      b. Reduce itching and protect lesions from air by the application of salves, ointments, lotions, and sterile dressings as ordered
      c. Protect from pressure by use of air mattress, bed cradle, and light loose clothing (avoid synthetic and woolen materials and use cotton fabrics)
   2. Patient has need for protection from secondary infection
      a. Use aseptic technique when caring for a patient with open lesions
      b. Administer antibiotics as ordered
      c. Encourage patient to avoid scratching and use gloves at night to limit the possibility of accidental scratching

   3. Patient needs emotional support
      a. Assist patient to understand the basis for the rash and the itch
      b. Allay fears that may be based on old wives' tales about shingles
      c. Encourage patient to express feelings

Hyperfunction of a spinal nerve

Example: ruptured nucleus pulposus or slipped disk, characterized by pressure and/or compression of nerves from a rupture, prolapse, or herniation of an intervertebral disk anywhere along the spinal column, commonly between fourth and fifth lumbar vertebrae
A. Assessment of patient
   1. Clinical manifestations
      a. Symptoms include radiating pain in area served by the nerves: cervical area, pain radiating to shoulder and down arm; lumbar area, pain radiating along sciatic nerve to buttock and leg; stiffness, tenderness, and muscle spasm in area of rupture; numbness and tingling in area served by nerve
      b. Pain and spasm are aggravated by activities such as coughing, straining, lifting, or bending that increase pressure on the nerve
   2. Diagnostic measures
      a. Neurologic examination to assess reflexes, sensory responses, and motor status
      b. Radiographic examination of the spinal column
         (1) Myelogram—injection of radiopaque liquid into spinal column to determine whether there is impingement on cord
         (2) Diskogram—injection of radiopaque liquid directly into the intervertebral disk to outline the disk
         (3) X-ray film of spine
      c. Electromyography to measure the electric activity of muscles
      d. History of onset of pain
B. Medical therapy—the physician may
   1. Reduce pain, pressure, and spasticity by ordering bed rest, bed board, and traction
   2. Prescribe muscle relaxants and analgesics
   3. Order physiotherapy as needed (heat, massage, exercise)

4. Intervene surgically to remove pressure and/or stabilize the spine (laminectomy, fusion)

C. Nursing diagnosis and intervention
1. Patient has need for comfort and relief from pain
   a. Administer analgesics and other medications as ordered
   b. Use a firm mattress and bed board under patient
   c. Make certain traction and/or braces are correctly applied and maintained
   d. Use fracture bedpan to avoid pressure when lifting
   e. Give frequent and extensive back care to relax muscles and promote circulation
2. Patient has need for special safety precautions
   a. Use side rails to prevent patient from falling
   b. Support patient's body alignment at all times
   c. Use log-rolling method to turn patient after surgery (refer to section on hypofunction of neural regulators for care of patients with spinal cord injuries, pp. 460-462)
   d. Protect patient from accidents caused by loss of sensation
   e. Maintain proper traction
   f. Observe carefully for signs of pressure sores
   g. Teach patient proper body mechanics
   h. Assess patient for changes in neurologic functioning
3. Patient has need for emotional support
   a. Allow patient to be dependent but foster independence
   b. Encourage patient to express feelings about altered functioning and self-image
   c. Encourage patient to verbalize fears about present condition and future disability
   d. Encourage patient to request pain medication as necessary

Hyperfunction in cerebrum

Example: epilepsy, characterized by the abnormal discharge of electric impulses from the nerve cells in the brain from idiopathic or secondary causes resulting in the typical manifestation of seizures

A. Assessment of patient
1. Clinical manifestation—type of seizure
   a. Generalized motor seizures (grand mal seizures) characterized by an aura; loss of consciousness; tonic and clonic movements; interruption of respirations; loss of bladder and bowel control
   b. Petit mal seizures characterized by brief transient loss of consciousness with or without minor motor movements of eyes, head, or extremities
   c. Jacksonian seizures (focal-motor seizures) characterized by disturbed sensations and interrupted motor functioning, beginning in a somewhat localized area of the body and progressing to other parts of the body; the areas affected by the seizure usually reflect the area of the brain involved
   d. Psychomotor seizures are characterized by a transient clouding of consciousness, behavioral alterations, and changes in affect and perception
2. Diagnostic measures
   a. Health history
   b. Radiographic examination of the skull to rule out possible causes of seizures
      (1) X-ray film of skull
      (2) Ventriculogram—injection of air or oxygen into the lateral ventricles
      (3) Cerebral angiogram—injection of radiopaque liquid into the cerebral arteries so that circulation can be visualized
   c. Electrodiagnostic examinations to identify possible causes of seizures and fix the location of the problem
      (1) Electroencephalogram—electrodes are applied to scalp to obtain a graphic record of brain activity
      (2) Echoencephalogram—ultrasound transmitted through skull to map position of intracranial structures
   d. Blood chemistries to determine status of electrolytes
B. Medical therapy—the physician may
1. Prescribe anticonvulsant medications; e.g., phenytoin (Dilantin)

2. Prescribe sedatives to reduce emotional stress; e.g., phenobarbital

C. Nursing diagnosis and intervention
   1. Patient has a need for special safety precautions
      a. Assist patient to identify aura
      b. Help patient to prepare and provide some protection before the seizure develops
      c. Provide protection for patient during and after the seizure (maintain airway, protect from injury)
      d. Encourage patient to carry and wear a medical alert tag
      e. Encourage patient to take medications even when seizure free
      f. Help the patient to plan a schedule that provides for adequate rest and a reduction of stress
      g. Instruct patient to refrain from excessive use of alcohol since it is contraindicated with the medications
      h. The nurse should observe and teach patient and family to observe aura, initial point of seizure, type of seizure, level of consciousness, loss of control of bladder and bowel, progression of seizure, and postseizure condition
   2. Patient needs emotional support
      a. Encourage patient to express feelings about illness and the necessary changes in life-style and self-image
      b. Assist patient and family to accept diagnosis and develop some understanding of the disease process
      c. Help patient to understand that medication must be taken continuously for the remainder of life
      d. Refer the patient for job counselling as needed
      e. Encourage patient and family to attend meetings of the local epilepsy association
      f. Refer the patient for genetic counselling if appropriate (age of patient, cause of seizures)

Hypofunction of neural regulators
Etiology and pathophysiologic processes

A. Localized or systemic stresses can result in inflammation, demyelinization, degeneration, and destruction of nerve cells
B. These stresses can also interfere with the production and utilization of the enzymes that act as catalysts in the transmission of neural impulses
C. The above changes can result in varying degrees of neural hypofunction
D. These types of hypofunction include a decrease, interruption, or absence of the capacity to receive and/or transmit and/or associate neural impulses
E. Because of the complexity of neural transmission, any interference can result in dysfunctions of
   1. Motor control; e.g., paresis, spastic paralysis, flaccid paralysis, sphincter control, motor aphasia, coordination
   2. Sensation; e.g., anesthesia; paresthesia; affective aphasia; impaired sight, hearing, taste, smell; proprioception
   3. Highest integrative functioning; e.g., perception, association, memory, mood, intellect, judgment, level of consciousness

Hypofunction of spinal nerves
Example: spinal cord injury, characterized by sudden impingements on the integrity of the spinal cord as a result of trauma
A. Assessment of patient
   1. Clinical manifestations
      a. The symptoms depend on the location (lumbar, thoracic, cervical) and extent of the damage (complete transection, partial transection, compression) and may be temporary or permanent
      b. The immediate symptoms of spinal cord injury include
         (1) Severe pain at the site of the injury resulting at times in an initial loss of consciousness
         (2) Spinal shock
            (a) The initial response of the body to any spinal cord injury that interrupts the transmission of impulses
            (b) This generalized tissue and neural reaction causes a disruption of the motor, sensory, and reflex activities below the site of the injury
            (c) The disruption of activities is initially unrelated to the extent of the injury and the degree of

permanent loss cannot be determined until this stage passes

c. The early symptoms of spinal cord injury include

(1) Flaccid paralysis (immobility accompanied by weak, soft, flabby muscles) below the level of injury

(2) Hypotonia caused by disruption of neural impulses results in bowel and bladder distention

d. The later symptoms of spinal cord injury include

(1) Reflex hyperexcitability (spastic paralysis)—the muscles below the site of injury become spastic and hyperreflexic

(2) A state of diminished reflex excitability (flaccid paralysis) below the site of injury follows the state of reflex hyperexcitability in all instances of total cord damage and may occur in some instances of partial cord damage

(3) In total cord damage, since both the upper and lower motoneurons are destroyed, the symptoms depend totally on the location of the injury; the loss of motor and sensory function present at this time is usually permanent

(a) Sacral region—paralysis (usually flaccid type) of lower extremities (paraplegia) accompanied by atonic (autonomous) bladder and bowel with impairment of sphincter control

(b) Lumbar region—paralysis of lower extremities that may extend to the pelvic region (usually flaccid type) accompanied by a spastic (automatic) bladder and loss of bladder and anal sphincter control

(c) Thoracic region—the same symptoms as lumbar region except the

paralysis extends to the trunk below the level of the diaphragm

(d) Cervical region—the same symptoms as thoracic region except the paralysis extends from the neck down and includes paralysis of all extremities (quadriplegia)

(4) In partial cord damage either the upper or the lower motoneurons or both may be destroyed, therefore, the symptoms depend not only on the location but on the type of neurons involved

2. Diagnostic measures

a. Lumbar puncture to determine whether there is an increase in cerebrospinal fluid pressure and to obtain a specimen of fluid for examination if pressure is not too high

b. Queckenstedt test to determine the failure of the cerebrospinal pressure to rise in response to timed compression of the jugular veins

c. Neurologic examination to assess variations in reflexes, sensory responses, and motor status above and below the site of injury

B. Medical therapy—the physician may

1. Evaluate degree of shock and treat as necessary (maintain respirations, intravenous fluids, Foley catheter, temperature control)

2. Maintain vertebral alignment by ordering

a. Bed rest with supportive devices (bed board, sand bags, etc.)

b. Bed rest with total immobilization

c. Traction (skeletal or skin traction; e.g., Crutchfield tongs, Buck's extension)

d. Corsets, braces, and other devices when mobility is permitted

3. Intervene surgically to reduce pain or pressure and/or stabilize the spine

4. Maintain elimination by use of stool softeners, cathartics, or enemas

5. Maintain nutrition by use of high protein diet with vitamin supplements

6. Prescribe muscle relaxants and, if necessary, tranquilizers

C. Nursing diagnosis and intervention
1. Patient has special safety needs
   a. Provide protection from devices being used for immobilization
   b. Maintain spinal alignment at all times; when turning patient use log rolling method and make certain enough help is available to move patient as a single unit
   c. Check safety locks on Stryker frames and Circ-O-lectric beds before turning patient (see Rehabilitation nursing, pp. 542-543, for additional care for patients on these turning devices)
   d. Keep side rails in place or use safety straps
   e. Maintain frequent observation of patient's respiratory and neurologic functioning
   f. Maintain surgical asepsis for patient with Crutchfield tongs or spinal surgery
   g. Provide special skin care to back and bony prominences
   h. Maintain body parts in functional position; prevent dysfunctional contractures
   i. Make certain all devices used are in operating condition and that they fit properly and are correctly applied
2. Patient has special elimination needs
   a. Maintain fluid intake
   b. Monitor intake and output
   c. Administer stool softeners and laxatives as ordered; increase bulk in diet
   d. Use Circ-O-lectric bed or tilt table to place patient in standing position as soon as tolerated
   e. Remove Foley catheter as soon as possible
   f. Start bladder and bowel retraining as soon as patient is able (see Rehabilitation nursing, pp. 552-554, for bowel and bladder retraining)
3. Patient needs emotional support
   a. Provide patient with simple explanations
   b. Encourage patient to verbalize and accept that hostility will surface
   c. Stay with patient when possible to provide assurance
   d. Allow patient to be independent when possible
   e. Include patient in decision-making process
   f. Help patient to adjust to change in body image and altered self-concept
   g. Accept periods of depression that occur
   h. Allow patient time to reorganize life-style
   i. Set realistic short term goals so that patient can achieve some success
4. Patient has specific need for rehabilitation (see Rehabilitation nursing for specific areas)
   a. Assist patient in carrying out activities of daily living
   b. Assist patient to develop weakened and unaffected muscle groups
   c. Stimulate and motivate patient to become involved in rehabilitation therapy

Hypofunction in cerebrum

Example: cerebral vascular accident (CVA or stroke), characterized by a reduction in the oxygen available to the brain cells caused by a sudden or gradual interruption in blood supply following a rupture of vessels, a blocking of vessels by thrombi or emboli, or other diseases or conditions affecting the vascular system

A. Assessment of patient
1. Clinical manifestations
   a. Symptoms are caused by injury or destruction of brain tissue and depend on the area of the brain involved and the extent of the involvement
   b. Symptoms may include changes in
      (1) Level of consciousness (syncope, dizziness, drowsiness, or unconsciousness)
      (2) Highest integrative functions (confusion, changes in affect, disorientation, memory lapse, poor judgment)
      (3) Intracranial pressure (intracranial pressure is increased causing nausea, headache, blurred vision, increasing rise in blood pressure, widening of pulse pressure, slowing of pulse, vomiting, unequal pupils)
      (4) Vital signs (rise in blood pres-

sure, rapid bounding pulse, stertorous or labored respirations, temperature may vary greatly or become fixed at extremely elevated or subnormal level)

    (5) Motor function (impairment of speech to motor aphasia, weakness to paralysis on side opposite the lesion, loss of bladder or bowel control, sluggish to absent reaction of pupil to light, alterations in superficial and deep reflexes)

    (6) Sensory function (changes in sight, smell, taste, touch, and hearing; anesthesia; hyperesthesia; hypoesthesia; paresthesia)

  c. Other primary nonvascular stresses that do not begin as vascular problems; e.g., tumors, infections, or compound skull fractures may cause any or all of the above symptoms

2. Diagnostic measures
  a. Lumbar puncture to check for elevation of fluid pressure and to observe for presence of blood in the cerebrospinal fluid
  b. Vital signs, especially blood pressure readings, to observe for changes
  c. X-ray film of skull to determine nature and extent of injury
  d. Cerebral angiogram—see explanation under hyperfunction
  e. Brain scans—to test for variations in rate of uptake of radioactive isotopes; used to differentiate between brain tumors and vascular malformations
  f. Echoencephalogram—see explanation under hyperfunction
  g. Neurologic examination to assess reflexes, sensory responses, and motor status

B. Medical therapy—the physician may
1. Maintain patient on complete bed rest with head slightly elevated
2. Order oxygen in low concentration as needed
3. Maintain patient's fluid and electrolyte balance
4. Initiate measures to maintain circula-

tion and respirations; e.g., IPPB, elastic stockings
5. Initiate therapy that is palliative, symptomatic, and supportive depending on the cause and extent of the stroke
6. Prescribe medications to
  a. Control blood coagulation time
  b. Reduce high blood pressure; e.g., methyldopa (Aldomet)
  c. Reduce headache and nuchal rigidity; e.g., aspirin and propoxyphene (Darvon)
  d. Reduce restlessness and anxiety; e.g., phenobarbital and tranquilizers
  e. Decrease intercranial pressure; e.g., hypertonic solutions by mouth or intravenously, and diuretics such as Lasix
  f. Prevent straining on bowel movements; e.g., dioctyl sodium sulfosuccinate (Colace) and glycerine suppositories
7. Intervene surgically to relieve pressure and control bleeding
8. Order physiotherapy and rehabilitation therapy as soon as patient's physical condition is stabilized

C. Nursing diagnosis and intervention
1. Patient needs to maintain effective respiratory function
  a. Assess patient's respiratory functioning (vital signs, type and rate of respirations, color, blood gases, etc.)
  b. Assess gag and swallowing reflexes
  c. Maintain patency of airway by positioning, suctioning, and inserting artificial airway
  d. Provide for drainage and expansion of lungs by placing patient in a low semi-Fowler's position with head turned to the side
  e. Provide oxygen as necessary
  f. Provide frequent oral hygiene
2. Patient needs special safety precautions
  a. Observe for level of consciousness
  b. Monitor vital signs
  c. Observe for signs of increasing intracranial pressure
  d. Use side rails to prevent patient from falling
  e. Protect patient from accidents caused by loss of sensation and

muscle weakness (see Rehabilitation nursing, p. 555)

f. Provide for frequent nursing observations since patient may be unable to signal for assistance

3. Patient needs to prevent complications
   a. Decubiti
      (1) Provide special care to back and bony prominences; keep patient clean and dry
      (2) Relieve pressure by use of mechanical and supportive devices
      (3) Turn patient every 2 hours
   b. Contractures and atrophy
      (1) Provide for active and passive range of motion and other exercises
      (2) Use footboards and other devices to prevent footdrop, flexion of fingers, abduction of hips, adduction of shoulders and arms
   c. Circulatory and respiratory problems
      (1) Provide elastic stockings for both legs
      (2) Encourage patient to breathe deeply and cough; administer intermittent positive pressure if necessary
      (3) Encourage patient to turn or turn patient from side to side frequently
      (4) Administer medications as ordered
   d. Fecal impaction and/or urinary tract problems
      (1) Maintain adequate hydration
      (2) Administer stool softeners and laxatives
      (3) Monitor intake and output
      (4) Observe for bladder and bowel distension
      (5) Provide natural bulk in diet if possible
      (6) If patient is incontinent, begin bladder and bowel training as soon as possible (see Rehabilitation nursing, p. 554)

4. Patient needs emotional support
   a. When necessary, orient patient to time, place, and person
   b. Assist patient and family to set realistic goals
   c. Provide patient with the means of retaining and regaining as much independence as possible (see Rehabilitation nursing, pp. 551-552)
   d. Encourage patient to communicate (see Rehabilitation nursing, pp. 555-556)
   e. Provide simple realistic explanations of all procedures and treatments
   f. Provide realistic encouragement and praise
   g. Accept patient's mood swings and emotional outbursts

5. Patient has special feeding needs
   a. Provide patient with tube feeding if gag and swallowing reflexes are depressed or absent
   b. Provide foods in a form that is easily swallowed
   c. Assist patient with feeding; e.g., use of padded spoon handle; feed on unaffected side of mouth; feed in as close to a sitting position as possible

Hypofunction in combined sites

Example: multiple sclerosis or disseminated sclerosis, a chronic, debilitating, progressive disease with periods of remission and exacerbation characterized by randomly scattered patches of demyelination in the brainstem, cerebrum, cerebellum, and spinal cord

A. Assessment of patient
   1. Clinical manifestations
      a. The demyelination causes an interruption in the transmission of neural impulses, which are slowed or blocked resulting in symptoms that vary in character, number, and duration, and include
         (1) Visual disturbances—diplopia, scotomas, nystagmus, blindness
         (2) Sensory impairment—paresthesia, numbness, tingling, altered position sense
         (3) Motor impairment—facial weakness, incoordination, intention tremors, ataxia, fatigability, spasticity, loss of sphincter control, dysphagia
         (4) Emotional alterations—

euphoria, depression, irritability, inappropriate emotional affect
  b. If areas of demyelination increase and periods of remission shorten, symptoms become more severe with frequent complications such as urinary tract infections, paraplegia, contractures, respiratory infections, decubiti, severe muscle spasms, mental deterioration
  2. Diagnostic measures
  a. No specific diagnostic tests
  b. History of symptoms
  c. Electrophoresis of cerebrospinal fluid to test for an elevation of gamma globulin
  d. Neurologic examination to assess changes in reflexes, sensory responses, and motor status
B. Medical therapy—the physician may
  1. Treat symptoms as they develop since there is no specific therapy for this disorder
  2. Prescribe a series of anti-inflammatory drugs such as adrenocorticotropic hormone (ACTH) or prednisone to see if symptoms are relieved
  3. Order physiotherapy and rehabilitation therapy as necessary
  4. Prescribe muscle relaxants such as methocarbamol (Robaxin)
C. Nursing diagnosis and intervention
  1. Patient needs to maintain as much independence as possible for as long as possible
  a. Encourage patient to use supportive devices to maintain ambulation
  b. Provide active and passive range of motion and other exercises
  c. Teach patient to use assistive devices in carrying out activities of daily living
  d. Assist family to understand why patient should be permitted and encouraged to do things
  e. Assist patient and family to plan and implement a bowel and bladder regimen
  2. Patient and family need emotional support
  a. Explain the disease process to both patient and family in understandable terms
  b. Do not encourage false hopes during periods of remission
  c. Spend time listening to both patient and family and encourage them to ventilate
  d. Attempt to refer patient and family to National Multiple Sclerosis Society
  e. Encourage patient to seek counselling and rehabilitation
  f. Explain to patient and family that mood swings and emotional alterations are part of the disease process
  g. Help patient reestablish a realistic self-image
  3. Patient has special safety needs
  a. Teach patient to compensate for problems with gait (walk with feet further apart to broaden base of support, use low heel shoes) and provide assistive devices when necessary (tripod cane, walker, wheelchair)
  b. Teach patient to compensate for loss of sensation by using a thermometer to test water temperature, avoiding constricting stockings, using protective clothing in cold weather, changing position often
  c. Teach patient to compensate for difficulty in swallowing by taking small bites, chewing well, using a straw with liquids, using foods of more solid consistency
  d. If patient is immobilized
    (1) Provide special skin care to prevent decubiti
    (2) Provide special attention to joints and attempt to avoid dysfunctional contractures

HORMONAL REGULATION

A. Types of hormonal problems
  1. Hyperfunction of endocrine glands—excessive production of hormones
  2. Hypofunction of endocrine glands—insufficient production of hormones
B. General etiology
  1. The endocrine glands of the body are closely interrelated by an intricate feedback mechanism that provides a system of checks and balances
  2. Malfunction in one gland may directly or indirectly stimulate functional changes in other glands because of this feedback mechanism

3. The production of hormones and their effect on the body are influenced by
   a. Heredity
   b. Age
   c. Race
   d. Sex
   e. Emotional factors
   f. Environmental factors
   g. Physical status
4. Problems with endocrine regulation may be primary or secondary
5. Localized or systemic trauma, neoplasms, degenerative changes, or inflammation can result in alterations in cell structure and functions

Hyperfunction of endocrine glands
Etiology and pathophysiologic processes

A. Localized or systemic trauma, neoplasms, degenerative changes, or inflammation can result in a proliferation, hypertrophy, and/or hyperplasia of cells in an endocrine gland
B. The resulting proliferation, hypertrophy, and/or hyperplasia causes the gland to produce and secrete an excessive amount of its hormone
C. The hyperfunction of an endocrine gland usually produces a systemic response that depends on the glands affected and the action of the hormone

Examples of hyperfunction
Excessive production of thyroid hormones

Example: hyperthyroidism (Graves' disease), characterized by an excessive concentration of thyroid hormones in the blood, overactivity and changes in the thyroid glands
A. Assessment of patient
   1. Clinical manifestations
      a. Increased appetite and loss of weight; increased activity, irritability, emotional lability and apprehension; increased systolic pressure and pulse rate; heat intolerance and hyperhidrosis; increased respiratory rate and some dyspnea; fine hand tremors and exophthalmos
      b. May occur at periods of high physiologic and psychologic stress although considered by some to be an autoimmune reaction

c. If untreated can progress to thyroid crisis and death
   2. Diagnostic measures
      a. Obtain family and personal health history—in particular look for recent stresses and/or changes in life-style
      b. Basal metabolic rate (BMR) to determine whether metabolism of oxygen is increased
      c. Radioactive iodine uptake test to determine whether ability of thyroid to pick up iodine is increased
      d. Blood studies to test for increase in T_3 (triiodothyronine), T_4 (thyroxine), PBI (protein-bound iodine)
B. Medical therapy—the physician may
   1. Prescribe antithyroid medications such as propylthiouracil and methimazole (Tapazole) to block the synthesis of thyroid hormone
   2. Prescribe antithyroid medications such as iodine to reduce the vascularity of the thyroid gland
   3. Administer radioactive iodine to destroy thyroid gland cells thereby decreasing the production of thyroid hormone
   4. Prescribe medications to relieve the symptoms related to the increased metabolic rate; e.g., digitalis, propranolol (Inderal), phenobarbital
   5. Order a well balanced, high calorie diet with vitamin supplement
   6. Intervene surgically—subtotal or total thyroidectomy depending on the underlying pathology
C. Nursing diagnosis and intervention
   1. Patient needs rest and relaxation
      a. Assign patient to private room with means for temperature control
      b. Schedule treatments so they do not interfere with patient's rest
      c. Provide for periods of uninterrupted rest
      d. Administer medications to promote sleep
      e. Use nursing measures such as warm milk, warm bath, backrub, etc. to establish a climate for rest
      f. Protect patient from stress-producing visitors
   2. Patient needs dietary management to meet metabolic demands

a. Provide diet high in calories, essential nutrients, and vitamins
b. Increase intake of carbohydrates for quick energy and proteins for tissue repair
c. Provide supplementary feeding between meals and before bedtime
d. Keep a close check on patient's weight

3. Patient needs emotional support
   a. Accept patient's behavior, set limits only when behavior creates a danger for the patient
   b. Understand that patient is upset by lability of mood and exaggerated response to environmental stimuli; take time to explain disease processes involved
   c. Assist family to see the relationship between disease process and patient's behavior
   d. Recognize that patient has difficulty with fine motor movements and provide assistance in a routine manner
   e. Explain all procedures, but give explanations in such a manner that it does not add to patient's anxiety

4. Patient needs safe administration of medications
   a. Administer iodine solution through a straw and make certain entire amount is ingested
   b. Observe patient closely for side effects of iodine, propylthiouracil, or other medications

5. Patient needs additional safety after thyroid surgery
   a. Observe for signs of respiratory distress and laryngeal stridor caused by tracheal edema (keep tracheotomy set available)
   b. Observe dressings at operative site and at back of neck and shoulders for signs of hemorrhage
   c. Keep patient's bed in semi-Fowler's position without pillows and teach patient to support head
   d. Observe for signs of tetany that can occur after accidental trauma to parathyroids
   e. Observe for signs of thyroid crisis; e.g., high fever, tachycardia, irritability, delirium, coma
   f. Encourage patient to adhere to medical regimen

Excessive production of pituitary hormones

Example: hyperpituitarism (acromegaly), characterized by an excessive concentration of pituitary hormones in the blood, overactivity and changes in the anterior lobe of the pituitary gland

A. Assessment of the patient
   1. Clinical manifestations
      a. Increased soft tissue and bone thickness; facial features become coarse and heavy with enlargement of lower jaw, lips, and tongue; hands and feet become enlarged
      b. May be accompanied by diabetes mellitus and hyperthyroidism
      c. Disease ultimately results in many systemic changes that are irreversible but the course progresses slowly
   2. Diagnostic tests
      a. Personal health history—patient usually relates changes in personal appearance
      b. X-ray films of long bones, skull (sella turcica area), and jaw to determine changes in structure
      c. Blood studies to test for increase in pituitary hormones (somatotropin)
B. Medical therapy—the physician may
   1. Prescribe medications to relieve symptoms of other endocrine imbalances resulting from pituitary hyperfunctioning
   2. Intervene surgically or use irradiation on the pituitary
C. Nursing diagnosis and intervention
   1. Patient needs emotional support
      a. Assist patient to accept the altered body image, which is irreversible
      b. Assist family to understand what the patient is experiencing
      c. Help patient to recognize that medical supervision will be required for duration of life
      d. Help patient to understand the basis for the change in sexual functioning
      e. Assist patient to express feelings
   2. Patient needs additional safety after hypophysectomy
      a. Encourage patient to follow established medical regimen
      b. Protect patient from stress situations

c. Protect patient from infection
d. Establish and maintain a schedule for hormone replacement
e. For nursing care of patients with cranial surgery observe for signs of increasing intracranial pressure and shock (see pp. 452, 460, and 462)

Hypofunction of endocrine glands
Etiology and pathophysiologic processes

A. Localized or systemic trauma, neoplasm, degenerative changes, or inflammation can result in a destruction, degeneration, and/or atrophy of cells in an endocrine gland
B. The resulting destruction, degeneration, and/or atrophy causes the gland to produce and secrete an insufficient amount of its hormone
C. The hypofunction of an endocrine gland usually produces a systemic response that depends on the glands affected and the action of the hormone

Examples of hypofunction
Insufficient production of insulin

Example: diabetes mellitus, a chronic, familial disease characterized by an absence or decrease in the production of insulin or a problem with its utilization that leads to abnormalities in the metabolism of carbohydrates, fats, and proteins
A. Assessment of patient
  1. Clinical manifestations
    a. Polyuria and polydipsia—water is not reabsorbed by the renal tubules as a result of the osmotic activity of glucose that causes increased urination, resulting in dehydration and thirst
    b. Weight loss and polyphagia—inability to utilize glucose results in tissue breakdown, starvation, and wasting, resulting in a substantial increase in appetite
    c. Hyperglycemia—increased blood sugar level draws fluid out of the cell resulting in cellular dehydration
    d. Glycosuria—the blood sugar level exceeds the renal threshold for glucose, thus it spills into the urine
    e. Ketosis—incomplete metabolism of fat causes an accumulation of acid substances (ketone bodies) in the blood and urine that are character-istic of diabetic metabolic acidosis; the metabolic acidosis results in acid-base and fluid and electrolyte imbalances
    f. Onset is usually abrupt in juvenile diabetes (see Pediatric nursing, pp 405-406, for discussion of this type) and insidious in the adult type diabetes
  2. Diagnostic measures
    a. Obtain family history (in particular, look for history of diabetes ethnic and cultural background information)
    b. Obtain personal history (in particular, look for history of overweight obstetric history, recent infections history of physical and emotional stress, and appearance of cardinal symptoms)
    c. Urine analysis to detect the presence of glucose and/or ketone bodies
    d. Fasting blood sugar to determine increase in blood glucose level after 8 to 12 hours of fasting
    e. Glucose tolerance tests to determine increase in blood and urine glucose levels after ingestion of large amounts of glucose
B. Medical therapy—the physician may
  1. Direct therapy toward maintaining balance in diet, activity, and available insulin depending on the condition of the patient and the philosophy of the physician
  2. Select a specific type of insulin depending on the condition and needs of the patient (see Pharmacology, p 236)
  3. Prescribe hypoglycemics for some patients—however these patients must have some functioning beta cells in the islets of Langerhans (more commonly prescribed for the adult with late developing mild diabetes)
  4. Attempt to manage mild uncomplicated diabetes by the use of diet
  5. Adjust insulin after considering the patient's physical and emotional stresses
C. Nursing diagnosis and intervention
  1. Patient needs emotional support
    a. Assist patient to accept diagnosis
    b. Encourage patient to express feelings about illness and the necessary changes in life-style and self-image

c. Assist patient and family to develop an understanding of the disease process

d. Explain all procedures to patient and use feedback to make certain all directions are understood

e. Allow patient time to assimilate what is being told and what is happening

f. Help patient with the administration of medication until self-administration is both physically and psychologically possible

g. Foster independence but permit necessary dependence

h. Assist patient to recognize the need for continuing health supervision

i. Assist patient to recognize the need for activities that promote and maintain health

j. Assist patient to understand the basis and need for dietary control

k. Assist patient to develop constructive ways to handle the stress encountered in daily living

2. Patient needs to be able to accurately assess physical status

a. Teach patient how to test urine for sugar and acetone

b. Assist patient to interpret urine test results and how to act on the basis of the interpretations

c. Teach patient and family the signs of impending diabetic coma (restlessness; hot, dry, flushed skin; thirst; rapid pulse; nausea; fruity odor to breath)

d. Teach patient to seek medical supervision if signs of illness or diabetic coma develop

e. Teach patients who are receiving insulin and their families the signs of impending hypoglycemia (headache; nervousness; diaphoresis; rapid thready pulse; slurred speech)

f. Teach patients receiving insulin to carry a readily available source of glucose

g. Assist patient to assess the relationship between dietary intake, insulin, and activity and the steps necessary to adjust them

3. Patient needs special safety precautions

a. Teach patient to avoid possible sources of infection

b. Teach patient how to care for legs, feet, and toenails

c. Teach patient how to administer insulin—use of sterile technique; rotation of injection sites; measurement of dosage; types and strengths of insulin; peak action periods

d. Teach patient to use dietary chart to make substitutions in diet (see Nutrition, pp. 175 and 181-185)

e. Encourage patient to wear medical alert tag

f. Encourage patient to continue medical supervision and follow-up care including visits to ophthalmologist and podiatrist

Insufficient production of thyroid hormone

Example: hypothyroidism, characterized by the absence of decreased production of thyroid hormone classified by duration and degree of thyroid failure and the time in life in which it occurs (cretinism—hypothyroidism in infants and young children; hypothyroidism without myxedema—mild degree of thyroid failure in older children and adults; hypothyroidism with myxedema—severe degree of thyroid failure in older children and adults)

A. Assessment of patient

1. Clinical manifestations

a. Apathy, lethargy, dull mental processes

b. Stolid mask-like facies, enlarged tongue, drooling, dry brittle hair, dry, puffy, thickened skin

c. Increase in weight

d. Constipation

e. Intolerance to cold, subnormal temperature and pulse

2. Diagnostic measures

a. Obtain family and personal history (especially, look for changes in personal appearance and personality)

b. Basal metabolic rate (BMR) to determine whether metabolism of oxygen is decreased

c. Radioactive iodine uptake test to determine whether ability of thyroid to pick up iodine is decreased

d. Blood studies to test for decrease in T_3 (triiodothyronine), T_4 (thyroxine), PBI (protein-bound iodine)

B. Medical therapy—the physician may

1. Prescribe thyroid hormone replacement therapy

2. Order a well balanced diet with adequate hydration and roughage
C. Nursing diagnosis and intervention
   1. Patient needs emotional support
      a. Assist patient to accept diagnosis
      b. Encourage patient to express feelings about illness and the necessary changes in life-style and body image
      c. Assist patient and family to develop an understanding of the disease process
      d. Assist patient and family to plan enough time to allow for delayed mental processes and slowed physical responses if they are present
   2. Patient needs special safety precautions
      a. Teach patient to take thyroid replacement as ordered and use feedback to check understanding of medical regimen
      b. Teach patient to take only those medications that have been prescribed or approved by the physician
      c. Teach patient and family to be alert for signs of complications (angina pectoris—chest pain, feeling of indigestion; cardiac failure—dyspnea, palpitations; myxedema coma—weakness, syncope, slow pulse rate, subnormal temperature, slow respirations, lethargy)
      d. Teach patient to seek medical supervision on a regular basis and when any signs of illness develop
      e. Help patient and family to recognize that patient's inability to adapt to cold temperature requires the use of additional protection and modification of outdoor activity in cold weather
      f. Teach patient to avoid constipation by the use of adequate hydration and roughage in the diet

PATIENTS WITH PROBLEMS IN SENSORIMOTOR FUNCTIONING

TYPES OF SENSORIMOTOR PROBLEMS

A. Alterations in reception and transmission of stimuli
B. Alterations in balance, locomotion, and muscular activity

BASIC CONCEPTS

A. Motor and sensory functioning is primarily dependent on the anatomic and physiologic integrity of the
   1. Peripheral receptor organs and nerves
   2. Spinal cord and brain
   3. Upper and lower motor neurons
   4. Bones and cartilage
   5. Muscles, tendons, and ligaments
B. Motor activity is essential to maintain muscle tone
C. The transmission of messages through both sensory and motor nerves is essential for perception and for voluntary and involuntary muscle activity
D. Knowledge and awareness of the external environment depend on interpretations of sights, smells, tastes, sounds, and feelings received through the senses
E. Interruption, interference, or distortion in the reception, transmission, or interpretation of stimuli can greatly disturb the ability to function

ALTERATIONS IN RECEPTION AND TRANSMISSION OF STIMULI
Etiology and pathophysiologic processes

A. Alterations in reception and transmission of stimuli can result from localized or systemic chemical, microbiologic, developmental, physiologic, and physical stresses
B. The type of alterations include
   1. Interference or distortions in the reception of stimuli; e.g., cataracts, excessive cerumen, ruptured tympanic membrane, paresthesia, tic douloureux
   2. Interruption, interference, or distortions in the transmission of stimuli; e.g., otosclerosis, retinoblastoma, detached retina, glaucoma, peripheral neuritis

Interference or distortions in the reception of stimuli

Example: cataract, an opacity of the crystalline lens or its capsule resulting from injury, exposure to heat, heredity, aging, or congenital factors that causes a diminution of sight
A. Assessment of patient
   1. Clinical manifestations
      a. Distortion of vision; e.g., haziness, cloudiness, diplopia
      b. Photophobia

c. Progressive loss of vision

d. The usual black pupil appears clouded and progresses to milky white appearance

2. Diagnostic measures

a. Ophthalmoscopic examination to visualize the opaque lens

b. Snellen and reading charts to determine visual acuity

B. Medical therapy—the physician may

1. Prescribe corrective lenses until cataract matures enough for removal

2. Order preoperative preparation with mydriatics and ophthalmic antibiotics

3. Intervene surgically to remove opaque lens

4. Prescribe corrective lenses (contact lenses or glasses)

5. Prescribe antiemetics, analgesics, and stool softeners postoperatively

C. Nursing diagnosis and intervention

1. Patient has specific safety needs

a. Instruct patient to prevent pressure on eyes by

   (1) Not touching or rubbing eyes

   (2) Not closing eyes tightly

   (3) Avoiding coughing, sneezing, or bending from waist (teach patient to open mouth when coughing)

   (4) Lying on back or unoperative side

   (5) Avoiding rapid head movements

   (6) Avoiding straining at stool

b. Instruct patient to request prescribed analgesics and antiemetics as required

c. Administer stool softeners

d. Provide side rails to assist in turning and preventing falls

e. Assist patient with ambulation because of distortions in depth perception

f. Provide an easily accessible call bell

2. Patient needs environmental modifications

a. Reduce amount of light and encourage use of sunglasses when eye patch is removed

b. Provide a quiet environment to promote rest

c. Avoid substances that might precipitate coughing or sneezing; e.g., pepper, talcum powder

3. Patient needs to prevent complications

a. Observe for signs of increased intraocular pressure; e.g., pain, restlessness, increased pulse rate

b. Observe for signs of infection; e.g., pain, changes in vital signs

c. Encourage deep breathing

4. Patient needs emotional support

a. Explain to patient that vision will still be impaired until corrective lenses are prescribed and obtained

b. Keep patient oriented; e.g., address patient when entering the room, explain all activities and procedures, redescribe surroundings, assist with feedings

c. Explain to patient that depth perception will be altered but assure patient that the corrective lenses will help to compensate for this distortion

ALTERATIONS IN BALANCE, LOCOMOTION, AND MUSCULAR ACTIVITY

Etiology and pathophysiologic processes

A. Alterations in balance, locomotion, and muscular activity can result from localized or systemic chemical, microbiologic, developmental, physiologic, and physical stresses

B. The type of alterations include

1. Generalized neuromuscular interference in which there is an intact muscle but disturbed neural stimuli as in paralysis agitans (Parkinson's syndrome), poliomyelitis, myasthenia gravis

2. Localized musculoskeletal interference in which there is an intact neural pathway but an interruption in the integrity of the musculoskeletal system as in fractures, sprains, myositis, arthritis

Generalized neuromuscular interference in which there is an intact muscle but disturbed neural stimuli

Example: paralysis agitans (Parkinson's syndrome), a progressive disorder in which there is a destruction of nerve cells in the basal ganglia of the brain, which results in a generalized degeneration of muscular function; the suspected causes include neurochemical imbalance (dopamine and acetylcholine), unknown virus, cerebrovascular disease, and chemical or physical trauma

A. Assessment of patient
1. Clinical manifestations
   a. Mild diffuse muscular pain and increasing difficulty in performing usual activities such as writing, dressing, and eating
   b. Generalized tremor commonly accompanied by "pill-rolling" movements of the thumb against the fingers; tremors are usually reduced by intentional movements
   c. Feelings of stiffness and rigidity, particularly of large joints
   d. Various disorders of locomotion; e.g., bent posture, difficulty in rising from a sitting position, shuffling propulsive gait, loss of rhythmic arm swing when walking
   e. Masklike facial expression with unblinking eyes
   f. Low-pitched, slow, poorly modulated, poorly articulated speech
   g. Drooling may be present because of difficulty in swallowing saliva
   h. Various autonomic symptoms; e.g., lacrimation, constipation, incontinence, decreased sexual capacity, excessive perspiration, and undue sensitivity to heat
   i. Defects in judgment and emotional lability may be present but intelligence is usually not impaired
2. Diagnostic measures
   a. No specific diagnostic tests are available, diagnosis is made on basis of history and presenting symptoms
   b. History often reveals the incidence of viral infections, encephalitis, arteriosclerosis, or physical or chemical trauma
   c. Present complaints demonstrate a slow progression of symptoms which may vary in degree, are seldom proportional to each other, are highly individualized, and which tend to increase with fatigue, excitement, and frustrations

B. Medical therapy—the physician may
1. Order a medical regimen that is palliative rather than curative in an attempt to reduce the symptoms
2. Prescribe levodopa (L-dopa), which may assist in restoring striatal dopamine deficiency and improve dyskinesia and rigidity
3. Prescribe anticholinergic agents that counteract the action of acetylcholine in the central nervous system
4. Order a physiotherapy program designed to reduce rigidity of muscles and prevent contractures
5. Prescribe medications to relieve related symptoms; e.g., antispasmodics, antihistamines, and analgesics to relieve muscular pains; sedatives to relieve restlessness or insomnia
6. Intervene surgically by using alcohol, freezing (cryosurgery), electric cautery, ultrasound, etc., to destroy the globus pallidus (to relieve rigidity) and/or the thalamus (to relieve tremor) portions of the brain

C. Nursing diagnosis and intervention
1. Patient has special safety needs
   a. Protect patient from falls by using
      (1) Side rails on bed
      (2) Safety rails or built up toilet seat
      (3) Safety seat in shower
      (4) Flat supportive shoes
      (5) Only anchored scatter rugs
   b. Teach patient or family to cut food into small bite-size pieces to prevent choking
   c. Suction when necessary to maintain adequate airway (usually advanced stages)
   d. Observe for toxic side effects of medications; e.g., pulse changes
2. Patient has specific rehabilitative needs
   a. Teach patient activities to limit postural deformities; e.g., use firm mattress without a pillow, periodically lie prone, keep head and neck as erect as possible, consciously think about posture when walking
   b. Teach patient activities to maintain gait as normal as possible; e.g., clasp hands behind back when walking, exercise with stationary bicycle, use low heeled shoes
   c. Teach and encourage daily physical therapy program to limit rigidity and prevent contractures; e.g., warm baths, passive and active exercises
   d. Teach and encourage patient to

use self-help devices to maintain as much independence as possible

e. Teach patient to partially control hand and arm tremors by grasping the arms of a chair while sitting

3. Patient needs emotional support

a. Recognize that lability of emotions is part of the disease process

b. Attempt to administer care when patient is able to emotionally accept it

c. Provide time for patient to perform as much of daily routine as possible

d. Encourage patient to use self-help devices

e. Avoid rushing patient since patient is unable to function under pressure

f. Encourage patient to follow rehabilitative and dietary regimens

g. Assure patient that intelligence will not be affected by disease

h. Encourage patient to continue taking medications even though results may be minimal

4. Patient has specific dietary needs

a. Limit foods high in pyridoxine (vitamin B_6) since it decreases the effectiveness of levodopa; e.g., dried beans, dry milk, salmon, tuna, pork, beef liver, and kidneys

b. Encourage small intake of alcohol since it promotes relaxation and reduces rigidity

c. Encourage the intake of a well balanced diet in small frequent amounts prepared so that it is easily masticated

d. Encourage an adequate intake of roughage and fluids to avoid constipation

Localized musculoskeletal interference in which there is an intact neural functioning but an interruption in the integrity of musculoskeletal system

Example: fracture of the tibia—fractures are breaks in the continuity of the bone that are either complete or incomplete, simple or compound, usually accompanied by localized tissue response and spasms of the muscle

A. Assessment of patient

1. Clinical manifestations

a. Loss of alignment or contour of extremity

b. Loss of motion in extremity

c. Pain and tenderness

d. Muscle spasm

e. May have impaired loss of sensation

f. Break may be visible, bone may have pierced the skin or may have a bruised or ecchymotic area around injury

2. Diagnostic measures

a. History of trauma or an obvious break without trauma

b. If break has occurred without trauma (pathologic fracture), extensive testing must be done to rule out causative factors such as osteoporosis, Cushing's syndrome, multiple myeloma, metastatic or primary bone tumors

c. X-ray films of bone

B. Medical therapy—the physician may

1. Place the patient in traction to reduce the fracture

2. Intervene surgically to reduce the fracture (open reduction)

3. Reduce fracture by manipulation (closed reduction)

4. Apply a cast to the part

5. Prescribe analgesics for pain

6. Prescribe methocarbamol (Robaxin) to reduce muscle spasm

7. Order involved part elevated

8. Order bed rest

9. Prescribe antibiotics and tetanus toxoid

10. Order a high protein diet

C. Nursing diagnosis and intervention

1. Patient needs emergency intervention when found at site of accident

a. Evaluate general physical condition

b. Treat for shock

c. Splint suspected fractures before moving patient, treat all suspected fractures as fractures until x-ray films are available

d. Cover open wound with sterile dressing if available

2. Patient has special safety needs

a. Observe for signs of circulatory impairment; e.g., change in skin temperature or color, numbness or tingling, unrelieved pain, decrease in pedal pulse, prolonged blanching of toes after compression

b. Protect cast from damage until dry

by elevating it on a pillow, handle with palms of hands only

c. Promote drying of cast by leaving uncovered

d. Maintain bed rest until cast is dry and ambulation is permitted

e. Observe for signs of hemorrhage and measure extent of drainage on cast when present

f. Observe for irritation caused by rough cast edges, and pad as necessary

g. Observe for swelling and notify physician if necessary

h. Observe for signs of emboli (fat or blood clot)

i. Administer analgesics judiciously and report unrelieved pain

j. Observe for signs of infection; e.g., elevated temperature, odor from cast, swelling

3. Patient has rehabilitative needs

a. Teach patient isometric exercises to promote muscle tone

b. Teach patient appropriate crutch walking technique (nonweight-bearing—three-point swing through, weight-bearing—four-point progressing to use of cane)

c. Encourage patient to elevate leg when sitting

d. Encourage high protein, high vitamin diet to promote healing

PATIENTS WITH PROBLEMS IN CARDIOPULMONARY FUNCTIONING

TYPES OF CARDIOPULMONARY PROBLEMS

A. Interference with intake of oxygen
B. Impairment of oxygen exchange
C. Interference with transportation of oxygen to body cells

BASIC CONCEPTS

A. A constant supply of oxygen in the environment is necessary for survival

B. A patent airway and an unobstructed respiratory tract are necessary for adequate oxygenation

C. The process of respiration is under neural (central nervous and autonomic) and chemical (oxygen, carbon dioxide, and pH) control

D. The process of inspiration and expiration depends on the maintenance of alternating positive and negative pressure within the lungs

E. Pulmonary ventilation depends on the ability of the lungs and the muscles of respiration to expand and contract

F. Gaseous exchange occurs in the alveoli and depends on the condition of the alveolar membrane, the oxygen pressure gradient, and the adequacy of the pulmonary capillary circulation

G. An adequate supply of hemoglobin in the red blood cells is necessary to pick up the oxygen from the lungs

H. Cellular respiration (internal respiration) depends on an adequate supply of hemoglobin, an effective cardiac output, and an efficient vascular network

I. Interference with the intake, exchange, or transportation of oxygen may directly or indirectly affect the function of other parts of the body

J. The nature of the effect is directly related to the cause, location, and degree of the interference

INTERFERENCE WITH INTAKE OF OXYGEN

Etiology and pathophysiologic processes

A. Interference with oxygen intake can result from localized or systemic chemical, microbiologic, developmental, and physical stresses

B. The types of interference include

1. Insufficient oxygen available in the environment; e.g., carbon monoxide poisoning, smoke poisoning, high altitudes

2. Disturbances in neural stimulation and muscular control of respirations; e.g., anxiety reactions, myasthenia gravis, poliomyelitis, Guillain-Barré syndrome

3. Obstructions within the respiratory tract; e.g., mucous plugs, foreign objects, edema or neoplasms of the larynx or bronchus

4. Interruptions in the integrity or expansion of lung tissue; e.g., penetrating chest wounds, crushing chest wounds, diaphragmatic hernia, ascites

Insufficient oxygen in the environment

Example: carbon monoxide poisoning—oxygen is replaced in the hemoglobin by the carbon monoxide molecule resulting in the stable compound of carboxyhemoglobin; this substance causes tissue anoxia and respiratory depression

A. Assessment of patient
   1. Clinical manifestations
      a. Headache
      b. Level of consciousness—lassitude, drowsiness, or coma
      c. Skin—cherry pink or cyanotic
   2. Diagnostic measures
      a. History of exposure to carbon monoxide; e.g., automobile exhaust, coal burning stove, gas heaters
      b. CBC and hemoglobin
      c. Few specific tests available
B. Medical therapy—the physician may
   1. Administer artificial respiration
   2. Order 100% oxygen until carboxyhemoglobin is reduced and respirations are normal
   3. Administer 50% glucose or mannitol intravenously for cerebral edema
C. Nursing diagnosis and intervention
   1. Patient needs emergency intervention when found at the source of carbon monoxide fumes
      a. Remove individual from immediate area
      b. Evaluate for cardiopulmonary function
      c. Institute cardiopulmonary resuscitation if necessary and maintain until additional help arrives
      d. Administer oxygen if available
   2. Patient needs to maintain ventilation and perfusion
      a. Maintain respirations with assistance, if necessary
      b. Maintain body temperature
      c. Observe vital signs with special concern for respirations
      d. Maintain oxygen flow at prescribed levels

Disturbances in neural stimulation and muscle control of respirations

Example: hyperventilation associated with anxiety reactions—hyperventilation is the rapid, prolonged deep breathing usually associated with anxiety whereby excessive carbon dioxide is expired and subnormal concentrations result in blood (hypocapnia)

A. Assessment of patient
   1. Clinical manifestations
      a. Presence of intermittent periods of abnormally rapid deep respirations
      b. Extreme anxiety approaching hysteria
      c. Syncope and lightheadedness
   2. Diagnostic measures
      a. Arterial blood gases to check for respiratory alkalosis (lowered pCO_2 and elevated pH)
      b. Determine whether patient's symptoms are related to environmental stimuli by reducing the stimuli and observing patient's response
B. Medical therapy—the physician may
   1. Administer carbon dioxide therapy by use of a paper bag for rebreathing expired air or by use of the gas itself
   2. Initiate psychotherapy after all physical causes have been ruled out
   3. Prescribe tranquilizers
C. Nursing diagnosis and intervention
   1. Patient needs emotional support
      a. Spend time with the patient
      b. Allow time and encourage verbalization of feelings
      c. Help patient to identify anxiety-producing situations and explore alternate methods of dealing with anxiety
      d. Provide activities that assist patient to rechannel feelings
      e. Encourage patient to participate in psychotherapy sessions
   2. Patient has special safety needs
      a. Assist patient to identify initial symptoms of hyperventilation
      b. Protect patient from falls and accidents

Obstructions within the respiratory tract

Example: cancer of the larynx, a malignant tumor that occludes the trachea and interrupts oxygen intake and speech

A. Assessment of patient
   1. Clinical manifestations
      a. Chronic hoarseness, cough, hemoptysis, dyspnea
      b. Presence of enlarged lymph nodes in cervical region
      c. Weight loss and sore throat
   2. Diagnostic measures
      a. History of hoarseness, weight loss, and sore throat
      b. Laryngoscopy with biopsy
      c. X-ray—barium swallow
B. Medical therapy—the physician may
   1. Radiate the area
   2. Order a series of chemotherapeutics;

e.g., methotrexate, bleomycin, fluorouracil
3. Intervene surgically
   a. Thyrotomy—removal of tumor from the larynx via an incision through the thyroid cartilage
   b. Total laryngectomy—removal of total larynx with construction of a permanent tracheostomy
   c. Radical neck dissection (used when tumor has metastasized into surrounding tissue and lymph nodes)—removal of larynx, surrounding tissue and muscle, lymph nodes, and glands with a permanent tracheostomy
4. Use chemotherapy, radiation, and surgery alone or in any combination
C. Nursing diagnosis and intervention for a patient with a total laryngectomy
   1. Patient needs emotional support before surgery
      a. Provide patient with time to discuss diagnosis and the ramifications of surgery
      b. Assist and encourage patient to express feelings
      c. Answer patient's questions as thoroughly and honestly as possible
      d. Arrange for individuals with laryngectomies to visit patient and discuss rehabilitative process
      e. Instruct patient as to method of communication that will be used postoperatively; e.g., slate board and chalk, pencil and paper, sign language
   2. Patient needs special safety measures after surgery
      a. Observe for obstruction of airway by mucous plugs, edema, or blood; e.g., air hunger, dyspnea, cyanosis, gurgling
      b. Observe for signs of hemorrhage; e.g., increased pulse rate, drop in blood pressure, cold clammy skin, appearance of blood on dressing
      c. Stay with patient but provide a bell or other system for patient to signal for help
      d. Provide at patient's bedside suction apparatus and catheters (additional laryngectomy tube and a surgical instrument set with additional hemostats should be immediately available should tube become dislodged or blocked)
      e. Prevent cross-infection and contamination of the wound by providing special oral hygiene, cleanliness at tracheal site, avoidance of people with respiratory infections, use of clean equipment
      f. In patients receiving radiation or chemotherapy, observe for signs of adverse reactions
   3. Patient needs help to psychologically adjust to laryngectomy
      a. Expect and accept a period of mourning but prevent withdrawal from reality by
         (1) Involving patient in laryngectomy care
         (2) Keeping channels of communication open
         (3) Supporting patient's strengths
         (4) Encouraging return to activities of daily living
         (5) Allowing patient time to write responses or use sign language
      b. Encourage patient to get involved in speech therapy and realistically support efforts and gains
      c. Teach patient the skills necessary to handle altered body functioning including
         (1) Method of tracheal-bronchial suctioning to maintain patency of airway emphasizing pressure, depth, frequency, and safety
         (2) Method of changing, cleaning, and securing laryngectomy tube
         (3) Care of skin around opening
         (4) Importance of providing humidified air for inspiration to prevent drying of secretions (can be achieved by use of moist dressing)
      d. Teach patient to avoid activities that may permit water or irritating substances to enter the trachea since the usual defensive mechanisms (glottis and cilia) are absent; patient should avoid showers, swimming, dust, hair spray, and other volatile substances
      e. Teach patient to avoid wearing

clothes with tight collars or constricting necklines

f. Teach patient that certain other activities will be interrupted; e.g., sipping through a straw, whistling, blowing the nose

Interruptions in the integrity or expansion of lung tissue

Example: a penetrating chest wound that extends through the skin, muscle, and pleura allowing air and/or blood to enter the pleural cavity causing a collapse of the lung tissue and a reduction in the lung capacity

A. Assessment of patient
1. Clinical manifestations
  a. Presence of a wound with a sucking sound on inspiration
  b. Presence of dyspnea, cyanosis, and symptoms of mild to profound shock depending on size of wound
  c. Mediastinal shift may occur toward the unaffected side caused by the pressure exerted by a pneumothorax or hemothorax causing a change in the site of the apical pulse and paradoxic respirations
2. Diagnostic measures
  a. Physical examination of the chest
  b. X-ray film of chest
B. Medical therapy—the physician may
1. Apply a pressure dressing over wound
2. Aspirate the pleural cavity to promote lung expansion
3. Establish a water sealed suction drainage
4. Reduce the oxygen demand by ordering bed rest and limitation of activity
5. Order oxygen as necessary
6. Restore blood volume and treat shock
7. Prescribe antibiotics and mild analgesics
8. Utilize respiratory therapy to promote lung expansion
C. Nursing diagnosis and intervention
1. Patient needs special safety measures
  a. Keep water sealed drainage below level of chest
  b. Keep a clamp readily available to close off tubes should the water seal be broken
  c. Make certain chest tubes are patent and suction is maintained
  d. Prevent tension on the drainage tubes

e. Observe patient for dyspnea and cyanosis
f. Monitor vital signs every 15 minutes until stable
g. Keep patient directly off affected side but turn frequently and encourage coughing
2. Patient needs emotional support
  a. Encourage patient to move and cough
  b. Teach patient to self-splint with hands and arms
  c. Explain purpose and functioning of chest tubes and water sealed drainage
  d. Administer oxygen and analgesics as ordered and as necessary
  e. Encourage patient to follow directions of respiratory therapists; e.g., blow bottles, IPPB

IMPAIRMENT OF OXYGEN EXCHANGE
Etiology and pathophysiologic processes

A. Impairment of oxygen exchange can result from localized or systemic chemical, microbiologic, developmental, and physical stresses that alter gaseous exchange at the alveolar membrane by interfering with ventilation, diffusion, or perfusion
B. The types of impairment include
1. Alterations in alveolar membrane
  a. Character of membrane; e.g., hyperplasia and fibrosis as seen in chronic bronchitis, recurrent pneumonitis, cystic lung disease; loss or lack of elasticity of membrane as seen in emphysema, hyaline membrane disease, neoplastic disease
  b. Reduction in the amount of membrane as seen in tuberculosis, neoplasms, abscesses
2. Alterations in the flow of oxygen across the alveolar membrane in the absence of change in the pulmonary structures as seen in pneumonia, pulmonary edema, pulmonary embolism (anemia also interferes with oxygen exchange but will be discussed under interference with transportation)

Alterations in the character of the alveolar membrane

Example: emphysema, a chronic destructive lung disease occurring as a sequela to chronic bronchitis, excessive smoking, or asthma; characterized by distended, inelastic, or destroyed alveoli and a bronchiolar obstruction and collapse; these alterations greatly impair the diffusion of gases through the alveolocapillary membrane

A. Assessment of patient
1. Clinical manifestations
   a. Dyspnea, orthopnea, expiratory wheezing, stertorous breathing sounds, cough
   b. Fatigue, weakness, hypoxia, anorexia, and weight loss
   c. Headache, impaired sensorium
   d. Barrel chest, cyanosis, and clubbing of fingers
   e. Distention of neck veins
   f. Edema of extremities
2. Diagnostic measures
   a. Check history for evidence of heavy smoking, chronic bronchitis, or asthma
   b. Pulmonary function tests such as tidal volume, vital capacity, and residual air to determine extent of respiratory damage
   d. Blood chemistries to check for pH, blood gases, CO_2-combining power
   e. Complete blood count and hematocrit to determine the presence of infection or polycythemia
   f. X-ray films of chest

B. Medical therapy—the physician may
1. Advise the elimination of smoking and other external irritants, such as dust, as much as possible
2. Prescribe antibiotics and cortisone to prevent and reduce inflammation
3. Prescribe bronchodilators to reduce muscular spasm
4. Prescribe mucolytics and expectorants to liquefy secretions and to facilitate their removal
5. Order oxygen at 2 to 3 L. if hypoxia is severe
6. Establish a respiratory therapy program to include IPPB, postural drainage, exercise, and blow bottles
7. Place the patient on a high protein, soft diet

C. Nursing diagnosis and intervention
1. Patient needs to facilitate respirations
   a. Teach patient proper use of nebulizer
   b. Teach or supervise patient's respiratory exercises such as pursed lip or diaphragmatic breathing
   c. Administer medications as ordered
   d. Maintain patient's fluid intake
   e. Carefully monitor patient for symptoms of carbon dioxide intoxication if oxygen is being administered
   f. Teach patient to adjust activities to avoid overexertion
2. Patient has special safety needs
   a. Teach patient to avoid people with respiratory infections
   b. Teach patient to maintain resistance by getting proper rest, eating proper food, dressing properly for existing weather conditions
   c. Teach patient to be alert to early symptoms of infection, hypoxia, hypercapnia, or adverse response to medications
   d. Encourage patient to continue with close medical supervision
3. Patient needs emotional support
   a. Encourage patient to express feelings about disease and therapy
   b. Accept patient's feelings about lifelong restrictions in activity
   c. Encourage patient to take an active role in planning therapy
   d. Encourage patient to take medications as ordered
   e. Support patient's efforts to give up smoking by providing diversional activities such as eating hard candies
   f. Encourage family to support patient's efforts to give up smoking

Reduction in the amount of alveolar membrane

Example: tuberculosis, a chronic infectious disease that progressively destroys lung tissue, characterized by formation of a tubercle that undergoes caseation and cavity formation before healing by the process of fibrosis

A. Assessment of patient
1. Clinical manifestations
   a. Fatigue, lassitude, and weight loss
   b. Cough productive of yellowish mucoid sputum and hemoptysis
   c. Indigestion and anorexia
   d. Late afternoon temperature elevation or "night sweats"
   e. Vague chest pain and dyspnea
   f. Pallor
2. Diagnostic measures
   a. X-ray examination of chest to de

termine presence of calcified lesions

b. Analysis of sputum and gastric contents for presence of acid-fast bacilli

c. Tuberculin testing such as tine, Heaf, or Mantoux to determine antibody response to tubercle bacillus; while these tests indicate prior exposure to the bacillus rather than an active disease state, a sudden change from negative to positive requires further testing and/or prophylactic therapy

3. Medical therapy—the physician may
   1. Determine and prescribe a program of combined antituberculin drugs such as INH, PAS, streptomycin, PZA
   2. Keep patient on bed rest until symptoms abate or therapeutic regimen is established
   3. Determine that a surgical resection of the involved lobe is necessary if symptoms such as hemorrhage develop or chemotherapy is unsatisfactory
   4. Place immediate contacts on prophylactic therapy (all cases and follow-up of contacts must be reported to public health agency)
   5. Place the patient on high carbohydrate, high protein, high vitamin diet with supplemental vitamin B_6

C. Nursing diagnosis and intervention
   1. Patient needs health teaching
      a. Teach patient to provide for scheduled rest periods
      b. Teach patient which foods to include in diet and the use of nutritious between-meal supplements
      c. Teach patient the importance of maintaining the drug program that has been established without variation
      d. Teach patient the proper techniques to prevent spread of infection
         (1) Frequent hand washing
         (2) Cover mouth when coughing
         (3) The proper use and disposal of tissues
         (4) The proper cleansing of eating utensils and disposal of food wastes
         (5) The use of isolation when the sputums are positive for the organism

   2. Patient has special need to limit complications; e.g., secondary infections, hemorrhage, development of drug-resistant strain of organism, side effects of drugs
      a. Encourage patient to participate in developing a schedule of activities and therapy and following the schedule once established
      b. Instruct patient to be alert to the early symptoms of hemorrhage such as hemoptysis, and to contact the physician immediately if any occur
      c. Instruct patient to be alert to the early symptoms of adverse drug reactions (e.g., neuritis, ringing in the ears, ataxia, dermatitis) and to contact the physician immediately if any occur
      d. Encourage patient to follow prescribed program for productive coughing and deep breathing
      e. Instruct patient to avoid any medications such as cough syrups without physician's approval
      f. Explain the need for and instruct the patient to continue follow-up care and supervision

   3. Patient has specific emotional needs
      a. Encourage patient to express feelings about disease and the many ramifications (stigma, isolation, fear) it creates
      b. Expect and accept patient's expression of hostility and depression
      c. Encourage patient to limit activities until physician gives approval for gradual increase
      d. Help patient plan a realistic schedule for taking the large number of necessary medications

Alterations in the flow of oxygen across the alveolar membrane in the absence of change in pulmonary structures

Example: pulmonary edema, an acute emergency condition characterized by a rapid accumulation of fluid in the alveolar spaces, a complication of valvular disease, left ventricular failure, circulatory overload, or congestive heart disease whereby blood backs up into the pulmonary circulation increasing pulmonary pressure and causing a filtering of fluid into the tissue spaces

A. Assessment of patient

1. Clinical manifestations
   a. Dyspnea, orthopnea, gurgling, wheezing, stertorous breathing sounds
   b. Cyanosis, air hunger, acute anxiety, apprehension, and restlessness
   c. Cough productive of pink frothy sputum
   d. Rapid thready pulse
2. Diagnostic measures
   a. Physical examination
   b. History of premonitory symptoms such as shortness of breath, paroxysmal nocturnal dyspnea, wheezing, and orthopnea
   c. Venous pressure and circulation time to measure cardiac output
B. Medical therapy—the physician may
   1. Administer morphine sulfate intravenously or subcutaneously
   2. Prescribe digitalization of the patient
   3. Prescribe diuretics intravenously or intramuscularly
   4. Prescribe bronchodilators such as aminophylline
   5. Order oxygen in high concentration or by IPPB as necessary
   6. Do a phlebotomy to remove aproximately 500 ml. of blood or order the application of rotating tourniquets to reduce the volume of circulating blood
   7. Begin cardiac monitoring
   8. Order blood chemistries and blood gases
C. Nursing diagnosis and intervention
   1. Patient needs to reestablish oxygen exchange
      a. Administer digitalis, bronchodilators, and diuretics as ordered
      b. Administer oxygen as ordered
      c. Support patient in a high- or semi-Fowler's position
      d. Carry out rotation of tourniquets as ordered and carefully observe patient's response
      e. Observe and record vital signs and cardiac monitoring
   2. Patient needs emotional support
      a. Stay with patient and provide a call bell even if you are just leaving for a moment
      b. Administer morphine sulfate as ordered to reduce anxiety
      c. Reassure patient by providing continuous presence of a staff member

and by giving brief explanations of all therapy
   d. Anticipate patient's needs to reduce the expenditure of energy
3. Patient needs to limit fluid intake
   a. Explain to patient why fluids are limited
   b. Carefully measure intake and output
   c. Administer all intravenous medications slowly
   d. Fluids offered to patient should be high in potassium to offset loss with diuretics

INTERFERENCE WITH TRANSPORTATION OF OXYGEN TO BODY CELLS

Etiology and pathophysiologic processes

A. Interference with transportation of oxygen can result from localized or systemic chemical, microbiologic, developmental, and physical stresses that affect the structure or function of the heart, vessels, blood, or blood-forming organs, thereby altering cellular (internal) respirations
B. The types of interference include
   1. Disturbances in the quantity and quality of blood; e.g., anemia, leukemia, polycythemia, bone marrow depression, other blood dyscrasias, and hypovolemic shock
   2. Disturbances in the effectiveness of the pumping action of the heart caused by alterations in electric stimulation as seen in cardiac arrhythmias and Adams-Stokes syndrome; changes in cardiac muscle as seen in myocardial infarction, myocarditis, and ventricular hypertrophy; impairment of valvular function as seen in mitral stenosis and aortic insufficiency; congenital malformation of the internal or external structure of the heart as seen in patent ductus arteriosus, patent foramen ovale, and transposition of the great vessels
   3. Disturbances in the structure, elasticity, and/or patency of other than coronary vessels resulting in alterations of blood flow as seen in peripheral vascular disease such as arteriosclerosis, atherosclerosis, thrombophlebitis, varicosities, and aneurysms

Disturbance in the quantity and/or quality of the blood

Example: anemia, an abnormal reduction or formation of the circulating red blood cells with a decrease in the total hemoglobin, which results in an interference with oxygen supply to the body cells; anemia is not a specific disease but is a manifestation of several different types of pathophysiology; e.g., marrow alterations or failure caused by toxic substances, nutritional deficiencies, tumor invasion, idiopathies; cell loss caused by bleeding or hemolysis; changes in cell structure or development caused by inherited or acquired factors (see Pediatric nursing, pp. 398-400, for additional information on the anemias)

A. Assessment of patient
  1. Clinical manifestations
    a. Symptoms depend on the severity and chronicity of the anemia, the age of the patient, and the underlying pathophysiology
    b. Symptoms are the result of tissue hypoxia (see Fundamentals of nursing, pp. 317-321)
    c. Pallor, dyspnea, increased rate of pulse and respiration, palpitations
    d. Easy fatigability, weakness, diaphoresis on exertion
    e. Restlessness, confusion, dizziness, headache, syncope, sensitivity to cold, and peripheral sensory motor changes
    f. Untreated, may progress to congestive heart failure or angina
  2. Diagnostic measures
    a. Complete blood studies including red blood count, hemoglobin, white blood count, platelet count, hematocrit, mean corpuscular volume (MCV), mean corpuscular hemoglobin (MCH), mean corpuscular hemoglobin concentration (MCHC), bilirubin, urobilinogen
    b. Bone marrow biopsy to examine cells active in blood cell production
    c. Gastric analysis to determine level of hydrochloric acid (intrinsic factor in pernicious anemia)
    d. Further diagnostic measures will be directed toward identifying primary cause of anemia; e.g., occult blood in stool, red blood cells in urine

B. Medical therapy—depending on the primary cause of the anemia, the physician may
  1. Order a high vitamin, high mineral, high protein diet
  2. Prescribe supplemental vitamins either orally or parenterally; e.g., B_{12}, iron, folic acid, vitamin C
  3. Prescribe appetite stimulants; e.g., wine, vitamin B_1
  4. Prescribe bone marrow stimulants; e.g., androgens
  5. Order oxygen as necessary
  6. Administer cell replacement therapy; e.g., blood transfusions, packed cells

C. Nursing diagnosis and intervention
  1. Patient needs to increase oxygen to cells
    a. Decrease oxygen needs by restricting activity
    b. Encourage periods of rest
    c. Administer oxygen as necessary
    d. Administer medications as ordered
    e. Keep warm but prevent overheating
  2. Patient has special safety needs
    a. Protect patient from falling
    b. Encourage patient to change position slowly
    c. Instruct patient to sit or lie down when dizzy
    d. Provide proper skin care
    e. Observe for reactions during transfusions
    f. Protect patient from injury caused by reduced sensorimotor response
  3. Patient needs health teaching
    a. Instruct patient to take medications as ordered
    b. Teach patient to follow established dietary regimen
    c. Instruct patient to avoid people with infectious diseases

Disturbance in the effectiveness of the pumping action of the heart

Example: myocardial infarction, an acute necrosis of an area of heart muscle caused by the interruption of the oxygen supply to the area resulting in altered functioning and reduced cardiac output

A. Assessment of the patient
  1. Clinical manifestations
    a. Sudden, severe, crushing or vicelike pain in the substernal region;

may radiate to the arms, neck, and back
b. Nausea and vomiting
c. Severe anxiety, dyspnea, pallor, cyanosis of extremities, circumoral pallor
d. Signs of shock; cold clammy skin, profuse diaphoresis, decreased blood pressure, rapid thready pulse

2. Diagnostic measures
a. Patient's health history including smoking and drinking habits, obesity, high cholesterol diet, physical and emotional stresses, chest pain, hypertension
b. Blood serum enzyme levels including serum glutamic-oxaloacetic transaminase (SGOT), lactic dehydrogenase (LDH), creatine phosphokinase (CPK) to determine tissue damage
c. Complete blood studies, particularly white blood cells and sedimentation rate, to determine presence of inflammatory process
d. Electrocardiogram and vectorcardiogram to determine any changes in the electric activity of the heart
e. Arterial blood gases particularly CO_2-combining power to identify amount of base bicarbonate available to combine with cations

B. Medical therapy—the physician may
1. Admit patient to coronary care unit
2. Prescribe morphine sulfate intravenously or subcutaneously to relieve pain and reduce apprehension
3. Place patient on bed rest with cardiac precautions to reduce demand for oxygen
4. Order oxygen as necessary
5. Order cardiac monitoring for continued surveillance of the heart's electric activity
6. Order frequent monitoring of vital signs including temperature, pulse (apical and radial), respirations, blood pressure, intake, and output
7. Prescribe one or more of the following medications to prevent or reduce complications: antiarrhythmic agents, digitalis, diuretics, anticoagulants, potassium salts, vasopressors or vasodilators, sedatives, and stool softeners
8. Start intravenous fluids at slow rate to keep vein open

9. Insert central venous pressure catheter to permit continuous monitoring
10. Order clear liquid diet as tolerated for first 48 hours progressing to soft low sodium, low caloric diet
11. Order blood studies as necessary to determine course of disease

C. Nursing diagnosis and intervention
1. Patient needs continuous observation of physical status
a. Observe cardiac monitor and immediately report changes in rate, conductivity, and rhythm
b. Observe for ventricular fibrillation and asystole and take appropriate life saving actions if they occur; e.g., cardiopulmonary resuscitation, electric defibrillation
c. Observe for other variations such as premature ventricular contractions close to a T-wave, ventricular tachycardia, and atrial fibrillation; if they occur administer prescribed medications and notify the physician
d. Observe patient's vital signs every 15 minutes until stable
e. Closely observe patient's intake and output
f. Measure central venous pressure as ordered
g. Observe for pulmonary congestion and dependent edema
h. Observe for pain and restlessness and administer medication as ordered
i. Observe for cyanosis and dyspnea and administer oxygen as necessary
j. Check laboratory tests for bleeding time before administering anticoagulants
k. If patient is receiving anticoagulants, observe for signs of bleeding
l. If patient is receiving digitalis, observe for signs of digitalis toxicity

2. Patient needs emotional support
a. Do not forget that there is a patient beyond the machinery
b. Recognize that patient is probably scared to death
c. Allow patient time to express feelings and fears
d. Explain all procedures to patient in simple direct terms
e. Encourage patient to ask questions

and answer them as honestly as possible

f. Encourage patient to follow the physician's orders and allow nursing staff to do the necessary care

g. Allow patient to be dependent but encourage independence when possible

h. Include patient in developing a plan of care

i. Help patient to accept and adjust to the necessary changes in lifestyle

j. Observe patient's emotional response to visitors and regulate visiting according to the observations

k. Encourage patient to stay on special diet

Disturbance in the structure, elasticity, and/or patency of vessels other than coronary vessels

Example: gangrene of the toes—gangrene occurs as a result of peripheral vascular disease, which interferes with the transportation of oxygenated blood to an area and the transportation of unoxygenated blood and wastes from an area; tissue anoxia progresses to tissue necrosis and removal of the part is often necessary

A. Assessment of patient
  1. Clinical manifestations
     a. Change in color, temperature, and sensation
     b. Pain that may be severe and continuous
     c. Absence or weakness of peripheral pulse
     d. Presence of ulcerative/necrotic lesion
  2. Diagnostic measures
     a. Patient's health history including smoking habits, type of employment, obesity, diabetes, age, history of exposure to severe cold, cramps, pain, difficulty in walking, change in sensation, slow healing sores on lower extremity
     b. Skin temperature studies
     c. Angiography to visualize the vascular system
     d. Oscillometry to measure pulse volume in larger arteries
     e. Exercise tolerance test to determine presence of intermittent claudication

f. Lumbar sympathetic block to determine arterial response to blocking of sympathetic nerve enervation

g. Phleborheogram to measure the flow of blood through vessels

h. Electrophoresis to measure lipoproteins in the blood

B. Medical therapy—the physician may
  1. Order patient positioned to increase arterial supply and venous return
  2. Prescribe vasodilators
  3. Administer sympathetic blocking agents such as ethyl alcohol or procaine
  4. Prescribe medication for pain
  5. Intervene surgically to increase circulation by doing a sympathectomy, bypass graft, or endarterectomy
  6. Intervene surgically to debride or amputate the involved parts
  7. Order physiotherapy as soon as patient is able to tolerate exercise

C. Nursing diagnosis and intervention
  1. Patient has special safety needs
     a. Protect limb from further damage by using bed cradle, tepid solutions, professional nail cutting, protective batting
     b. Provide special skin care to prevent infection and breakdown
     c. Handle limb with extreme caution
     d. Protect from falling
     e. Avoid weight-bearing
     f. Position limb as ordered
     g. Observe for temperature, color, and pedal pulses in extremity
  2. Patient needs emotional support
     a. Encourage patient to express feelings
     b. Explain all procedures in simple terms
     c. Assist patient to accept change in body image
     d. Encourage patient to care for self when possible
     e. Assist patient to set realistic plans for discharge and aftercare
     f. Encourage patient to follow physician's orders and remain under medical supervision
     g. Encourage patient to avoid smoking
  3. Patient needs health teaching
     a. Teach patient about rest and posture

b. Teach patient how to care for feet; e.g., avoid restrictive clothing or tight shoes, visit the podiatrist regularly, avoid extremes in temperature including heating pad or hot water bottle, special skin care
c. Teach patient special exercises to improve circulation; e.g., Buerger-Allen exercises, walking, etc.

PATIENTS WITH PROBLEMS IN NUTRITION AND ELIMINATION

TYPES OF NUTRITION AND ELIMINATION PROBLEMS

A. Hyperactivity within the gastrointestinal and urinary systems
1. In movement of nutrients and wastes through the gastrointestinal and urinary tracts as in regional enteritis, ulcerative colitis, dysentery, irritable bowel syndrome, and cystitis
2. In secretory functions of structures involved in digestion and absorption as in esophagitis, gastritis, pancreatitis, and peptic ulcer
B. Hypoactivity within the gastrointestinal and urinary systems
1. In movement of nutrients and wastes through the intestinal and urinary tracts as in achalasia, diaphragmatic hernia, pyloric obstruction, obstruction of the small intestine, cancer of the bowel, volvulus, adhesions, renal calculi, stricture of the ureters, and pyelonephritis
2. In secretory functions of the gastrointestinal tract as in cancer of the stomach, cirrhosis of the liver, cholelithiasis, and cancer of the pancreas
3. In secretory and excretory functions of the nephron as in glomerulonephritis, glomerulonephrosis, cancer of the kidney, renal failure, and uremia (see Pediatric nursing for material on nephritis and nephrosis)
C. Malabsorption within the gastrointestinal system (see Pediatric nursing for material on celiac disease)

BASIC CONCEPTS

A. Autoregulatory processes within the gastrointestinal and urinary tracts function to keep substances moving at a slow enough pace for digestion and absorption to take place, yet quick enough to provide nutrients and remove wastes
B. Movement of substances throughout the tracts depends on
1. Autonomic stimulation
2. Intermural and intramural stimulation
3. Mechanical stimulation
4. Chemical stimulation
C. Any interference in autonomic, intramural, mechanical, or chemical stimulation may directly or indirectly cause functional changes in the gastrointestinal or urinary tract
D. Stimulation of the parasympathetic system containing cholinergic and adrenergic fibers results in increased tonic contractions and increased velocity of excitatory waves along the walls of the gastrointestinal and urinary tracts, increased intensity and rate of rhythmic contractions, and localized secretion of digestive juices in the gastrointestinal tract
E. The rate of motility and secretory functions and their effect on digestion, absorption, and elimination are influenced by
1. Heredity
2. Age
3. Life-style
4. Sex
5. Emotional factors
6. Physical status
F. Alterations in gastrointestinal and urinary tract motility and secretion can be caused by stress such as trauma, inflammation, infection, neoplasms, congenital abnormalities, degenerative changes, psychosocial factors, chemical irritants, parasites, and mechanical factors
G. Psychosocial factors such as anxiety, emotional upset, fear of pain, and voluntary inhibition of impulses to defecate or void may also result in alterations of the functions of the gastrointestinal and urinary tracts
H. Secretory functions within the gastrointestinal system are dependent on
1. Autonomic stimulation
2. Mechanical stimulation
3. Chemical stimulation
I. The 3 major types of food contributing to cellular life (fats, proteins, carbohydrates) require the same chemistry of digestion, namely hydrolysis

J. Interferences with the production of secretions essential to hydrolysis (hydrochloric acid, enzymes) will cause disturbances in the rate and quantity of the basic nutrients absorbed (amino acids, glucose, and fatty acids)

K. Interference with the quality of chyme (fat, protein, carbohydrate, pH), the degree of stimulation present in the small intestine, and movement of food through the duodenum will influence the rate of emptying of the stomach

L. Interference with the gastric mucosa will result in disturbances in absorption (active transport and diffusion) thereby affecting the rate and quantity of basic nutrients absorbed

M. The large intestine is responsible for the reabsorption of water and the collection and elimination of the solid waste products of digestion that have not been absorbed

N. The kidneys remove the waste products of metabolism, nitrogenous products, drugs, toxins, and other foreign substances that have been absorbed from the digestive tract

O. The kidneys are responsible for the formation of urine, control of its volume and concentration, thereby governing and maintaining the body's fluid and electrolyte balance

HYPERACTIVITY WITHIN THE GASTROINTESTINAL AND URINARY SYSTEMS
Etiology and pathophysiologic processes

A. Hyperactivity causes a decreased digestion, absorption and assimilation, and an increased output of nutrients, wastes, electrolytes, and water

B. Hyperactivity may be caused by a variety of local and systemic microbiologic, chemical, mechanical, physical, psychosocial, and psychologic stresses

C. Inflammatory and infectious processes that increase local pressure and/or release toxins will irritate nerve endings (receptors) and may result in moderate distention and increased secretion and motility within the gastrointestinal and urinary tracts

D. Mucosal irritation, excessive distention, and/or the presence of specific chemicals in the gastrointestinal system produce local or systemic responses by way of reflex mechanisms to the intramural plexus and the central nervous system

E. Hyperstimulation of the parasympathetic nerves (cranial via the vagus and sacral to the distal half of the large intestine) results in increased smooth muscle tone, increased motility, and relaxation of sphincters

F. Clinical manifestations depend on the location of the interference in the gastrointestinal and urinary tracts, the degree of involvement, the tissue involved, and the effectiveness of compensatory mechanisms of the body

G. In addition, clinical manifestations in the gastrointestinal tract also depend on the degree of hypersecretion, the nature of the substance being secreted in excess, the tissue involved, and the effectiveness of compensatory mechanisms in the body

Hypermotility
Small intestine

Example: regional enteritis, characterized by chronic inflammatory changes involving any part of the alimentary tract but usually involving demarcated segments of the small bowel

A. Assessment of patient
   1. Clinical manifestations
      a. Ulceration of the intestinal submucosa accompanied by congestion, thickening of the small bowel, and fissure formations
      b. Enlargement of regional lymph nodes
      c. Fibrosis and narrowing of intestinal wall
      d. Abscesses and fistulas to abdominal wall, bladder, and vagina
      e. Pain in lower right quadrant, cramping, and spasms
      f. Nausea, flatulence, and borborygmus
      g. Fever, weight loss, and anemia
      h. Diarrhea with fluid and electrolyte disturbances
   2. Diagnostic measures
      a. History of intestinal problems for a long period with remissions and exacerbations
      b. Exacerbations that appear to be related to emotional upsets or dietary indiscretions especially with

milk, milk products, and fried or fatty foods

c. Age of patient—usually occurs in young adults but can occur at any age

d. Gastrointestinal x-ray series to detect and outline congested, thickened, fibrosed, and narrowed appearance of the intestinal wall; abscesses and fistulas; partial bowel obstruction; ulceration of mucosa

e. Proctosigmoidoscopy is performed to exclude other pathology such as ulcerative colitis, diverticulitis

f. Stools are examined to determine presence of blood, fat, protein, parasites, or ova

g. Blood studies are used to determine general condition of patient but are not specific for the disorder

h. Fecal fat test is performed to indicate fat content in feces, an abnormal amount of which is significant in malabsorptive disorders or hypermotility

i. D-xylose tolerance test is performed to determine absorptive ability of upper intestinal tract

j. Shilling test is valuable to determine the extent of intestinal functioning in relation to absorption of vitamin B_{12}

B. Medical therapy—the physician may

1. Institute a dietary regimen that maintains nutrition, relieves diarrhea and pain

   a. Nothing by mouth in presence of vomiting

   b. Clear fluid diet progressing to bland, low residue, low fat but increased in calories, proteins, vitamins (especially vitamin K), and carbohydrates

   c. Hyperalimentation may be ordered when oral intake is inadequate

2. Prescribe antiemetics to reduce vomiting and/or nausea; e.g., Tigan, Compazine, Gravol

3. Prescribe vitamins to correct a low intake of folic and ascorbic acid and decrease extent of anemia; e.g., oral folic and ascorbic acid

4. Prescribe minerals to correct anemia; e.g., iron and calcium (iron given with hydrochloric acid to facilitate its absorption)

5. Prescribe anticholinergics to relieve cramplike pain and diarrhea; e.g., Donnatal, Pro-Banthine, Belladonna

6. Prescribe potassium to replace electrolyte lost in persistent diarrhea

7. Prescribe hydrophilic mucilloids to decrease the fluidity and number of stools; e.g., Metamucil

8. Prescribe antidiarrheics to control and decrease diarrhea; e.g., Kaolin, Lomotil

9. Prescribe anti-inflammatories to bring about remission during exacerbation; e.g., prednisone, ACTH

10. Prescribe anti-infectives to control suppurative complications; e.g., Sulfasuxidine, Neomycin

11. Intervene surgically (resection of diseased part) if patient does not respond to medical therapy or if complications such as obstruction, abscesses, or fistulas occur

C. Nursing diagnosis and intervention

1. Patient needs assistance with improving and maintaining nutritional status

   a. Offer clear liquids hourly as ordered once patient ceases to experience nausea and vomiting

   b. Encourage high caloric, high protein, high carbohydrate diet supplemented with vitamins and potassium as ordered

   c. Assist with hyperalimentation therapy if ordered

   d. Offer small, frequent feedings considering patient preference, types of foods allowed, and esthetic factors

   e. Closely monitor intake and output

   f. Weigh daily for determining progress in weight gain pattern

2. Patient has additional safety needs

   a. Observe for signs of complications such as elevated temperature, increasing nausea and vomiting, abdominal rigidity

   b. Assess patient for signs of toxicity especially during steroid therapy; e.g., electrolyte disturbance, gastrointestinal bleeding, fluid retention, emotional changes

   c. In hyperalimentation, initiate surgical aseptic measures to prevent infection at site of catheter insertion; observe and regulate rate of flow; observe for complications

such as atelectasis, infection, and metabolic disturbances (reflex hypoglycemia)
  d. Administer anticholinergics as ordered observing for signs of overdose; e.g., dry mouth, dizziness, flushing, and urinary retention
  e. Teach the patient to avoid taking laxatives and salicylates that irritate intestinal mucosa
  f. Teach the patient how to effectively take antidiarrheics and mucilloid drugs and the observations to make during their use
  g. Teach skin care if perineal area is irritated
  h. Teach patient the importance of seeking help early when exacerbations occur
  3. Patient needs emotional support
  a. Keep patient informed about procedures, approaches in care, and general progress
  b. Encourage verbalization of feelings
  c. Discuss ways of dealing more effectively with the stress of pressures encountered in daily living
  d. Realistically support patient's body image and ego strengths
  e. Involve patient and family in planning care related to both exacerbative and remissive stages of the disease process
  f. Communicate concern and awareness regarding patient's discomfort and emotional lability during exacerbations of this chronic illness

Large intestine

Example: ulcerative colitis, characterized by a chronic inflammation and ulcerations of the colon and rectum
A. Assessment of patient
  1. Clinical manifestations
  a. Passage of bloody, purulent, mucoid, watery stools
  b. Colon shows cryptic abscess formation accompanied by hyperemia and edema of wall
  c. Weakness, debilitation, dehydration, and anemia
  d. Low grade fever
  e. Hemorrhages in the mucosa and submucosa of the colon
  f. If untreated, may result in excessive losses of water and electrolytes, malabsorption of nutrients with resultant dehydration and malnutrition, blood loss, acid-base imbalance, and death
  2. Diagnostic measures
  a. Physical examination and history to determine precipitating factors (bacterial invasion, an autoimmune response, allergies, emotional upsets) and extent of illness
  b. Proctoscopy to examine for granular mucous membrane with small abscesses and hemorrhages scattered throughout the rectosigmoid area
  c. Stool examinations to determine presence of pathogens and blood
  d. Barium enema to detect and outline ulcerated areas in the colon
B. Medical therapy—the physician may
  1. Institute diet therapy
  a. Unrestricted fluid intake; high protein, high caloric diet; avoidance of food allergens, especially milk
  b. Parenteral electrolytes, vitamins, and nutrients as required
  2. Prescribe blood and parenteral iron to alter the anemic state
  3. Prescribe sedatives, analgesics, tranquilizers as required
  4. Prescribe anticholinergic drugs or opiates to decrease frequency of stools and cramps
  5. Prescribe antiemetics if nausea and vomiting are present
  6. Prescribe corticosteroids parenterally, orally, or via retention enemas to decrease inflammatory changes and related symptomatology
  7. Prescribe antibacterials to reduce infection
  8. Intervene surgically when no response is evident to medical treatment, when course of the disease is downhill, when massive hemorrhage or colonic obstruction occurs, or when cancer is suspected; a temporary ileostomy, a partial colectomy, or a total colectomy with a permanent ileostomy may be performed
C. Nursing diagnosis and intervention
  1. Patient needs assistance with maintaining nutritional status
  a. Identify importance of maintaining an environment conducive to eat-

ing—free of malodors and irritating external stimuli

b. Serve small frequent feedings of a high protein, high caloric, low residue, bland nature

c. Teach patient about importance of diet in controlling and/or minimizing symptoms

d. Involve patient in dietary selection recognizing preferences as much as possible

e. Initiate accurate administration and recording of fluid, electrolyte, or blood replacements as ordered by the physician

2. Patient needs symptomatic relief
   a. Administer medications accurately and promptly as ordered by the physician
   b. Observe for effects of medications on related symptomatology
   c. Plan nursing care to allow for complete bed rest and maximum number of rest periods
   d. Institute comfort measures such as use of warm, powdered bedpan; sheepskin under buttocks; and gentle, thorough perineal care as required

3. Patient needs to be protected against complications
   a. Observe carefully for signs of complications; e.g., rectal bleeding, fever, dehydration
   b. Administer antibiotics as ordered by the physician
   c. Encourage fluid and food intake as ordered
   d. Instruct patient to report symptoms such as increasing pain, chills, nausea, board-like abdomen

4. Patient needs emotional support
   a. Keep patient and family informed about care and procedures
   b. Encourage verbalization of feelings, especially expressions of fears
   c. Institute measures to assure patient privacy
   d. Implement health teaching related to preoperative and postoperative care, the disease process, ileostomy care if applicable
   e. Encourage patient and appropriate family members to participate in planning care and making arrangements for continuity of health care once patient is discharged

f. Realistically support the patient's strengths

g. Help patient accept the chronicity of the health problem

5. Patient needs help in acceptance of ileostomy
   a. Allow time for patient to express feelings and ask questions about ileostomy
   b. Teach patient the special care necessary for the stoma and the skin as soon as possible
   c. Provide for a visit by a member of an "Ostomy Club" to discuss with the patient the problems of continuous drainage and odor
   d. Teach the patient how and when to change the ileostomy bag and explain that the bag should be changed immediately if skin irritation occurs

Urinary bladder

Example: cystitis, characterized by inflammation of the bladder wall usually caused by an ascending bacterial infection (*E. coli* most common)

A. Assessment of patient
   1. Clinical manifestations
      a. Urgency, frequency, burning, and pain on urination
      b. Nocturia
      c. Bearing down on urination
      d. Pyuria and hematuria
   2. Diagnostic measures
      a. History of above symptoms
      b. Clean catch urine specimen for culture and sensitivity
      c. Urinalysis

B. Medical therapy—the physician may
   1. Prescribe chemotherapeutic and antibiotic agents; e.g., sulfonamides, penicillin, tetracycline
   2. Prescribe antispasmodics to soothe the irritable bladder; e.g., Pyridium
   3. Order diet directed toward maintaining an acid urine; e.g., cranberry juice
   4. Order the intake of additional fluids to dilute the urine

C. Nursing diagnosis and intervention
   1. Patient needs increased hydration
      a. Encourage patient to drink additional fluids
      b. Monitor intake and output with attention to character of urine
   2. Patient needs health teaching
      a. Teach patient proper perineal care

b. Teach patient to seek medical attention at the first sign of symptoms

c. Teach patient to take medications as directed

Hypersecretion
Upper gastrointestinal tract

Example: peptic ulcer, characterized by ulceration of the gastric mucosa extending below the epithelium; in peptic ulcers, gastric juices, especially pepsin and hydrochloric acid, create inflammatory changes, lowered pain threshold, and vascular engorgement

A. Assessment of patient
1. Clinical manifestations
   a. Problem may be acute or chronic; gastric or duodenal; or may occur as a stress ulcer following burns, trauma, or surgery
   b. Several factors seem to influence the development of peptic ulcers
      (1) A source of irritation such as increased hydrochloric acid secretion in the presence of a decrease of alkaline mucus
      (2) Breakdown in local tissue resistance and defense mechanisms as a result of poor epithelial blood supply, failure of epithelium to regenerate
      (3) Influence of personality, hormonal, and hereditary factors
      (4) Overstimulation of secretory mechanisms
      (5) Failure of mechanisms that function to inhibit secretions
      (6) Use of drugs such as cortisone, aspirin, phenylbutazone
   c. Aching, gnawing epigastric pain
   d. Nausea, regurgitation, and vomiting
   e. Dyspepsia and eructation when stomach is empty
   f. Sense of fullness or hunger
   g. Weakness
   h. Occurrence of coffee-ground vomitus
   i. Complications may result such as pyloric or duodenal obstruction, hemorrhage, or perforation
2. Diagnostic measures
   a. Physical assessment of abdomen to determine sounds, degree of peristalsis, presence of bruit, size of various organs, presence of excessive amounts of fluid or air
   b. Health history including personal habits and life-style, characteristics of pain, relief of pain, changes in stool, food intolerance
   c. Barium swallow (upper gastrointestinal series) to expedite diagnosis of pathologic conditions of the stomach
   d. Gastric biopsy to diagnose abnormalities of the gastric mucosa
   e. Gastric endoscopy to directly visualize gastric mucosa for disease processes and obtain biopsy
   f. Gastric analysis to diagnose gastric pathology from a study of the gastric secretions obtained following basal analysis; stimulation analysis using histamine or Histalog; nocturnal analysis; hypoglycemic analysis or insulin tolerance test; or tubeless analysis (Diagnex Blue Test)
   g. Cytologic studies to distinguish between benign and malignant lesions
   h. Stool specimens to determine presence of occult blood

B. Medical therapy—the physician may
1. Institute measures to neutralize or buffer hydrochloric acid, inhibit acid secretion, and decrease the activity of pepsin and hydrochloric acid such as
   a. Radiation and gastric hypothermia to suppress gastric secretions
   b. Diet regulation through the use of bland foods and restriction of irritating substances such as nicotine, caffeine, alcohol, spices, gassy foods
   c. Prescribe antacids to reduce acidity
2. Order type and cross-match so that blood will be available should gastric hemorrhage occur
3. Prescribe sedatives, tranquilizers, anticholinergics, and analgesics for pain and restlessness
4. Prescribe antiemetics for nausea and vomiting
5. Order bed rest to reduce physical activity
6. Encourage patient to seek counselling or psychotherapy to explore the emotional components of the illness
7. Intervene surgically if medical therapy is inadequate, complications like

hemorrhage occur, the pylorus obstructs, or the lesion is thought to be precancerous; a partial gastric resection, excision of ulcer, vagotomy, or pyloroplasty may be performed

C. Nursing diagnosis and intervention

1. Patient needs physical and emotional rest
   a. Assist patient to understand the importance of complete bed rest
   b. Reduce physical activity
   c. Attend to needs promptly to lessen unfavorable stimuli
   d. Implement a regular, smooth plan of care avoiding noise, rush, confusion, and impatience
   e. Encourage visitors and activities that keep patient diverted and occupied but not fatigued
   f. Separate from any usual tension-producing situations, if possible
   g. Administer and assess effects of sedatives, tranquilizers, antacids, anticholinergics, and special dietary foods such as milk and cream
   h. Plan listening time in patient's care plan to pick up clues about anxieties or problems

2. Patient has additional safety needs
   a. Observe for circulatory and respiratory complications as a result of heavy sedation primarily during the acute stage
   b. Utilize side rails while patient is sedated
   c. Encourage turning and deep breathing frequently while heavy sedation is being given
   d. Refrain from administering drugs such as salicylates, phenylbutazone, steroids, and ACTH that are normally contraindicated
   e. Teach prevention of recurrences through such means as modified styles of living, working, eating; regularity in activities of daily living; consistency of medical supervision; symptoms to report; drug therapy
   f. Observe for complications such as gastric hemorrhage, perforation, drug toxicity
   g. Encourage hydration to reduce anticholinergic side effects and dilute the hydrochloric acid in the stomach

3. Patient needs relief from pain and assistance with healing of the ulcerated gastric mucosa
   a. Administer drugs such as Amphojel, Maalox, nonsystemic antacids that lower acidity of gastric secretions and neutralize hydrochloric acid
   b. Instruct patient to take hourly feedings of milk alternately with antacids as ordered
   c. Advise against the use of sodium bicarbonate, which alters acid-base balance
   d. Administer anticholinergic drugs such as Banthine and Donnatal to decrease gastric motility and secretions
   e. Encourage ingestion of diet as ordered
   f. Administer small, frequent, attractive feedings to keep stomach contents diluted and the work of the gastrointestinal tract to a minimum
   g. Teach avoidance of spicy foods, fried foods, nicotine, caffeine, alcohol, etc.

4. Patient needs assistance with re-establishing appropriate dietary life-style and nutritional status
   a. Explain to patient that dietary regulations depend on acuteness of illness, symptoms, and response to ulcer therapy; e.g., Sippy diet to usual diet of a bland, nonirritating, low fiber, nongasforming nature with elimination of alcohol, caffeine, nicotine, carbonated drinks, meat extracts, soups, and gravies
   b. Teach importance of adequate calories and basic foods eaten slowly in a pleasant environment
   c. Teach family about meal planning, cooking, and foods to avoid, paying attention to cultural and religious influences
   d. Instruct patient regarding the rationale for small, frequent, bland feedings, and need to keep weight under control by using skim milk, decreased animal fats

5. Patient needs emotional support
   a. Allow patient to be dependent in acute stages but encourage increasing independence

b. Teach patient importance of avoiding anxiety-producing situations
c. Allow ample time for patient to express feelings and concerns
d. Offer guidance in matters of adjusting for work, home situations, rest requirements
e. Help patient to understand the disease process
f. Assist patient to set realistic goals and plans for convalescence
g. Teach importance of avoiding ulcerogenic drugs such as salicylates but possibility of taking substitutes such as Tylenol or Ascriptin
h. Encourage regular medical supervision and counselling as required

Glands associated with digestion

Example: acute pancreatitis, characterized by inflammation with or without edema of pancreatic tissues, suppuration, abscess formation, hemorrhage, or necrosis depending on the severity of the disease and the cause; acute pancreatitis is commonly associated with gallstones, alcoholism, carcinoma, or acute trauma to the pancreas or abdomen

A. Assessment of patient
  1. Clinical manifestations
    a. Abrupt onset of pain in the central, epigastric area that may radiate to shoulder, chest, and back described as aching, burning, stabbing, or pressing; elevated temperature; abdominal tenderness; nausea and vomiting; tachycardia, hypotension, shock; changes in character of stools may occur
    b. Severity of symptoms depend on the cause of the problem; amount of fibrous replacement of normal duct tissue; degree of autodigestion of organ; type of associated biliary disease, if present; and the amount of interference in blood supply to the pancreas
    c. Symptoms may be exaggerated by the development of complications such as pseudocysts, abscesses, pancreatic fistulas, and hyperglycemia
  2. Diagnostic measures
    a. History of biliary, hepatic, or gastric disorders; duodenal spasms and reflux; metabolic disturbances; abdominal trauma; neurogenic or emotional factors; onset and relief of pain; alcohol and drug ingestion (opiates, steroids, thiazides, oral contraceptives, and oral hypoglycemics)
    b. Examination of stool specimens to determine degree of digestion of fat and protein
    c. Pancreatic scanning to determine presence of mass
    d. Splenoportography, which helps to determine presence of tumors of the body and tail of the pancreas by injecting dye into the splenic vein
    e. Exocrine pancreatic function tests to measure enzyme levels and hence assist in determining the degree of inflammatory change or destruction; e.g., secretin stimulation test, duodenal aspiration, duodenal secretion test, serum amylase and lipase
    f. White blood count and differential to evaluate the severity of the acute episode
    g. Serum bilirubin and alkaline phosphatase to determine whether an associated biliary problem exists
    h. Prothrombin time to determine whether there is altered blood coagulability
    i. Sulkowitch test to measure urinary calcium levels
    j. Urine test to determine presence of glucose
B. Medical therapy—the physician may
  1. Prescribe antacids to neutralize gastric secretions; barbiturates and tranquilizers to reduce emotional tension, promote rest and relaxation; and narcotics for pain
  2. Order bed rest to decrease metabolic demands and promote healing
  3. Prescribe cardiotonics (digitalis) to lessen strain on the heart caused by increased metabolic demands and altered circulatory volume
  4. Order frequent monitoring of vital signs
  5. Institute nasogastric suction to control nausea and remove gastric hydrochloric acid
  6. Regulate diet according to patient's condition: nothing by mouth; parenteral administration of fluid, electro-

lytes, and other nutrients; diet low in fats and proteins with restriction of stimulants such as caffeine and alcohol

7. Prescribe antiemetics to alleviate nausea and vomiting
8. Prescribe anticholinergics to suppress vagal stimulation, decrease gastric motility and duodenal spasm, and decrease pancreatic output
9. Prescribe carbonic anhydrase inhibitors such as Diamox to reduce volume and bicarbonate concentration of pancreatic secretions
10. Order monitoring of intake and output
11. Prescribe antibiotics to prevent secondary infections and abscess formation
12. Intervene surgically if patient fails to recover, develops persistent jaundice or bleeding; type of surgery is determined by the cause; e.g., biliary tract surgery, removal of gallstones, drainage of cysts

C. Nursing diagnosis and intervention
   1. Patient needs relief of pain and promotion of comfort and rest
      a. Administer frequent, thorough mouth care when patient is intubated with nasogastric tube
      b. Apply lubricant to external nares to prevent irritation and eventual breakdown of mucous membranes
   2. Patient needs assistance with re-establishing nutritional status
      a. Maintain nothing by mouth during the acute stage of the illness
      b. Closely monitor intravenous feedings until oral feedings can be tolerated
      c. Assist patient in ingestion of small feedings of low fat, gaseous-free fluids progressing to diet as tolerated and prescribed
      d. Teach patient and family the importance of dietary discretion, especially the avoidance of alcohol, coffee, spicy foods, heavy meals, while recognizing religious and cultural factors
   3. Patient has additional safety needs
      a. Observe for electrolyte imbalances manifested by such symptoms as tetany, irritability, jerking, muscular twitching, mental changes, and psychotic behavior
      b. Observe for signs of adynamic ileus; e.g., nausea and vomiting, abdominal distention
      c. Be alert for hyperglycemic states
      d. Administer antibiotics as ordered to prevent secondary infections
      e. Institute use of cool, moist vapor to minimize drying of mucous membranes
      f. Teach importance of taking medications containing amylase, lipase, and trypsin in controlling pancreatic insufficiency
      g. Encourage adoption of a life-style that allows for emotional stability, rest, follow-up medical care
      h. Use semi-Fowler's position and encourage deep breathing and coughing to promote deeper respiration and prevent respiratory problems
   4. Patient needs emotional support
      a. Help patient to understand the disease process
      b. Encourage the verbalization of feelings
      c. Help patient to recognize limitations while focusing on strengths
      d. Help patient set realistic goals for convalescent period
      e. Teach patient and family about prevention of recurrences and/or control of symptoms; e.g., diet therapy, drug therapy, avoiding foods and substances such as alcohol and caffeine, regular medical supervision, rest requirements

HYPOACTIVITY WITHIN THE GASTROINTESTINAL AND URINARY SYSTEMS
Etiology and pathophysiologic processes

A. Hypostimulation of the parasympathetic nerves results in decreased smooth muscle tone, decreased motility and distention in the digestive tract as well as flaccidity of the bladder in the urinary tract
B. Hypostimulation of the sympathetic nerves results in increased intensity and rate of rhythmic contractions of the gut wall and dilation of sphincters
C. Interferences with reflexes that normally initiate movements in the colon and urinary tract will result in prolonged storage of fecal matter and urine
D. A decrease in secretions may be the re-

sult of trauma, psychosocial factors, inflammation, infection, neoplasms, and degenerative changes

E. Trauma may cause loss of blood supply and eventual nerve damage, which produces hypomotility in the gastrointestinal and urinary tracts

F. Neoplasms tend to cause compression of pelvic organs resulting in a decreased evacuation of the lower digestive and urinary tracts

G. Degenerative processes produce atrophy in the urinary system and the gastrointestinal mucosa resulting in alterations in the amount of secretions and excretions, changes in motility manifested by increasing pressure, distention, constipation, suppression, and retention

H. Clinical manifestations of interferences with the movement of substances through the urinary and gastrointestinal systems depend on the completeness of the obstruction, the degree of interruption in the blood supply, the type of lesion, the length and level of involvement, and the effectiveness of the body's adaptive processes

I. Clinical manifestations of interferences with secretory functions of the urinary and gastrointestinal systems depend on the location of the interference, the degree of hyposecretion of the structure involved, the nature of the substance being secreted, the tissues involved, and the effectiveness of the body's adaptations

J. Simultaneous stimulation of the duodenum by sympathetic as well as parasympathetic nerves reduces secretions by inhibiting the duodenal glands causing the initial portion of the duodenum to become vulnerable to acidic digestive juices from the stomach

K. Decreased esophageal peristalsis interferes with ingestion of nutrients and elicits manifestations such as choking, coughing, regurgitation, spitting up, pain

L. Hypomotility in the churning, mixing, and emptying of the stomach elicits such manifestations as pain associated with distention, heartburn (pyrosis), nausea and vomiting, localized tenderness, eructation, hematemesis

M. Interferences with absorption of nutrients in the small intestine elicit such manifestations as loss of weight, anemia, fatigue, general malnutrition, changes in bowel habits, and stool consistency

Hypomotility
Small intestine

Example: intestinal obstruction, characterized by interference with the passage of gas, fluids, and residue through the intestines as a result of a partial or complete obstruction; the obstruction can be caused by mechanical factors such as closure or narrowing of intestinal lumen caused by inflammation, trauma, neoplasms, adhesions, strangulated hernia, volvulus, intussusception; mesenteric arterial or venous occlusion; or paralytic ileus

A. Assessment of patient
  1. Clinical manifestations
     a. Pain that is wavelike in character
     b. Increased peristalsis, distension caused by fluid and gas, and an alteration in the capacity of bowel to absorb fluid
     c. Nausea, vomiting, and critical electrolyte imbalance progressing to dehydration, acidosis, and shock
     d. Increased bacterial growth
     e. May pass blood and mucus but little or no flatus or fecal matter
     f. Fecal vomiting may occur if the obstruction is in the ileum
     g. The cardinal manifestations of complete small bowel obstruction (a surgical emergency) are distension, pain, vomiting, absolute constipation
     h. Complications include intestinal perforation, peritonitis, release of endotoxins into the circulation, and subsequent endotoxic shock
  2. Diagnostic measures
     a. History of flatulence, character of stools, pain, vomiting, distention, and constipation
     b. Abdominal x-ray film to detect presence of gas in bowel or abdominal cavity
     c. Barium swallow to outline the upper gastrointestinal tract for identification of abnormalities on x-ray film
     d. Barium enema to rule out abnormalities in the lower gastrointestinal tract
     e. White blood count and differential to detect infectious response

f. Hemoglobin and hematocrit to detect red blood cell and fluid loss
g. SMA 12 to evaluate electrolyte levels

B. Medical therapy—the physician may
1. Prescribe small doses of Demerol or other synthetics to relieve pain without masking symptoms of complications (morphine is not given since it decreases intestinal motility)
2. Insert a nasogastric tube and order continuous drainage and nothing by mouth to relieve and/or prevent distention and stop vomiting
3. Order necessary electrolytes for replacement by parenteral therapy
4. Order necessary parenteral therapy to maintain hydration
5. Order daily blood chemistries to determine levels of electrolytes
6. Order frequent monitoring of vital signs and intake and output
7. Prescribe antibiotics to reduce possibility of infection
8. Intervene surgically on an emergency or elective basis to relieve the cause of the obstruction

C. Nursing diagnosis and intervention
1. Patient needs relief of pain and promotion of comfort and rest
a. Administer frequent, thorough mouth care when patient is intubated with nasogastric tube
b. Apply lubricant to external areas to prevent irritation and damage to mucous membrane
c. Administer analgesics as needed for pain but as sparingly as possible to prevent masking of complications
d. Assure patency of gastrointestinal tube
e. Allow for prolonged, planned rest periods in plan of care
f. Maintain as nonstimulating an environment as possible
g. Assist with turning and bathing since patient is physically exhausted from pain, nausea, and vomiting
2. Patient needs assistance with re-establishing fluid and electrolyte balance and nutritional status
a. Administer intravenous fluids as ordered
b. Carefully note character and type of drainage from intestinal tube

c. Accurately monitor intake and output, especially noting emesis or drainage from intestinal tube
3. Patient has additional safety needs
a. Observe for preoperative complications such as intestinal perforation, peritonitis, shock; e.g., increasing pain, elevated temperature, rigidity of abdomen, decrease in quality of vital signs
b. Observe for postoperative complications such as paralytic ileus, duodenal fistula, further obstruction or peritonitis; e.g., increasing temperature and distention
c. Use low-Fowler's position to facilitate breathing and drainage
d. Teach patient to breathe through the nose and refrain from swallowing air
e. Observe amount and type of urinary output to determine urinary retention problems
4. Patient needs emotional support
a. Encourage verbalization of feelings and concerns
b. Reassure patient that intubation with intestinal tube is required to relieve symptoms
c. Allow patient to be dependent in acute stages, but increasingly independent and self-assertive as recovery progresses
d. Help patient and family to understand the disease process and treatment plan
e. Assist patient and family to set realistic goals for recovery and convalescence
f. Assist patient to accept surgical intervention performed and any adjustment in self-image and self-esteem; e.g., cecostomy, resection of bowel
g. Following resection of the bowel, teach patient importance of avoiding constipation, use of dietary modifications rather than laxatives to stimulate bowel evacuation, importance of regular medical supervision, necessity of gradual resumption of activities

Large intestine

Example: cancer of the bowel, characterized by the insidious growth of a malignant tumor that may project into the lumen or encircle the bowel resulting in stenosis, ulcerations, necrosis, and/or perforations

A. Assessment of patient
1. Clinical manifestations
   a. Contributory factors to colon pathology include carcinogens such as food additives, microorganisms, and bowel stasis
   b. Manifestations vary with location and size of the growth and commonly include alteration of bowel habits (constipation and/or diarrhea); abdominal cramping; passage of blood in the stool (melena); flatulence; distention; dyspepsia; borborygmi; pencil-shaped stools (descending colon pathology); and general decline in health such as weakness, anorexia, weight loss, anemia, dyspnea on exertion, lassitude, and apathy
   c. Rectal bleeding usually prompts the patient to seek medical help since other early symptoms are few and vague
   d. Metastasis depends on extent of the invasion, permeation of vascular or lymphatic system, and proximity of lesion to lymphatic flow
   e. Complications include obstruction, perforation with peritonitis, abscess and fistula formation, hemorrhage, dehydration, and shock
2. Diagnostic measures
   a. Health history including relationship of symptoms to foods, fluids, activity, defecation patterns, bleeding, pain; and preexisting conditions such as ulcerative colitis, benign lesions, granulomas, polyps (all thought to be precancerous)
   b. History of presence of blood and mucus in the stool caused by irritating effect of dry stool on gastrointestinal mucosa
   c. History of anorexia and nausea caused by reflex mechanisms initiated by distention
   d. Digital examination of rectum to detect any palpable masses
   e. Proctosigmoidoscopy to directly visualize bowel to determine presence of abnormalities and to perform a biopsy
   f. Stool examination to test for occult blood
   g. Cytologic examination to detect for malignant cells
   h. Hemoglobin to detect anemia
   i. Alkaline phosphatase and SGOT levels to detect metastasis to liver
   j. Serum carcinoembryonic antigen (C.E.A.) measure to screen for carcinoma of colon

B. Medical therapy—the physician may
1. After establishing the diagnosis, prepare the patient for surgery by
   a. Prescribing antibiotics to reduce bacteria in bowel
   b. Ordering type and cross-match and blood transfusions to correct anemia
   c. Ordering vitamin supplements to improve nutritional status
   d. Inserting a Cantor or Miller-Abbott tube with suction to decompress the colon
2. Intervene surgically to remove mass and restore bowel function; e.g., hemicolectomy, resection of transverse colon, or abdominal perineal resection
3. Order radiation in nonsurgical situations in an attempt to relieve symptoms or postoperatively to limit metastases
4. Prescribe chemotherapy orally or parenterally in an attempt to reduce the lesion and limit metastases
5. Postoperatively
   a. Prescribe antibiotic therapy to reduce infection
   b. Order parenteral fluids and electrolytes to maintain levels
   c. Order frequent monitoring of vital signs and intake and output
   d. Prescribe cholinergics to stimulate peristalsis
   e. Order Cantor or Miller-Abbott tube clamped for regular increasing periods
   f. Order sips of water progressing to clear liquid diet as tolerated
   g. Remove Cantor or Miller-Abbott tube after patient has tolerated clamping for extended periods and bowel sounds have returned
   h. Order progressive low residue diet as tolerated
6. If colostomy has been performed
   a. Order colostomy irrigations as required
   b. Order irrigations of perineal incision if present and the application

of enzymes such as streptokinase to liquefy protein matter and promote drainage

C. Nursing diagnosis and intervention

1. Patient has additional safety needs preoperatively
   a. Monitor patency of Cantor or Miller-Abbott tube to ensure that accumulated air and fluid are decreased and distention is minimized; instill or irrigate tube with normal saline as ordered
   b. Implement measures for mechanical cleansing and intestinal antisepsis preoperatively; e.g., enemas, colonic irrigations, antibacterial therapy such as neomycin or sulfonamides
   c. Observe vital signs, increasing abdominal pain, nausea and vomiting to detect early signs of complications
   d. Administer chemotherapeutic drugs if ordered and observe for significant side effects such as stomatitis (ulceration of mouth), dehydration, nausea and vomiting, diarrhea, leukopenia

2. Patient needs emotional support preoperatively
   a. Allow ample listening time to encourage verbalization of feelings especially those related to recovery, concerns about self-image, resumption of role in family unit and social groups
   b. Help patient to understand the disease process
   c. Preoperatively teach the patient; e.g., concept of postoperative dependency during acute stage, possible adjustments to body changes if colostomy is to be performed, types of supportive measures used such as parenteral therapy, etc.

3. Patient needs assistance with reestablishing fluid and electrolyte balance and nutritional status
   a. Maintain accurate intake and output, measuring emesis or intestinal tube drainage
   b. Note character of drainage from decompression tube
   c. Administer electrolyte and parenteral replacement as ordered in sit-

uations of bleeding, vomiting, and/or obstruction
   d. Carefully note patient's tolerance to introduction of oral fluids and foods while intestinal tube is clamped
   e. Encourage gradual resumption of eating from fluids to full diet once tube is removed paying particular attention to patient preferences if possible
   f. Teach patient and family dietary modifications including low residue, nongas-forming foods, avoidance of stimulants, adequate fluid intake

4. Patient needs rest, comfort, and relief of pain
   a. Provide rest periods while giving care
   b. Administer mouth care frequently, particularly when nasogastric tube is in place
   c. Administer narcotics as ordered and observe for effects produced
   d. Position patient in side-lying position postoperatively since it is uncomfortable to lie on back
   e. Offer frequent back care and change of linen to keep patient more relaxed and comfortable in a dry, clean environment

5. Patient has special safety needs postoperatively
   a. Observe for complications such as infection and bleeding
   b. Promote effective elimination preventing constipation and straining once dietary intake is increased
   c. Encourage deep breathing and coughing exercises to prevent pulmonary complications
   d. Encourage bed rest to allow healing of pelvic floor and decrease possibility of perineal hernia when abdominal perineal resection has been performed
   e. Implement surgically aseptic care of perineal wound to prevent abscess formation and promote wound healing when abdominal perineal resection has been performed

6. Patient needs special emotional support postoperatively if colostomy has been performed

a. Recognize that the patient with a colostomy may experience sadness, withdrawal, depression, and suicidal thoughts as a result of body image changes

b. Assess patient's reaction to the colostomy recognizing that a great deal will depend on how patient sees it affecting life-style; patient's physical and emotional status; patient's social and cultural background; patient's place and role in the family

c. Encourage patient's involvement in colostomy care as soon as physical and emotional status permits

d. Encourage visiting by family members stressing patient's increased need for love and acceptance

e. Recognize that the patient with a cecostomy or colostomy is especially sensitive to gestures, odors, facial expressions, and amount of attention given

f. Teach patient and family care of colostomy, measures to facilitate acceptance and adjustment, resumption of activities, and the need for regular medical supervision

g. Teach patient that colostomy drainage can be controlled by following a regular irrigation schedule and dietary modifications

h. Arrange for follow-up care with community agencies as required; e.g., Public Health, Home Care Program, Cancer Society, "ostomy" resource person, etc.

Urinary system

Example: renal calculi, characterized by the formation of stones in the urinary tract; stones may be composed of calcium phosphate, uric acid or oxalate; they tend to recur and may cause obstruction, infection, and/or hydronephrosis

A. Assessment of patient
  1. Clinical manifestations
     a. Severe pain in kidney area radiating down the flank to the pubic area
     b. Sweating, pallor, nausea and vomiting
     c. Hematuria; pyuria may occur if infection is present
     d. Frequency and urgency of urination

  2. Diagnostic measures
     a. History of onset and type of pain
     b. History of prior or associated health problems; e.g., gout, parathyroidism, immobility, dehydration, urinary tract infections
     c. Urinalysis to determine pH, uric acid, red blood cells, and infection
     d. Flat plate of the kidneys, ureter, and bladder (KUB), and intravenous pyelogram (IVP) to determine presence of stones
     e. Sulkowitch urine test to determine level of calcium in urine

B. Medical therapy—the physician may
  1. Prescribe narcotics for pain
  2. Prescribe antispasmodics to reduce the renal colic
  3. Prescribe allopurinol or sulfinpyrazone to reduce uric acid excretion
  4. Prescribe antibiotics to reduce infecfection
  5. Order monitoring of intake and output, forced fluids, and straining of urine
  6. Order diet depending on type of stone (see section on Nutrition, p. 180)
  7. Intervene surgically if stone is not passed or complications are present; e.g., nephrolithotomy, litholapaxy, etc.

C. Nursing diagnosis and intervention
  1. Patient needs relief from pain and promotion of rest
     a. Administer medications as ordered
     b. Permit patient to set own pattern of activity
     c. Plan care to provide patient with periods of undisturbed rest
  2. Patient has specific nursing needs related to diagnosis
     a. Strain all urine
     b. Monitor intake and output
     c. Force fluids
     d. Administer medication as ordered
  3. Patient needs emotional support and health teaching
     a. Encourage patient to accept medication for pain
     b. Provide as much privacy as possible
     c. Encourage patient to remain on diet
     d. Teach patient to read labels on food preparation for the presence of contraindicated additives such as calcium or phosphate

Hyposecretion
Accessory organs of digestion

Example: cirrhosis of the liver, characterized by diffuse inflammation, fibrosis, and destruction of liver cells eventually resulting in a nodular lobular structure that impedes blood flow, causes vascular insufficiency and subsequent portal hypertension; the term *cirrhosis* is used in reference to 3 main types of liver disease—portal (most common type), postnecrotic, and biliary

A. Assessment of patient
   1. Clinical manifestations
      a. Early symptoms include anorexia, indigestion, lassitude, flatulence, nausea and vomiting, fatigue, constipation or diarrhea, and fever
      b. Intermediate symptoms include congestion of gastrointestinal tract and spleen, dyspepsia, gradual weight loss, spider nevi, ascites, headache, and peripheral neuritis
      c. Late symptoms include abdominal pain, anemia, ascites, edema (peripheral, ankle, and sacral) avitaminosis, depression, wasting, jaundice, gynecomastia and testicular atrophy, amenorrhea, esophageal varices, bleeding tendencies, delirium, coma
   2. Diagnostic measures
      a. History of chronic alcoholism will be found in 60% to 90% of the patients; liver damage is primarily a result of malnutrition especially of dietary protein
      b. History of other predisposing causes such as toxic or viral hepatitis, cardiac disease, drugs (sulfonamides and barbiturates), chemicals (mercury and carbon tetrachloride), and obstruction in the biliary tract
      c. Age of patient—most common in people 45 to 65 years of age
      d. Cholecystogram to directly visualize the gallbladder
      e. Cholangiograms (intravenous and operative) to visualize biliary ductal system
      f. Percutaneous transhepatic cholangiogram to differentiate extrahepatic from intrahepatic obstructive jaundice, detect hepatic pathology and presence of calculi
      g. Serum bilirubin to measure both in-
direct and direct serum bilirubin levels
      h. Fecal and urine urobilinogen to determine level of excretion and extent of hepatic interference
      i. Albumin-globulin ratio to assess protein metabolism (total proteins decreased with severe liver damage)
      j. Galactose tolerance test to determine glycogenic functions of the liver
      k. Tests related to fat metabolism such as serum cholesterol, serum phospholipids to assess liver function (values decreased in severe liver disease and increased in biliary obstruction)
      l. Serum flocculation tests such as thymol turbidity and cephalin flocculation to measure function of liver cells and reflect balance of protein fractions not specific to liver disease
      m. Blood ammonia levels to determine extent of intestinal absorption of nitrogenous substance after protein breakdown and to assess liver function
      n. Hippuric acid and Bromsulphalein tests to determine liver's ability to detoxify harmful substances from blood
      o. Tests related to serum enzyme measure such as SGOT and SGPT, which measure extent of liver disease; LDH, which is increased in liver damage; cholinesterase, which is decreased in cirrhosis; alkaline phosphatase, which reflects patency of biliary channels
      p. Examination of duodenal drainage to differentiate types of jaundice and assist with diagnosis
      q. Liver biopsy to detect and diagnose growths in liver tissue
      r. Liver scan to determine presence of mass
      s. Splenoportal venography to directly visualize portal venous system to diagnose hepatic disease
      t. Tests to determine prothrombin and coagulation times, which are increased in liver disease

B. Medical therapy—the physician may
   1. Order complete bed rest progressing

to bed rest with activity as liver tests begin returning to normal limits and fever decreases

2. Order adequate diet with protein and caloric quantities compatible with liver's ability to metabolize foodstuffs ordered (as liver function decreases protein will be restricted)

3. Order tube feedings or hyperalimentation if patient's condition necessitates it

4. Restrict ingestion or contact with toxic agents; e.g., alcohol completely withdrawn

5. Prescribe supplemental vitamins to compensate for liver's inability to store vitamins A, B complex, D, and K

6. Prescribe stool softeners to reduce straining

7. Prescribe bile salts to assist with vitamin A absorption and vitamin K synthesis

8. Prescribe folic acid to correct deficiency and anemia

9. Institute measures to prevent and/or treat complications
   a. Restrict sodium intake when fluid retention occurs
   b. Prescribe antipruritic agents to control or reduce pruritus and prevent trauma to skin through scratching
   c. Institute drug therapy with caution (since liver degrades many drugs): antiemetics (Dramamine); vitamin K injectable, vasopressin for esophageal varices; diuretics (thiazides, Lasix, Aldactone) for edema; antiemetics (Tigan) for nausea
   d. Perform paracentesis to remove excess amounts of fluid in the peritoneal cavity
   e. Order whole blood transfusions to overcome blood loss as a result of bleeding tendencies and rupture of esophageal varices
   f. Institute gastric lavage with ice water, intravenous injection of vasopressin, esophagogastric tamponade with Sengstaken-Blakemore tube to control esophageal hemorrhage

10. Intervene surgically as indicated by presenting symptomatology; e.g., ligation of varices, splenectomy, esophagogastric resection, or a splenorenal or portacaval anastomosis to relieve portal hypertension

C. Nursing diagnosis and intervention
1. Patient needs comfort and rest
   a. Plan for regular, prolonged rest periods to conserve energy and decrease metabolic demands on the liver
   b. Assist patient to understand importance of rest for recovery
   c. Encourage visitors and activities that keep patient diverted but not fatigued
   d. Plan listening time to pick up clues about patient's anxieties or problems

2. Patient has additional safety needs
   a. Maintain a safe, accident-free environment depending on physical status; e.g., bleeding tendencies, stupor, mental confusion
   b. Apply gentle pressure to injection sites
   c. Observe for complications such as melena, hematemesis, coma, ascites
   d. Recognize signs of behavioral and/or personality changes
   e. Apply oil-based lotions and antipruritic agents to relieve pruritus
   f. Use soapless bathing, careful handling, and frequent turning to maintain intact integument in presence of edema and pruritus
   g. Discourage straining at stool, vigorous blowing of nose, and sneezing because of tendency to bleed
   h. Prepare patient for paracentesis by encouraging patient to empty bladder prior to procedure and support patient in sitting position
   i. Assess patient's vital signs before, during, and after paracentesis; observe for signs of shock
   j. When a Sengstaken-Blakemore tube is passed, maintain patency and irrigate as ordered; observing character of drainage; deflate balloon periodically as ordered; observe vital signs and monitor for respiratory distress

3. Patient needs assistance with establishing dietary modifications and maintaining nutritional status
   a. Encourage small, frequent palatable meals as ordered in an esthetic

environment considering patient preferences if possible
  b. Assist with hyperalimentation or tube feedings as ordered for severe nausea and vomiting
  c. Provide oral hygiene prior to meals and between feedings
  d. Offer protein supplements (Sustagen) between meals as ordered
  e. Administer antiemetics to control nausea; vitamin supplements and B complex to enhance utilization of food
  f. Teach patient importance of well balanced diet, dietary restrictions, withdrawal from toxic substances such as alcohol and drugs
4. Patient needs emotional support
  a. Help patient and family to understand the disease process, care, and procedures
  b. Encourage verbalization of feelings, fears, and concerns
  c. Avoid making moral judgments about the patient with alcohol problems
  d. Recognize that patient may become withdrawn and depressed as a result of changes in body image
  e. Utilize community agencies and services to assist patient adjustment and provide for continuity of care; e.g., Public Health Nurse, Alcoholics Anonymous
  f. Teach patient regarding need for rest, altered life-style, continued medical supervision, avoidance of substances toxic to the liver
  g. Encourage patient and family to participate in planning care and making arrangements for the prolonged convalescent and rehabilitative phase of recovery
  h. Realistically support and strengthen patient's body image and ego strengths
  i. Communicate concern regarding patient's discomfort and emotional lability

Glands associated with digestion

Example: cancer of the pancreas, characterized by malignant growth from the epithelium of the ductal system producing cells that block the ducts causing chronic pancreatitis, fibrosis, obstruction, and jaundice; tends to metastasize by direct extension to duodenal wall, splenic flexure of colon, posterior stomach wall, and common bile duct

A. Assessment of patient
  1. Clinical manifestations
    a. Vague symptoms such as weight loss, ascites, anxiety, depression, anorexia, and nausea usually precede severe pain and jaundice
    b. Diarrhea and steatorrhea, clay-colored stools and dark urine
  2. Diagnostic measures
    a. History of chronic pancreatitis, diabetes mellitus, and alcoholism
    b. Age of patient—more common in middle-aged men than women
    c. Physical examination usually demonstrates presence of right upper quadrant mass
    d. Cytologic examination of duodenal secretion to determine presence of malignant cells
    e. Pancreatic scanning to detect and outline pancreatic tumors
    f. Serum bilirubin and alkaline phosphatase levels to determine whether biliary ducts are obstructed
    g. Glucose tolerance test to detect or rule out diabetes mellitus
    h. Serum amylase and serum lipase levels to determine degree of secretion of enzymes
B. Medical therapy—the physician may
  1. Have the patient prepared for surgical intervention by ordering red blood cell and blood volume replacement and medications to correct coagulation problems and nutritional deficiencies
  2. Order chemotherapy and radiation when surgery is not possible to provide comfort, or in conjunction with surgery to limit metastasis
  3. Order medications to control diabetes if present
  4. Order drug therapy such as pancreatic enzymes, bile salts, and vitamin K to correct deficiencies
  5. Order analgesics and tranquilizers for pain
  6. Intervene surgically (treatment of choice, although postsurgical prognosis is grim), Whipple's procedure (removal of head of the pancreas, duodenum, portion of stomach, and the

common bile duct) or a cholecystoje-
junostomy may be performed
C. Nursing diagnosis and intervention
1. Patient needs emotional support
   a. Assist patient to understand disease
      process
   b. Allow for ample listening time in
      plan of care
   c. Encourage verbalization of feelings
      related to recovery, concerns about
      self-image, prognosis
   d. Teach patient preoperatively re-
      garding postoperative dependency
      during acute stage and types of
      supportive measures that will be
      used
   e. Keep patient and family informed
      about care and procedures
   f. Offer realistic reassurance regard-
      ing general progress
   g. Support and strengthen patient's
      body image and ego strengths
   h. Assist patient and family to com-
      municate and set realistic goals and
      plan for convalescence
2. Patient needs relief of pain and promotion of comfort
   a. Administer analgesics as ordered
      before pain reaches peak
   b. Use soapless bathing and antiprurit-
      ic agents to relieve pruritus of skin
3. Patient needs to be protected against
   complications preoperatively and postoperatively
   a. Observe patient for complications
      such as peritonitis, gastrointestinal
      obstruction, jaundice, hypergly-
      cemia, hypotension
   b. Observe stools for undigested fat
   c. Frequently monitor vital signs ob-
      serving for wound hemorrhage
      caused by coagulation deficiency
   d. Administer vitamin K parenterally
      as ordered
   e. Encourage coughing, turning, and
      deep breathing since ambulation
      postoperatively is postponed
   f. Assist with IPPB therapy as re-
      quired
   g. Monitor urinary output
   h. Observe for chemotherapeutic and
      radiation side effects; e.g., skin ir-
      ritation, anorexia, nausea and vom-
      iting
   i. Maintain skin markings of radia-
      tion therapist

4. Patient needs assistance with re-establishing as optimal a level of nutrition
   as possible
   a. Encourage frequent and supple-
      mental feedings as tolerated
   b. Control nausea and vomiting be-
      fore feedings, if possible
   c. Administer vitamin supplements,
      bile salts, and pancreatic enzymes,
      as ordered
   d. Provide oral hygiene and main-
      tain an esthetic environment es-
      pecially at mealtime

Hyposecretion and hypoexcretion in the urinary system

Example: acute renal failure, characterized
by a sudden and almost complete loss of
glomerular and/or tubular function, usually
follows direct trauma to the kidneys or overwhelming physiologic stress such as burns,
septicemia, nephrotoxic drugs and chemicals,
hemolytic blood transfusion reaction, severe
shock, or renal vascular occlusion; acute
renal failure may cause death from acidosis,
potassium intoxication, pulmonary edema or
infection; may progress from the anuric or
oliguric phase through the diuretic phase to
the convalescence phase (which can take
6 to 12 months) to recovery of function; or
may progress to chronic renal failure (chronic renal failure may develop as a separate
entity and does not have to be a sequela of
acute failure)
A. Assessment of patient
   1. Clinical manifestations
      a. Sudden dramatic drop in urinary
         output appearing a few hours after
         the causative event; oliguria—uri-
         nary output less than 400 ml. but
         more than 100 ml. per 24 hours;
         anuria—urinary output less than
         100 ml. per 24 hours
      b. Other symptoms are the result of
         fluid, electrolyte, and waste reten-
         tion
      c. Lethargy and drowsiness, which
         can progress to stupor and coma
      d. Irritability, restlessness, and head-
         ache, which can progress to muscle
         twitching and convulsions
      e. Circumoral numbness, tingling of
         extremities, and muscle weakness,
         which can include the myocardium
         and can progress to cardiac ar-
         rhythmias, cardiac arrest

f. Anorexia, nausea, and vomiting, which can progress to dehydration and electrolyte imbalance

g. Skin pallor, anemia, and increased bleeding time, which can progress to epistaxis and internal hemorrhage

h. Ammonia (urine) odor to breath and perspiration, which can progress to uremic frost on skin and pruritus

i. Generalized edema, hypervolemia, hypertension, and increased venous pressure, which can progress to pulmonary edema and congestive heart failure

j. In addition, respirations are deep and rapid as a compensatory response to the developing metabolic acidosis

2. Diagnostic measures

a. Blood chemistries to determine serum levels; of particular significance are creatinine, potassium, and urea nitrogen, which increase, and calcium and sodium, which decrease

b. Blood gases to determine serum levels; of particular significance are the blood pH and the CO_2-combining power, which are both decreased

c. Hematocrit is decreased as a result of hypervolemia

d. Blood count to determine whether anemia and leukocytosis are present

e. Urinalysis to determine presence of red blood cells, albumin, or casts and a decrease in specific gravity

f. Other diagnostic measures are used when patient's history or signs and symptoms cloud the underlying cause of the renal failure; e.g., IVP, flat plate of the abdomen, KUB, PSP

B. Medical therapy—the physician may

1. Direct treatment toward correcting the underlying cause of renal failure; e.g., treat shock, eliminate drugs and toxins, treat transfusion reactions, restore integrity of urinary tract, etc.

2. Maintain patient on complete bed rest

3. Restrict fluid intake but replace fluid lost

4. Order high carbohydrate, low protein, high fat diet with restricted intake of sodium and potassium

5. Order frequent monitoring of vital signs and intake and output

6. Order packed cells, electrolytes, and glucose IV as necessary

7. Order exchange resins to decrease serum potassium

8. Prescribe antibiotics to reduce possibility of infection

9. Order peritoneal dialysis or hemodialysis

10. Intervene surgically if kidney transplant is a viable alternative

C. Nursing diagnosis and intervention

1. Patient needs to maintain fluid and electrolyte balance

a. Monitor intake and output at frequent intervals

b. Limit fluid intake as ordered

c. Weigh patient daily

d. Observe for signs of overhydration; e.g., dependent, pitting, sacral, or periorbital edema; rales or dyspnea; headache, distended neck veins, and hypertension

e. Observe for signs of hyperkalemia and hyponatremia

f. Administer electrolytes as ordered by the physician

2. Patient has specific safety needs

a. Provide periods of undisturbed rest to conserve energy and oxygen

b. Protect patient from injury caused by bleeding tendency, possibility of convulsions, and clouded sensorium

c. Protect patient from cross-infection

d. Observe for early signs and symptoms of complications; e.g., hemorrhage, convulsions, cardiac problems, pulmonary edema, etc.

e. Provide special skin care frequently to prevent breakdown and remove uremic frost

f. Monitor vital signs and intake and output at frequent intervals; record and report any deviations immediately

g. Administer antibiotics as ordered

3. Patient needs assistance with establishing dietary modifications and maintaining nutritional status

a. Encourage intake of diet as ordered and record amount consumed

b. Allow patient as much choice as possible in the selection of food while recognizing that little variation is possible

c. Provide mouth care before, after, and between meals

d. Administer dietary and electrolyte supplements as ordered

e. Administer antiemetics to control nausea and antacids to reduce gastrointestinal irritation

4. Patient has specific needs related to peritoneal or hemodialysis

a. Explain procedure to patient and family; answer questions related to the procedure

b. Take vital signs and weigh patient before procedure is begun

c. Use surgical asepsis in preparation of site (abdomen or radial vessels)

d. Assure patient that a staff member will be present at all times

e. If indwelling catheter is not in place, have patient void before procedure is started

f. Once the procedure is instituted by the physician, monitor the patient's response and add dialysate as prescribed

g. Monitor vital signs every 15 minutes

h. During peritoneal dialysis keep an accurate flowchart

i. During hemodialysis observe site for clotting; check clotting time and administer heparin as prescribed by the physician

j. During both procedures check tubes for patency

k. Since both procedures are long, provide back care to promote comfort and diversional activities to help pass the time

PATIENTS WITH PROBLEMS IN FLUID AND ELECTROLYTE BALANCE

TYPES OF FLUID AND ELECTROLYTE PROBLEMS

A. Factors affecting fluid volume and electrolyte concentration

B. Pathophysiologic changes within the fluid and electrolyte control system

BASIC CONCEPTS

A. Fluid is the major component of the internal and external environment of all body cells

B. All body fluid contains electrolytes although the type and concentration vary

C. There is a constant exchange of fluid and electrolytes between the extracellular (interstitial and intravascular) and intracellular compartments

D. Fluid and electrolyte exchange occurs by a variety of processes; e.g., osmosis, diffusion, active transport, and filtration

E. The exchange processes depend on the condition of the membrane, the volume and pressure of intracellular and extracellular fluid, and the concentration of electrolytes on either side of the membrane

F. Body fluids are obtained by ingestion and oxidation and are normally lost via the urinary system, respiratory system, skin, and gastrointestinal system

G. Since the relationship between fluid volume and electrolyte concentration is reciprocal, any alterations in either one will cause alterations in the other

H. Electrolytes are lost via body fluid; e.g., sodium via gastrointestinal tract and skin, potassium via urinary system and lower gastrointestinal tract, chlorides via upper gastrointestinal tract, and calcium via gastrointestinal and urinary tract

I. An alteration in any one electrolyte concentration will cause alterations in other electrolyte concentrations

J. Even slight variations in fluid volume or electrolyte concentration will result in alterations in body functioning; e.g., hyperkalemia, which causes cardiac irritability; increased hydrogen ion concentration, which causes metabolic acidosis

K. Fluid and electrolyte balance is regulated mainly by hormonal and renal mechanisms

L. Acid-base balance is maintained by the blood buffers, respiration, and the kidneys

M. Fluid and electrolyte problems occur as frequent adaptations to a wide variety of stress in humans

FACTORS AFFECTING FLUID VOLUME AND ELECTROLYTE CONCENTRATION

Etiology and pathophysiologic processes

A. Fluids and electrolytes can be depleted by nausea and vomiting (hypermotility of gastrointestinal tract), loss of blood (hemorrhage), destruction of tissue (burns, radiation), environmental temperature

(high fever, external heat), inadequate fluid and food intake (starvation), and iatrogenic factors (medications such as diuretics, drainage such as gastrointestinal suction or T-tube drainage, fluid loss such as in surgery)
B. Fluids and electrolytes can be increased by reabsorption of fluid from lower gastrointestinal tract, increased fluid intake, and portal hypertension; localized fluid increase (edema) can occur as a result of decreased osmotic pressure, insufficient venous return, and an obstruction in the lympathic system
C. Fluids and electrolytes can be shifted to other compartments or trapped in a compartment and although they are not depleted on a total body basis they are inaccessible and unavailable for body use; e.g., generalized edema, ascites, and small bowel obstruction

Fluid and electrolyte depletion

Example: thermal burns that cause cell destruction and result in depletion of fluid and electrolytes; the extent of the fluid and electrolyte loss in burns is directly related to the extent and degree of the burn (first or second degree, loss is slight to moderate, especially if less than 15% of body surface is involved; third degree, with destruction of underlying tissue, loss is usually severe, especially if more than 2% of the body surface is involved)
A. Assessment of patient
  1. Clinical manifestations
    a. Condition of skin will determine depth and extent of the injury
      (1) Depth
        (a) First degree—erythema, edema, and pain
        (b) Second degree—erythema, pain, vesicles with oozing
        (c) Third degree—charred or pearly white, dry skin, absence of pain
      (2) Extent of trauma can be estimated by rule of nines or Lund and Browder chart
      (3) Classification of second and third degree burns
        (a) Minor burns—no burns involving hands, face, or genitalia; total burn area does not exceed 15% and third degree burns do not exceed 2% of body area
        (b) Major burns—total burn area is between 15% and 30% of body but third degree burns do not exceed 10% of body area
        (c) Critical burns—total burn area exceeds 30% of body surface; this classification is also used if patient has a preexisting chronic health problem, is under 18 months of age or over 50 years of age, or has additional injuries
      (4) Pulmonary injury should be suspected if 2 of the following factors are present and expected if 3 or all 4 are present
        (a) Hair in nostrils is singed
        (b) The patient was trapped in a closed space
        (c) The face, nose, and lips are burned
        (d) The initial blood sample contains carboxyhemoglobin
      (5) Presence of symptoms of hypovolemic shock caused by circulatory failure resulting from seepage of water, plasma, proteins, and electrolytes into burned area
      (6) Presence of symptoms of neurogenic shock (symptoms similar to hypovolemic shock) caused by the fright, terror, hysteria, and pain involved in the situation
      (7) Hematuria, oliguria, or anuria may be present or may develop in the first 24 hours
      (8) Disorientation and confusion may be present
  2. Diagnostic measures
    a. Blood samples for hemoglobin, hematocrit, electrolytes, type and cross-match, blood gases, pH, complete blood count, proteins—to determine fluid and electrolyte status
    b. Urinalysis for hematuria, sugar, and acetone—to determine kidney function

c. Hourly urinary output—to determine fluid replacement needed

B. Medical therapy—the physician may
1. Order tetanus toxoid immediately
2. Start intravenous replacement therapy at a rate of 250 ml. per hour to achieve an intake of between 6000 and 7000 ml. for the first 24 hours (half of total intravenous solutions will be an electrolyte solution such as Ringer's lactate and half will be plasma or plasma substitute)
3. Reduce total intravenous solutions during second 24 hours depending on patient's urinary output, blood work, and central venous pressure
4. Insert Foley catheter and monitor hourly urinary output and specific gravity to observe kidney functioning and determine fluid replacement
5. Insert central venous pressure and order hourly reading to monitor circulating fluid volume
6. Order vital signs monitored every 15 minutes
7. Order frequent serum electrolytes and blood gases to observe for levels and to assist in deciding replacement therapy
8. Order IPPB and continuous oxygen to assist with respirations
9. Perform a tracheostomy if laryngeal edema occurs
10. Prescribe Demerol for pain and restlessness
11. Prescribe intraveneous and topical antibiotics to limit infection (Keflin and penicillin intravenously; Sulfamylon Ointment)
12. Order patient placed on reverse isolation
13. Permit patient nothing by mouth except for mineral water for first 24 to 48 hours; after this period place patient on high protein, high carbohydrate, high fat, high vitamin diet as tolerated
14. Order daily Hubbard tank baths after fifth day and dressings with antibiotic ointment and Kling dressing
15. Intervene surgically to perform debridement and skin grafts to promote healing and limit contractures

C. Nursing diagnosis and intervention
1. Patient needs close monitoring of vital signs and fluid and electrolyte balance
   a. Observe vital signs, central venous pressure, intake and output, and specific gravity as ordered; notify physician if deviations occur or if output falls below 30 ml. or rises above 50 ml. per hour
   b. Maintain patency of Foley catheter
   c. Make certain blood electrolytes and gases are performed and results are available
   d. Administer fluid and electrolytes as ordered
   e. Observe for signs of electrolyte imbalance (calcium, potassium, and sodium) and metabolic acidosis
2. Patient needs to maintain respiratory functioning
   a. Administer oxygen as ordered
   b. Suction as needed
   c. Administer IPPB as ordered
   d. Observe for signs of tracheal edema (dyspnea, stridor)
   e. Elevate head of bed
   f. Encourage patient to cough and deep breathe
3. Patient has special safety needs
   a. Maintain reverse isolation
   b. Use sterile technique (irrigating drainage tubes, dressings, and bed linens)
   c. Administer tetanus toxoid as ordered
   d. Administer intravenous and topical antibiotics as ordered
   e. Observe for signs of infection (rising temperature and white blood cell count, odor)
   f. Support joints and extremities in functional position
   g. Support patient while turning
   h. Keep room temperature as constant as possible
   i. Observe for symptoms of Curling's (stress) ulcer
4. Patient has special nutritional needs
   a. Administer vitamins as ordered
   b. Encourage progressive diet as ordered and tolerated
   c. Give small frequent high protein, high carbohydrate, high fat, high vitamin feedings
   d. Observe for symptoms of negative nitrogen balance as healing occurs
5. Patient needs emotional support
   a. Give medication for pain as ordered and particularly before dressing change

b. Allow patient time to express feelings

c. Explain all procedures

d. Stay with patient as much as possible

e. Provide periods of rest and periods of diversional activity

f. Encourage patient to assist with moving to reduce need for external pressure

g. Explain how healing occurs and what will be done with burned areas

h. Remove mirrors from room when patient has facial burns

i. Accept and expect patient to express negative feelings about burns

j. Explain need for staff wearing gowns and masks

k. Give realistic reassurance

l. Prepare patient for prolonged period of rehabilitation

m. Attempt to have same staff member do dressings and administer care

Fluid and electrolyte increase

Example: cirrhosis of the liver resulting in portal hypertension (see area on Hypoactivity within the gastrointestinal system in the section on Patients with problems in nutrition and elimination, pp. 492-497)

PATHOPHYSIOLOGIC CHANGES WITHIN THE FLUID AND ELECTROLYTE CONTROL SYSTEM

Etiology and pathophysiologic processes

A. Fluid and electrolyte balance can be depleted or increased by alterations in the ductless glands producing the hormones, which are directly or indirectly involved in the body's fluid and electrolyte control system; e.g., posterior pituitary—antidiuretic hormone (ADH), adrenal cortex—aldosterone and cortisone, anterior pituitary—adrenocorticotropic hormone (ACTH), and ovaries—estrogen

B. Severe fluid and electrolyte imbalance will result when internal or external factors interrupt the function of the posterior pituitary and/or adrenal cortex; if the production of ADH or aldosterone is greatly reduced synthetic hormones must be administered or death will result

C. Since the kidney has the major responsibility for controlling fluid and electrolyte balance in the body, any factor that interrupts the nephron's filtration or reabsorption ability will result in severe fluid and electrolyte imbalance and ultimate death

Hormonal alterations causing imbalance

Dysfunctions of the adrenal cortices that interrupt or increase the production of both mineralocorticoids and glucocorticoids result in either Addison's disease (hypoproduction) or Cushing's syndrome (hyperproduction)

Example: Addison's disease results from destruction or atrophy of the adrenal cortex; therapy in Addison's disease often causes symptoms related to Cushing's syndrome

A. Assessment of patient
1. Clinical manifestations
   a. Symptoms of hyperkalemia such as nausea, abdominal cramps, diarrhea, numbness and tingling of extremities, irregular pulse rate
   b. Symptoms of hypoglycemia such as nervousness, headache, trembling, and diaphoresis
   c. Symptoms of hyponatremia such as muscular weakness, dehydration, fatigue, and hypotension
   d. Emotional changes such as apprehension, anxiety, irritability, and depression
   e. Bronzelike pigmentation of the mucous membranes and skin especially at the elbows, knees, and beltline caused by the overproduction of ACTH and melanocyte-stimulating hormone (MSH)
   f. Anorexia, vomiting, and weight loss
   g. Symptoms of Addisonian crisis (hypotension, shock, coma, and vasomotor collapse) may be present
2. Diagnostic measures
   a. Blood chemistries to observe for increases in potassium (hyperkalemia), urea nitrogen, and magnesium (hypermagnesemia); and decreases in sodium (hyponatremia), glucose (hypoglycemia), and CO_2-combining power
   b. Hematology and differential cell count to observe for increases in eosinophils (eosinophilic leukocytosis), lymphocytes (lymphocy-

tosis), and hematocrit; and decreases in absolute white blood cell count (leukopenia)
c. Urine studies to measure 17-ketosteroids (17-KS), 17-hydroxycorticosteroids (17-OHCS), or 17-ketogenic steroids (17-KGS) for evaluating adrenal function
d. Hormonal response tests to determine whether disease is caused by primary adrenocortical insufficiency or is secondary to pituitary insufficiency
   (1) 8-hour intravenous ACTH test to measure urinary steroid output after administration of ACTH; if output fails to rise, problem is primary adrenocortical insufficiency (Addison's), if output rises slowly (normal response is rapid rise), problem is secondary to pituitary insufficiency
   (2) Plasma cortisol ACTH test to measure plasma cortisol level before and 30 minutes after administration of ACTH; if level fails to rise, problem is primary adrenocortical insufficiency (Addison's), if level rises (which is also the normal response), problem is secondary to pituitary insufficiency
   (3) Thorn test to measure eosinophil count before and after administration of ACTH; if count remains the same, problem is primary adrenocortical insufficiency (Addison's)
e. X-ray film to determine whether calcification is present in the area of the adrenal glands
B. Medical therapy—the physician may
   1. Prescribe corticosteroid drugs for replacement therapy
      a. Glucocorticoid (cortisone or hydrocortisone) to correct metabolic imbalance
      b. Mineralocorticoid (fludrocortisone acetate or desoxycorticosterone acetate) to correct electrolyte imbalance, hypotension, and maintain plasma volume levels
   2. Order adequate fluids, monitoring of intake and output and daily weights

   3. Order high carbohydrate, high protein diet governing intake of potassium and sodium by patient needs
   4. Order daily testing of urine for sugar and acetone
   5. If the patient is in Addisonian crisis
      a. Replace hormones by prescribing intravenous hydrocortisone
      b. Restore circulating blood volume and treat shock by ordering intravenous glucose, saline, plasma, whole blood, or serum albumin
      c. Reverse hypotension by prescribing vasopressors (Aramine, Levophed)
      d. Prevent or combat infection, which is often the precipitating cause of the crisis, by prescribing antibiotics and ordering reverse isolation
      e. Order absolute bed rest
      f. Order monitoring of vital signs, particularly blood pressure and temperature
      g. Insert nasogastric tube if patient is vomiting
      h. Order oxygen as necessary
C. Nursing diagnosis and intervention
   1. Patient needs assistance in maintaining fluid and electrolyte balance
      a. Administer steroids as ordered
      b. Observe for signs of sodium and potassium imbalance
      c. Monitor intake and output and weigh daily
      d. Encourage adequate diet and fluid intake
      e. Administer antiemetics to prevent fluid and electrolyte loss by vomiting
   2. Patient has special safety needs
      a. Put patient in a quiet room avoiding contact with patients having infectious diseases
      b. Limit the number of visitors
      c. Monitor vital signs four times a day; be alert for elevation in temperature (infection, dehydration), alterations in pulse rate (hyperkalemia), alterations in blood pressure
      d. Administer steroids with milk or an antacid to limit ulcerogenic factor of the drug
      e. Use side rails and assist patient in and out of bed to prevent falls
      f. Keep patient warm by use of bed socks, warm robe, and maintaining a consistent temperature

3. Patient needs emotional support
    a. Encourage patient to express feelings
    b. Provide patient with simple explanations for all procedures
    c. Provide for periods of rest by scheduling tests and treatments around rest periods, disconnecting telephone, limiting visitors, reducing stress
    d. Help patient to understand the lifetime need for medication
    e. Help patient to understand that there is a need to conserve psychologic and physiologic energy
    f. Expect and accept patient's anger about disease and necessary changes in life-style
    g. Assist patient to accept altered body image
    h. Assist patient and family to understand that emotional changes are related to disease process and drug therapy
4. Patient needs health teaching
    a. Teach patient the importance of taking hormones as ordered
    b. Teach patient to seek immediate medical attention in the event of physiologic or psychologic stress that may produce Addisonian crisis
    c. Teach patient to obtain and wear a medical alert tag
    d. Teach patient to carry an emergency kit containing intramuscular and additional oral hormones
    e. Teach patient and family to observe for symptoms of exacerbations and crisis and to take appropriate actions
    f. Teach patient to avoid chilling, avoid contact with people with infections, and adequately treat all injuries regardless of how minor they may appear

Alterations in nephron's filtration or reabsorption ability

Example: renal failure resulting in fluid and electrolyte imbalance (see areas on hyposecretion and hypoexcretion in the urinary system in the section on Patients with problems in nutrition and elimination, pp. 501-503)

PATIENTS WITH PROBLEMS OF THE REPRODUCTIVE ORGANS

TYPES OF PROBLEMS WITH THE REPRODUCTIVE ORGANS

A. Inflammatory conditions
B. Benign neoplastic conditions
C. Malignant neoplastic conditions

GENERAL ETIOLOGY AND PHYSIOLOGIC PROCESSES

A. Problems of the reproductive organs can interfere with the reproductive process
B. Problems in either the reproductive or urinary systems frequently coexist, extend, or are transmitted because of their proximity
C. The contiguous nature of the reproductive tract in both the male and the female permits extension of an external infectious process to internal structures
D. There is a direct relationship between hormones, age, sex, sexual activity, and specific problems with certain reproductive organs
E. Emotional problems such as distorted self-image and concern over sexual functioning often accompany problems in the reproductive system
F. Since cancer of the breast and reproductive organs is the leading cause of death in females, these diagnoses may create fear and a feeling of hopelessness in the patient
G. The function of specific reproductive organs is initiated, maintained, and terminated by endocrine secretions
H. Because of the tubular nature of both the male and female reproduction systems, factors that constrict the tubes interfere with the movement of the ovum or sperm

Inflammatory conditions

A. Assessment of patient
    1. Clinical manifestations
        a. Pelvic inflammatory disease—an acute or chronic extension of infectious process into the female pelvic cavity (see Streptococcal and gonococcal infections of the female organs of reproduction in chapter on Maternal health, p. 367)
        b. Epididymitis—an acute or chronic inflammation of the epididymis in

the male, which occurs as a sequela of urinary tract infections, venereal disease, prostatitis, or postoperative prostatectomy; symptoms include chills, fever, scrotal pain, edema, erythema and tenderness, groin pain, swollen and tender epididymis, pyuria and bacteriuria, elevated white blood count
2. Diagnostic measures
   a. History and physical examination
   b. Culture and smear of vaginal or urethral discharge
   c. Urine analysis including culture and sensitivity
B. Medical therapy—the physician may
   1. Prescribe medication to control pain and fever
   2. Prescribe specific antibiotics depending on the organism identified
   3. Maintain the patient on complete bed rest
   4. Order scrotal support for male patients
   5. Identify and notify sexual contacts and Department of Health if venereal disease is present
C. Nursing diagnosis and intervention
   1. Patient needs to limit infection and prevent complications
      a. Explain why antibiotics must be taken as ordered
      b. Maintain bed rest and explain reason for it to patient
      c. Encourage patient to maintain good personal hygiene
      d. Encourage patient to maintain fluid intake
   2. Patient needs emotional support
      a. Explain diagnosis to patient
      b. Answer patient's questions regarding future sexual functioning
      c. If venereal disease is present, explain to patient why identification and notification of sexual contacts are vital

Benign neoplastic conditions
A. Assessment of patient
   1. Clinical manifestations
      a. Benign prostatic hypertrophy—a slow enlargement of the prostatic gland common in males over 40 years of age, which chokes the urethra and interferes with micturition; symptoms include frequency, urgency, nocturia, difficulty in ini-

tiating stream, decrease in force of stream, cystitis; symptoms may progress to total urinary retention
      b. Endometrial hyperplasia—an increase in the endometrial lining of the uterus associated with hormonal changes; this condition is a major cause of dysfunctional uterine bleeding in women approaching menopause; an aberrant growth of endometrial tissue to pelvic areas outside of the uterus is known as endometriosis; symptoms include menorrhagia, metrorrhagia, dysmenorrhea, backache; endometriosis may cause infertility, abdominal discomfort, and pain
   2. Diagnostic measures—directed toward differentiating between benign and malignant neoplastic conditions and include
      a. History and physical examination
      b. Radiographic examinations; e.g., hysterosalpingogram, intravenous pyelogram
      c. Cystoscopic, rectal, or pelvic examinations and uterine curettage (D & C) for visualization, palpation, and/or obtaining biopsies and smears for cytologic studies
B. Medical therapy
   1. In benign prostatic hypertrophy, the physician may
      a. Attempt to reestablish emptying of bladder by ordering a hot bath to induce voiding or by inserting an indwelling catheter or a cystotomy tube
      b. Prescribe urinary antiseptics and medications for reduction of pain and anxiety
      c. Have patient prepared for surgical removal of prostate gland by means of a suprapubic, transurethral, perineal, or retropubic prostatectomy
      d. Postoperatively, order maintenance of drainage; forced fluids; medications for pain, antibiotics, and stool softeners
   2. In endometrial hyperplasia, the physician may
      a. Intervene surgically to remove excess endometrial tissue; D & C if localized in uterus; hysterectomy and salpingo-oophorectomy may be

necessary if it extends outside uterus

b. Prescribe hormonal therapy to
    (1) Regulate menses
    (2) Keep endometrial tissue quiescent by simulating the pregnant state

C. Nursing diagnosis and intervention
  1. Benign prostatic hypertrophy
    a. Patient needs to maintain urinary output
      (1) Use nursing measures to facilitate voiding (see elimination area in Fundamentals of nursing, pp. 324-326) before catheters are inserted or after they have been removed
      (2) Observe for or initiate measures to maintain patency of catheters
      (3) Irrigate catheters as ordered
      (4) Encourage increased fluid intake (2400 to 3000 ml. per day)
    b. Patient needs to prevent infection
      (1) Use sterile technique when necessary; e.g., insertion of urinary catheter, irrigations, dressing changes
      (2) Maintain integrity of closed drainage systems
      (3) Administer antiseptics, bacteriostatics, and antibiotics as ordered
    c. Patient has special safety needs
      (1) See section on general preoperative and postoperative care, pp. 449-451
      (2) In acute urinary retention, decompress the bladder slowly via Foley catheter (not more than 800 to 1200 ml. at a time) to prevent shock and and hematuria
      (3) Observe for signs of hemorrhage; e.g., change in vital signs, nature of drainage, pain, symptoms of shock, frank bleeding
      (4) Avoid postoperative complications by encouraging patient to deep breathe and cough and to exercise muscles in lower extremities
    d. Patient needs emotional support
      (1) Explain to patient why voiding is interrupted
      (2) Teach patient preoperatively what can be expected postoperatively; e.g., presence of catheters, bloody drainage, bladder spasms, pain
      (3) Accept and encourage patient to express concerns about sexual functioning
      (4) Provide patient as much privacy as possible
      (5) Administer medication for pain as ordered
  2. Endometrial hyperplasia
    a. Patient has special safety needs after D & C
      (1) See section on general preoperative and postoperative care, pp. 449-451
      (2) Observe for hemorrhage; e.g., check for signs of shock, vaginal bleeding, and vaginal pack
      (3) Check patient's output; make certain patient is emptying bladder
    b. Patient needs emotional support
      (1) Provide patient with as much privacy as possible
      (2) Explain procedures to patient
      (3) Provide patient time to talk about feelings
      (4) Administer analgesics as ordered
    c. See area under malignant neoplastic conditions for nursing care of patient after a hysterectomy, pp. 512-513

Malignant neoplastic conditions

A. Assessment of patient
  1. Clinical manifestations
    a. Cancer of the prostate gland—a slow, malignant change in the prostate gland, which produces symptoms similar to those found in benign prostatic hypertrophy; tends to spread by direct invasion of surrounding tissues and metastases to the bony pelvis and spine
    b. Cancer of the cervix—a slow, malignant change in the tissue forming the neck of the uterus (cervix); most common form of genital tract malignancy in women; the fact that it produces few symptoms until later stages and if diagnosed early has an extremely high cure

rate make yearly Papanicolaou smears a necessity for all women over 30 years of age; appears to be related to sexual activity; the earliest signs are spotting after intercourse and vaginal discharge; tends to spread by direct invasion of surrounding tissues and metastases to the lungs, bones, and liver

c. Cancer of the breast—a slow, malignant change in the mammary tissue; frequently begins as a hard, non-tender, relatively fixed nodule found most often in the upper outer quadrant of the breast; can often be detected during monthly self-examination in an early stage when there is a better chance for survival; leading cause of death in women; occurring in 1 out of 15 women, much rarer in men; later breast signs include dimpling of the skin, inversion and discharge from the nipple, asymmetry of the breasts, changes in color of the skin over the site, and swelling of the lymph nodes under the arm; tends to spread by direct invasion of surrounding tissues and metastases to axillary lymph nodes, lung pleura, liver, and bone

2. Diagnostic measures—see material under benign neoplastic conditions, pp. 509-510; in addition
   a. Elevated serum acid phosphatase is found in 60% of men with cancer of the prostate
   b. Papanicolaou cytologic findings of Class V are considered conclusive of cervical cancer; Papanicolaou cytologic findings of Class I, II, III, or IV require further studies before a conclusive diagnosis can be determined
   c. Xeromammogram, thermogram mammogram, and xerogram are used to determine the character of suspicious lumps in the breasts; however, a biopsy and frozen section are considered the only conclusive diagnostic tools

B. Medical therapy
   1. In cancer of the prostate gland see material under benign prostatic hypertrophy, pp. 509-510
      a. The type of surgical intervention depends on the extent of the lesion,
      the physical condition of the patient, and the patient's full awareness of the outcome (impotency follows radical prostatectomy)
      b. Radical prostatectomy, done by perineal or retropubic approach, removing the seminal vesicles and a portion of the bladder neck
      c. Radiation therapy alone or in conjunction with surgery may be ordered preoperatively or postoperatively to reduce the lesion and limit metastases
      d. Diethylstilbestrol (estrogen) may be ordered to reduce the size of inoperative lesions or postoperatively to limit metastases
      e. Orchiectomy may be done to limit production of testosterone
   2. Cancer of the cervix
      a. The type of surgical intervention depends on the extent of the lesion and the physical condition of the patient
      b. Hysterosalpingo-oophorectomy (panhysterectomy) to remove total uterus, fallopian tubes, and ovaries is usually done; in advanced lesions the parametrial tissue and lymph nodes may also be removed
      c. Radiation therapy alone or in conjunction with surgery may be ordered to reduce the lesion and limit metastases
   3. Cancer of the breast
      a. The type of surgical and medical intervention depends on the extent of the lesion and the physical condition of the patient
      b. The physician may perform one of the following procedures
         (1) Lumpectomy—removal of lump and a fourth to a third of breast (only used for early, minute, peripheral lesions)
         (2) Simple mastectomy—removal of breast only
         (3) Radical mastectomy—removal of breast, pectoral muscles, pectoral fascia and nodes (pectoral, subclavicular, apical, and axillary); this procedure may be modified
      c. Radiation therapy alone or in conjunction with surgery may be ordered preoperatively or postopera-

tively to reduce the lesion and limit metastases

d. Estrogen may be ordered for postmenopausal women; androgens for premenopausal women; corticosteroids (prednisone) used for those patients with metastases to brain or liver

e. An oophorectomy, adrenalectomy, and/or a hypophysectomy may be done to control metastases

f. The physician may order chemotherapy
  (1) Alkylating agents
    (a) Cyclophosphamide (Cytoxan)
    (b) Chlorambucil (Leukeran)
    (c) Triethylenethiophosphoramide (Thio-TEPA)
  (2) Antimetabolites
    (a) 5-Fluorouracil (5-FU, Fluorouracil)
    (b) Methotrexate (Amethopterin, MTX)
  (3) Other drugs
    (a) Adriamycin (Doxorubicin)
    (b) Vincristine (Oncovin)

C. Nursing diagnosis and intervention
1. Cancer of the prostate (see Nursing diagnosis and intervention under Benign prostatic hypertrophy, pp. 509-510)
a. Additional emotional needs include
  (1) Explain to patient that development of secondary female sexual characteristics will occur and are a result of the medication and not the surgery
  (2) Allow time and opportunity for patient to express feelings about impotency
  (3) Support patient's male image
  (4) Explain situation to patient's family and include them in planning
  (5) Assist patient and family in dealing with diagnosis of cancer

b. See area under Cancer of the cervix for nursing care of patients receiving internal radiation therapy and cancer of the breast for patients receiving external radiation therapy (pp. 512-513)

2. Cancer of the cervix
a. Patient needs emotional support
  (1) Assist patient and family in dealing with diagnosis of cancer
  (2) Allow and encourage patient to express feelings and concerns about change in self-image and sexual functioning
  (3) Support patient's feminine image
  (4) If patient is receiving or is to receive internal radiation therapy, explain the side effects that may occur and the procedures involved, especially the need for isolation during treatment

b. Patient has special elimination needs
  (1) Maintain patency of urinary catheter that has been inserted prior to surgery to decompress bladder and reduce stress on operative site
  (2) Observe for reestablishment of bowel sounds
  (3) Maintain accurate intake and output
  (4) Following removal of urinary catheter, note amount of output and pattern of voiding, catheterize for residual urines if ordered and whenever necessary for urinary retention

c. Patient has general preoperative and postoperative needs (see section on General preoperative and postoperative care, pp. 449-451)

d. The patient receiving internal radiation therapy has special safety needs
  (1) Instruct patient in maintaining proper positioning (supine and side-lying)
  (2) Inspect implant for proper position
  (3) Provide low residue diet and prevent bowel and urinary distention to avoid displacement of radioactive substance and irradiation of adjacent tissues
  (4) Explain to patient and family that visitors and staff will be

limited in the amount of time they can spend in the room to avoid their overexposure to radiation

3. Cancer of the breast
   a. Patient needs emotional support
      (1) Assist patient and family to cope with diagnosis of cancer and altered body image by encouraging them to talk with staff and with each other
      (2) Administer medication for pain as ordered
      (3) Listen and accept patient's anger and depression and don't attempt to minimize it
      (4) Assist patient to identify feelings and encourage discussion of them
      (5) Support patient's feminine image
      (6) Do not avoid talking about physical appearance and, when patient is ready, discuss the use of prosthesis
      (7) Use agencies such as "Reach for Recovery" to help patient with physical and emotional readjustment
      (8) If patient is receiving cobalt therapy or the antineoplastics, inform, explain, and assist the patient to accept the side effects that may occur; e.g., nausea, vomiting, hair loss, anorexia, diarrhea, stomatitis, malaise, itching
   b. Patient has special safety needs
      (1) Provide preoperative and postoperative nursing care (see section on General preoperative and postoperative care, pp. 449-451)
      (2) Observe for hemorrhage by checking all areas of the dressing, the drainage unit, and vital signs
      (3) Maintain functioning of portable vacuum drainage unit by assuring patency of tube, emptying when necessary, and supporting to avoid tension at site of insertion
      (4) Encourage good posture and provide assistance with ambu-lation until patient adjusts to altered balance
      (5) Prevent or reduce lymphedema by elevating and supporting hand above elbow and elbow above shoulder
      (6) If patient is receiving radiation therapy
         (a) Observe for signs of radiation burns (erythema, desquamation)
         (b) Avoid removal of skin markings drawn by the radiologist
         (c) Instruct patient to use only ointments or emollients prescribed by physician
   c. Patient has special rehabilitation needs
      (1) Encourage patient to gradually increase participation in activities of daily living
      (2) Initiate active exercise postoperatively when the physician permits
      (3) Teach patient and/or family to care for operative site; e.g., observe for infection, bathe operative area, change dressings, etc.
      (4) Instruct patient to care for hand and affected side; e.g., if possible avoid even minor injury, treat all injuries immediately, do not permit affected arm to be used for injections or blood pressure
      (5) Instruct patient as to types of prosthesis and where to obtain them
      (6) Teach and encourage patient to perform monthly self-examination of remaining breast and to return to physician at regular intervals

REVIEW QUESTIONS FOR MEDICAL-SURGICAL NURSING

Mrs. Evans, with a history of upper abdominal pain, nausea, and vomiting, is admitted to the hospital for a diagnostic work-up to confirm a possible diagnosis of cancer of the pancreas. She has a history of hypertension and is on an antihypertensive medication. Questions 1 through 11 refer to this situation.

1. As you are admitting Mrs. Evans to her room she asks you, "Do you think I have anything serious—like cancer?" Your best reply is
   1. "Why don't you discuss this with your doctor."
   2. "Don't worry, we won't know until all the test results are back."
   3. "What makes you think you have cancer?"
   4. "I don't know if you do, but let's talk about it."

2. A complete blood count, urinalysis, and x-ray film of the chest are ordered for Mrs. Evans prior to surgery. She asks why these tests are done. Your best answer would be
   1. "Don't worry, these tests are strictly routine."
   2. "They are ordered for all patients having surgery."
   3. "I don't know but the doctor ordered them."
   4. "They determine that it is safe to proceed with surgery."

3. Preoperative nursing care is mainly directed toward
   1. Teaching and answering all questions
   2. Maintaining proper nutritional status
   3. Recording accurate vital signs
   4. Alleviating the patient's anxiety

A progressive ambulation schedule is to be instituted for Mrs. Evans the morning after surgery. Morphine sulfate 10 mg. has been ordered q.4h. p.r.n. for pain.

4. You are getting Mrs. Evans out of bed. Have her sit on the edge of the bed with her feet dangling first because her expected adaptation will be
   1. Respiratory distress
   2. Initial hypertension
   3. Abdominal pain
   4. Postural hypotension

5. A significant influence on Mrs. Evans' perception of pain is her
   1. Overall physical status
   2. Intelligence and economic status
   3. Present age and sex
   4. Previous experience and cultural values

6. Early symptoms of morphine overdose are
   1. Profuse sweating, pinpoint pupils, and deep sleep
   2. Slow respirations, dilated pupils, and restlessness
   3. Slow pulse, slow respirations, stupor
   4. Slow respirations, constricted pupils, and deep sleep

7. On the second postoperative day the patient complains of pain in her right calf. You would
   1. Elevate the extremity
   2. Apply warm soaks
   3. Notify the physician
   4. Chart the symptoms

Mrs. Evans had difficulty voiding and an indwelling catheter was inserted. Irrigations have been ordered for once each shift.

8. Mrs. Evans' catheter is irrigated regularly primarily to
   1. Dilute the urine
   2. Prevent infection
   3. Maintain patency
   4. Stimulate the bladder wall

9. The solution of choice for maintaining patency of an indwelling catheter is
   1. Isotonic saline
   2. Hypotonic saline
   3. Sterile water
   4. Genitourinary irrigant

10. When irrigating Mrs. Evans' catheter a safety precaution is
    1. Avoidance of undue force when instilling
    2. Obtaining and using sterile equipment
    3. Aspiration to assure return flow
    4. Warming the solution to body temperature

11. When irrigating the patient's catheter you would avoid which one of the following?
    1. Using sterile aseptic technique
    2. Allowing solution to flow in by gravity
    3. Having irrigating solution at room temperature
    4. Aspirating irrigating solution with an aseptic syringe

12. In the recovery room, while caring for a patient who has received a general anesthesia, the nurse would notify the doctor if
    1. The patient pushes out the airway
    2. The respirations are regular but shallow
    3. The systolic blood pressure drops from 130 mm. to 100 mm.
    4. The patient has snoring respirations

13. Which of the following nursing actions during the immediate postoperative period has the highest priority?
    1. Checking vital signs every 15 minutes
    2. Maintaining a patent airway
    3. Recording intake and output
    4. Observing for hemorrhage

14. You are caring for a patient in the recovery room who has had a nasogastric tube inserted. The patient vomits 30 ml. of bile colored fluid. You would
    1. Administer an antiemetic
    2. Check the patency of the tube
    3. Elevate the head of the bed
    4. Encourage the patient to breathe deeply

15. When positioning the patient who is recovering from general anesthesia, it is important for the nurse to
    1. Keep the head turned to the side
    2. Place the patient in a Trendelenburg position
    3. Elevate the head of the bed
    4. Position the patient flat on the back

16. In suctioning a tracheostomy, the nurse must remember that it is important to
    1. Initiate suction as the catheter is being withdrawn slowly
    2. Insert catheter until cough reflex is stimulated
    3. Untie the neck tapes while cleansing the skin edges of the wound
    4. Remove the inner cannula before inserting the suction catheter

17. Mr. James has had abdominal surgery and a Penrose drain inserted. As you are caring for him in the recovery room, you notice that the dressing has become soiled with a brownish-red drainage. You would
   1. Change the dressing
   2. Reinforce the dressing
   3. Apply an abdominal binder
   4. Remove the tape and apply Montgomery straps

Mrs. Thompson has had an abdominal resection. Postoperatively, she suddenly complains of numbness in her right leg and a "funny feeling" in her toes. Questions 18 through 21 refer to this situation.

18. As her nurse, your first reaction is to
   1. Elevate her legs and tell her to stay in bed
   2. Rub her legs to start circulation and place a warm blanket on her
   3. Tell her she has been staying in bed too much and encourage ambulation
   4. Tell her to remain in bed and notify her physician
19. Mrs. Thompson was convalescing from abdominal surgery when she developed thrombophlebitis. Nurses must be aware of which of the following signs that indicate this complication?
   1. Severe pain on extension of extremity
   2. Pitting edema of lower extremities
   3. Intermittent claudication
   4. Warm, tender area on leg
20. An anticoagulant drug, Dicumarol, has been ordered by the doctor for Mrs. Thompson. Which of the following drugs would you expect the physician to order if symptoms of overdose of Dicumarol are observed?
   1. Imferon
   2. Heparin
   3. Vitamin K
   4. Protamine sulfate
21. Patients on anticoagulant therapy usually have daily blood work done. Which of the following tests would be most specific for calculating daily dosage of anticoagulant?
   1. Prothrombin time
   2. Clotting time
   3. Bleeding time
   4. Sedimentation rate
22. The main postoperative complication that the nurse should observe for after a patient has a laminectomy is
   1. Atony of the bladder
   2. Pain referred to the flanks
   3. Compression of the cord
   4. Cerebral edema
23. Shock is
   1. Failure of peripheral circulation
   2. An irreversible phenomenon
   3. Always caused by decreased blood volume
   4. A fleeting reaction to tissue injury
24. On a large medical ward, you discover a patient with a history of a recent myocardial infarction unconscious on the floor of the room. The nurse would *first*
   1. Help the patient back to bed
   2. Check the blood pressure
   3. Check the carotid pulse
   4. Call for assistance
25. A patient who is in asystole requires nursing attention because the heart is
   1. Beating very rapidly
   2. Not beating
   3. Beating irregularly
   4. Beating slowly
26. During a cardiac arrest, the nurse and the arrest team must keep in mind the
   1. Time the patient is anoxic
   2. Heart rate of the patient before arrest
   3. Age of the patient
   4. Emergency medications available
27. As the cells are deprived of oxygen in the patient with cardiac arrest, metabolic acidosis develops. The medication used to combat this type of metabolic acidosis is
   1. Potassium chloride
   2. Calcium gluconate
   3. Sodium bicarbonate
   4. Regular insulin
28. To initiate cardiopulmonary resuscitation the first thing the nurse would do is to
   1. Clear the airway
   2. Give four full lung inflations
   3. Compress the lower sternum 15 times
   4. Check for a radial pulse
29. A precardiac thump may be effective in restarting the heartbeat in cases of witnessed cardiac arrest. The fleshy side of the clenched fist is used to deliver a sharp blow to the
   1. Apex of the heart
   2. Xiphoid process
   3. Midsternum
   4. Xiphisternal junction
30. In performing external cardiac compression in adults, the nurse exerts downward vertical pressure on the lower sternum by placing
   1. The heels of each hand side by side, extending the fingers over the chest
   2. The heel of one hand on the sternum and the heel of the other hand on top of it and interlocking the fingers
   3. The fingers of one hand on the sternum and the fingers of the other hand on top of them
   4. The fleshy part of the clenched fist on the lower sternum
31. While performing external cardiac compression on an adult, it is essential to exert a vertical downward pressure which depresses the lower sternum at least
   1. ½ inch to ¾ inch
   2. ¾ inch to 1 inch
   3. 1 inch to 1½ inches
   4. 1½ inches to 2 inches
32. Where there is only one person to perform cardiopulmonary resuscitation the rate of ventilation to cardiac compression is
   1. 1:5
   2. 1:10
   3. 2:15
   4. 4:15
33. When performing cardiopulmonary resuscitation with 2 people, the rate of ventilation to cardiac compression is
   1. 1:5

2. 1:10
3. 2:15
4. 4:15

34. To prepare the skin area for placement of the electrodes for cardiac monitoring, the nurse
   1. Uses a scrubbing motion while cleansing the skin
   2. Shaves the chest of both male and female patients
   3. Makes sure the area is moistened with normal saline before applying the electrodes
   4. Applies electrode paste only if the skin becomes excoriated

35. That portion of the cardiac monitor which sets an alarm if the heart rate goes above or below a certain predetermined setting is called the
   1. Oscilloscope
   2. Voltmeter
   3. Pacemaker
   4. Synchronizer

36. When ventricular fibrillation occurs in a coronary care unit, the first person reaching the patient would
   1. Initiate cardiopulmonary resuscitation
   2. Defibrillate the patient
   3. Administer sodium bicarbonate intravenously
   4. Administer oxygen

37. Mr. Daniels is unconscious when admitted to the emergency room. After a diagnosis of heroin overdose, nalorphine hydrochloride (Nalline) is administered. The planned effect of the drug is to
   1. Stimulate cortical sites controlling consciousness and cardiovascular function
   2. Accelerate metabolism of heroin and stimulate respiratory centers
   3. Compete with narcotics for receptors controlling respiration
   4. Decrease analgesia and the comatose state induced by heroin

38. Within an hour Mr. Daniels is responding. Close observation of his status is indicated because
   1. The combined action of nalorphine hydrochloride and heroin causes cardiac depression
   2. Nalorphine hydrochloride may cause neuropathy and convulsions
   3. Narcotic effect may cause return of symptoms after the nalorphine hydrochloride is metabolized
   4. Hyperexcitability and amnesia may cause the patient to thrash about and become abusive

39. A patient is admitted to your ward from the emergency room in acute respiratory distress resulting from an asthmatic attack. The patient should be placed in which position to facilitate maximum air exchange?
   1. High-Fowler's
   2. Semi-Fowler's
   3. Orthopneic
   4. Supine with pillows

40. A nurse will use an Ambu bag in the Intensive Care Unit when
   1. The patient is in ventricular fibrillation
   2. A surgical incision with copious drainage is present
   3. Respiratory output must be monitored at intervals
   4. There is a respiratory arrest

41. An emergency measure for an asthmatic attack is to administer Adrenalin 1:1000 hypodermically. Since this effect is not immediate, it may be supplemented by
   1. CO_2 inhalations
   2. Morphine 30 mg. intramuscularly
   3. Digitalis 30 mg. orally
   4. Aminophylline 225 mg. intravenously

Mrs. Gray, a 34-year-old mother of 5 children, has been diagnosed as having rheumatoid arthritis. Mrs. Gray is being admitted to the hospital because of a recent flare-up of symptoms. She has been on aspirin and steroid therapy for the past year. Questions 42 through 44 refer to this situation.

42. Daily blood work is ordered for Mrs. Gray during the first 3 days of her hospitalization. Which one of the following symptoms may be indicative of complications of the prolonged use of medications?
   1. Elevated sedimentation rate
   2. Leukopenia
   3. Elevated C-reactive protein
   4. Hypochromic, normocytic anemia

43. Mrs. Gray's husband asks the nurse whether his wife will be an invalid. Recognizing the individuality of responses to disease, the best answer would be
   1. "The progression is slow, so she will spend her young life with little problems."
   2. "Deformities will occur, but she will not be an invalid."
   3. "With continuous treatment, the disease progression can be controlled."
   4. "There will be periods when she is confined to bed rest and times when she can have fairly normal activity."

44. Which one of the following diversional activities would meet the nursing objectives for Mrs. Gray during remissions?
   1. Watching selected television shows
   2. Swimming with the family
   3. Teaching sewing classes
   4. Short hikes with the family

45. Which of the following would you expect to develop as a result of whole body irradiation? Increased
   1. Red blood cell production
   2. Susceptibility to infection
   3. Tendency for pathologic fractures
   4. Blood viscosity

Mr. Bloom, a 56-year-old baker, was admitted to the hospital 5 weeks ago with a fractured skull and concussion. Two weeks after admission, he exhibited evidence of increasing intracranial pressure. Questions 46 through 52 refer to this situation.

46. Mr. Bloom has been receiving dexamethasone (Decadron) during the past 3 weeks for control of cerebral edema. The planned effect of the drug on his problem is to
   1. Increase fluid removal from tissues

2. Reduce cerebrospinal fluid secretion by the choroid plexus
3. Increase elasticity of the ventricle walls
4. Suppress production of antibodies

47. While Mr. Bloom is receiving dexamethasone (Decadron), the nurse is testing his urine for sugar and acetone every 4 hours because the drug
   1. Lowers the renal threshold for glucose
   2. Mobilizes liver stores of glycogen
   3. Accelerates protein breakdown and liberates excess glycogen
   4. Has a glucose component, which raises the blood sugar level

48. Mr. Bloom is receiving Maalox while he is receiving dexamethasone. The antacid is prescribed because dexamethasone is a drug that
   1. Is irritating to the gastric mucosa
   2. Stimulates gastric production of hydrochloric acid
   3. Increases acidity of the stomach and slows emptying time
   4. Increases pepsin-induced erosion of the gastric mucosa

49. Mr. Bloom has several loose bowel movements and the physician changes his antacid prescription to Amphojel. The change is made because
   1. Maalox and dexamethasone act synergistically to increase fluid content of the intestine
   2. Amphojel increases the bulk of feces and slows peristalsis
   3. Amphojel neutralizes larger amounts of the hydrochloric acid that causes diarrhea
   4. Maalox contains a magnesium component that stimulates peristalsis

50. Mr. Bloom complains about the chalky taste of Amphojel. He states that he would rather take bicarbonate of soda that he takes at home. The nurse would tell him it is not advisable to take bicarbonate of soda regularly. Her statement is based on knowledge that bicarbonate of soda
   1. Causes distention by producing carbon dioxide in the stomach
   2. Is absorbed from the stomach and the sodium component causes ankle edema
   3. Is absorbed from the stomach and may cause alkalosis
   4. Causes rebound hyperacidity after initial neutralization of hydrochloric acid

51. The nurse notes that Mr. Bloom's face has a rounded appearance. She recognizes the change as "moon face," which occurs during glucocorticoid therapy and is primarily related to the drug
   1. Slowing excretion of sodium and water in the kidneys, so that fluid is retained in tissues
   2. Causing breakdown of protein stores, so that amino acids are utilized to build new cells in superficial tissues
   3. Accelerating catabolism of protein and glycogen; the process supplies components for fat stores in tissues
   4. Decreasing the metabolic rate; the resultant weight gain is first evident in facial tissues

52. The physician states he plans to gradually reduce Mr. Bloom's dexamethasone dosage and to continue him on a lower maintenance dosage during the new few weeks. The reason for gradual dosage reduction is to allow
   1. Production of adrenocorticotropic hormone (ACTH)
   2. Return of cortisone production by the adrenal glands
   3. Time to observe for return of increased intracranial pressure
   4. Building of glycogen and protein stores in liver and muscle

53. A patient is admitted to the hospital with a history of convulsive disorders. The nurse should automatically place at the bedside
   1. A sphygmomanometer
   2. Oxygen equipment
   3. A padded tongue blade
   4. A rubber or plastic airway

54. Mrs. Green is 55 years of age and a known diabetic. She is to receive NPN insulin, 40 units each morning. You have NPN insulin 100 U = 1 ml. and a regular syringe available. To give 40 units you would withdraw
   1. 6 minims
   2. 12 minims
   3. 20 minims
   4. 40 minims

55. Mrs. Green has developed symptoms of diabetic acidosis. The insulin used in this emergency would be
   1. Protamine zinc
   2. Globulin
   3. NPH
   4. Regular

56. Glucagon is given as a follow-up to 50% dextrose in the treatment of hypoglycemia because
   1. Provides more storage of glucose
   2. Increases blood sugar levels
   3. Stimulates release of insulin
   4. Inhibits glycogenesis

57. In which of the following instances would there be a need to increase the insulin dosage? The patient
   1. Has the prodromal symptoms of a cold
   2. Ate a dish of ice cream for dessert
   3. Had to walk a mile when she ran out of gas
   4. Was emotionally upset after a fight with her husband

Mrs. August, a 44-year-old female, is admitted to the hospital with a tentative diagnosis of hyperthyroidism. Questions 58 through 64 refer to this situation.

58. The nurse would expect Mrs. August to exhibit
   1. Nervousness, weight loss, increased appetite
   2. Protruding eyeballs, slow pulse, sluggishness
   3. Increased appetite, slow pulse, dry skin

4. Loss of weight, gastrointestinal disturbances, listlessness

59. Diagnostic tests to confirm this diagnosis include
    1. Radioactive iodine uptake and T_3
    2. Protein bound iodine and SMA 12
    3. T_4 and x-ray films
    4. Basal metabolism rate and pO_2

60. Mrs. August would probably be placed on a
    1. High caloric diet with supplementary feeding
    2. High protein diet with supplementary nourishment
    3. Regular diet with nourishment between meals
    4. Soft, easily digested, nourishing diet

61. The major nursing problem in caring for Mrs. August would be
    1. Providing an adequate diet
    2. Keeping the bed linen neat
    3. Providing sufficient rest
    4. Modifying hospital routines

62. Mrs. August was ordered propylthiouracil, the purpose of which is to
    1. Interfere with the synthesis of thyroid hormone
    2. Produce atrophy of the thyroid gland
    3. Increase the uptake of iodine
    4. Decrease the secretion of thyroid-stimulating hormone

63. The doctor decided that Mrs. August should have a subtotal thyroidectomy. In preparation for surgery, Lugol's iodine was ordered. Lugol's iodine is given to
    1. Maintain the function of the parathyroid glands
    2. Decrease the total basal metabolic rate
    3. Block the formation of thyroxin by the thyroid gland
    4. Decrease the size and vascularity of the thyroid gland

64. Postoperatively the nurse should be alert to observe for signs of "thyroid storm." These include
    1. Loss of consciousness
    2. Elevated serum calcium
    3. Rapid heart action and tremors
    4. Sudden drop in pulse rate

Mr. Saul, a 68-year-old retired civil service employee, is admitted to the hospital via the emergency service. He was found unconscious a half hour previous to the admission. The physical examination revealed right hemiplegia. Tentative diagnosis: cerebral vascular accident. Questions 65 through 68 refer to this situation.

65. In observing Mr. Saul, the nurse should check for signs of increased intracranial pressure. Which one of the following combinations of symptoms would be indicative of increased intracranial pressure?
    1. Rapid, weak pulse; rising blood pressure; elevated temperature; stupor
    2. Rapid, weak pulse; fall in blood pressure; low temperature; restlessness
    3. Slow bounding pulse; normal blood pressure; intermittent temperature; lethargy

4. Slow bounding pulse; fall in blood pressure; temperature below 97°; stupor

66. Since Mr. Saul is unconscious, you would expect him to
    1. Be unable to react to painful stimuli
    2. Be incontinent
    3. Be capable of spontaneous motion
    4. Demonstrate carphology

67. Mr. Saul regains consciousness and has expressive aphasia. As a part of the long-range planning, the nurse would
    1. Help the family to accept the fact that Mr. Saul cannot participate in verbal communication
    2. Wait for Mr. Saul to verbalize his needs regardless of how long it may take
    3. Begin associating words with physical objects
    4. Help Mr. Saul accept this disability as permanent

68. Urinary retention and overflow, a frequent problem with the stroke patient, is evidenced by
    1. Decrease in total amount of urine voided
    2. Frequency from inability to empty bladder
    3. Continual incontinence
    4. Oliguria and edema

69. Neostigmine bromide (Prostigmine) is used for the diagnosis of myasthenia gravis because this drug will cause a temporary
    1. Increase in symptoms
    2. Drying of the mouth and throat
    3. Decrease in blood pressure
    4. Increase in muscle strength

70. Which one of the following conditions predisposes the individual to Parkinson's disease?
    1. Pulmonary emphysema
    2. Arteriosclerosis
    3. Pancreatitis
    4. Essential hypertension

71. L-dopa appears to be a useful method in treating Parkinson's disease because it can
    1. Replace the dopamine in the brain cells
    2. Cause regeneration of injured thalamic cells
    3. Increase acetylcholine production
    4. Cross the blood-brain barrier

72. A patient immobilized in a body cast may develop renal calculi as a complication because
    1. He has more difficulty urinating in a supine position
    2. He may be drinking a great deal of milk
    3. Lack of muscle action and normal tension causes calcium withdrawal from the bone
    4. Fracture healing requires more calcium and hence increases total calcium metabolism

Mrs. Kraft, a 45-year-old woman, is admitted to the hospital for elective surgery. She has a history of closed-angle chronic glaucoma and has been using 2% pilocarpine eyedrops 4 times a day for the past year. Questions 73 through 76 refer to this situation.

73. The chief aim of medical treatment in chronic glaucoma is
    1. Controlling intraocular pressure

2. Dilating the pupil to allow for an increase in visual field
3. Resting the eye to reduce pressure
4. Preventing secondary infections that may add to the visual problem

74. Which of the following ocular symptoms would Mrs. Kraft most likely exhibit?
   1. A complete loss of forward vision
   2. Attacks of acute pain
   3. Impairment of peripheral vision
   4. Constant blurred vision

75. The anesthesiologist prescribed Demerol 50 mg. and atropine 0.4 mg. preoperatively. The nurse would
   1. Withhold the atropine since it is contraindicated
   2. Give the medication as ordered
   3. Administer the pilocarpine 30 minutes before the atropine
   4. Get the anesthesiologist to change the order

76. The patient with glaucoma needs assistance in learning to accept the disease because
   1. There is usually restriction in the use of both eyes
   2. Lost vision cannot be restored
   3. Total blindness is inevitable
   4. Surgery will only temporarily help the problem

Mr. Ray, a 67-year-old retired plumber, fell and could not get up. His daughter called an ambulance and he was brought to the emergency room where it was found he had a fracture of the neck of the left femur. Mr. Ray was admitted to the orthopedic unit, put in Buck's extension, and prepared for surgery the next day. Questions 77 through 80 refer to this situation.

77. On examination of Mr. Ray, the nurse would expect to find
   1. Shortening of the affected extremity with internal rotation
   2. Shortening of the affected extremity with external rotation
   3. Abduction with external rotation
   4. Adduction with internal rotation

78. Following a fracture of the neck of the femur, the desirable position for the limb is
   1. External rotation with flexion of the knee and hip
   2. External rotation with extension of the knee and hip
   3. Internal rotation with extension of the knee
   4. Internal rotation with flexion of the hip and knee

79. The chief reason for applying Buck's extension traction is to
   1. Help reduce the fracture and to relieve muscle spasm and pain
   2. Keep patient from turning and moving in bed
   3. Prevent contractures from developing
   4. Maintain the limb in a position of external rotation

80. When Mr. Ray is ready to walk with crutches after the hip pinning, he will probably be taught
   1. Four-point crutch walking
   2. Two-point crutch walking
   3. Swing-through gait
   4. Three-point crutch walking

Mr. Boise, a 45-year-old tunnel guard, is diagnosed as having emphysema. He has cyanosis of his lips and fingernails and is short of breath. Questions 81 through 87 refer to this situation.

81. While waiting for the examining physician to arrive, Mr. Boise would be most comfortable in which of the following positions?
   1. Moderate Fowler's supported with pillows
   2. Semirecumbent with one pillow
   3. Sitting on the edge of the bed
   4. Supine with his head slightly elevated

82. As you are admitting Mr. Boise, you observe that he is experiencing difficulty in breathing. You know that this is caused by
   1. Spasm of the bronchi that traps the air
   2. A too rapid expulsion of the air from the alveoli
   3. An increase in the vital capacity of the lung
   4. Difficulty in expelling the air trapped in the alveoli

83. At home, Mr. Boise has been taking aminophylline for control of his asthma. The planned effect of the drug is to
   1. Increase the ventilation-perfusion ratio of the bronchioles
   2. Stimulate chemoreceptor control of bronchial dilation
   3. Dilate the bronchial and coronary arteries
   4. Dilate the smooth muscles of the bronchi

84. The physician ordered that O_2 be given to Mr. Boise in low concentration and intermittently rather than in high concentration and continuously to prevent
   1. Depression of the respiratory center
   2. Decrease in red blood cell formation
   3. Rupture of emphysematous bullae
   4. Excessive drying of respiratory mucosa

85. Deep breathing exercises help in which one of the following ways?
   1. Counteracting respiratory acidosis
   2. Expanding the alveoli
   3. Increasing blood volume
   4. Decreasing the partial pressure of oxygen

86. Mr. Boise has been advised to use an isoproterenol hydrochloride (Isuprel) inhaler for intermittent periods of bronchial constriction. Because the drug affects beta adrenergic receptors, the nurse would tell him he may have
   1. Slow pulse, headache, muscle tension
   2. Facial flushing, tingling in his fingers, dizziness
   3. Rapid pulse, dizziness, pounding of his heart
   4. Coldness of fingers and toes, muscle cramps, headache

87. The nurse also will tell Mr. Boise that the problems occurring with use of the inhaler will be lessened by
   1. Limiting use of the drug to the time required for relief of dyspnea
   2. Using rapid, shallow (panting) respirations while using the inhalant

3. Interrupting the spray of inhalant while continuing normal breathing patterns
4. Gradually decreasing pressure on the spray control after initial relief is obtained

88. Mr. Jones, a 48-year-old man, with a long history of chronic obstructive lung disease is admitted to the hospital for a segmental resection of the right lower lobe. Intermittent positive pressure breathing is given preoperatively to
   1. Encourage respiration at a faster rate than that established by respiratory center control
   2. Provide more adequate lung expansion than could be achieved by unassisted breathing
   3. Force air through the infected secretions that had accumulated in the lung bases
   4. Remove air and fluid from the pleural cavity

89. Immediately following Mr. Jones' arrival in the recovery room, the nurse should undertake which of the following measures in relation to the closed chest drainage apparatus?
   1. Secure the chest catheter to the wound dressing with a sterile safety pin
   2. Mark the time and the fluid level on the side of the drainage bottle
   3. Raise the drainage bottle to bed level to check patency of the system
   4. Add 3 to 5 ml. of sterile saline to the water seal

90. The purpose of the water in the closed chest drainage bottle is to
   1. Facilitate emptying bloody drainage from the chest
   2. Foster removal of chest secretions by capillarity
   3. Prevent entrance of air into pleural cavity
   4. Decrease the danger of sudden change in pressure in tube

91. Mr. Louis is receiving an anticoagulant for pulmonary embolism. Which of the following drugs is contraindicated for patients receiving anticoagulants?
   1. Vasodilan
   2. Chloral hydrate
   3. Thorazine
   4. Aspirin

92. Which of the following actions would the nurse initiate with Mr. Louis as a measure to prevent further emboli?
   1. Encourage deep breathing and coughing
   2. Use of the knee gatch when positioning the patient
   3. Limit the fluid intake of the immobilized patient
   4. Encourage patient to move his legs while confined to bed

93. Which of the following postoperative patients have the *least* likelihood of developing pulmonary embolism? The patient with a(n)
   1. Prostatectomy
   2. Hysterectomy
   3. Saphenous vein ligation
   4. Appendectomy

94. Patients with peripheral vascular disease are instructed to stop smoking because the nicotine
   1. Dilates the peripheral vessels causing a reflex constriction of visceral vessels
   2. Constricts the peripheral vessels and increases the force of flow
   3. Constricts the collateral circulation, dilating the superficial vessels
   4. Constricts the superficial vessels, dilating the deep vessels

95. In chronic occlusive arterial disease, often the precipitating cause for ulceration and gangrenous lesions is
   1. Poor hygiene
   2. Stimulants such as coffee, tea, or cola drinks
   3. Emotions
   4. Trauma from mechanical, chemical, or thermal sources

96. Common symptoms of Buerger's disease are
   1. Burning pain precipitated by cold exposure, fatigue, blanching of skin
   2. Easy fatigue of part, continuous claudication
   3. General blanching of skin, intermittent claudication
   4. Intermittent claudication, local blanching of skin, burning pain after exposure to cold

97. The important characteristics when assessing the peripheral pulse would be
   1. Contractility and rate
   2. Color of skin and type of spasms
   3. Amplitude, symmetry, and rhythm
   4. Local temperature, visible pulsations

98. Atherosclerosis is best described as
   1. A loss of elasticity, thickening and hardening of the arteries
   2. Development of atheromas within the myocardium
   3. A mobilization of free fatty acid from adipose tissue
   4. Development of fatty deposits within the intima of the arteries

Mr. Gold, a 42-year-old insurance broker, is admitted to the hospital with a diagnosis of coronary occlusion. Questions 99 through 109 refer to this situation.

99. The pain of coronary occlusion is caused primarily by
   1. Arterial spasm
   2. Irritation of nerve endings in cardiac plexus
   3. Ischemia of the heart muscle
   4. Blocking of the coronary veins

100. Diagnostic tests specific for myocardial infarction include
   1. Paul-Bunnell Test, serum potassium
   2. LDH, CPK, SGOT
   3. Sedimentation rate, SGPT
   4. Serum calcium, APPT

101. Morphine sulfate, 15 mg. q.4h. p.r.n. was ordered for Mr. Gold. Caution should be exercised in administering this drug because
   1. Mr. Gold may become addicted
   2. Morphine's accumulative effect may result in shock

3. The development of tolerance is likely
4. Cardiac pain is antagonistic to morphine

102. In addition to its cardiotonic action, the digitalis preparations also promote diuresis. As a result Mr. Gold can be depleted of
    1. Calcium
    2. Phosphates
    3. Potassium
    4. Sodium

103. Mr. Gold complains of severe nausea and his heartbeat is irregular and slow. The nurse would recognize these symptoms as toxic effects of
    1. Lanoxin
    2. Lidocaine
    3. Morphine sulfate
    4. Meperidine hydrochloride

104. In addition to a decreased apical rate, which one of the following symptoms would be an indication to withhold digitoxin?
    1. Decreased urinary output
    2. Tachycardia
    3. Chest pain
    4. Diplopia

105. Mr. Gold was placed on strict bed rest and a 1500 calorie bland diet. The primary rationale for his diet is
    1. To reduce metabolic work load associated with digestion and to control gastric acidity
    2. To reduce metabolic work load associated with digestion and to avoid pressure from a volume of food
    3. To reduce his weight and to control gastric acidity
    4. To reduce his weight and to avoid pressure from a volume of food

106. During the acute period of Mr. Gold's illness the best method of making his bed would be to
    1. Remake the bed by changing the top linen and only the necessary bottom linen
    2. Change the linen from top to bottom without lowering the head of the bed
    3. Slide him onto a stretcher, remake the bed, then slide him back to the bed
    4. Lift rather than roll him from side to side while changing the linen

107. Mr. Gold was given oxygen. The primary therapeutic action in this case is to
    1. Prevent dyspnea
    2. Prevent cyanosis
    3. Increase oxygen concentration to heart cells
    4. Increase oxygen tension in the circulating blood

108. Two days after admission Mr. Gold develops a temperature of 101.2°F. The nurse should realize that this elevation indicates
    1. Possible infection
    2. Tissue necrosis
    3. Pulmonary infarction
    4. Pneumonia

109. Mr. Gold expresses concern with how long the heart takes to heal. You can answer that myocardial necrosis usually heals within
    1. 3 to 4 weeks
    2. 6 to 8 weeks
    3. 10 to 14 weeks
    4. At least 24 weeks

110. One of the more common complications of myocardial infarction is
    1. Cardiac arrhythmia
    2. Anaphylactic shock
    3. Cardiac enlargement
    4. Hypokalemia

111. The lethal arrhythmia that often requires immediate intervention by the nurse is
    1. Atrial fibrillation
    2. Auricular flutter
    3. Second degree heart block
    4. Ventricular fibrillation

112. The greatest danger of premature ventricular contractions is that they can lead to ventricular fibrillation if they strike on the
    1. P wave
    2. P-R interval
    3. R wave
    4. T wave

113. A patient is admitted to the coronary care unit with ventricular fibrillation. The nurse should prepare for
    1. An intramuscular injection of Lanoxin
    2. An intravenous line for emergency medications
    3. Immediate defibrillation
    4. Elective cardioversion

114. A patient is admitted to the coronary unit and placed on a cardiac monitor. The doctor says there is ventricular irritability evidenced on the screen. The medication you might expect to administer is
    1. Lanoxin
    2. Lidocaine
    3. Lasix
    4. Levophed

115. Which of the following findings always occurs in bundle branch block?
    1. Absence of P waves
    2. Widening of QRS complex to 0.12 second or greater
    3. Inverted T waves
    4. Sagging S-T segment

116. In charting notes describing a patient's heart rate, the nurse uses the term *bradycardia*. This describes
    1. A grossly irregular heart rate
    2. A heart rate of over 90 per minute
    3. A heartbeat that has regular "skipped" beats
    4. A heart rate of under 60 per minute

117. Cardioversion is a procedure that is utilized to convert certain arrhythmias to normal rhythm. In addition to atrial fibrillation, which of the following arrhythmias is an indication for cardioversion?
    1. Ventricular fibrillation
    2. Premature ventricular contraction
    3. Ventricular tachycardia
    4. Ventricular standstill

118. To overcome the potential danger of inducing ventricular fibrillation during cardioversion, it is essential for
    1. The energy level to be set at its maximum level

2. The synchronizer switch to be in the "on" position
3. The skin electrodes to be applied after the T wave
4. The alarm system of the cardiac monitor to be functioning simultaneously

119. The monitor shows a PQRST wave for each beat and indicates a rate of 120. The rhythm is regular. The nurse can note that the patient is experiencing
   1. Atrial fibrillation
   2. Ventricular fibrillation
   3. Sinus tachycardia
   4. Sinus bradycardia

Mrs. Johnson, a 64-year-old housewife, is admitted to the hospital with a diagnosis of hypertension. Questions 120 through 126 refer to this situation.

120. Mrs. Johnson is receiving methyldopate hydrochloride (Aldomet) intravenously for control of hypertension. Her blood pressure before the infusion started was 150/90. Fifteen minutes after the infusion is started her blood pressure rises to 180/100. The response to the drug would be described as a(n)
   1. Synergistic response
   2. Individual hypersensitivity
   3. Allergic response
   4. Paradoxic response
121. To assess the effectiveness of methyldopate hydrohcloride (Aldomet) in lowering blood pressure levels, the nurse would take Mrs. Johnson's pulse and blood pressure
   1. One half hour after giving the drug
   2. Immediately after she gets out of bed
   3. After she has been supine for 5 minutes
   4. Prior to giving the drug
122. Mrs. Johnson is also receiving hydrochlorothiazide (Diuril). The planned therapeutic effect of the drug is to
   1. Decrease circulating blood volume
   2. Stimulate chemoreceptor control of sodium excretion
   3. Depress aldosterone-induced reabsorption of sodium
   4. Increase glomerular filtration
123. Mrs. Johnson's serum potassium level is low and she is placed on a cardiac monitor. She is to receive 40 mEq. potassium chloride in 1000 ml. 5% D/W intravenously. The nurse analyzes the monitor pattern to obtain a baseline for evaluating progress. The monitor pattern would show
   1. Shortening of the QRS complex
   2. Elevation of the S-T segment
   3. Increased deflection of the Q wave
   4. Lowering of the T wave
124. Mrs. Johnson's intravenous medication inadvertently runs in rapidly. The physician prescribes insulin added to a 10% D/W solution. The rationale for the prescription is
   1. Glucose and insulin increase the metabolic rate and accelerate potassium excretion
   2. Potassium moves into body cells with glucose and insulin
   3. Increased potassium causes a temporary slowing of pancreatic production of insulin

4. Increased insulin accelerates excretion of glucose and potassium
125. Mrs. Johnson's condition has improved and methyldopa (Aldomet) is being given orally. When explaining why orthostatic hypotension occurs, the nurse would base her response on knowledge that the drug causes vasodilation by
   1. Depleting acetylcholine
   2. Decreasing adrenal release of epinephrine
   3. Stimulating histamine release
   4. Interrupting norepinephrine release
126. When discussing the plan for taking methyldopa (Aldomet) at home, the nurse would tell Mrs. Johnson that orthostatic hypotension may be modified by
   1. Lying down for ½ hour after taking the drug
   2. Avoiding tasks that require high energy expenditure
   3. Wearing support hose continuously
   4. Sitting on the edge of the bed for a short time before arising
127. Mrs. Harvey has an acute episode of congestive heart failure and she is receiving furosemide (Lasix). The physician has prescribed aspirin for her arthritic pain. When Mrs. Harvey asks why she is not receiving the same aspirin dosage she usually takes, the nurse's response would be based on knowledge that
   1. Aspirin in large dosage after an acute stress episode increases the bleeding potential
   2. Use of furosemide and aspirin concomitantly increases formation of uric acid crystals in the nephron
   3. Competition for renal excretion sites by the drugs causes increased serum levels of aspirin
   4. Aspirin accelerates metabolism of furosemide and decreases the diuretic effect
128. The symptoms that Mrs. Harvey most likely presented on admission are
   1. Dyspnea, edema, fatigue
   2. Weakness, palpitations, nausea
   3. Fatigue, vertigo, and headache
   4. A feeling of distress when breathing
129. Mrs. Harvey has edema during the day and it disappears at night. The patient states it is not painful and is located in the lower extremities. The nurse should suspect
   1. Pulmonary edema
   2. Right sided heart failure
   3. Myocardial infarction
   4. Lung disease
130. The patient with congestive heart failure develops ascites because of
   1. Loss of colloidal proteins
   2. Rapid diffusion of solutes and solvents into plasma
   3. Rapid osmosis from tissue spaces to cells
   4. Loss of cellular constituents in blood
131. A patient is admitted to the coronary care unit with a diagnosis of acute pulmonary edema. The nurse should be prepared for
   1. Postural drainage
   2. Inhalation therapy

3. Rotating tourniquets
4. Phlebotomy

132. The rotating tourniquet technique is effective for
   1. Decreasing arterial flow of blood to the body
   2. Restricting visceral flow in the internal body cavities
   3. Decreasing venous flow of blood to the heart
   4. Increasing the flow of blood through the capillaries

133. When rotating tourniquets are used the nurse should remember that
   1. The automatic tourniquets occlude arterial blood flow
   2. The tourniquets are simultaneously applied to all 4 limbs
   3. The tourniquets are rotated every 15 minutes
   4. The tourniquets are rotated 2 at a time

134. In caring for a patient who is being mechanically ventilated and is having central venous pressure monitored, the nurse understands that
   1. The patient should not be taken off the ventilator for the central venous pressure readings
   2. The fluid level in the manometer fluctuates with each respiration
   3. Blood should not be easily aspirated from the central venous pressure line
   4. The zero mark on the manometer should be at the level of the diaphragm

135. The medication most frequently used to relieve anxiety and apprehension in the patient with pulmonary edema is
   1. Atarax
   2. Sodium phenobarbital
   3. Chloral hydrate
   4. Morphine sulfate

136. Intravenous digitalis preparations are used to treat patients with acute pulmonary edema associated with left-sided heart failure. Which of the following preparations is administered intravenously?
   1. Digoxin
   2. Gitalin
   3. Deslanoside
   4. Digitalis leaf

137. If the patient is receiving aminophylline intravenously to relieve pulmonary edema, the nurse would observe the patient for
   1. Decreased pulse rate
   2. Increased urinary output
   3. Hypotension
   4. Visual disturbances

138. An example of a rapidly acting diuretic that can be administered intravenously to patients with acute pulmonary edema is
   1. Spironolactone
   2. Ethacrynic acid
   3. Chlorothiazide
   4. Chlothalidone

Mr. Smith, a 36-year-old father of 2 children, was admitted to the hospital after an episode of vomiting "coffee-ground" material. The tentative diagnosis was peptic ulcer. Questions 139 through 148 refer to this situation.

139. Eighty-five percent of all peptic ulcers occur in the
   1. Pyloric portion of the stomach
   2. Lesser curvature of the stomach
   3. Cardiac portion of the stomach
   4. Esophageal junction

140. The doctor ordered Pro-Banthine for Mr. Smith. Pro-Banthine is an anticholinergic drug whose main action is to
   1. Neutralize gastric acidity
   2. Increase gastric motility
   3. Reduce the pH of gastric contents
   4. Delay gastric emptying

141. Patients with peptic ulcers usually describe the pain associated with it as
   1. A dull ache radiating to the left side
   2. An intermittent colicky flank pain
   3. A generalized abdominal pain intensified by moving
   4. A gnawing sensation relieved by food

142. While caring for Mr. Smith the nurse would *immediately* report which of the following observations?
   1. Tachycardia, sweating, and cold extremities
   2. Complaints of thirst and warm flushed skin
   3. Nausea, weakness, and headache
   4. Dyspepsia, distention, and diarrhea

143. Which of the following foods would be permitted for a patient with a healing peptic ulcer?
   1. Sliced oranges, pancakes with syrup, coffee
   2. Applesauce, cream of wheat, milk
   3. Orange juice, fried eggs, sausage
   4. Tomato juice, raisin bran cereal, tea

144. The most common complication of peptic ulcer is
   1. Perforation
   2. Hemorrhage
   3. Pyloric obstruction
   4. Esophageal varices

Mr. Smith has not responded to conservative therapy and a vagotomy and partial gastrectomy have been scheduled.

145. Mr. Smith was returned to the unit from the recovery room with intravenous solutions running and a nasogastric tube in place. Later that evening you note that there has been no nasogastric drainage for 1½ hours. Physician's orders state "irrigate nasogastric tube p.r.n." Which of the following actions would you employ? Insert
   1. 30 ml. of normal saline and withdraw slowly
   2. 15 ml. of distilled water and disconnect suction for 30 minutes
   3. 20 ml. of air and clamp off suction for 1 hour
   4. 50 ml. of saline and increase pressure of suction

146. Intravenous orders for Mr. Smith state that he is to receive 1000 ml. of fluid every 8 hours. If the equipment you are using de-

livers 15 gtt./ml. you would regulate the flow at
1. Approximately 60 gtt./min.
2. Approximately 15 gtt./min.
3. Approximately 23 gtt./min.
4. Approximately 31 gtt./min.

147. During the convalescent period the nurse sets up a health teaching program designed specifically to meet Mr. Smith's needs. This plan would include
    1. A thorough explanation of the dumping syndrome and how to limit or prevent it
    2. A warning to avoid *all* gas-forming foods
    3. Encouragement to resume his previous eating habits as soon as possible
    4. An explanation of the therapeutic effect of a high roughage diet

148. The emotional response that most frequently contributes to psychosomatic illnesses is
    1. Anxiety
    2. Depression
    3. Fear
    4. Rage

Mr. Dunham, a college senior and the first of his family to attend college, is admitted to the hospital with an exacerbation of colitis. He is thin, pale, and dehydrated. He is placed on a residue free, bland, high protein diet, and vitamins B, C, and K parenterally. An intravenous solution containing electrolytes is also started. Questions 149 through 161 refer to this situation.

149. The type of person who most frequently develops ulcerative colitis is
    1. Hard driving and immature
    2. Sensitive and dependent
    3. Quick-tempered and hostile
    4. Unassuming and secure

150. Although ulcerative colitis can be caused by multiple stresses, it is most commonly associated with
    1. Psychologic stress
    2. Chemical stress
    3. Endocrinologic stress
    4. Physical stress

151. Mr. Dunham is receiving vitamins parenterally because
    1. Intestinal absorption may be inadequate
    2. More rapid action results
    3. They are ineffective orally
    4. They increase colon irritability

152. Which of these food combinations would be the best on his residue free diet?
    1. Lean roast beef, buttered white rice with egg slices, white bread with butter and jelly, tea with sugar
    2. Creamed soup and crackers, omelet, mashed potatoes, roll, orange juice, coffee
    3. Stewed chicken, baked potato with butter, strained peas, white bread, plain cake, milk
    4. Baked fish, macaroni with cheese, strained carrots, fruit jello, milk

153. Mr. Dunham's diet is designed to reduce
    1. Gastric acidity
    2. Colon irritation
    3. Electrolyte depletion
    4. Intestinal absorption

154. Chemical irritation to the gastrointestinal tract is minimized by which dietary alteration?
    1. Low salt content
    2. Low cellulose content
    3. High protein content
    4. No coffee or seasonings

155. High protein is necessary in Mr. Dunham's diet to
    1. Correct anemia
    2. Slow peristalsis
    3. Improve muscle tone
    4. Repair tissues

156. Mr. Dunham is to receive 2000 ml. of intravenous fluid in 12 hours. The drop factor is 10 gtt./1 ml. The nurse would regulate the flow so that the number of drops per minute is approximately
    1. 48 to 50
    2. 30 to 32
    3. 27 to 29
    4. 40 to 42

The doctor has ordered daily stool examinations. Mr. Dunham is also scheduled for a sigmoidoscopy and barium enema.

157. Stool examinations are ordered to determine
    1. Culture and sensitivity
    2. Occult blood and organisms
    3. Ova and parasites
    4. Fat and undigested food

158. Specific nursing responsibility in preparing Mr. Dunham for his diagnostic procedures includes
    1. Administering soapsuds enemas till clear
    2. Giving castor oil the afternoon before
    3. Withholding food and fluid for 8 hours
    4. Assuring his understanding of what is to happen

159. The physician decides to perform an ileostomy on Mr. Dunham. In caring for him postoperatively, he asks what effect the surgery will have on his sexual relationships. The nurse would tell him that
    1. Sexual relationships must be curtailed
    2. He should tell his partner about his surgery prior to sexual activity
    3. He will be able to resume normal sexual relationships
    4. The surgery will temporarily decrease his sexual impulses

160. In caring for the patient with an ileostomy the nurse would
    1. Expect the stoma to start draining on the third postoperative day
    2. Explain that the drainage can be controlled with daily irrigations
    3. Anticipate that emotional stress can increase intestinal peristalsis
    4. Encourage the patient to eat foods high in residue

161. Which of the following types of sports should be avoided in the patient with an ileostomy?
    1. Track
    2. Swimming
    3. Skiing
    4. Football

Mrs. Palecek was admitted to the hospital with a diagnosis of acute cholecystitis, biliary colic, and possible obstructive jaundice. Questions 162 through 168 refer to this situation.

162. In addition to pain in the right upper quadrant, what other manifestations might the nurse expect Mrs. Palecek to have?
   1. Intolerance of foods high in lipids
   2. Vomiting of "coffee-ground" emesis
   3. Gnawing pain when the stomach is empty
   4. Melena

163. Mrs. Palecek had an interference in bile utilization caused by cholecystitis. The ejection of bile into the alimentary tract is controlled by which of the following hormones?
   1. Cholecystokinin
   2. Secretin
   3. Gastrin
   4. Hepatokinin

164. A patient with obstruction of the common bile duct may show a prolonged bleeding and clotting time because
   1. The extrinsic factor is not absorbed
   2. Vitamin K is not absorbed
   3. The ionized calcium level falls
   4. Bilirubin accumulates in the plasma

165. Vitamin K was administered to Mrs. Palecek prior to surgery. Vitamin K is used in the formation of
   1. Bilirubin
   2. Prothrombin
   3. Thromboplastin
   4. Cholecystokinin

166. Mrs. Palecek was prone to upper respiratory complications as are all patients who have had biliary tract surgery. This is because of the
   1. Proximity of the incision to the diaphragm
   2. Length of time required for surgery
   3. Lowering of resistance caused by bile in the blood
   4. Invasion of the bloodstream by infection from the biliary tract

167. To promote healing of the large incision, Mrs. Palecek's physician would order daily doses of which of these vitamins?
   1. Ascorbic acid
   2. Mephyton
   3. Vitamin B_{12} complex
   4. Vitamin A

168. When Mrs. Palecek is ready to be discharged, the dietician instructs her to remain on her prescribed diet for several more weeks. Afterward, she asks her nurse, "Will I have to stay away from fat for the rest of my life?" Which of the following responses would be most appropriate?
   1. "You'll have to remain on a fat-free diet from now on to avoid problems."
   2. "It's too early to say. Later, when we see whether your operation is successful, we'll know the answer."
   3. "Only your doctor can answer that. Why don't you ask him about it before you are discharged from the hospital."
   4. "After you have fully recovered from surgery, you'll probably be able to eat a normal diet, avoiding excessive fat."

Mr. Leonard is an alcoholic and has cirrhosis of the liver. Questions 169 through 181 refer to this situation.

169. Mr. Leonard is brought to the emergency room having protracted clonic convulsions. He is given diazepam (Valium), which decreases central neuronal activity and
   1. Dilates the tracheobronchial structures
   2. Relaxes peripheral muscles
   3. Slows cardiac contraction
   4. Provides amnesia for the convulsive episodes

170. In what way does excessive alcohol intake lead to cirrhosis?
   1. Malnutrition
   2. Alters fatty metabolism and storage in liver
   3. Toxification of tissues
   4. Produces obstruction of portal system

171. The patient with cirrhosis has a "swollen appearance" as a result of the edema and ascites. The ascites is caused by
   1. Portal obstruction
   2. Kidney malfunction
   3. Decreased production of potassium
   4. Shift of protein from cells

172. Mr. Leonard's serum albumin level is low and the physician has prescribed 50 ml. salt-poor albumin intravenously. Albumin replacement is expected to
   1. Decrease tissue fluid accumulation; decrease the hematocrit level
   2. Decrease ascites; decrease the blood ammonia level
   3. Increase capillary perfusion; decrease the blood pressure level
   4. Decrease venous stasis; decrease the blood urea nitrogen level

173. While Mr. Leonard is receiving the albumin, the planned therapeutic effect will be greater if the infusion is required to run
   1. Slowly and fluid intake is withheld
   2. Rapidly and fluids are encouraged liberally
   3. Slowly and fluids are encouraged liberally
   4. Rapidly and fluid intake is withheld

174. Mr. Leonard is having delirium tremens and is given paraldehyde (Paral) intramuscularly. Elimination of the drug can be assessed by monitoring
   1. Urination
   2. Salivation
   3. Diaphoresis
   4. Breathing

175. Mr. Leonard is receiving neomycin sulfate (Mycifradin) orally. The purpose for administration of the drug is to
   1. Protect against infection while immune mechanisms are deficient
   2. Suppress ammonia-forming bacteria in the intestinal tract
   3. Increase urea digestive activity of enteric bacteria
   4. Protect regenerative nodules in the liver from invading bacteria

176. What complication is most likely to occur when a patient has portal hypertension?
    1. Perforation of the duodenum
    2. Hemorrhage from esophageal varices
    3. Liver abscess
    4. Intestinal obstruction
177. The symptoms of portal hypertension are largely caused by
    1. Infection of the liver parenchyma
    2. Lack of hydrochloric acid in the stomach
    3. Obstruction of the portal circulation
    4. Obstruction of the bile ducts
178. When bleeding esophageal varices occur in the cirrhotic patient a Sengstaken-Blakemore tube is frequently inserted. The patient should be maintained in which position following the insertion?
    1. Prone
    2. Right lateral
    3. High-Fowler's
    4. Supine
179. A patient with known liver damage begins to develop slurred speech, confusion, drowsiness, and tremors. With these symptoms of impending hepatic coma, the diet would be limited to
    1. 20 g. protein, 2000 calories
    2. 80 g. protein, 1000 calories
    3. 100 g. protein, 2500 calories
    4. 150 g. protein, 1200 calories
180. Immediately before an abdominal paracentesis, the nurse should ask the patient to void because
    1. A urine specimen must be obtained at this time to check level of nonprotein nitrogen
    2. A full bladder increases the danger of puncturing the bladder
    3. An empty bladder will decrease the intra-abdominal pressure
    4. A full bladder decreases the amount of fluid in the abdominal cavity
181. Mr. Leonard, participating in an alcohol abstinence program, has a cold when he comes to the clinic. He tells the nurse he plans to use elixir of terpin hydrate for his cough. The nurse would advise him not to take it while he is taking disulfiram (Antabuse) because it will cause
    1. Abdominal cramps and muscle twitching
    2. Epigastric pain and headache
    3. Jitteriness and nausea
    4. Dizziness and violent vomiting
182. Mrs. Carter has hepatitis and her children are being given gamma globulin to provide passive immunity, which
    1. Stimulates production of short-lived antibodies
    2. Stimulates the lymphatic system to produce large numbers of antibodies
    3. Provides antibodies that neutralize the antigen
    4. Accelerates antigen-antibody union at hepatic sites
183. The physician has prescribed phenobarbital sodium (Luminal) for Mrs. Carter. The nurse will tell Mrs. Carter to contact the physician if she notices

    1. Decreased tolerance to common foods constipation
    2. Diarrhea, rash on the upper part of her body
    3. Anal pruritus, orthostatic hypotension
    4. Loss of appetite, persistent lethargy

Mr. Thomas, 62 years of age, is admitted to the hospital complaining of nausea, vomiting, weight loss of 20 pounds in 2 months, and periods of constipation and diarrhea. A diagnosis of carcinoma of the colon was made. Questions 184 through 190 refer to this situation.

184. A sigmoidoscopy was performed as a diagnostic measure. The nurse should place the patient in which position for this examination?
    1. Prone
    2. Lithotomy
    3. Sims
    4. Knee-chest
185. As part of the preparation of a patient for a sigmoidoscopy, the nurse
    1. Should withhold all fluids and foods for 24 hours before the examination
    2. Should explain to the patient that he will have to swallow a chalk-like substance
    3. Will have to administer an enema the morning of the examination
    4. Will have a container available for collection of a stool specimen
186. If Mr. Thomas has carcinoma of the descending portion of the colon, the operative procedure that would probably be performed is a(n)
    1. Cecostomy
    2. Ileostomy
    3. Colectomy
    4. Colostomy
187. Neomycin sulfate was given preoperatively to
    1. Decrease the possibility of urinary infection postoperatively
    2. Increase the production of vitamin K
    3. Destroy intestinal bacteria
    4. Decrease the incidence of any secondary infection
188. The doctor performed a colostomy. Postoperative nursing care should include
    1. Having the patient change his own dressing
    2. Keeping the skin around the opening clean and dry
    3. Limiting fluid intake
    4. Withholding all fluids for 72 hours
189. After surgery, the most effective way of helping Mr. Thomas accept his colostomy would be to
    1. Give him literature containing factual data about colostomies
    2. Point out to him the number of important people who have had colostomies
    3. Begin to teach him self-care of his colostomy immediately
    4. Contact a member of Colostomies Inc. to speak with him
190. A person who has a permanent colostomy
    1. Needs special clothing
    2. Has to limit his activities

3. Will have to dilate the stoma periodically
4. Needs to be on a bland, low residue diet

191. The diet for a person with a colostomy should be
    1. As close to normal as possible
    2. Rich in protein
    3. Low in fiber content
    4. High in carbohydrate

192. In teaching Mr. Thomas to care for his colostomy, the nurse should advise him to irrigate it at the same time every day and to choose a time
    1. When he can be assured of uninterrupted bathroom use at home
    2. That approximates his usual daily time for elimination
    3. About halfway between the 2 largest meals of the day
    4. About 1 hour before breakfast

193. If, during the irrigation, Mr. Thomas complains of abdominal cramps, the nurse should
    1. Lower the container of fluid
    2. Discontinue the irrigation
    3. Clamp the catheter for a few minutes
    4. Advance the catheter about 1 inch

194. When performing a colostomy irrigation the catheter should be inserted in the stoma
    1. 2 inches
    2. 4 inches
    3. 6 inches
    4. 8 inches

195. When doing a colostomy irrigation the height of the container with the solution should be no more than
    1. 18 inches
    2. 6 inches
    3. 10 inches
    4. 12 inches

196. The skin surrounding the colostomy opening can be protected with
    1. Petroleum jelly
    2. Alcohol
    3. Aluminum paste
    4. Mineral oil

Mrs. Graham has a diagnosis of possible bowel obstruction. She complains of nausea, is vomiting dark bile material, and has severe crampy, intermittent, abdominal pain. Her physician suspects the bowel obstruction is caused by an intussusception. Questions 197 through 200 refer to this situation.

197. An intussusception is
    1. Kinking of the bowel onto itself
    2. Telescoping of a proximal loop of bowel into a distal loop
    3. A band of connective tissue compressing the bowel
    4. A protrusion of an organ or part of an organ through the wall that contains it

198. A flat plate of the abdomen was ordered. The nurse recognizes that the patient should receive
    1. Nothing by mouth for 8 hours
    2. A low soapsuds enema
    3. No special preparation
    4. A laxative the evening before the x-ray film

199. Surgery was performed. Mrs. Graham was found to have a perforated appendix with localized peritonitis rather than an intussusception. In view of this finding, how would you position Mrs. Graham postoperatively?
    1. Semi-Fowler's
    2. Trendelenburg
    3. Sims
    4. Dorsal recumbent

200. Four days after surgery Mrs. Graham had not passed any flatus and there were no bowel sounds. Despite the fact that her abdomen became increasingly more distended, there was little discomfort. Paralytic ileus was suspected. In this condition there is an interference caused by
    1. Impaired blood supply
    2. Impaired neural functioning
    3. Perforation of the bowel wall
    4. Obstruction of the bowel lumen

Miss Stewart was admitted to the hospital with complaints of hematuria, frequency, urgency, and pain on urination. She stated she has had this problem for several days. Questions 201 and 202 refer to this situation.

201. The admitting diagnosis would most likely be
    1. Cystitis
    2. Pyelitis
    3. Nephrosis
    4. Pyelonephritis

202. Women are more susceptible to this condition *primarily* because of
    1. Poor hygiene practices
    2. Length of the urethra
    3. Continuity of the mucous membrane
    4. Inadequate fluid intake

Mr. Carson is hospitalized with severe right flank pain, general weakness, and fever. He has a history of recurrent urinary tract infection and the formation of renal calculi is suspected. The physician orders a 200 mg. calcium diet for 3 days to be monitored with urinary calcium tests. Questions 203 through 206 refer to this situation.

203. In caring for patients with renal calculi, the *most* important nursing action is to
    1. Record blood pressure
    2. Strain all urine
    3. Limit fluids at night
    4. Administer analgesics every 3 hours

204. What background knowledge helps you understand the reasons for this strict 200 mg. calcium diet?
    1. Excessive calcium intake has little influence on renal stone formation
    2. The thyroid hormone controls the serum levels of calcium and phosphorus
    3. If calcium excretion is lowered on the test diet, hyperparathyroidism can be identified as the cause of the calculi
    4. If calcium excretion is still elevated on the test diet, dietary influences can be ruled out

205. Mr. Carson's calcium balance studies following his test diet are negative. His diet order

is increased to 400 mg. calcium—a general low calcium diet level. Which of the following foods would be allowed on his diet?
1. Vanilla ice cream with chocolate syrup and nuts
2. Salmon loaf with cheese sauce
3. Chocolate pudding
4. Roast beef with baked potato

206. The name of the procedure for the removal of a bladder stone is
1. Cystolithiasis
2. Cystolithopexy
3. Cystometry
4. Cryoextraction

You are assigned to care for Mr. Burn who has a diagnosis of benign prostatic hypertrophy. Questions 207 through 216 refer to this situation.

207. The night nurse reported that Mr. Burn is complaining of inability to void. You find that his bladder is distended. Your nursing intervention would be directed toward
1. Forcing fluids to induce voiding
2. Encouraging him to use a urinal
3. Applying firm pressure over the pubic area
4. Assisting him into a warm tub bath

208. The definitive diagnosis of this condition is arrived at by
1. Biopsy of prostatic tissue
2. Pap smear of prostatic fluid
3. Rectal examination
4. Serum phosphatase studies

209. While caring for Mr. Burn the nurse is aware that benign prostatic hypertrophy
1. Usually becomes malignant
2. Predisposes to hydronephrosis
3. Is a congenital abnormality
4. Causes an elevated acid phosphatase

210. Which of the following tests might be ordered to estimate the effect of Mr. Burn's illness on the kidneys?
1. PSP, urea clearance, urine concentration
2. Sulkowitch, catecholamines, urine dilution
3. Bence-Jones protein, urine concentration, albumin
4. Microscopic porphyrins, urinalysis

211. Mr. Burn went to surgery for a suprapubic prostatectomy. After the surgery, in addition to the placement of a Foley catheter, the nurse would expect the patient to have
1. A rectal incision and a ureteral catheter
2. A ureterostomy with gravity drainage
3. A nephrostomy tube with tidal drainage
4. An abdominal incision and a cystostomy tube

212. The most significant complication immediately following this surgery is
1. Hemorrhage
2. Impotence
3. Urinary incontinence
4. Spasms

213. Mr. Burn had just returned from the recovery room following the suprapubic prostatectomy. You discover he has pulled out the urethral catheter. You would
1. Check for bleeding by irrigating the suprapubic tube

2. Have the male nurse reinsert a new catheter
3. Notify the doctor immediately
4. Take no immediate action if the suprapubic tube was draining

214. In implementing postoperative care for Mr. Burn an important action to prevent secondary bladder infection would be to
1. Observe for signs of uremia
2. Attach the catheter to suction
3. Clamp off the connecting tubing
4. Change the dressings frequently

215. Intermittent irrigations (tidal drainage) were ordered for Mr. Burn. This was carried out for the primary purpose of
1. Maintaining the patency of the tube
2. Administering electrolyte solutions
3. Restoring the muscular function of the bladder
4. Flushing out blood clots

216. Mr. Burn complains of pain in the operative area. The initial response of the nurse would be to
1. Administer the prescribed analgesic
2. Take vital signs before administration of analgesic
3. Inspect drainage tubing for occlusion
4. Encourage intake of fluids to dilute urine

217. Personality changes associated with patient with kidney damage may be caused by
1. A consistently elevated BUN
2. Hypernatremia
3. Limited fluid intake
4. Hyperkalemia

218. If the patient with renal failure does not respond to treatment, dialysis may be performed to remove waste products from the blood. The main indication for dialysis is
1. Increase in blood pressure
2. High and rising potassium levels
3. Ascites
4. Acidosis

219. In caring for the patient who is receiving peritoneal dialysis, the nurse would
1. Maintain the patient in a flat, supine position during the entire procedure
2. Notify the physician if there is a deficit of 200 ml. in the drainage fluid
3. Apply firm manual pressure to the lower abdomen if fluid is not draining properly
4. Remove the cannula at the end of the procedure and apply a dry, sterile dressing

220. The patient who is on hemodialysis for chronic renal failure is especially prone to develop
1. Peritonitis
2. Renal calculi
3. Bladder infection
4. Serum hepatitis

221. In caring for the patient who has had an arteriovenous shunt inserted for hemodialysis the nurse would
1. Notify the doctor if she hears bruit in the cannula
2. Use strict aseptic technique when giving shunt care
3. Cover the entire cannula with an Ace bandage

4. Take the blood pressure every 4 hours on the arm that contains the shunt

Mrs. Curran is admitted to the burn unit with second and third degree burns. Questions 222 through 224 refer to this situation.

222. The major objective during the early post-burn phase is to
1. Prevent infection
2. Replace blood loss
3. Restore fluid volume
4. Relieve pain

223. The relationship between body surface area and fluid loss is
1. Directly proportionate
2. Inversely proportionate
3. Equal
4. Unrelated

224. The rate of fluid replacement for a patient with severe burns during the first 48 hours is considered satisfactory if the urinary output is approximately
1. ½ intake
2. $\frac{1}{10}$ intake
3. ⅓ intake
4. Equal to intake

225. Of the following, which is *most* important in maintaining the fluid and electrolyte balance of the body?
1. Urinary system
2. Respiratory system
3. Antidiuretic hormone (ADH)
4. Aldosterone

226. Which of the following body fluids comprise 40% to 50% of the total body weight?
1. Intracellular
2. Extracellular
3. Intravascular
4. Interstitial

227. The most important electrolyte of intracellular fluid is
1. Calcium
2. Sodium
3. Potassium
4. Chloride

228. A patient arrives in the emergency room and is weak, pale, and complains that he's had diarrhea for 2 weeks. The nurse finds that his blood pressure is 100/60 and while the cuff is inflated she observes spasms of his hand. While awaiting the physician's arrival, she would prepare equipment for administration of 5% dextrose in saline intravenous solution and for replacement of
1. Potassium chloride
2. Magnesium
3. Calcium
4. Bicarbonate

Mrs. Loft, 42 years of age, is admitted to the hospital with a tentative diagnosis of chronic adrenal insufficiency. Questions 229 through 235 refer to this situation.

229. A room assignment contraindicated for Mrs. Loft would be one
1. With an elderly CVA patient
2. With a middle-aged woman with pneumonia
3. That is private and away from the nurses' station
4. Next to a 17-year-old girl with a fractured leg

230. Mrs. Loft complains of weakness and dizziness on arising from bed in the morning. The nurse realizes that this is most probably caused by
1. Postural hypertension
2. A hypoglycemic reaction
3. A lack of potassium
4. Increased extracellular fluid volume

231. After a Thorn test showed an increased eosinophil count, Mrs. Loft was advised that she had Addison's disease. It is *most important* that the nurse discuss with her the need for
1. Frequent visits to the doctor
2. Restriction of physical activity
3. A special low salt diet
4. Hormonal replacement therapy

232. Mrs. Loft was placed on cortisone 10 mg. orally three times a day. In teaching Mrs. Loft about her medication and diet the nurse would tell her to
1. Add a little extra salt to her food
2. Limit the caloric intake to 1200 calories
3. Omit protein foods at each meal
4. Restrict her daily intake of fluids

233. In the event a patient with Addison's disease neglects to continue the hormonal therapy, an adrenal crisis may occur. Usually the predominating symptom is
1. Hypertension
2. A high body temperature
3. Muscle spasms
4. Diarrhea

234. Patients on prolonged cortisone therapy may exhibit adaptations caused by its glucocorticoid and mineralocorticoid actions. The nurse aware of this would observe for
1. Hypoglycemia and anuria
2. Weight gain and moon face
3. Anorexia and hyperkalemia
4. Hypotension and fluid loss

235. In observing a patient for cortisone overdose, the nurse should be particularly alert to
1. Behavioral changes
2. Severe anorexia
3. Hypoglycemia
4. Anaphylactic shock

236. Cushing's syndrome is caused by functioning bilateral tumors of the adrenal cortex. Which of the following symptoms are commonly seen in Cushing's syndrome?
1. "Buffalo hump," obesity, and hypertension
2. Dehydration and menorrhagia
3. Pitting edema and frequent colds
4. Migraine headache and dysmenorrhea

237. A patient who is scheduled to have a bilateral adrenalectomy would most likely receive which of the following drugs on the day of surgery and in the immediate postoperative period?
1. Regular insulin
2. ACTH
3. Solu-Cortef
4. Pituitrin

238. Mrs. Garvin has cancer of the cervix. She is hospitalized for internal radiation therapy with radium. Upon return to her room, the nurse would
    1. Immediately place Mrs. Garvin in high Fowler's position to prevent dislodging of radium
    2. Check Mrs. Garvin's voiding and catheterize if necessary since a distended bladder may interrupt the path of radiation
    3. Check that Mrs. Garvin is on a low residue diet to prevent bowel movements and the possibility of dislodging radium
    4. Stay with the patient for half an hour to watch for symptoms of radiation sickness

239. In caring for Mrs. Garvin after the radium implant, the nurse would
    1. Collect and store urine for examination by nuclear medicine
    2. Wear a lead apron when giving care
    3. Restrict visitors to a 10-minute stay
    4. Avoid giving intramuscular injections into the gluteal muscle

240. An early symptom of cancer of the cervix that should have brought Mrs. Garvin to the gynecologist was
    1. Bloody spotting after intercourse
    2. Foul smelling discharge
    3. Abdominal heaviness
    4. Pressure on the bladder

241. Which one of the following operative procedures would result in surgical menopause?
    1. Bilateral oophorectomy
    2. Partial hysterectomy
    3. Bilateral salpingectomy
    4. Tubal ligation

242. Mrs. Butler has a radical mastectomy and the physician plans chemotherapy 2 weeks after the surgery. The delay in instituting the plan for drug therapy is because the drugs
    1. Interfere with cell growth and delay wound healing
    2. Cause vomiting that endangers the integrity of the large incisional area
    3. Decrease red blood cell production and the resultant anemia would add to postoperative fatigue
    4. Increase edema in areas distal to the incision by blocking lymph channels with destroyed lymphocytes

243. Mrs. Butler's pathology report shows metastatic adenocarcinoma. She is to receive Adriamycin, which modifies growth of cancer cells by
    1. Preventing folic acid synthesis
    2. Changing the osmotic gradient in the cell
    3. Inhibiting RNA synthesis by binding DNA
    4. Increasing the permeability of the cell wall

244. Because of problems occurring in 80% of the patients receiving Adriamycin, the nurse will observe Mrs. Butler for evidence of
    1. Nausea or vomiting, tachycardia
    2. Hair loss, erythema of the oral mucosa
    3. Decreased appetite, necrosis at the intravenous site
    4. Low blood pressure, decreased vital capacity

Mrs. Lamb is 39 years of age and has 3 children ages 12, 9, and 5 years of age. She was admitted to the hospital with the diagnosis of severe metrorrhagia and menorrhagia of 1-year duration. She was found to have a submucous myoma that had grown over the past 6 months. Mrs. Lamb was told that a hysterectomy was necessary. Questions 245 through 248 refer to this situation.

245. The term metrorrhagia refers to
    1. Periods of bleeding between menstrual periods
    2. Severe bleeding during each menstrual period
    3. Presence of blood in vaginal discharge
    4. Spotting or staining after intercourse

246. Following the operative procedure (total hysterectomy), Mrs. Lamb develops abdominal distention. Which of the following measures would most likely provide immediate relief?
    1. Restriction of oral intake, frequent change of position
    2. Ambulation, bicarbonated drink
    3. Insertion of a rectal tube, heat to abdomen
    4. Nasogastric intubation, administration of cholinergic agents

247. Mrs. Lamb is recovering from the hysterectomy. Which of the following signs would be indicative of a developing thrombophlebitis?
    1. Reddened area at ankle
    2. Pruritus on calf and thigh
    3. Pitting edema of the ankle
    4. A tender, reddened area on leg

248. As the nurse walks into Mrs. Lamb's room on the fifth postoperative day, the patient asks for sanitary pads because she feels like she is going to have her period. Your response would be based on your knowledge of which of the following statements?
    1. Mrs. Lamb will have a surgical menopause
    2. It will take several weeks before Mrs. Lamb will have a normal menstrual flow
    3. Mrs. Lamb is showing signs of psychosomatic responses
    4. The postoperative appearance of frank vaginal bleeding is expected

CHAPTER 12

Rehabilitation nursing

Rehabilitation is the process of assisting people to attain their full potential—physically, psychologically, socially, and economically. Rehabilitation is particularly concerned with establishing function where none exists and restoring function that is lost while expanding, maintaining, and supporting the limited function remaining.

The concepts of nursing care and rehabilitation are synonymous. Assisting the patient and the family to help themselves is now and always has been an integral component of the services that nurses provide. Many factors influence an individual's adaptation to an illness or disability. In this section, these many factors are explored and emphasis is given to the personal and community resources available for assistance.

One of the major goals of rehabilitation is for the patient to become as independent as possible as soon as possible. To accomplish this goal, the patient must be assisted to master certain activities of daily living, particularly those concerned with the personal needs that occur each day. Since the role of the nurse is to teach, support, and supervise the mastery of these tasks, emphasis has been given to the specific nursing skills involved.

The central figure of the rehabilitation team is the patient. It is the responsibility of the nurse to teach and motivate the patient and family during the entire rehabilitative process. For the sake of clarity, the principles of motivation and the teaching-learning process have been presented separately. However, in reality, these processes are totally dependent on each other and do not occur separately.

Today, with the increase in the aged population, improved medical care saving and maintaining life, the stresses associated with increased urbanization, and high speed, congested transportation, the nurse must be prepared to care for patients with a multiplicity of health problems. Nursing care, by necessity, must emphasize the many aspects of rehabilitation.

BASIC CONCEPTS

A. Immediate or potential rehabilitation needs are exhibited in all health problems
B. The patient is the primary rehabilitator—professional health team members only assist the patient and family with the process of self-rehabilitation
C. Rehabilitation is not an isolated process; it involves the patient, the family, the health team, the community, and society
D. The rehabilitation process is concerned with all levels of prevention—primary, secondary, and tertiary
E. Health problems that cause disabilities are socially significant because of the number of people affected, the economic cost and loss, the distress of personal suf-

fering, and the conditions in society that increase their incidence

INFLUENCING FACTORS

A. Age—developmental milestones
1. Infant—the infant must adapt to a totally new environment; the stress from this culture shock is compounded for the infant with a congenital defect
2. Child—maturation involves physical, functional, and emotional growth; it is an everchanging process that produces stress; disabilities will provide additional factors that may quantitatively or qualitatively affect maturation
3. Adolescent—the adolescent is experiencing a physical, psychologic, and social growth spurt; the individual is asking: "Who am I?" on the way to developing a self-image; limitations provide additional stress during identity formation
4. Adult—in society the adult is expected to be independent and productive, to provide for self and family; if one cannot assume this role totally or partially, it can cause additional stress
5. Aged—our society tends to venerate youth and deplore old age; all aged persons are experiencing multiple stresses (loss of loved ones, change in usual life style, loss of physical vigor, and, for many, the thought of approaching death) at a time when their ability to adapt is compromised by the anatomic, physiologic, and psychologic alterations that occur during the aging process
B. Age at onset
1. Infancy—developmental tasks may be interfered with and the lag that occurs is often impossible to overcome
2. Childhood—limitations prevent interaction with peers and disrupt the independence versus dependence struggle
3. Adolescence—adolescents place great value on health and physical attractiveness; conformity with peers is important; adolescents react to disabilities that influence a developing self-image or "being different"
4. Adulthood—adults have reached the peak years of independence and productivity; disease is usually viewed by the adult as a threat to personal integrity while in "the prime of life"
5. Senescence—the stresses of aging revolve around dependence—physical, emotional, and financial; these limitations may be resented by some ready to enjoy their "golden years," while others may look forward to the relief death brings
C. Type of onset
1. Hereditary—genetic traits decided at conception can impair function and cause an individual to exhibit the disease at birth or have the tendency to develop it later in life
2. Congenital—present at the time of birth but not necessarily caused by genes; frequently related to events affecting the fetal environment during pregnancy or at the time of birth
3. Insidious—no early symptoms of its development are exhibited
4. Acquired—develops after birth any time during the life cycle
5. Traumatic—an unexpected, abrupt injury at any time during the life cycle
D. Type of condition
1. Acute illness—caused by a health problem that produces signs and symptoms abruptly, runs a short course and from which there is usually a full recovery; an acute illness may leave an individual with a loss of a body part or function and may develop into a long-term illness
2. Chronic illness—caused by a health problem that produces signs and symptoms over a period of time, runs a long course, and from which there is only partial recovery
   a. Exacerbation—a period of time when a chronic illness becomes more active and there is a recurrence of pronounced signs and symptoms of the disease
   b. Remission—a period of time when a chronic illness is controlled and signs and symptoms are reduced or not obvious
   c. Degenerative—a continuous deterioration or increased impairment of a person's physical state
3. Terminal illness—an illness that has no cure and death is inevitable in the near future
4. Primary health problem—an original

condition developing independently of another health problem
5. Secondary health problem—a condition or disorder that develops as a direct result of another health problem
E. General physical condition
1. Quantitative and qualitative level of physical state
2. Balance between necessary rest and desired activity
3. Nutritional status of the individual
F. Personal resources
1. Level of self-esteem—an attitude that reflects the individual's perception of self-worth; it is a personal subjective judgment by one's self
2. Experiential background—knowledge derived from one's own actions, observations, or perceptions; maturation, culture, and environment influence the individual's experiential foundation
3. Intelligence
a. Genetic intellectual potential
b. Amount of formal and informal education
c. Level of intellectual development; e.g., child versus adult
d. Ability to reason, conceptualize, and translate words into actions
4. Level of motivation—an internal desire or incentive to accomplish something
5. Values—factors that are important to the individual
6. Religion—a deep personal belief in a higher force than humanity
G. Extent of actual or perceived change in body image
1. Obvious reminder of disability to self and others
a. Loss of a body part
b. Need for a prosthesis; e.g., breast, leg, eye
c. Need for hardware; e.g., pacemaker, braces, hearing aid, wheel chair
d. Extent of disability or limitation
e. Need for medication
2. Value placed on loss by self or society
a. "No longer whole," "a cripple"
b. Type of loss—perceptions of body part or function as being good, pleasing, repulsive, clean, dirty, etc.
(1) Symbols of sexuality—breast, uterus, prostate, heart
(2) May lack social acceptability

—colostomy, mental illness, incontinence, cancer, tuberculosis
(3) Impairment of senses and/or ability to communicate—laryngectomy, stroke, deafness, blindness
(4) Altered body image resulting from anatomic changes—amputation of limb or breast, colostomy
H. Degree of physical or psychologic dependence
1. Physical
a. Independence—activity need not be restricted
b. Slight dependence—mild limitations
c. Increased dependence—moderate limitations
d. Extensive dependence—activity markedly restricted
e. Total dependence—needs complete physical care
2. Psychologic—a continuum from minimum dependence to total dependence, reliant upon individual's adaptation at a particular time
I. Patient's and family's stage of adaptation
1. Self-protection—disbelief, denial, avoidance, and/or intellectualization
2. With developing awareness of implications of illness the individual defends the self further—anger, depression, and/or joking
3. With developing realization of implications of illness the individual reorganizes self-feelings and restructures relationships with family and society
4. As the losses are resolved, the individual begins to accept the consequences of the illness and acknowledges feelings about the self and further changes that must be made
J. Attitudes of patient, family, professional health workers, friends, and community
1. Basic concepts—attitudes
a. Are learned through identification, imitation, and conditioning
b. Do not necessarily follow knowledge of facts
c. Are emotionally charged feelings
d. Are always present in the individual
e. Reflect themselves in behavior

f. Have a penetrating effect on other people
2. Stigma attached to certain illnesses; e.g., fear, hopelessness, social unacceptability
3. Role expectations altered; e.g., "no longer a man (woman)," "cripple"
K. Availability of professional health workers
1. Variety of health professionals; e.g., graduate nurse, physician, physical therapist, occupational therapist, nutritionist, social worker, inhalation therapist
2. Accessibility of professional health workers
   a. Distribution of facilities—rural areas have fewer, less sophisticated facilities than urban areas
   b. Disparity of quality of health care—achieved standards of care are unevenly distributed throughout the country
3. Economic factors
   a. Personal ability to pay for service
   b. Extent of insurance coverage
   c. Availability of health reserves; e.g., social service, voluntary agencies, public services
4. Personal factors influencing the use of available health workers by the individual
   a. Education and experiential background—ignorance concerning health needs and resources
   b. Pride—unwilling to accept assistance
   c. Attitudes of indifference and apathy
   d. Religious beliefs; e.g., Catholic—anti-abortion, anti-contraception; Christian Scientist—anti-medical intervention
   e. Cultural beliefs; e.g., "the male must be strong," "the hospital is a place to die"
L. Patient's level of needs
1. Need to survive—physiologic needs for air, food, water, etc.
2. Need for safety and comfort—physical and psychologic security
3. Interpersonal needs—social needs for love, acceptance, status, and recognition
4. Intrapersonal needs—self-esteem, self-actualization

M. Patient's previous history
1. Health history
   a. Physiologic—what physical adaptations were manifested in the past
   b. Psychologic—what psychologic methods of adaptation were exhibited in the past
2. Sociocultural history
   a. Religion—particular denomination, specific belief; e.g., agnostic, atheist, "energy force"
   b. Ethnic group
   c. Occupation
   d. Economic status
   e. Family members and their personal resources
   f. Race
   g. Educational background
   h. Environment—urban versus rural, private home versus apartment
   i. Social status
N. Health resources
1. Government agencies
   a. Definition—associations functioning at the international, national, state, and local levels, providing a variety of services to meet the health, education, and welfare needs of the people; these programs are funded by the government and services are rendered by professionals
   b. Examples of government agencies
      (1) International—World Health Organization
      (2) National
         (a) United States—Department of Health, Education and Welfare; United States Public Health Service
         (b) Canada—Department of National Health and Welfare
      (3) State or provincial
         (a) United States—state health departments
         (b) Canada—provincial departments of health
      (4) Local—county or city department of health, fire department, police department
2. Voluntary agencies
   a. Definition—organizations consisting of lay and professional persons dedicated to the prevention and

solution of health problems by providing educational, research, and service programs; these agencies are dependent on voluntary donations for funds, are often concerned with specific health problems, and are national organizations that function through state and/or provincial and local chapters

b. Examples of voluntary agencies
   (1) International—Rockefeller Foundation; international branches of professional organizations
   (2) National—The American Heart Association, The American Cancer Society, National Multiple Sclerosis Society
   (3) State and/or provincial—chapters of national organizations
   (4) Local—branches of national voluntary organizations, community hospitals, volunteers (a league of women supporting a community hospital, a Girl Scout troop visiting a nursing home, a church group visiting an orphanage)

3. Crises intervention groups
   a. Services of crises intervention groups
      (1) Provide assistance for people in crises—clients' previous methods of adaptation are inadequate to meet present needs
      (2) The focus of some groups is specific; e.g., poison control, drug addiction centers, suicide prevention; while others are general; e.g., walk-in mental health clinics, hospital emergency rooms
      (3) Depending on the community's needs and facilities, these services can be offered by the government; e.g., state hospitals, Department of Health; or voluntary organizations; e.g., community hospitals, community drug councils
      (4) Some crises intervention groups provide service over the phone; e.g., poison control, suicide prevention cen-

ters; while others provide services for the physically present; e.g., hospital emergency rooms, walk-in mental health clinics

b. Crises intervention group success factors
   (1) The client or family is seeking help
   (2) The client is provided an immediate opportunity to explore feelings
   (3) The client is assisted in investigating alternative approaches to solving the problem
   (4) Information is provided about other health resources where the client may receive additional assistance

4. Self-help groups
   a. Services of self-help groups
      (1) Groups organized by patients or their families to provide services that are not adequately supplied by previous organizations
      (2) Meets needs of patients and families with chronic problems requiring intervention over an extended period of time
      (3) The focus of some groups is specific; e.g., Gamblers Anonymous; while others deal with a range of problems; e.g., Association for Children with Learning Disabilities
      (4) Some organizations are nonprofit; e.g., Alcoholics Anonymous; while others are profit-making; e.g., Weight Watchers International, Inc.
      (5) Provides services to people who frequently are not accepted by society (the individual who is a drug addict, an alcoholic, a child abuser, mentally ill, obese, or brain injured)
   b. Self-help group success factors
      (1) All members are accepted as equals
      (2) All members have experienced similar problems
      (3) They deal with behavior and

changes in behavior rather than the underlying causes of the behavior

(4) A ready supply of human resources is available
    (a) Personal resources
    (b) Assistance from peers
    (c) Finally, extension of self to others

(5) Each member has identified the problem and wants help in meeting needs—self-motivation

(6) The group has a ritual and language specific to the group and specific to the problems

(7) Leadership of the group remains with the membership

(8) Group interaction
    (a) Identification with peers —a sense of belonging
    (b) Group expectations— discipline required of members
    (c) Small steps are encouraged and, when attained, reinforced by the group

(9) As a member achieves success within the group, the individual will frequently start to receive reinforcement from outside the group

5. Progressive patient care—based on the precept that different levels of patient needs require different kinds of services and facilities; approaches to patient care can be specialized and individualized by providing progressive care—care designed to meet the patient's needs in an appropriate, continuous, and dynamic pattern
  a. Acute hospital care—the general hospital provides care for the short-term ill patient undergoing treatment for a health problem
    (1) Intensive care—provides services and equipment to meet the needs of the acutely ill patient undergoing intensive treatment for a health problem; e.g., intensive care unit, coronary care unit, burn unit, psychiatric unit
    (2) Intermediate care—provides services for the moderately ill patient who is overcoming a health crisis but still has special needs that cannot be adequately met in a general unit; e.g., intermediate care unit, progressive coronary care unit, isolation units
    (3) Self-care—provides services for the patient and family who need little assistance with health care but have a greater need for teaching, motivation, and control over own care
  b. Extended care facilities—the extended care facility provides services to persons who require either short- or long-term convalescence; these patients need a wide range of services beyond acute care (nursing care, physical therapy, social and psychologic services) extended care facilities can be self-contained or function as an extension of a hospital that utilizes its facilities when needed; the expense of extended care services is usually less than hospital care because of larger nursing units, less building support systems, increased paramedical personnel, and smaller range of services
  c. Long-term services—facilities provide services over an extended period of time and most deal with chronic or long-term health problems
    (1) Nursing home—where a person goes to live, either for an extended period of time or for permanent residency; the resident is generally well but aged and can function fairly independently; however, for physical or psychosocial reasons, requires the medical and nursing services and environmental facilities offered by the nursing home
    (2) Adult facility—a residence where an individual goes to live; meals and recreational programs may often be supplied; however, medical and nursing supervision are generally not provided on a full-time basis
    (3) Rehabilitation center—an in-

stitution that provides multiple services and facilities that assist a patient and family to make an adjustment to living; the patient can obtain an optimal level of health by developing personal abilities to their fullest potential and utilizing the following resources

(a) Medical and nursing—total health assessment and planning, physical therapy, occupational therapy, and speech therapy

(b) Psychosocial—personal counselling, social service, and psychiatric service

(c) Vocational—work evaluation, vocational counselling, vocational training, trial employment in sheltered workshops, terminal employment in sheltered workshops, and placement

(4) Continued patient care—includes those facilities and services that are available for people with health needs who are living at home

(a) Outpatient or ambulatory care—diagnosis, treatment, and follow-up care are provided by patient care facilities for people on an outpatient basis; e.g., emergency room, outpatient clinics, mobile health units

(b) Home care—provides comprehensive care for people who do not need to be hospitalized and yet require more care than an outpatient facility can provide; e.g., public health nurses, homemaker services, medical home care programs

(c) Community resources—special services provided by organizations to meet specific client needs; e.g., Meals on Wheels, FISH

(d) Day-care facilities—provide supervised activities and other services to individuals on a daily basis; individual comes to the center for the day and returns home in the evening

NURSE'S ROLE

A. Responsibilities

1. Know and understand self as a person, including personal attitudes, values, and exhibited behavioral responses

2. Understand the pathophysiologic and psychosocial processes involving the patient's and family's health problem

3. Encourage and preserve the patient's individuality, self-identity, and inalienable right to be the center of the health team

4. Utilize the problem-solving approach (collect and assess data, define needs and establish nursing care, institute nursing intervention and evaluate responses to intervention) to meet patient needs in achieving full potential

5. Utilize the team approach when orchestrating the rehabilitation process (especially the complex services available in the community) to provide coordination and continuity of care

6. Utilize teaching and motivation skills to assist the patient to move from dependence to independence

B. Basic concepts

1. Nursing rehabilitation is a basic component of all nursing care of persons with a health problem

2. Nursing rehabilitation is a dynamic process that must be started early and continued without interruption for as long as necessary

3. Rehabilitation takes place within the context of a person's whole life—within the self, the family, the community, and society; therefore, nursing care must focus on humanity as an open system

4. The patient is the prime rehabilitator and must assume the responsibility; health professionals can only assist the patient to adapt

5. The rehabilitative process has multiple

facets; physical, psychologic, and sociocultural factors exert powerful influences on the restorative process
6. Time and space are powerful tools that may help or hinder the rehabilitative process
7. Disabilities resulting from physiologic or psychologic health problems may be compensated for or corrected to varying degrees; some disabled persons need not be handicapped, others may only make modest gains toward independence, while still others may only prolong a progressive degenerative process
C. Teaching-learning process (motivation and the teaching-learning process are interrelated and do not occur independently)
1. Definitions
   a. Teaching is communication especially structured and sequenced to produce learning
   b. Learning is the activity by which knowledge, attitudes, and skills are acquired, resulting in a change in behavior; goals of learning
      (1) Understanding or acquiring knowledge—cognitive learning; e.g., What is diabetes and how does it affect me?
      (2) Feeling or developing attitudes—affective learning; e.g., What does this health problem mean to me?
      (3) Doing or developing psychomotor skills—conative learning; e.g., How do I give myself an injection?
2. Principles of the teaching-learning process and related nursing approaches
   a. Learning occurs best when there is a felt need or readiness to learn
      (1) Identify the patient's emotional or motivational readiness—is the person ready to put forth the effort necessary to learn
      (2) Identify the patient's experiential readiness—does the person have the necessary background of experience, skills, attitudes, and ability to learn what is needed
      (3) Determine the patient's level of adaptation—it is usually

difficult to teach during the beginning stages of adaptation because the patient is expressing denial, anger, and/or depression; once the initial defensive compensatory reactions have passed, the individual is more receptive to teaching
      (4) Assess the patient's level of human needs; the patient whose physical and safety needs are not met will not be concerned with interpersonal and intrapersonal needs
      (5) Specific signs of the patient's readiness to learn
         (a) The patient is adapting to the initial crisis
         (b) The patient has a developing awareness of the health problem and its implications
         (c) The patient is asking direct questions
         (d) The patient is presenting clues that indicate indirect seeking of information
         (e) The patient's physical condition or behavior invites the nurse to intervene through teaching
      (6) Once a need is recognized, readiness is determined, and the time and place are appropriate, develop a plan and teach
   b. The method of presentation of material influences the patient's ability to learn
      (1) A tentative teaching plan should be developed and communicated to all members of the health team
      (2) Information presented should be organized, accurate, and concise; e.g., simple to the complex, general to the specific
      (3) Appropriate teaching methods should be instituted
         (a) Concepts are best taught with lectures, audiovisual materials, and discussion
         (b) Attitudes are taught by

exploring feelings, role
models, discussions, and
atmosphere of acceptance
- (c) Skills are taught by illustrations, models, demonstration, return demonstration, and practice
- (4) Teaching tools should be used when indicated; e.g., models, film strips, illustrations
- (5) The patient and family should be encouraged to ask questions, which should be answered directly
- (6) Opportunities should be provided for evaluation
c. Learning is made easier when material to be learned is related to what the learner already knows
- (1) Find out what the patient knows about the problem
- (2) Begin the teaching program at the patient's level of understanding
- (3) Avoid the use of technical terminology; use simple terms or ones with which the patient feels comfortable
d. Learning is purposeful; short- and long-term goals are important because they identify the behavior to be attained
- (1) With the patient, set short- and long-term goals
- (2) Goal should meet the following criteria
  - (a) Specific—state exactly what is to be accomplished
  - (b) Measurable—set a minimum acceptable level of performance
  - (c) Realistic—the goal must be potentially achievable
e. Learning is an active process and takes place within the learner
- (1) Utilize a teaching approach that includes the learner; e.g., programmed instruction books, discussion, questions and answers, return demonstration
- (2) Provide opportunities for the patient to practice motor skills
- (3) Encourage self-directed activities

f. Every individual has capabilities and strengths (physical strengths, emotional maturity, a supportive family) that can be utilized to help the patient learn
- (1) Identify the patient's personal resources
- (2) Build on the identified strengths
- (3) Utilize these personal resources when and where appropriate
g. Energy and endurance levels will affect the patient's ability to learn and perform
- (1) During instructions, balance teaching with sufficient rest periods
- (2) Provide teaching at opportune times; e.g., earlier in the day rather than at night, after periods of rest
- (3) Present instruction in a manner the patient can comprehend and at a pace that can be maintained
- (4) Be flexible and adjust plan according to patient's rest and activity needs
h. Learning does not always progress on a straight line forward and upward; the patient may experience plateaus and remissions with a resulting change in adaptation and needs
- (1) Accept patient's feelings regarding lack of progress
- (2) Point out progress that has been made
- (3) Be patient and do not cause additional stress for the patient
- (4) Try alternative approaches for achieving goals
- (5) Identify short-term objectives for meeting goals
- (6) Alter long-term goals as necessary
i. Learning from previous experience can be transferred to new situations
- (1) When teaching something new, relate the commonalities or similarities of previously learned experiences
- (2) Base the plan of instructions on the foundation of the patient's knowledge

(3) Once the known is reinforced, then the unknown can be explored and the differences taught

D. Motivation
 1. Definition—motivation is the process of stimulating a person to assimilate certain concepts or behavior
 2. Principles of motivation and related nursing approaches
   a. People are complex products of self, family, and culture; the nurse must care for the patient as a unified being
     (1) Respect the patient as a person
     (2) Accept the patient's feelings without minimizing them
     (3) Assist the patient and family in accepting that the person's individuality and wholeness continue despite the changed physical or emotional state
     (4) Involve the person in deciding what to do and how to do it
     (5) The person must take precedence over the purpose of the lesson
   b. Learning is fostered when the plan of instruction is designed to operate within the individual's personal attitude and value system
     (1) Provide an atmosphere that allows for acceptance of differing value systems
     (2) Let the patient explore personal values, attitudes, and feelings concerning the health problem and its implications
     (3) Explore with the family the possibilities of carrying out instruction and how to individualize it so it is acceptable and practical for the patient and family
   c. A motivated learner assimilates what is learned more rapidly than one who is not motivated
     (1) The patient needs an opportunity to explore and discover personal learning needs and feelings concerning them
     (2) Awareness of a need to know can cause mild anxiety, which in itself is motivating
     (3) Motivation that is too intense

may reduce the effectiveness of learning
     (4) Determine patient's readiness for learning
   d. Intrinsic motivation (stimulated from within the learner) is preferable to extrinsic motivation (stimulated from outside the learner)
     (1) Identify those factors that are essential for the individual to have a feeling of meaningful achievement; e.g., being able to care for own health needs, respect and appreciation from others, acquiring new knowledge, receiving a reward
     (2) Satisfaction with learning progress promotes additional learning; therefore, design nursing care that will assist the patient in attaining that feeling of meaningful achievement
     (3) Encourage the patient to participate as a member of the health team and to be self-directed
   e. Information is learned more readily when it is relevant and meaningful to the learner
     (1) Help the patient interpret why the information is important and how the information gained will be useful
     (2) Relate the information by building the teaching plan on the patient's foundation of knowledge, experience, attitudes, and feelings
   f. Learning motivated by success or rewards is preferable to learning by failure or punishment
     (1) Help patient to set realistic goals within the motivation zone (goals set too high may be too challenging while goals set too low may lead to no action)
     (2) Focus on a patient's strengths and abilities rather than on failures and disabilities
     (3) Select learning tasks in which the patient is likely to succeed
     (4) Assist the patient to master or feel successful at one stage

of instruction before moving
on to the next
(5) Errors must be accepted as
part of the learning process
(6) Tolerance for failure is best
taught through providing a
backlog of success that com-
pensates for experienced failure
g. Planned reinforcement is essential
for learning; operant conditioning
is based on the theory that satisfaction motivates learning and that
those events that occur together
are associated
(1) For each patient identify and
utilize those factors that are
stimulants or incentives for
action; e.g., praise, smile, rewards, rest, specific privileges,
being able to care for self
(2) Provide visible reinforce-
ments; e.g., progress charts,
graphs
(3) Repetition is a form of reinforcement; therefore, repeated
activities tend to become habitual
(a) Provide opportunities for
the patient to practice
old and new skills
(b) Review information previously taught before in-
troducing new informa-
tion
(4) Involve the patient in groups
with people with the same
health problems but at various
stages of convalescence
(a) To be successful it is
helpful for the patient to
associate with successful
people
(b) Individuals can often
learn more by teaching
than in any other way
h. Evaluation of performance aids in
learning
(1) Purpose of evaluation
(a) Involves measuring behavior and interpreting
the results with regard to
what degree the set goals
are being attained
(b) Reinforces correct behavior

(c) Assists the learner to
realize how to change in-
correct behavior
(d) Helps the teacher to determine the adequacy of
the teaching
(2) Together the teacher and
learner should observe and
evaluate the learner's response in light of the desired
behavior
(3) Explain the "whys" of a good
or poor evaluation
(4) Value judgments, especially
"poor" or "inadequate," must
relate to the performance
rather than the individual

ACTIVITIES OF DAILY LIVING
A. Overview
1. Definitions
a. Activities of daily living are those
self-care activities that have to be
mastered for the patient to care
for personal needs that must be
met each day
b. Contracture—a condition in which
a muscle loses its ability to relax
to its original position; it may be
acquired or congenital
c. Hemiplegia—paralysis of one side
of the body and sometimes of the
face on the opposite side of the
affected extremities
d. Paraplegia—loss of power and sensation in the legs only, loss of sexual function and bowel and bladder control caused by trauma or
severance of the spinal cord in
the lumbar region
e. Paresis—partial or incomplete paralysis or weakness
f. Quadriplegia—loss of motor power
in the arms and legs, loss of sensation below the level of the lesion,
loss of sexual function and bladder
and bowel control caused by severance of the spinal cord at the
fifth or sixth cervical vertebra
g. Spasticity—a state of muscular
rigidity or alternating contraction
and relaxation with exaggeration
of the reflexes
2. Patient goal in activities of daily living—to care for routine daily needs
with minimal dependence on others

3. Role of the nurse—to teach, support, and supervise the patient while performing these activities
   a. Determine what the patient can do by observing performance
   b. Select activities within a patient's limitations and move from gross motor activities (bathing, combing hair) to finer motions (buttoning, eating with utensils)
   c. Ascertain what approaches could be used to accomplish a task
   d. Teach and encourage the patient to exercise the muscles necessary to perform the motions involved in the activity
   e. Determine what self-help devices, if any, may assist the patient in these daily activities
   f. Encourage the patient to do everything independently within the framework of the individual's disability
   g. Have the patient perform and practice the activity in a real life situation

B. Bed activities (constitute the basic preparation for self-care because they consist of gross body movement involved with sitting, transfer, and locomotion; they are also important for preventing the complications of immobility and inactivity)
   1. Active positioning
      a. Patient mobility
         (1) Rolling over
         (2) Sitting up in bed
         (3) Moving forward and backward while sitting
         (4) Moving sideways and placing legs off bed
      b. Assistive devices that promote mobility in bed
         (1) Bed frame itself
         (2) Side rails
         (3) Overhead trapeze
         (4) Pull ropes
         (5) Bradford frame—flat metal and canvas frame with an opening in the canvas to facilitate elimination
         (6) Whitman frame—a curved Bradford frame
         (7) Balkan frame—overhead bars used for traction and/or a trapeze

2. Passive positioning
   a. Passive movement of patient between supine and prone positions, e.g., log rolling, use of a "pull" or draw sheet
   b. Assistive devices for passive positioning
      (1) Types of turning frames
         (a) Stryker or Foster frames—allows for horizontal turning of patient
         (b) Circ-O-lectric bed—allows for vertical turning of patient; the patient can be placed in a variety of positions (Trendelenburg, prone, standing, and supine); one nurse can turn the patient with the electric motor providing the power; attachments permit application of traction and other accessories
      (2) Purposes of frames
         (a) Hyperextention
         (b) Immobilization
         (c) Correction of deformities
         (d) Facilitation of turning
         (e) Relief of pressure
         (f) Promotion of body functions (circulation, respiration, elimination)
      (3) General considerations concerning use of frames
         (a) Turning is done all in one piece
         (b) Frames are narrow and, therefore, for safety purposes the patient cannot sit up, roll over, or reach out to the side; extremely obese and disoriented patients should not be placed on a frame
         (c) Since only the prone and supine and, on the Circ-O-lectric bed, the vertical position can be used, strict attention must be paid to prevention of decubiti
         (d) Before releasing pivot pins, secure all bolts and straps to ensure patient safety

(e) These frames have wheels so that the patient can be moved about the room or taken to a recreation area for a change in surroundings; wheels should be locked prior to turning the patient

(f) To avoid disturbance of body alignment the patient's clothing should facilitate removal; e.g., shirts opening down the back

(g) When turning the Circ-O-lectric bed, do so slowly so that the patient's cerebral circulation can adjust to the new position; observe for signs of hypotension

(4) Tilt table—a board about 2 feet in width and 6 feet in length, padded with foam rubber, on which a person can be maintained in a straight position anywhere between horizontal and vertical by being strapped to the board around the chest, pelvic region, thighs, and below the knees; purposes include

(a) Overcome orthostatic hypotension

(b) Prevent loss of calcium from long bones

(c) Prevent formation of urinary calculi

(d) Prevent genitourinary infection

(e) Improve circulation, nutrition, and morale

C. Transfer
1. Definitions
   a. Transfer refers to methods of movement of the patient from one surface to another; e.g., bed to wheelchair, wheelchair to commode
   b. Weight-bearing transfers—carried out by patients who have at least one stable lower extremity; e.g., hemiplegia, unilateral lower extremity amputation, patients with fractured hips
   c. Nonweight-bearing transfers—carried out by patients who do not have a stable lower extremity; e.g., paraplegics not wearing braces, patients with double lower extremity amputations

2. Nursing responsibilities
   a. Assess patient's abilities; e.g., sitting tolerance, balance, weight-bearing potential, strength, motivation, understanding of principles of transfer
   b. Identify need for and selection of assistive devices; e.g., slide board, trapeze, wheelchair with a removable arm, hydraulic lift
   c. Select most appropriate transfer method and teach and assist the patient with this new technique
   d. Provide for patient safety; e.g., encourage use of low heeled shoes; lock wheelchair brakes during transfer; remove hazards—scatter rugs, slippery floors, stepstools; ensure adequate assistance
   e. Communicate individualized transfer techniques by instructing the patient and family and informing the entire health team

3. Principles
   a. Maintain correct proximity and visual relationship of wheelchair to bed; e.g., paraplegia—place wheelchair lateral or perpendicular to bed; hemiplegia—place wheelchair at a 30° angle to the bed on the unaffected side
   b. Movement through a 90° angle can be accomplished by pivoting while bearing weight on upper extremities and one leg
   c. The patient's abilities and disabilities must be considered when deciding appropriate transfer technique and need for assistive devices; e.g., hemiplegia—place wheelchair on side opposite affected extremities; paraplegia—may use trapeze, slide board, wheelchair with removable arm
   d. Transfers on the same level are easier than with variation in heights that require a push-up technique
   e. Before pivoting on a weight-bearing transfer, make sure that the patient's knees are "locked" (this

is accomplished by full leg extension or by the nurse standing in front of the patient and placing knee against one of the patient's knees)

f. The nurse should know and utilize all the principles of body mechanics (see Nursing fundamentals, pp. 327-329)

D. Locomotion (the act of moving from one place to another)

1. Ambulation—walking carried out in an upright position with some degree of weight-bearing on one or both legs; important because it
   a. Transports body from one place to another
   b. Helps to maintain self-esteem and independence
   c. Assists in preventing deformity
   d. Helps maintain body functions; e.g., improves circulation, helps maintain muscle tone, aids in elimination, and improves respiration

2. Preparation for ambulation
   a. Determine direct body maintenance ability; e.g., can patient maintain proper body alignment especially when erect
   b. Determine weight-bearing and balance ability of the upper extremities; muscle demands of assistive walking include
      (1) Flexors of the fingers and thumbs—ability to grasp the walking aid
      (2) Dorsiflexors of the wrist—ability to keep the hands in the correct position on the handpiece
      (3) Extensors of the forearms—ability to bear the weight of the body when lifted from the floor
      (4) Flexors of the arms—ability to move the walking aid forward
      (5) Depressors and downward rotators of the shoulder girdle—ability to support the body when it leaves the floor
   c. Determine weight-bearing and balance ability of the lower extremities; e.g., can the patient bear weight and keep balanced on one or both lower extremities

d. Determine step ability; e.g., can the patient take steps with either or both lower extremities by placing one foot in front of the other
e. Strengthen upper extremities with bed exercises prior to ambulation
f. Provide activities that will promote good posture and balance; e.g., dangle before standing, encourage holding chest high and body, including hips and knees, in full extension
g. Determine gait pattern best suited to meet the individual's needs
h. Proper selection and correct fit of the particular walking aid, if required
i. Provide for patient safety; e.g., firm and well-fitting shoes, eliminate obstructions such as throw rugs and stepstools, extra personnel to provide assistance
j. People who have walked normally at one time and understand the pattern of normal walking (normal walking involves moving alternate arms and legs, flexing the hip and knees, and bearing weight on the feet moving from heels to toes) will grasp the initials of the techniques of crutch walking more quickly than those who have never learned to walk; teaching should be based on a patient's experiential background; e.g., a person with an amputation, a stroke, or a fracture versus a person with cerebral palsy or a congenital deformity
k. Teach ambulation by discussion, illustrations, demonstrations, and return demonstration
l. When assisting a disabled person to walk, go up and down stairs, or get in and out of bed, help on the unaffected side
m. If possible, teach at least two gaits to anticipate situations and different needs; e.g., safety and speed

3. Ambulating with assistive devices
   a. Crutches—underarm metal or wooden mechanical aid with double uprights and hand bars
      (1) Purposes of crutches
         (a) Support body weight, assist weak muscles, and provide joint stability

(b) Relieve pain
(c) Prevent further injury
(d) provide for improvement of function
(e) Allow for greater patient independence
(2) Selection of crutches
  (a) Measurement for proper length—measure distance from anterior fold of axilla to point 6 inches out from heel
  (b) Axillary bar must be 2 inches below axilla and may or may not be padded
  (c) Hand bar should allow almost complete extension of arm with the elbow flexed, about 30° when the patient places weight on the hands
  (d) Rubber crutch tip should be in good condition, about 5.1 to 7.6 cm. (2 to 3 inches) in height, with a circumference of 3.8 to 4.4 cm. (1½ to 1¾ inches)
(3) Types of crutch walking—choice of particular gait depends on the patient's ability to bear weight and to take steps with either or both of the lower extremities
  (a) Four-point alternate crutch gait
    (1) Right crutch, left foot, left crutch, right foot
    (2) Equal but partial weight-bearing on each limb
    (3) A slow but stable gait; there are always 3 points of support on the floor
    (4) The patient must be able to manipulate both extremities and get one foot ahead of the other; e.g., polio, arthritis, cerebral palsy
  (b) Two-point alternate crutch gait

    (1) Right crutch and left foot simultaneously
    (2) There are always 2 points of support on the floor
    (3) This is a more rapid version of the four-point gait and requires more balance and strength; e.g., bilateral amputation
  (c) Three-point gait
    (1) Advance both crutches and the weaker lower extremity simultaneously, then the stronger lower extremity
    (2) A fairly rapid gait but requires more balance and strength in the arms and the good lower extremity
    (3) Used when one leg can support the whole body weight and the other lower extremity cannot take full weight-bearing; e.g., fractured hip
  (d) Swing crutch gaits
    (1) Swing-to gait
      (a) Place both crutches forward, then lift and swing body *up to* crutches, place crutches in front of body and continue
      (b) There are always 2 points of support on the floor
      (c) This technique is indicated for any patient with adequate power in the upper arms
    (2) Swing-through gait
      (a) Place both crutches forward, then lift and swing body *through* crutches, place crutches in

front of body and
continue
(b) A very difficult
gait because as
the patient swings
through the
crutches, it neces-
sitates rolling the
pelvis forward
and arching the
back in order to
get the center of
gravity in front
of the hips
(c) Indicated for the
patient who has
power in the
trunk and upper
extremities, ex-
cellent balance,
self-confidence,
and a dash of
daring; e.g., bi-
lateral amputa-
tion, paraplegic
with braces
(e) Tripod crutch gaits
(1) Tripod alternate gait
(a) Right crutch, left
crutch, drag the
body and legs
forward
(b) The patient con-
stantly maintains
a tripod position
—both crutches
are held fairly
widespread out
front while both
feet are held to-
gether in the
back
(c) Necessary for the
individual who
cannot place one
extremity ahead
of the other; e.g.,
flaccid paralysis
from polio-
myelitis, spinal
cord injuries
(2) Tripod simultaneous
gait
(a) Place both
crutches forward,
drag the body
and legs forward

(b) Because the tri-
pod must have a
large base, the
patient's body
must be inclined
forward suffi-
ciently to keep
the center of
gravity in front
of the hips
(f) Common errors made in
crutch walking are
(1) Using the body in
poor mechanical fash-
ion
(2) Hiking hips with ab-
duction gait (com-
mon in amputee)
(3) Lifting crutches
while still bearing
down on them
(4) Walking on ball of
foot with foot turned
outward and flexion
at hip or knee level
(5) Hunching shoulders
(crutches usually too
long) or stooping
with shoulders
(crutches usually too
short)
(6) Looking downward
while ambulating
(7) Bearing weight un-
der arms should be
avoided to prevent
injury to the nerves
in the brachial plex-
us; damage to these
nerves can cause pa-
ralysis and is known
as crutch palsy
b. Canes—a singular piece of wood
or metal designed to aid the ambulating patient who does not need
crutches but needs the assistance
of an additional support
(1) Purposes of a cane
(a) Improve stability
(b) Maintain balance
(c) Prevent further injury
(d) Provide security while
developing confidence in
ambulating
(e) Relieve pressure on
weight-bearing joints
(f) Assist in increasing speed

of ambulation with less fatigue

(g) Provide for greater mobility and independence

(2) Types of canes

  (a) Standard cane with its C-curve handle

  (b) T top cane, J cane, and ortho cane are variations of the shape of a standard cane

  (c) Crab cane, quad cane, and four-legged cane have extra prongs at the end of the shaft providing extra contact points on the floor

  (d) Lofstrand crutch—a lightweight cane with a forearm support; the forearm bar and cuff stabilize the wrists, make walking easier and safer, and allow the patient to release the handbar without dropping the cane

(3) Selection of a cane

  (a) Useful for patients with a lower limb disability

  (b) Patient must be able to bear weight on the afflicted extremity

  (c) Patient must be able to use upper extremity opposite the affected lower extremity

  (d) Measurements to determine length of cane

    (1) The highest point of the cane should be about level with the great trochanter

    (2) The handpiece should allow 30° of flexion at the elbow with the wrist held in extension

(4) Techniques for ambulating with a cane

  (a) Hold in the hand opposite to the affected extremity

  (b) The cane and the affected extremity should be advanced simultaneously and then the un-

affected leg should be advanced

(c) The cane should be kept close to the body

(d) When climbing, the patient should step up with the unaffected extremity and then place the cane and the affected lower extremity on the step; when descending the procedure is reversed

(5) Common errors made in using a cane

  (a) Leaning the body over the cane

  (b) Shortening the stride on the unaffected side

  (c) Inability to develop a normal walking pattern

  (d) The abnormal gait pattern tends to persist after the cane is no longer needed

c. Walkers—lightweight and sturdy assistive devices that have a wide four-point base of support

(1) Purposes of walkers

  (a) Maintain balance

  (b) Provide additional support because of wide area of contact with floor

  (c) Allow for some ambulatory independence

(2) Types of walkers

  (a) Standard walker has 3 sides and 4 points of contact with the floor

  (b) Walkerette and Rollator have wheels or runners on some or all of the points so that the patient does not have to lift the device

  (c) Walkers with accessories to meet patient's specific needs; e.g., brakes, adjustable crutches attached to the horizontal bars, seats

(3) Selection of a walker

  (a) A walker should not be used unless the patient will never be able to ambulate with a cane or crutches

  (b) Measurements for a

walker are the same as for a cane

(c) The patient must have strong elbow extensors and shoulder depressors and partial strength in the hands and wrist muscles

(d) The patient needs maximum support to ensure security and enhance confidence

(e) Use is usually limited to the home because it cannot be used on steps

(4) Techniques for ambulating with a walker

(a) Lift device off the floor and place forward a short distance, then advance between the walker

(b) Two-wheeled walkers—raise back legs of device off the floor, roll walker forward and then advance to it

(c) Four-wheeled walkers—push device forward on floor and then walk to it

(5) Common errors in using a walker

(a) Arms are kept rigid and do not swing through to counter-balance the position of the lower extremity

(b) Tending to lean forward with abnormal flexion at the hips

(c) Affected leg not encouraged to swing through; the patient tends to step forward with good leg and shuffle affected leg up to the bar

d. Braces and splints—assistive mechanical devices of varying lengths and designs depending on the patient's needs; they consist of 2 lateral bars attached to a shoe or foot plate, joints and hinges that correspond with the joints of the extremity, and straps, belts, and linings for securing the brace to the patient; an orthosis is a device commonly known as a brace

(1) Purposes of braces and splints

(a) A support that protects weakened muscles

(b) Prevents and corrects anatomic deformities

(c) Aids in controlling involuntary muscle movements

(d) Immobilizes and protects a diseased or injured joint

(e) Provides for improvement of function

(2) Types of braces and splints—literally hundreds of different kinds of braces, each specifically designed to meet the patient's individual needs

(3) Selection of a brace or splint depends on

(a) Type of disability

(b) Severity of disability

(c) Parts of the body involved

(d) Age and mentality of the patient

(e) Emotional and physical readiness

(f) The device is serving a real need

(g) Correct measurements—these are individual and depend on anatomy, pathology present and predicted, and the resulting desired functions

(4) General considerations concerning use of braces and splints

(a) Equipment should be kept in good repair; e.g., oil joints, replace straps when worn, wash with saddle soap

(b) Adequate shoes; e.g., keep in good repair, heels low and wide, high top to hold the heel in the shoe

(c) Skin should be examined daily for evidence of pressure points

(d) Check alignment of braces; e.g., leg braces—joints should coincide with body joints; back brace—upright bars in center of back, brace should grip pelvis and trocanter firmly, lacing should begin from the bottom

e. Prosthetics
  (1) Definitions
    (a) Prosthesis—an artificial substitute for a missing extremity or organ
    (b) Amputation—surgical removal of an extremity because of ischemia, trauma, revision of congenital deformities, or prevention of metastasis of a tumor
  (2) Purposes of a prosthesis
    (a) Prevent excessive atrophy
    (b) Manipulate and transport objects (upper extremity prosthesis)
    (c) Provide for weight-bearing and assist in ambulation (lower extremity prosthesis)
    (d) Provide a cosmetic effect (helps to conceal the lack of a limb, eye, or breast)
  (3) Selection of a prosthesis depends on
    (a) Physical condition—range of motion, strength of musculature, condition of stump site of amputation
    (b) Psychologic factors—stage of adaptation, level of needs, experiential background, personal resources
    (c) Social and vocational factors—present job, career desires, family- and community-related needs
    (d) Considerations concerning an upper extremity prosthesis
      (1) Mastery of an upper extremity prosthesis is more complex than that of a lower extremity prosthesis
      (2) The patient must do bilateral shoulder exercises to prepare for fitting the prosthesis
      (3) The artificial arm cannot be used above the head or behind the back because of the harnessing
      (4) There is no artificial hand that can duplicate all the fine movements of the fingers and thumb of the normal hand although the development of electronic limbs does not negate this possibility for the future
      (5) There must be a reeducation of the remaining upper extremity to compensate as much as possible for what has been lost
      (6) There is a loss of sensory feedback; therefore, the patient must use visual control at all times (a blind person could not adequately use a functional prosthesis)
  (4) Nursing care of the patient with an amputation
    (a) Support the patient psychologically
      (1) Accept feelings of shock and grief
      (2) Encourage patient and family to explore feelings
      (3) Explain various phases of rehabilitation
    (b) Build up the patient's nutritional status—preparation for wound healing and energy expenditure in exercises and ambulation
    (c) Instruct and encourage patient to exercise to

strengthen the remaining muscles

(d) Watch for signs and symptoms of hemorrhage and infection

(e) Prevent contractures

   (1) Elevating the stump on a pillow decreases edema and lessens pain in the immediate postoperative period; however, the pillow should be removed as soon as danger of hemorrhage has passed (about 24 hours)

   (2) Keep patient's extremities close to the body to prevent abduction deformity

   (3) Encourage patient to move stump

   (4) Place the patient with a lower extremity amputation in a prone position twice daily to stretch the flexor muscles

   (5) Start range of motion exercises to the stump after about 10 days

   (6) Encourage the patient not to sit in any one position for prolonged periods of time since this inactivity can cause hip flexion contractures

(f) Provide and teach good care of the stump

   (1) Stump shrinkage (a change in size and shape of stump) is caused by reduction of subcutaneous fat by pressure of constrictive bandage and socket of prosthesis as well as disuse atrophy occurring in the involved muscles; maximum shrinkage usually takes, a minimum of 1 to 1½ years and sometimes longer

   (2) Keep the stump clean —wash with mild soap but do not soak, use clean bandages and socks

   (3) Physical preparation for a prosthesis

      (a) Apply compression bandage to prevent edema and promote stump shrinkage

      (b) Massage the stump to soften the scar, decrease tenderness, and improve vascularity

      (c) Teach and encourage the patient to do stump-conditioning exercises to harden the stump (push stump against pillow and then progress to harder surfaces)

(g) With the physical therapist, assist the patient with a lower extremity amputation to learn crutch walking (see Rehabilitation nursing, pp. 544-546)

(h) For patients fitted with a prosthesis immediately after surgery, ambulation instruction is begun on the first postoperative day

(i) Explain and discuss phantom limb phenomenon with the patient

   (1) Phantom limb—a physiologic reaction of the nerves in the stump causing an unpleasant feeling that the limb is still there; this response may or may not be precipitated by a psychologic overlay

   (2) Phantom limb pain —when the unpleas-

ant feelings become painful or disagreeable

(3) Characteristics of phantom limb—sensations may be constant, intermittent, and of varying severity

(4) Approaches that may help relieve phantom limb—have the patient look at the stump or close eyes and put the stump through range of motion as if the full limb were still there; if the patient continues to have severe pain of long duration, the medical therapy may include

(a) Injecting the nerve endings in the stump with alcohol to give temporary relief

(b) Surgical revision of the stump

4. Locomotion on wheels—the patient is propelled or self-propelled on wheels or casters in a sitting position

a. Purposes of wheelchair

(1) Support the body

(2) Decrease cardiac workload

(3) Promote independence and stimulate activities

(4) Provide mobility for those who cannot ambulate or those who can ambulate but whose ambulation is unsteady, unsafe, or too strenuous

b. Selection of a wheelchair depends on

(1) Nature of the patient's disability

(2) Present and predicted physical measurements; e.g., height, weight

(3) The user's capabilities; e.g., sitting balance, function of the upper extremities, power of propulsion

(4) Environmental conditions of operating area; e.g., indoor

versus outdoor, architectural conditions

(5) Functions and services expected; e.g., needs for light weight, collapsible, durable chair

(6) Safety and appearance; e.g., design, workmanship, and quality of material

c. General considerations in the use of wheelchairs

(1) The patient must adapt to living in a sitting position

(2) There is a large variety of wheelchairs depending on the patient's needs; e.g., front-wheel or rearwheel drive, commode chairs, 1-arm drive chairs—for patient with multiple defects or hemiplegia

(3) There are hundreds of accessories to meet the patient's specific needs; e.g., removable arms, lap boards, knobs on the handrims, extra long leg panels, battery or motor propulsion

(4) Specific devices are necessary for patient safety; e.g., wheel brakes, arm locks, seat belts, swing foot rests

(5) There are a variety of other wheeling devices; e.g., prone self-propelled stretchers, scooters, rolling stands, crawlers

(6) Prolonged sitting in one position can cause flexion contractures of the hips and knees and ischial decubiti (encourage the patient to change body positions, use padded cushions and exercise such as push-ups every hour to relieve pressure)

(7) Some patients become too dependent on a wheelchair because of the comfort and lack of effort required

E. Self-care—the ability to carry out unassisted the ordinary activities of personal care

1. Self-care activities include

a. Dressing

b. Eating

c. Miscellaneous hand activities; e.g.,

writing, opening letters, using the telephone
   d. Toilet activities
     (1) Personal appearance
     (2) Personal hygiene
     (3) Bowel and bladder elimination
2. Nursing responsibilities
   a. Determine what self-care activities the patient can handle
   b. Determine the patient's potential abilities, those additional activities that could be accomplished as a result of rehabilitation procedures
   c. Determine the methods by which the patient can achieve the full potential of personal abilities
     (1) Physical conditioning of affected and unaffected body parts to increase their strength and range of motion
     (2) Instruction in self-care methods to circumvent the disability
     (3) Use of assistive devices as necessary
     (4) Use of adaptive equipment and modifications of clothing and living arrangements
3. Bowel and bladder function
   a. Bowel function
     (1) Goal of bowel management is to establish a scheduled pattern of bowel evacuation
     (2) Nursing responsibilities in reestablishing bowel function are to
       (a) Understand what the individual's bowel functioning means to the patient and family
       (b) Involve the patient, family, and entire health team in the development of a plan of care
       (c) Review the patient's bowel habits prior to illness as well as the current pattern of elimination
       (d) Supply diet adequate in bulk, roughage, and bowel-stimulating properties
       (e) Encourage sufficient fluid intake—2000 to 3000 ml. per day

       (f) Encourage the patient to be as active as possible to develop the tone and strength of muscles that can be used
       (g) Establish a specific and definite time for the bowel movement; regularity is the most important aspect of bowel reeducation
         (1) Exact time depends on patient's schedule
         (2) Depends on patient's past pattern
         (3) Consider scheduling evacuation after a meal to utilize the gastrocolic reflex (peristaltic wave in colon induced by entrance of food into fasting stomach)
       (h) Determine if the patient is aware of need or act of defecation; e.g., feeling of fullness or pressure in rectum, flatus, rumbling in stomach
       (i) Provide privacy for the patient during toileting activities
       (j) Encourage the patient to assume a position most nearly the physiologic position for defecation (sitting the patient up frequently assists in preparing for this)
       (k) Utilize assistive measures to induce defecation by
         (1) Teaching the patient to bear down and contract abdominal muscles (the Valsalva maneuver should be avoided by people with cardiac problems)
         (2) Teaching the patient to lean forward to increase intra-abdominal pressure by compressing abdomen against the thighs

(3) Digital stimulation

(4) Use suppository if necessary

(5) Enemas should be used only as a last resort

(1) Provide for adaptation of equipment as necessary; e.g., elevated toilet seat, grab bars, padded back rest

(m) Teach the family the bowel training program

b. Bladder function

(1) Goal of bladder management is to empty the bladder regularly and completely

(2) Definitions

(a) Neurogenic bladder—any disturbance in bladder functioning caused by a lesion of the nervous system

(b) Spastic (reflex or automatic) bladder—a bladder disorder caused by a lesion of the spinal cord above the bladder reflex center in the conus medullaris; there is a loss of conscious sensation and cerebral motor control; the bladder empties automatically when the detrusor muscle is sufficiently stretched (about 500 ml.)

(c) Flaccid (atonic nonreflex or autonomous) bladder —a bladder disorder caused by a lesion of the spinal cord at the level of the sacral conus or below; the bladder continues to fill, becomes distended, and periodically overflows; the bladder muscle does not contract forcefully and, therefore, does not empty except with a conscious effort

(3) Nursing responsibilities in reestablishing function

(a) Understand what the individual's bladder func-

tioning means to the patient and family

(b) Involve the patient, family, and entire health team in the development of a plan of care

(c) Review the patient's bladder habits prior to illness as well as the current pattern of elimination

(d) Encourage activity

(e) Encourage sufficient fluid intake

(1) 3000 to 5000 ml. per 24-hour period

(2) Drink a glass of water with each attempt to void

(3) Reduce amount of fluid as the day progresses and restrict fluid after 6 P.M. to limit amount of urine in bladder during the night

(f) Provide for privacy during toileting activities

(g) Encourage the patient to assume as normal a position as possible for voiding

(h) Establish a voiding schedule

(1) Begin trial voiding at the time the patient is most often incontinent

(2) Attempt voiding every 2 hours all day and 2 to 3 times during the night

(3) Time intervals between voiding should be shorter in the morning than later in the day

(4) As the patient's ability to maintain control improves, lengthen time between attempts at voiding

(5) Time of intervals is not as important as regularity

(i) Determine whether the patient is aware of need or act of urination; e.g., fullness or pressure, flushing, chilling, goose pimples, cold sweats

(j) Utilize assistive measures to induce urination by teaching the patient to
  (1) Use the Credé maneuver—manual expression of the urine from the bladder with moderate external pressure, downward and backward, from the umbilicus to over the suprapubic area
  (2) Bend forward to increase intra-abdominal pressure
  (3) Stimulate "trigger points"—those areas that, for the individual, will instigate urination; e.g., stroke thigh, pull pubic hair, touch meatus

(k) Record intake, output, voiding times, and times of incontinence

(l) Provide for adaptive equipment as necessary; e.g., elevated toilet seats, commode, urinals, drainage systems

(m) Teach the family the bladder training program

c. Functional disorders of the bladder and the bowel
  (1) Definition—disturbances in bladder and bowel functioning unrelated to neurologic disorders or motor and sensory defects; most often these problems are a result of mismanagement or inadequate nursing care in patients with hemiplegia, arthritis, fractured hip, lower extremity amputation, and cardiopulmonary problems
  (2) Nursing responsibilities in caring for the potentially incontinent patient

(a) Provide adequate fluid intake

(b) Provide diet with enough roughage for sufficient quantity of bowel content and proper consistency for evacuation

(c) Avoid preoccupation with elimination

(d) Avoid overt encouragement of incontinence; e.g., routine use of diapers, Chux, and other depersonalizing devices

(e) Stimulate normal elimination by exercise and activity

(f) Help patient develop regular bowel and bladder patterns

(g) Respect the individual; e.g., provide for privacy, individuality of routine, avoidance of delay, encourage the patient to make decisions

(h) Utilize physical and psychologic techniques to stimulate elimination; e.g., running water, place patient's hands in warm water, place patient in as normal a position as possible for elimination

(i) Create an environment that keeps sensory monotony to a minimum; e.g., orient to time and place, use radio and television selectively, increase patient's social contacts, provide visual stimulus, extend environment beyond patient's room

(j) Provide for self-esteem; e.g., encourage patient to wear own clothes, do self-care activities, make decisions

(k) Accept and explore patient's feelings of fear, anger, and depression; a disabled person has few avenues by which to express anger; incontinence is often used in this manner

F. Nursing responsibilities for patients in whom sensation is diminished or absent
1. Test temperature of bath water to avoid burns; teach patient to test water temperature in any water-related activity
2. Avoid bumps and bruises when involved in activities; utilize techniques to prevent pressure and examine skin for signs of pressure from positioning, braces, or splints
3. Use a footboard to stimulate pressure sensation and proprioception
4. Provide opportunity for patient to touch, grasp, and manipulate objects of different sizes, weights, and textures to stimulate tactile sensation
5. Encourage patient to be aware of all body segments; look at both extremities, comb both sides of hair, shave both sides of chin, put make-up on both sides of face
6. Protect affected limbs by proper positioning during transfer and using a sling when indicated
7. Teach the patient to use unaffected extremities to manipulate, move, and stabilize affected ones

G. Problems in communication resulting from physiologic disorders
1. Communication is the sending and receiving of ideas and information
2. Problems with communication can result from
   a. Disorders of respiration—amount of air available for speech is diminished; e.g., Guillain-Barré syndrome, poliomyelitis
   b. Disorders of phonation—disorders affecting the ability of the vocal cords to vibrate adequately; e.g., laryngitis, polyps, cancer
   c. Disorders of resonation—disorders causing voice and air pressure to go out through the nose; e.g., cleft palate
   d. Disorders of articulation—inadequate use of palate, tongue, teeth, mouth, and lips to make variety of sounds; e.g., myasthenia gravis, multiple sclerosis, parkinsonism, and cerebral vascular accidents

3. Aphasia—the brain is unable to fulfill its communicative functions because of damage to its input, integrative, or output centers; it is a disturbance of language function and may involve impairment of the ability to read, write, speak, or interpret messages
   a. Expressive aphasia—the patient has difficulties making own thoughts known to others; speaking and writing are most affected
   b. Receptive aphasia—the patient has difficulty understanding what others are trying to communicate; interpretation of speech and reading are most affected
   c. Expressive-receptive aphasia—the patient has equal difficulty in speaking, writing, interpreting speech, and reading
   d. Nursing approaches for patients with aphasia; the nurse should
      (1) Be aware of own reactions to the speech difficulty
      (2) Evaluate extent of patient's ability to understand and express self at a simple level
      (3) Include health team, especially the speech therapist, in planning patient care
      (4) Involve the family as much as possible
      (5) Convey to the patient that there is a problem with communication, not with intelligence
      (6) Try to eliminate anxiety and tension related to communication attempts; e.g., be consistent, give the patient time to respond, employ a calm, accepting, and deliberate manner
      (7) Help the patient set attainable goals
      (8) Stimulate patient's communication without pushing to point of frustration
      (9) Keep distractions at a minimum since they interfere with the reception and integration of messages; e.g., one-to-one conversations rather than group conversations, shut off radio when speaking
      (10) Speak slowly, clearly, and in

short sentences and do not raise voice

(11) Use alternate means of communication; e.g., gestures, writing, picture board

(12) Involve the patient in social interactions; e.g., encourage socialization, do not anticipate all needs, ask questions and expect answers, do not ignore patient in group conversations

(13) Make a definite transition between tasks to prevent or reduce confusion

(14) Be alert for clues and gestures when speech is garbled; e.g., continue to listen, nod, and make occasional neutral statements, let patient know when you cannot understand

(15) Provide for periodic re-evaluation to demonstrate to the patient and health team the effect and nature of progress

THE PATIENT—A MEMBER OF THE COMMUNITY

A. Nursing responsibilities for discharge
1. Plan for patient's discharge from either an acute care setting or a community setting at first contact
2. Obtain knowledge of the impact of the health problem on the patient, the family unit, and interrelationships of importance (job, school, church)
3. Identify patient's and family's personal resources; e.g., education, vocation, economic status, physical abilities, avocational interests
4. Evaluate environment for promoting and inhibiting factors and indicate any necessary changes to provide for space, safety, comfort, or ease in accomplishing common activities of daily living
5. Identify need for and availability of community resources that may assist the patient and family
6. Promote continuance of health education and development of good health practice

B. Rehabilitation can be considered successful when
1. The individual has been discharged to the home or a place that provides maximum opportunities within capabilities for social relationships with family and friends

2. The individual's potentials have been developed to their fullest
3. The individual has satisfactorily resolved how to meet independence, vocational, and economic needs

REVIEW QUESTIONS FOR REHABILITATION NURSING

Mr. Andrews, 57 years of age, had a cerebral vascular accident. Three weeks after his stroke he had left-sided paresis but was able to ambulate fairly well with a cane. He was very frustrated and angry because of his expressive aphasia. Questions 1 through 5 refer to this situation.

1. A person with expressive aphasia has difficulty with
   1. Following instructions
   2. Recognizing the words for familiar objects
   3. Speaking and/or writing
   4. Understanding speech and/or writing
2. Mr. Andrews gets very frustrated and upset when he tries to communicate with the nurse. To help alleviate this frustration the nurse should
   1. Face the patient and raise her voice so that he can see and hear her better
   2. Limit his contact with other patients to limit the frustration
   3. Anticipate his needs so that he does not have to ask for help
   4. Give patient plenty of time to speak and respond so he does not have to formulate a response under pressure
3. Although Mr. Andrews has regained control of his bowel movements, he is still incontinent of urine. To help Mr. Andrews reestablish bladder function the nurse should encourage him to
   1. Assume his normal position for voiding
   2. Void every 3 hours and attempt to hold urine between set times
   3. Drink a minimum of 4000 ml. of fluid equally divided among the hours he is awake
   4. Attempt to void more frequently in the afternoon than in the morning
4. Mr. Andrews is using a cane specifically to
   1. Prevent further injury to weakened muscles
   2. Maintain balance and improve stability
   3. Relieve pressure on weight-bearing joints
   4. Aid in controlling involuntary muscle movements
5. When teaching Mr. Andrews to ambulate with a cane the nurse should instruct him to
   1. Hold it in the hand on the same side of the affected lower extremity
   2. Lean the body toward the cane when ambulating
   3. Advance the cane and the affected extremity simultaneously
   4. Shorten the stride on the unaffected extremity

Ann Varney, a 14-year-old junior high school student, was just diagnosed as having diabetes mellitus. She is a cheerleader, receives excellent grades, and is the only member of the family with diabetes. Mrs. Varney told the nurse that her sister died of diabetes at 21, several years before Ann was born, and that she was afraid that Ann would die too. Questions 6 through 10 refer to this situation.

6. A basic concept of rehabilitation is
   1. Rehabilitation is a specialty area with unique methods for meeting the patient's needs
   2. Rehabilitation is not necessary for most patients because they will return to their usual activities following hospitalization
   3. Rehabilitation needs, immediate or potential, are exhibited by all patients with a health problem
   4. Rehabilitation needs are best met by the patient's family and community resources
7. Ann exhibited a need for cognitive learning when she asked
   1. "What is diabetes?"
   2. "How do I give myself an injection?"
   3. "When do I test my urine for S and A?"
   4. "Can I still be a cheerleader?"
8. When teaching Ann about diabetes and giving herself insulin, the very first step for the nurse would be to
   1. Begin the teaching program at Ann's present level
   2. Find out what Ann knows about her health problem
   3. Set specific and realistic short- and long-term goals
   4. Collect all the equipment needed to demonstrate giving an injection
9. When promoting affective learning (developing attitudes), the nurse must remember the influence of the
   1. Patient's personal resources
   2. Type of onset of the disease
   3. Nurse's own attitude towards the disease itself
   4. Physical and emotional stress of adolescence
10. A week after the physician spoke with Ann's parents, Mrs. Varney was still slightly anxious and asked the nurse for more information about diabetes. She should recognize that Mrs. Varney is
    1. Too upset to learn new information
    2. Transferring attitudes about her sister to her daughter
    3. Exhibiting readiness for learning
    4. Expressing her attitudes through her behavior

Miss Daley, a 24-year-old secretary, is pregnant for the first time. She discussed the pregnancy with her boyfriend who told her everything would work out fine. Two days later she received a letter from him with $500 and the news that he had left town. Miss Daley was very upset, felt that she was at the end of her rope, and called the crisis intervention center for help. Questions 11 through 15 refer to this patient.

11. Miss Daley was experiencing a crisis situation because
    1. She was experiencing a great deal of stress
    2. Her boyfriend left her when she was pregnant
    3. She was going to have to raise her child alone
    4. Her past methods of adapting were ineffective for this situation
12. Crisis intervention groups are successful because
    1. The client is encouraged to talk about herself
    2. The client is assisted to investigate alternative approaches to solving the identified problem
    3. The crisis intervention worker is a psychologist and understands behavior patterns
    4. The client is supplied with a workable solution to her problems
13. When talking with Miss Daley, the crisis intervention worker should
    1. Respect her and involve her in deciding what she will do and how she will do it
    2. Restate the problem putting it in the proper perspective
    3. Explain to her that the center has helped many other people with the same problem
    4. Explore her religious and cultural beliefs so that your instructions are within her value system
14. Miss Daley has decided to go through with the pregnancy and keep the baby. Now the crisis intervention worker's primary responsibility is to
    1. Support her for making a wise decision
    2. Make an appointment for her to see a physician for prenatal care
    3. Explore other problems she may be experiencing
    4. Provide information about other health resources where she may receive additional assistance
15. Miss Daley is now excited and looking forward to caring for her baby. Her decision to attend prenatal child care classes is an example of
    1. Extrinsic motivation
    2. Operant conditioning
    3. Intrinsic motivation
    4. Behavior modification

Mrs. Ryan, 82 years of age, has severe painful arthritis. She was admitted to a nursing home when she became incontinent and her family could no longer care for her. Questions 16 through 18 refer to this situation.

16. Mrs. Ryan's condition would indicate that a primary consideration in her care would be her need for
    1. Immobilization of joints
    2. Bladder re-education
    3. Control of pain
    4. Motivation and teaching
17. Since Mrs. Ryan's admission to the nursing home she has not been incontinent. While exploring with Mrs. Ryan her past and present elimination patterns the patient told the nurse that she has been very angry because she has been bedridden and never gets to go anywhere or see anyone. The nurse deducted that the patient's incontinence at home was
    1. An expression of hostility
    2. A method to determine her family's love for her

3. A physiologic response expected with elderly bedridden patients
4. A way of maintaining control
18. When caring for Mrs. Ryan the nurse should
    1. Frequently ask if she needs the bedpan to void
    2. Create an environment that prevents sensory monotony
    3. Limit her fluid intake in the evening
    4. When not in the room put on the television or radio

John, a 21-year-old physical education major in college, sustained a spinal cord injury while practicing on the trampoline. Three days after the injury the physician explained to him that he had paraplegia and what this diagnosis entails. Questions 19 through 23 refer to this situation.

19. Paraplegia means
    1. Paresis of both lower extremities
    2. Paralysis of one side of the body
    3. Upper and lower extremities are paralyzed
    4. Both lower extremities are paralyzed
20. When caring for John, the initial responsibility of the nurse is to
    1. Prevent contractures
    2. Protect the patient from flexion or hyperextension of the spine
    3. Prevent urinary tract infections
    4. Prepare the patient for vocational rehabilitation
21. Considering the diagnosis, the nurse knows she must encourage John to drink a lot of fluid to prevent
    1. Urinary tract infections
    2. Fluid and electrolyte imbalance
    3. Dehydration
    4. Constipation
22. John was placed on a Circ-O-lectric bed primarily to
    1. Promote mobility
    2. Prevent loss of calcium from long bones
    3. Prevent pressure sores
    4. Promote orthostatic hypotension
23. Three weeks after his injury, John explained to the nurse that he must get out of the hospital soon to practice for the upcoming intercollegiate gymnastic tournament. In light of what the patient is saying, the nurse should realize that John is
    1. No longer able to adapt
    2. Extremely motivated to get well
    3. Verbalizing a fantasy
    4. Exhibiting denial

Following a car accident, Harry Martin, a 26-year-old high school math teacher, was diagnosed as having quadraplegia. He was critically ill and needed specific services and equipment to have his needs met; therefore, he was admitted to the hospital's intensive care unit. Questions 24 through 28 refer to this situation.

24. Harry was placed on a Stryker frame because it
    1. Allows for horizontal turning of the patient
    2. Promotes body functions
    3. Allows for vertical turning of the patient
    4. Helps prevent deformities
25. Before releasing the pivot pins and turning the Stryker frame, the nurse should
    1. Tell the patient to hold on to the bottom part of the frame
    2. Observe the patient for signs of hypotension
    3. Secure all bolts and straps to ensure patient safety
    4. Get another nurse since this procedure requires 2 people
26. Two weeks after his accident Harry's physical condition had stabilized. He was overcoming his initial health crisis but he still had special needs that could not be met on a general unit; therefore, Harry was transferred to the Intermediate Care Unit. Progressive patient care means
    1. Providing specialized nursing care using an episodic approach
    2. Utilizing a variety of services and facilities to provide specialized care depending on a patient's individual needs
    3. Transferring patients from an area of greater intensive care to an area of lesser intensive care
    4. Providing total nursing care by using the latest techniques and technology
27. Three weeks after his injury Harry was placed on a tilt table for 1 hour while the head of the table was elevated to a 20° angle. Each day the angle was gradually increased. The tilt table was used to
    1. Facilitate turning
    2. Prevent pressure sores
    3. Promote hyperextension of the spine
    4. Prevent loss of calcium from the bones
28. The majority of patients with quadraplegia use wheelchairs because
    1. They usually are not and never will be functional walkers
    2. It assists them in overcoming orthostatic hypotension
    3. Their lower extremities are paralyzed but they have the strength in the upper extremities for self-propulsion
    4. It prepares them for bracing and crutch walking

Jimmy is a 7-year-old boy with cerebral palsy. He has no speech problems; however, he does need braces and self-help appliances to provide self-care. Although Jimmy's vision and hearing are fine, he does have a slight general sensory loss in both legs regarding position, pain, and temperature. Questions 29 through 33 refer to this situation.

29. In preparing Jimmy for crutch walking the nurse must determine
    1. The weight-bearing ability of Jimmy's upper and lower extremities
    2. Whether Jimmy has the power in his trunk to drag his legs forward when erect
    3. Whether Jimmy's body functions (i.e., respiration, circulation, elimination) can tolerate an erect position
    4. The ability of Jimmy's depressors and downward rotators of the shoulder girdle to support his body weight when it leaves the floor

30. It was decided that Jimmy would be taught the four-point alternate crutch gait. This gait was probably chosen because
    1. There are always 2 points of support on the floor
    2. Jimmy has more power in the upper extremities than the lower extremities
    3. It provides for equal but partial weight-bearing on each limb
    4. Jimmy has no power or step ability in the lower extremities

31. In light of his slight sensory loss in the legs, Jimmy and his mother should be taught to
    1. Keep braces in good repair and pad them well
    2. Check alignment of braces (brace joints should coincide with body joints)
    3. Select shoes that have heels that are wide and low
    4. Examine skin for evidence of pressure points

32. When teaching Jimmy to ambulate with crutches, the nurse should remember
    1. Learning progresses on a line forward and upward
    2. Because of his age, Jimmy's experiential background is limited
    3. Learning is a result of adequate teaching
    4. Jimmy must first understand normal walking patterns

33. Because of Jimmy's diminished sensation in the legs, he should be taught the following safety precautions
    1. Test temperature of water in any water-related activity
    2. Set the clock 2 times during the night to awaken and change position
    3. Tighten straps and buckles more than usual on braces when ambulating
    4. Look down at lower extremities when crutch walking to determine proper positioning of legs

Mrs. O'Reilly, 62 years of age, has been admitted to the hospital after having had a cerebrovascular accident resulting in a left hemiplegia. Questions 34 through 37 refer to this situation.

34. Left hemiplegia can be identified by the following observations
    1. Paralysis of the left lower extremity
    2. Paralysis of the left arm, left leg, and left side of the face
    3. Paralysis of the left arm and left side of the face
    4. Paralysis of the left arm, left leg, and right side of the face

35. When the nurse brought in Mrs. O'Reilly's dinner tray, she was staring blankly at the wall and stated that she felt like half a person. The nursing care of Mrs. O'Reilly should be directed at
    1. Including her in all decisions
    2. Helping her explore her feelings
    3. Distracting her from self-pity
    4. Preventing contractures and decubiti

36. Mrs. O'Reilly has been incontinent of feces. When establishing a bowel training program, the nurse must remember that the most important factor is the

1. Patient's previous habits in the area of diet and use of laxatives
2. Timing of elimination to take advantage of the gastrocolic reflex
3. Use of medication to induce elimination
4. Planning with the patient a definite time for attempted evacuations

37. In aiding Mrs. O'Reilly to develop independence, the nurse can motivate the patient by
    1. Demonstrating ways she can regain independence
    2. Establishing long-range goals for the patient
    3. Reinforcing success in tasks accomplished
    4. Pointing out her errors and helping her correct them

Mrs. Brice, a 73-year-old widow, lives with her daughter. While picketing for senior citizens' rights at the state legislature, she fell and fractured her right hip. Mrs. Brice was admitted to the hospital where the fracture was reduced and a nail was inserted. Questions 38 through 42 refer to this situation.

38. During the day the nurse put up Mrs. Brice's side rails specifically
    1. As a safety measure because of the patient's age
    2. Because all patients over 65 years of age should use side rails
    3. Because aged people are often disoriented for several days after anesthesia
    4. To be used as hand holds and to facilitate patient mobility

39. While assisting Mrs. Brice to transfer from the bed to a wheelchair, the nurse should remember
    1. When performing a weight-bearing transfer, the patient's knees should be slightly bent
    2. Transfers to and from the wheelchair will be easier if the bed is higher than the wheelchair
    3. The transfer can be accomplished by pivoting while bearing weight on both upper extremities and not on the legs
    4. To maintain appropriate proximity and visual relationship of wheelchair to bed

40. To prepare Mrs. Brice for crutch walking, the nurse should encourage the patient to
    1. Sit up straight in a chair to develop back muscles
    2. Keep the affected limb in extension and abduction
    3. Do exercises in bed to strengthen her upper extremities
    4. Use the trapeze to strengthen the biceps muscles

41. When assisting Mrs. Brice to ambulate, the nurse should be standing
    1. In front of the patient
    2. Behind the patient
    3. On the left side of the patient
    4. On the right side of the patient

42. Mrs. Brice is being discharged from the hospital; however, she needs assistance with several activities of daily living and needs to learn how to use a cane since her daughter

works full-time and cannot care for her mother. The most appropriate place for Mrs. Brice to go to convalesce would be
1. Her own home with visits from the public health nurse
2. A nursing home
3. An adult facility
4. An extended care facility

Mr. Ray, a 32-year-old salesman, is attending his first meeting of Alcoholics Anonymous because he finally realized and admitted that he is an alcoholic. Questions 43 through 47 refer to this situation.

43. Self-help groups such as Alcoholics Anonymous are successful because they meet the patient's need
1. To be trusted
2. To grow
3. To be independent
4. To belong
44. Self-help groups assist their members to
1. Deal with behavior and changes in behavior
2. Identify with their peers
3. Set long-term goals
4. Identify the underlying cause of their behavior
45. An insidious disease
1. Is attained after birth and is caused by genes
2. Runs a short acute course
3. Does not exhibit early symptoms of its advent
4. Is present at birth and is not caused by genes
46. For patients with alcoholism, the primary rehabilitator is the
1. Nurse
2. Physician
3. Entire health team
4. Patient
47. The most important factor in Mr. Ray's rehabilitation is
1. His emotional or motivational readiness
2. The qualitative level of his physical state
3. His family's accepting attitude
4. The availability of community resources

Mr. Jones is 55 years of age, has severe diabetes, and has had a midthigh amputation of his right leg because of a gangrenous leg ulcer. Questions 48 through 52 refer to this situation.

48. To prevent contractures of the hip, the nurse would
1. Place pillows under the stump
2. Encourage Mr. Jones to lie in the prone position several times daily
3. Remove pillows from under the stump and elevate the head of the bed
4. Encourage Mr. Jones to sit in a chair as much as possible
49. To promote early and efficient ambulation when Mr. Jones is allowed out of bed, he should be encouraged to
1. Keep hip in extension and abduction
2. Keep hip in extension and adduction
3. Keep hip in flexion and adduction
4. Keep right shoulder raised when swinging stump
50. Stump shrinkage is an important step in the healing process. There are two factors that contribute to stump shrinkage: one is atrophy of the muscles and the other is
1. Postoperative edema
2. Development of skin turgor
3. Reduction of subcutaneous fat
4. Loss of tissue and bone during operation
51. In helping Mr. Jones prepare his stump for a prosthesis, the nurse should encourage him to
1. Abduct the stump when ambulating
2. Hang the stump off the bed frequently
3. Soak the stump in warm water twice a day
4. Periodically press the end of the stump against a pillow
52. When preparing Mr. Jones for dinner, it is the nurse's responsibility to
1. Remove the pillow under the stump and raise the head of the bed
2. Check Mr. Jones' urine for sugar and acetone
3. Get Mr. Jones out of bed and into a chair
4. Make sure that Mr. Jones uses sugar substitutes

Bibliography

ANATOMY AND PHYSIOLOGY

Anderson, W. A. D., editor: Pathology, ed. 6, St. Louis, 1971, The C. V. Mosby Co.

Anthony, C. P., and Kolthoff, N. J.: Textbook of anatomy and physiology, ed. 9, St. Louis, 1975, The C. V. Mosby Co.

Guyton, A. C.: Textbook of medical physiology, ed. 4, Philadelphia, 1971, W. B. Saunders Co.

Mountcastle, V. B., editor: Medical physiology, ed. 13, St. Louis, 1974, The C. V. Mosby Co.

PHYSICAL SCIENCE

Chemistry

Arnow, L. E.: Introduction to physiological and pathological chemistry, ed. 9, St. Louis, 1976, The C. V. Mosby Co.

Conn, E. E., and Stumpf, P. K.: Outlines of biochemistry, ed. 3, New York, 1972, John Wiley & Sons, Inc.

Horrobin, D. F.: Biochemistry, endocrinology, and nutrition, New York, 1971, G. P. Putnam's Sons.

Laughlin, A.: Roe's principles of chemistry, ed. 12, St. Louis, 1976, The C. V. Mosby Co.

Lehninger, A.: Biochemistry, New York, 1975, Worth Publishers, Inc.

Linstromberg, W. W.: Organic chemistry: a brief course, ed. 2, Lexington, Mass., 1970, D. C. Heath & Co.

Orten, J. M., and Neuhaus, O. W.: Biochemistry, ed. 9, St. Louis, 1975, The C. V. Mosby Co.

White, A., Handler, P., and Smith, E.: Principles of biochemistry, ed. 5, New York, 1973, McGraw-Hill Book Co.

Physics

Berne, R. M., and Levy, M. N.: Cardiovascular physiology, ed. 3, St. Louis, 1977, The C. V. Mosby Co.

Flitter, H. H.: Physics in nursing, ed. 7, St. Louis, 1976, The C. V. Mosby Co.

Guyton, A. C.: Textbook of medical physiology, ed. 4, Philadelphia, 1971, W. B. Saunders Co.

Haldane, J. B. S.: On being the right size. In Newman, J. R., editor: The world of mathematics, vol. 2, New York, 1956, Simon & Schuster, Inc.

Hewitt, P. G.: Conceptual physics, ed. 2, Boston, 1974, Little, Brown and Co.

Horrobin, D. F.: Physics, chemistry and biology, New York, 1971, G. P. Putnam's Sons.

Klotz, I. M.: Energy changes in biochemical reactions, New York, 1967, Academic Press, Inc.

Patton, A. R.: Biochemical energetics and kinetics, Philadelphia, 1965, W. B. Saunders Co.

Weidner, R. T., and Sells, R. L.: Elementary physics: classical and modern, Boston, 1975, Allyn & Bacon, Inc.

MICROBIOLOGY

Barrett, J. T.: Textbook of immunology, ed. 2, St. Louis, 1974, The C. V. Mosby Co.

Burnett, G. W., and Schuster, G. S.: Pathogenic microbiology, St. Louis, 1973, The C. V. Mosby Co.

Jawelz, E., Melnick, J. L., and Adelberg, E.: A review of medical microbiology, ed. 10, Los Altos, 1972, Lange Medical Publications.

Smith, A. L.: Principles of microbiology, ed. 7, St. Louis, 1973, The C. V. Mosby Co.

Volk, W. A., and Wheeler, M. F.: Microbiology, ed. 3, Philadelphia, 1973, J. B. Lippincott Co.

NUTRITIONAL SCIENCE

Bogert, L. J., Briggs, G., and Calloway, D.: Nutrition and physical fitness, ed. 10, Philadelphia, 1975, W. B. Saunders Co.

Davidson, S., Passmore, R., Brock, J. F., and Truswell, A. S.: Human nutrition and dietetics, ed. 6, New York, 1975, Longman, Inc.

Guthrie, H. A.: Introductory nutrition, ed. 3, St. Louis, 1975, The C. V. Mosby Co.

Guthrie, H. A., and Braddock, K. S.: Programmed nutrition, St. Louis, 1975, The C. V. Mosby Co.

Robinson, C. H.: Normal and therapeutic nutrition, ed. 14, New York, 1972, The Macmillan Co.

Williams, S. R.: Essentials of nutrition and diet therapy, St. Louis, 1974, The C. V. Mosby Co.

Williams, S. R.: Self-study guide for nutrition and diet therapy, St. Louis, 1974, The C. V. Mosby Co.

Williams, S. R.: Nutrition and diet therapy, ed. 3, St. Louis, 1977, The C. V. Mosby Co.

Williams, S. R.: Nutrition and diet therapy: a learning guide for students, St. Louis, 1977, The C. V. Mosby Co.

Williams, S. R.: Review of nutrition and diet therapy, St. Louis, 1973, The C. V. Mosby Co.

BEHAVIORAL SCIENCE

Engel, G. L.: Grief and grieving, A.J.N. **64:**93-98, 1964.

Erikson, E.: Identity: youth and crisis, New York, 1968, W. W. Norton & Co., Inc.

Friedman, J. L., Carlsmith, J. M., and Sears, D. O.: Social psychology, Englewood Cliffs, N.J., 1970, Prentice-Hall, Inc.

Freud, S.: A general introduction to psychoanalysis, Garden City, N.Y., 1943, Garden City Publishing Co.

Hammond, P. B.: An introduction to cultural and social anthropology, New York, 1971, The Macmillan Co.

Kagan, J.: Psychology: an introduction, New York, 1968, Harcourt Brace Jovanovich.

Kaluger, G., and Kaluger, M. F.: Human development: the span of life, St. Louis, 1974, The C. V. Mosby Co.

Peplau, H. E.: Interpersonal relations in nursing, New York, 1952, G. P. Putnam's Sons.

Peterson, M.: Understanding defense mechanisms, A.J.N. **72:**1651-1674, 1972.

Selye, Hans: The stress syndrome, A.J.N. **65:**97-99, 1965.

Smith, D. W., and Bierman, E. L., editors: The biologic ages of man, Philadelphia, 1973, W. B. Saunders Co.

Sullivan, H. S.: The interpersonal theory of psychiatry, New York, 1953, W. W. Norton & Co., Inc.

PHARMACOLOGY

Goodman, L. S., and Gilman, A., editors: The pharmacological basis of therapeutics, ed. 5, New York, 1970, The Macmillan Co.

Goth, A.: Medical pharmacology, ed. 8, St. Louis, 1976, The C. V. Mosby Co.

Hartshorn, E. A.: Handbook of drug interactions, ed. 2, Hamilton, 1973, Drug Intelligence Publications.

Johns, M. P.: Pharmacodynamics and patient care, St. Louis, 1974, The C. V. Mosby Co.

Modell, W., editor: Drugs of choice 1976-1977, St. Louis, 1976, The C. V. Mosby Co.

Reilly, M. J., editor: American hospital formulary service, vols. 1 and 2, Washington, D.C., 1975, American Society of Hospital Pharmacists.

HISTORY AND TRENDS IN NURSING

American Nurses' Association: A position paper, New York, 1965, American Nurses' Association.

Brown, E. L.: Nursing for the future, New York, 1948, Russell Sage Foundation.

Bullough, V. L., and Bullough, B.: The emergence of modern nursing, New York, 1969, The Macmillan Co.

Campbell, G.: Community colleges in Canada, Toronto, 1971, Ryerson Press.

Canadian Nurses' Association: The leaf and the lamp, Ottawa, 1968, Canadian Nurses' Association.

Committee on Grading of Nursing Schools: Nursing schools today and tomorrow, New York, 1934, The Committee.

Committee for the Study of Nursing Education: Nursing and nursing education in the United States, New York, 1923, The Macmillan Co.

DeYoung, L.: The foundations of nursing, ed. 3, St. Louis, 1976, The. C. V. Mosby Co.

Dolan, J. A.: Nursing in society, Philadelphia, 1973, W. B. Saunders Co.

Gibbon, J. M., and Mathewson, M. L.: Three centuries of Canadian nursing, Toronto, 1947, The Macmillan Co.

Good, S., and Kerr, J.: Contemporary issues in Canadian law for nurses, Toronto, 1973, Holt, Rinehart and Winston.

Innis, M. Q.: Nursing education in a changing society, Toronto, 1970, University of Toronto Press.

Lenburg, C. B., ed.: Open learning and career mobility in nursing, St. Louis, 1975, The C. V. Mosby Co.

Marshall, H. E.: Adelaide Nutting—pioneer of modern nursing, Baltimore, 1972, Johns Hopkins University Press.

Montag, M. L.: Community college education for nursing, New York, 1959, McGraw-Hill Book Co.

Montag, M. L.: The education of nursing technicians, New York, 1951, G. P. Putnam's Sons; reprinted by John Wiley & Sons, Inc., 1971.

Nutting, M. A., and Dock, L. L.: A history of nursing, New York, 1935, G. P. Putnam's Sons.

Roberts, M. M.: American nursing, New York, 1954, The Macmillan Co.

Stewart, I. M.: The education of nurses, New York, 1943, The Macmillan Co.

Stewart, I. M., and Austin, A. L.: A history of nursing, New York, 1962, G. P. Putnam's Sons.

Weir, G. M.: Survey of nursing education in Canada, Ottawa, 1932, Canadian Nurses' Association.

Woodham-Smith, C.: Florence Nightingale, New York, 1951, The McGraw-Hill Book Co.

FUNDAMENTALS OF NURSING

Berni, R., and Readey, H.: Problem-oriented medical record implementation, St. Louis, 1974, The C. V. Mosby Co.

Byrne, M. L., and Thompson, L. F.: Key concepts for the study and practice of nursing, St. Louis, 1972, The C. V. Mosby Co.

'uerst, E. V., Wolff, L., and Weitzel, M. H.: Fundamentals of nursing, ed. 5, Philadelphia, 1974, J. B. Lippincott Co.

Gragg, S. H., and Rees, O. M.: Scientific principles in nursing, ed. 7, St. Louis, 1974, The C. V. Mosby Co.

arvis, C. M.: Vital signs, Nursing '76, 6:31-37, April, 1976.

Marram, G. D., Schlegel, M. W., and Bevis, E. O.: Primary nursing, St. Louis, 1974, The C. V. Mosby Co.

Matheney, R. V., Nolan, B. T., Hogan, A. E., and Griffin, G. J.: Fundamentals of patient-centered nursing, ed. 3, St. Louis, 1972, The C. V. Mosby Co.

McCaffery, M.: Nursing management of the patient with pain, Philadelphia, 1972, J. B. Lippincott Co.

Mitchell, P. H.: Concepts basic to nursing, New York, 1973, McGraw-Hill Book Co.

Murray, M.: Fundamentals of nursing, Englewood Cliffs, N.J., 1976, Prentice-Hall, Inc.

Rines, A., and Montag, M. L.: Nursing concepts and nursing care, New York, 1976, John Wiley and Sons.

Saxton, D. F., and Hyland, P. A.: Planning and implementing nursing intervention, St. Louis, 1975, The C. V. Mosby Co.

Vitale, B., Schultz, N., and Nugent, P.: A problem-solving approach to nursing care plans, St. Louis, 1974, The C. V. Mosby Co.

White, D. T., Rubino, E. and DeLorey, P. E.: Fundamentals: the foundations of nursing, Englewood Cliffs, N.J., 1972, Prentice-Hall, Inc.

FAMILY-CENTERED NURSING

Parent-child nursing

Alexander, M., and Brown, M.: Pediatric physical diagnosis for nurses, New York, 1974, McGraw-Hill Book Co.

Barnard, K. E., and Erickson, M. L.: Teaching children with developmental problems, St. Louis, 1976, The C. V. Mosby Co.

Barnett, H.: Pediatrics, ed. 14, New York, 1968, Appleton-Century-Crofts.

Chinn, P.: Child health maintenance: concepts in family-centered care, St. Louis, 1975, The C. V. Mosby Co.

Chinn, P., and Leitch, C.: Child health maintenance: a guide to clinical assessment, St. Louis, 1974, The C. V. Mosby Co.

Erikson, E.: Childhood and society, ed. 2, New York, 1963, W. W. Norton & Co., Inc.

Helfer, R., and Kempe, C., editors: The battered child, Chicago, 1968, University of Chicago Press.

Jacoby, F.: Nursing care of the patient with burns, St. Louis, 1976, The C. V. Mosby Co.

Krugman, S., and Ward, R.: Infectious diseases of children and adults, ed. 5, St. Louis, 1973, The C. V. Mosby Co.

Marlow, D. R.: Textbook of pediatric nursing, ed. 4, Philadelphia, 1975, W. B. Saunders Co.

Money, J.: Sex errors of the body, ed. 4, Philadelphia, 1975, W. B. Saunders Co.

Nelson, W. E., Vaughan, V. C., and McKay, R. J.: Textbook of pediatrics, ed. 10, Philadelphia, 1975, W. B. Saunders Co.

Petrillo, M., and Sanger, S.: Emotional care of hospitalized children, Philadelphia, 1972, J. B. Lippincott Co.

Scipien, G., and others: Comprehensive pediatric nursing, New York, 1975, McGraw-Hill Book Co.

Shirkey, H., editor: Pediatric therapy, ed. 5, St. Louis, 1975, The C. V. Mosby Co.

Steele, S.: Nursing care of the child with a long-term illness, New York, 1971, Appleton-Century-Crofts.

Whaley, L.: Understanding inherited disorders, St. Louis, 1974, The C. V. Mosby Co.

Maternal nursing and reproductive problems

Abramson, H.: Resuscitation of the newborn infant, ed. 3, St. Louis, 1973, The C. V. Mosby Co.

Brody, S.: Patterns of mothering, New York, 1956, N.Y. International University Press, Inc.

Calderone, M.: Manual of family planning and contraceptives, Baltimore, 1970, Williams & Wilkins Co.

Chabon, I.: Awake and aware: participating in childbirth through psychoprophylaxis, New York, 1966, Dell Publishing Co.

Duvall, E. M.: Family development, Philadelphia, 1971, J. B. Lippincott Co.

Eiger, M., and Olds, S.: Complete book of breast-feeding, New York, 1973, Bantam Books.

Ewy, D., and Ewy, R.: Preparation for childbirth—a lamaze guide, Boulder, Colo., 1970, Pruett Publishing Co.

Flanagan, G. L., First nine months of life, New York, 1962, Simon & Schuster Inc.

Gusberg, S. B.: Gynecologic cancer, Baltimore, 1970, Williams & Wilkins Co.

Guttmacher, A.: Planning your family, New York, 1964, The Macmillan Co.

Hellman, L., and Pritchard, J.: Williams' obstetrics, ed. 14, New York, 1971, Appleton-Century-Crofts.

Howells, J. G.: Modern perspectives in psycho-obstetrics, New York, 1971, Brunner/Mazel.

Iorio, J.: Childbirth: family-centered nursing, ed. 3, St. Louis, 1975, The C. V. Mosby Co.

Kaplan, H.: The new sex therapy, New York, 1974, Brunner/Mazel.

Korones, S.: High risk newborn infants, ed. 2, St. Louis, 1976, The C. V. Mosby Co.

Lipkin, G. B.: Psychosocial aspects of maternal-child nursing, St. Louis, 1974, The C. V. Mosby Co.

Masters, W. H., and Johnson, V.: Human sexual responses, Boston, 1966, Little, Brown and Co.

Moore, K. L.: Before we are born—basic embryology and birth defects, Philadelphia, 1974, W. B. Saunders Co.

Moore, M. L.: The newborn and the nurse, Philadelphia, 1972, W. B. Saunders Co.

Pannor, R.: The unmarried father, New York, 1971, Springer Publishing Co.

Pierog, S., and Ferrara, A.: Approaches to medical care of the sick newborn, ed. 2, St. Louis, 1976, The C. V. Mosby Co.

Read, G. D.: Childbirth without fear, New York, 1953, Harper & Row, Publishers.

PSYCHIATRIC NURSING

Arieti, S., editor: American handbook of psychiatry, New York, 1966, Basic Books, Inc.

Arieti, S.: Interpretation of schizophrenia, New York, 1974, Basic Books, Inc.

Ayd, F. J.: The chemical assault on mental illness, A.J.N. **65:**70-93, 1965.

Basic Systems Inc.: Anxiety recognition and intervention, A.J.N. **65:**129-152, 1965.

Duran, F. A., and Errion, G. D.: Perpetuation of chronicity in mental illness, A.J.N. **70:**1707-1709, 1970.

Eisenberg, J., and Abbott, R. D.: The monopolizing patient in group therapy, Perspectives of Psychiatric Nursing Care **6**(2):66-69, 1968.

Elwell, R.: Community mental health centers, A.J.N. **70:**1014-1025, 1970.

Goldin, P., and Russell, B.: Therapeutic communication, A.J.N. **69:**1928-1930, 1969.

Hofling, C., and Keys, J.: Basic psychiatric concepts in nursing, ed. 3, Philadelphia, 1974, J. B. Lippincott Co.

Huey, F. L.: In a therapeutic community, A.J.N. **71:**926-933, 1971.

Kaplan, B., editor: The inner world of mental illness, New York, 1964, Harper and Row.

Kolb, L. C.: Modern clinical psychiatry, ed. 8, Philadelphia, 1973, W. B. Saunders Co.

Matheney, R., and Topalis, M.: Psychiatric nursing, ed. 6, St. Louis, 1974, The C. V. Mosby Co.

Mereness, D., and Taylor, C.: Essentials of psychiatric nursing, ed. 9, St. Louis, 1974, The C. V. Mosby Co.

Phinney, R. P.: The student of nursing and the schizophrenic patient, A.J.N. **70:**790-792, 1970.

Russaw, E.: Nursing in a narcotic detoxification unit, A.J.N. **70:**1720-1723, 1970.

Schwartz, M. S., and Shockley, E. L.: The nurse and the mental hospital, New York, 1956, Russell Sage Foundation.

Ulett, G. A.: A synopsis of contemporary psychiatry, ed. 5, St. Louis, 1972, The C. V. Mosby Co.

Weiss, E., and English, S. P.: Psychosomatic medicine, Philadelphia, 1957, W. B. Saunders Co.

MEDICAL-SURGICAL NURSING

Anderson, W. A. D., editor: Pathology, ed. 6, St. Louis, 1971, The C. V. Mosby Co.

Anthony, C. P., and Kolthoff, N. J.: Textbook of anatomy and physiology, ed. 9, St. Louis, 1975, The C. V. Mosby Co.

Barber, J. M., Stokes, L. G., and Billings, D. M.: Adult and child care—a client approach to nursing, ed. 2, St. Louis, 1977, The C. V. Mosby Co.

Bergersen, B. S.: Pharmacology in nursing, ed. 13, St. Louis, 1976, The C. V. Mosby Co.

Brunner, L. S., and others: The Lippincott manual of nursing practice, Philadelphia, 1974, J. B. Lippincott Co.

Burke, S. R.: The composition and function of body fluids, ed. 2, St. Louis, 1976, The C. V. Mosby Co.

Carini, E., and Owens, G.: Neurological and neurosurgical nursing, ed. 6, St. Louis, 1974, The C. V. Mosby Co.

Ganong, W. F.: Review of medical physiology, ed. 7, Los Altos, Calif., 1975, Lange Medical Publications.

Johns, M.: Pharmacodynamics and patient care, St. Louis, 1974, The C. V. Mosby Co.

Krupp, M. A., and Chatton, M. J.: Current medical diagnosis and treatment, Los Altos, Calif., 1974, Lange Medication Publications.

Luckman, J., and Sorensen, K. C.: Medical-surgical nursing—a psychophysiological approach, Philadelphia, 1974, W. B. Saunders Co.

Metheny, N. M., and Shively, W. D., Jr.: Nurse's handbook of fluid balance, ed. 2, Philadelphia, 1974, J. B. Lippincott Co.

Saxton, D. F., and Hyland, P. A.: Planning and implementing nursing intervention, St. Louis, 1975, The C. V. Mosby Co.

Shafer, K. N., and others: Medical-surgical nursing, ed. 6, St. Louis, 1975, The C. V. Mosby Co.

Sproul, C. W., and Mullanney, P. J., editors: Emergency care—assessment and intervention, St. Louis, 1974, The C. V. Mosby Co.

Tilkien, S. M., and Conover, M. H.: Clinical implications of laboratory tests, St. Louis, 1975, The C. V. Mosby Co.

Tucker, S. M., and others: Patient care standards, St. Louis, 1975, The C. V. Mosby Co.

Williams, S. R.: Nutrition and Diet Therapy, ed. 3, St. Louis, 1977, The C. V. Mosby Co.

REHABILITATION

Aguilera, D. C., and Messick, J. M.: Crisis intervention: theory and methodology, ed. 2, St. Louis, 1974, The C. V. Mosby Co.

Christopherson, V. A., Coulter, P. P., and Wolanin, M. O.: Rehabilitation nursing—perspectives and applications, New York, 1974, McGraw-Hill Book Co.

Hall, J. E., and Weaver, B. R.: Nursing of families in crisis, Philadelphia, 1974, J. B. Lippincott Co.

Maslow, A. H.: Motivation and personality, ed. 2, New York, 1970, Harper & Row, Publishers.

Redman, B. K.: The process of patient teaching in

nursing, ed. 3, St. Louis, 1976, The C. V. Mosby Co.

Reinhardt, A. M., and Quinn, M. D., editors: Family-centered community nursing—a sociocultural framework, St. Louis, 1973, The C. V. Mosby Co.

Rusk, H. A.: Rehabilitation medicine, ed. 3, St. Louis, 1971, The C. V. Mosby Co.

Sorenson, L., and Ulrich, P.: Ambulation guide for nurses, Minneapolis, 1974, Sister Kenny Institute.

Steinberg, F. U., editor: Cowdry's care of the geriatric patient, ed. 5, St. Louis, 1976, The C. V. Mosby Co.

Index